Regulation of Hepatic Metabolism

Intra- and Intercellular Compartmentation

Regulation of Hepatic Metabolism
Intra- and Intercellular Compartmentation

Edited by

Ronald G. Thurman

University of North Carolina School of Medicine
Chapel Hill, North Carolina

Frederick C. Kauffman

University of Maryland School of Medicine
Baltimore, Maryland

and

Kurt Jungermann

Georg-August Universität
Göttingen, Federal Republic of Germany

PLENUM PRESS • NEW YORK AND LONDON

Library of Congress Cataloging in Publication Data

Main entry under title:

Regulation of hepatic metabolism.

Includes bibliographies and index.
1. Liver. 2. Metabolism — Regulation. 3. Cell compartmentation. I. Thurman, Ronald G. II. Kauffman, Frederick C. III. Jungermann, Kurt. [DNLM: 1. Cell Compartmentation. 2. Liver — metabolism. WI 702 R344]
QP185.R44   1986   612′.35   85-30084
ISBN 0-306-42137-2

© 1986 Plenum Press, New York
A Division of Plenum Publishing Corporation
233 Spring Street, New York, N.Y. 10013

Printed in the United States of America

Contributors

William F. Balistreri, Children's Hospital, Research Foundation, University of Cincinnati, Cincinnati, Ohio 45229

Jeffrey Baron, The Toxicology Center, Department of Pharmacology, The University of Iowa, College of Medicine, Iowa City, Iowa 52242

Gunnar Bengtsson, Research Laboratories of the Finnish State Alcohol Company, Alko Ltd., SF-00101 Helsinki 10, Finland. *Present address*: National Institute of Forensic Toxicology, N-0372 Oslo, Norway

Britton Chance, The Johnson Research Foundation, University of Pennsylvania, Philadelphia, Pennsylvania 19104

Wolfgang Gerok, Medizinische Universitätsklinik, D-7800 Freiburg, Federal Republic of Germany

Jorge J. Gumucio, Veterans Administration Hospital, University of Michigan, Ann Arbor, Michigan 48109

Dieter Häussinger, Medizinische Universitätsklinik, D-7800 Freiburg, Federal Republic of Germany

Sungchul Ji, Department of Pharmacology and Toxicology, College of Pharmacy, Rutgers University, Piscataway, New Jersey 08854

Kurt Jungermann, Institut für Biochemie, Universität Göttingen, D-3400 Göttingen, Federal Republic of Germany

Norbert Katz, Institut für Biochemie, Universität Göttingen, D-3400 Göttingen, Federal Republic of Germany

Frederick C. Kauffman, Department of Pharmacology and Experimental Therapeutics, University of Maryland School of Medicine, Baltimore, Maryland 21202

Thomas T. Kawabata, The Toxicology Center, Department of Pharmacology, The University of Iowa College of Medicine, Iowa City, Iowa 52242

A.V. LeBouton, Department of Anatomy, College of Medicine, University of Arizona, Tucson, Arizona 85724

John J. Lemasters, Laboratories for Cell Biology, Department of Anatomy, School of Medicine, University of North Carolina at Chapel Hill 27514

Kai O. Lindros, Research Laboratories of the Finnish State of Alcohol Company, Alko Ltd., SF-00101 Helsinki 10, Finland

Franz M. Matschinsky, Department of Biochemistry and Biophysics, Diabetes Research Center, University of Pennsylvania, Philadelphia, Pennsylvania 19104

Bjørn Quistorff, Department of Biochemistry, University of Copenhagen, 2200 Copenhagen, Denmark

Jan A. Redick, The Toxicology Center, Department of Pharmacology, The University of Iowa College of Medicine, Iowa City, Iowa 52242

P.D.I. Richardson, Medical Department, Astra Pharmaceuticals Ltd., Home Park Estate, Kings Langley, Hertfordshire WD4 8DH, United Kingdom

Mikko Salaspuro, Research Laboratories of the Finnish State School Alcohol Company, Alko Ltd., SF-00101 Helsinki 10, Finland

Dieter Sasse, Institute of Anatomy, University of Basel, CH-4056 Basel, Switzerland

Fred J. Suchy, Children's Hospital, Research Foundation, University of Cincinnati, Cincinnati, Ohio 45229

Ronald G. Thurman, Department of Pharmacology, School of Medicine, University of North Carolina at Chapel Hill, North Carolina 27514

Hannu Väänänen, Research Laboratories of the Finnish State Alcohol Company, Alko Ltd., SF-00101 Helsinki 10, Finland

Jeffrey M. Voigt, The Toxicology Center, Department of Pharmacology, The University of Iowa College of Medicine, Iowa City, Iowa 52242

P.G. Withrington, Department of Pharmacology, The Medical College of St. Bartholomew's Hospital, London EC1M 6BQ, England

Preface

The liver is an exceptionally complex and diverse organ that functions both as an exocrine and an endocrine gland. It secretes bile, which contains many constituents in addition to bile salts, and it synthesizes and releases many substances in response to the body's demands, including prohormones, albumin, clotting factors, glucose, fatty acids, and various lipoproteins. It has a dual blood supply providing a rich mixture of nutrients and other absorbed substances via the portal vein and oxygen-rich blood via the hepatic artery. This functional heterogeneity is accompanied by cellular heterogeneity. The liver contains many cell types including hepatic parachymal cells, Küpffer cells, Ito cells, and endothelial cells. The most abundant cell type, the parenchymal cells, are biochemically and structurally heterogeneous. The cells in the oxygen-rich areas of the portal triad appear more dependent on oxidative metabolism, whereas those around the central vein (pericentral, perivenous, or centrolobular areas) are more dependent upon an anaerobic mechanism. Throughout this volume the latter three terms are used synonymously by various authors to indicate the five to eight layers of cells radiating from the central vein.

Structural and metabolic heterogeneity of hepatic parenchymal cells has been demonstrated by a variety of approaches, including histochemical, ultrastructural, and ultramicrobiochemical studies. This microheterogeneity is linked to the physiological functions of the liver and its response to injurious substances. For example, it has long been appreciated that many drugs and chemicals damage different regions of the liver lobule with a great deal of specificity. Mechanisms responsible for these phenomena remain obscure. Many drugs with allyl groups damage hepatocytes around the portal triad (periportal regions). In contrast, acetaminophen, ethanol, and halogenated hydrocarbons damage cells near the central vein. Mechanisms regulating the expression of different biochemical properties of hepatocytes in different regions of the liver lobule remain poorly defined; however, recent data indicate that zonation of metabolism is under short- and long-term control.

The purpose of the work described in this volume is two-fold: first, to describe the application of recently developed methods to investigate the role of inter- and intracellular compartmentation in hepatic function and toxicity and second, to present work that relates metabolic microheterogeneity to liver function. The book is divided into five sections. The first deals with modern anatomical concepts of hepatic cellular heterogeneity. In addition to discussing cellular heterogeneity, these chapters deal with current understanding of the hemodynamics of the liver and its innervation. This discussion is followed by several chapters which detail state-of-the-art methods that are currently being applied in studies of hepatic biochemical microheterogeneity. Recent applications of these methods are highlighted. The third section of this book is comprised of chapters by recognized authorities who evaluate metabolic zonation in liver function and disease. A final chapter summarizes advantages and limitations of the approaches that have been taken to investigating hepatic intracellular heterogeneity and identifies research areas that we feel require immediate and long-term attention. The intention of this volume is to emphasize metabolic zonation as a new dimension in hepatic function and regulation. The thorough treatment of new methods and their application in defining metabolic microheterogeneity of the liver is aimed at stimulating new initiatives in this exciting area of research.

Ronald G. Thurman
Frederick C. Kauffman
Kurt Jungermann

Contents

II. Methods

Chapter 3

Histology and Histochemistry

Dieter Sasse

Chapter 4

Immunohistochemistry

Jeffrey Baron, Jeffrey M. Voigt, Thomas T. Kawabata, and Jan A. Redick

Chapter 5

Quantitative Histochemical Measurements within Sublobular Zones of the Liver Lobule

Frederick C. Kauffman and Franz M. Matschinsky

Chapter 6

Separation of Functionally Different Liver Cell Types

Kai O. Lindros, Gunnar Bengtsson, Mikko Salaspuro, and Hannu Väänänen

Contents

Chapter 7

New Micromethods for Studying Sublobular Structure and Function in the Isolated, Perfused Rat Liver

John J. Lemasters, Sungchul Ji, and Ronald G. Thurman

Chapter 8

Redox Scanning in the Study of Metabolic Zonation of Liver

Bjørn Quistorff and Britton Chance

III.   Distribution of Metabolic Functions

Chapter 9

Metabolism of Carbohydrates

Kurt Jungermann and Norbert Katz

Chapter 12

Lobular Oxygen Gradients: Possible Role in Alcohol-Induced Hepatotoxicity

Ronald G. Thurman, Sungchul Ji, and John J. Lemasters

Chapter 13

Biotransformation and Zonal Toxicity

Ronald G. Thurman, Frederick C. Kauffman, and Jeffrey Baron

Chapter 14

Protein Synthesis and Secretion

A. V. LeBouton

Chapter 15

Bile Acid Metabolism

Jorge J. Gumucio, William F. Balistreri, and Fred J. Suchy

IV. Induction of Liver Cell Heterogeneity

Chapter 16

Zonal Signal Heterogeneity and Induction of Hepatocyte Heterogeneity

Kurt Jungermann

V. Speculations and Directions for the Future

I

Liver Structure

Liver Structure and Innervation

Dieter Sasse

1. INTRODUCTION

The problems one encounters in any attempt to describe the architecture of the liver date back to the beginnings of light microscopy itself. For most other organs, it is not very difficult to establish conformity between the structural and functional units, and in such cases the proposed nomenclature makes use of the suffix "-on." Thus, the nephron is the structural and functional unit of the kidney, the neuron of nervous tissue, the chondron of cartilage, and so on. The term "hepaton" was used years ago, but it has never really been accepted because the structural units are difficult to recognize and because the liver has two quite separate functions. As an organ of excretion, it is connected by the bile duct to the gut, for which it serves as a gland comparable to the pancreas, whereas its type of microcirculation is similar to that of an endocrine organ that also acts in a heterotopic position. This chapter demonstrates that despite our increased knowledge, fundamental problems persist when hepatic structures are described in terms of their functional aspects.

DIETER SASSE • Institute of Anatomy, University of Basel, CH-4056 Basel, Switzerland.

2. LIVER STRUCTURE

2.1. Development

In man, the first anlage of the liver appears at the end of the third week as a diverticulum arising in a pocketlike evagination of the gut distal to the precursor of the definitive stomach. This hepatic bud increases in size and then shows a division into a large cranial and a smaller caudal diverticulum. The cranial diverticulum gives rise to the parenchymatous tissue of the liver and the hepatic ducts; the caudal portion develops into the gallbladder and cystic duct. Soon the epithelial cells of the cranial diverticulum begin migrating forward and invade the horizontally oriented ventral mesentery, a mesenchymal plate called the septum transversum (Fig. 1).

Thus, present from the beginning are the two cellular components from which the differentiated liver parenchyma is also built up: the entodermal liver epithelium, which gives rise to the true parenchymal cells, and the mesenchymal tissue of the septum transversum, from which the fibrocytes and the sinusoidal cells originate. The fibrocytes form the connective tissue of Glisson's capsule, which underlies the peritoneal mesothelium and extends into the portal spaces to form a common sheet around the afferent blood vessels and the bile ducts.

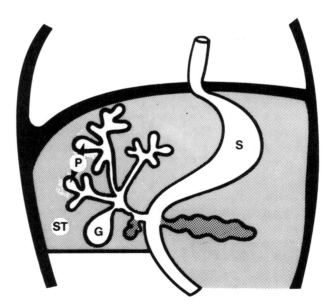

Figure 1.   Schematic drawing of liver development. Distal to the stomach (S), out of the cranial position the parenchymatous tissue (P) and out of the distal portion the gallbladder (G) invade the septum transversum (ST). The anlagen of the pancreas are also marked.

The sinusoidal cells form the walls of the sinusoidal capillaries that lie in the lacunae between the columns of hepatocytes. At first, they receive blood from the vitelline and umbilical veins, but after birth, they receive blood from the afferent liver vessels, the hepatic artery and the portal vein. Together, the epithelial and the mesenchymal cells contribute to the normal functions of the organ.

2.2. General Histology

The parenchymal cells of the liver make up 80% of its volume and 60% of its total cell number[1] (for further data, see Table I). In histological sections, the liver cells appear irregularly polygonal and form a wall-like structure (muralium) of anastomosing plates. In all mammals, these plates are only one cell thick and are bent so as to surround the lacunae, thus forming the "labyrinthus hepatis"[2] (Fig. 2).

Since the liver not only receives the blood coming from the intestinal tract (ingestive function) but also produces bile (glandular secretory function), the organization of each liver cell must meet each of these functions. The parenchymal cell possesses both perisinusoidal surfaces, covered with microvilli, and surfaces that make contact with adjacent cells. The latter show diverticuli of the plasma membrane, which, together with the contiguous cell, form the bile canaliculus.

In the lacunar meshwork of the liver cell plates, the sinusoids lead the mixed blood of the terminal branches of the hepatic artery and the portal vein to the terminal hepatic venule. The sinusoidal walls are formed by cells of the retic-

Table I. Volumetric Composition of the Liver Parenchyma[a]

Hepatocytes	77.8 ± 1.15
Nuclei	7.6 ± 0.50
Cytoplasm	70.2 ± 1.13
Sinusoidal cells	6.3 ± 0.49
Endothelial cells	2.8 ± 0.19
Nuclei	0.44 ± 0.08
Cytoplasm	2.36 ± 0.08
Kupffer cells	2.1 ± 0.31
Nuclei	0.39 ± 0.07
Cytoplasm	1.71 ± 0.07
Fat-storing cells	1.4 ± 0.19
Nuclei	0.28 ± 0.04
Cytoplasm	1.12 ± 0.04
Spaces	15.9 ± 0.75
Disse space	4.9 ± 0.35
Sinusoidal lumen	10.6 ± 0.45
Biliary canaliculi	0.43 ± 0.05

[a] Data from Blouin.[21] Values are percentages ± S.E.

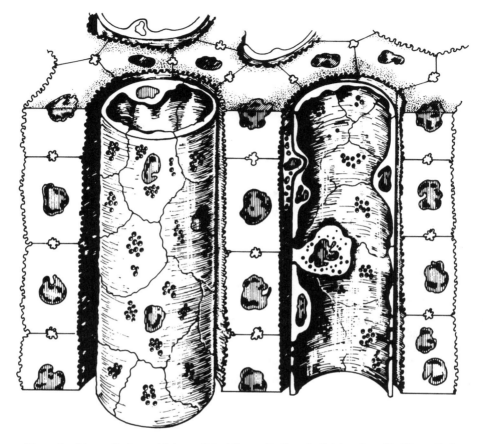

Figure 2.   Liver-cell plates with intercellular bile canaliculi, and adjoining sinusoids. The wall of the right sinusoid shows endothelial cells, a Kupffer cell bulging into the lumen, and a perisinusoidal fat-storing cell. Schematic drawing according to Elias.[2]

uloendothelial system. In addition to the endothelial cells proper (which are modified reticulum cells), these include Kupffer cells, fat-storing cells, and pit cells. A perisinusoidal space, the space of Disse, remains between the lining cells and the hepatocytes, and this communicates with the lumen of the sinusoid through numerous fenestrations with pores of 0.1 μm in diameter. The space of Disse also contains the reticular network, which acts as scaffolding for the parenchymatous organ.

2.3. Ploidy

Under the light microscope, liver cells are seen to contain large, usually spherical nuclei of varying sizes, and binucleate cells are frequently present.

This observation has led to numerous investigations beginning in the 1920s. It was found that the nuclei of the hepatocytes fall into different size classes, which bear a specific numerical relationship to one another. Calculation of the nuclear volumes in liver cells of rat and mouse produces a curve with several peaks, to which the maxima of the frequencies are related as 1 : 2 : 4 : 8.[3] The relationship of nuclear size to ploidy is not a direct one, since DNA represents only 28.8% of the contents of rat liver nuclei.[4] Many investigations, however, suggest that doubling of the DNA content in liver nuclei is roughly reflected by a doubling of nuclear volume.[5]

In contrast to the liver in fetal or newborn animals, where roughly all parenchymal cells are mononucleate and diploid, hepatic parenchyma of the adult shows both polyploid nuclei and multinucleate cells. Binuclearity is the most common type of the multinucleate condition. According to the data given by Münzer,[6] the number of binucleate cells ranges from 10 to 25% in rodents, swine, monkeys, and man.

Polyploidy and binucleation show variations with regard to species, age, mitotic activity, endocrine regulation, and spatial distribution within the liver parenchyma. Nevertheless, it is possible to observe certain principles. The data of Alfert and Geschwind,[7] Nadal and Zajdela,[8] Carriere,[4] and James *et al.*[9] indicate the sequence of events in the normal rat liver shown in Fig. 3. After birth, the liver parenchyma consists almost entirely of diploid mononuclear cells.

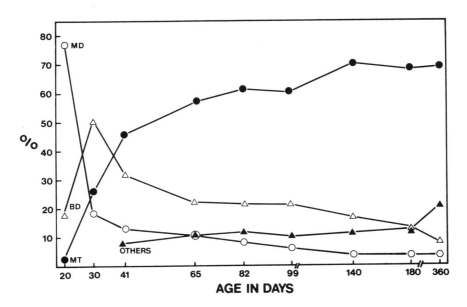

Figure 3. Relative frequencies (in percentages) of the various cell types in rat liver parenchyma. (MD) Mononuclear diploid cells; (BD) binuclear diploid cells; (MT) mononuclear tetraploid cells. After James et al.[9]

The binucleate cells with two diploid nuclei are the first polyploid cells to appear in the young rat. These cells reach their maximum during the second postnatal month and then decrease in number to 10% in the adult animal. The decrease of binucleate cells with two diploid nuclei is accompanied by a drastic increase of mononucleate tetraploid cells, which make up 60–70% of the liver cells in the adult animal. At the same time, the number of cells with two tetraploid nuclei is augmented, and these form 10% of the total cell population in the adult animal. Further cells with octoploid nuclei develop more slowly, and their number amounts finally to 10–20% of the total.

Divergent results have been published concerning the spatial distribution pattern of hepatocytes with different ploidy classes. According to Geller,[10] in areas adjacent to the terminal hepatic venules, around the portal spaces, and around the terminal afferent vessels that arise in this area, diploid and binucleate cells with two diploid nuclei are particularly numerous. Cells with tetraploid and octoploid nuclei are present in a broad intermediate zone. These findings demonstrate that the different zones of the acinus do not correlate with the ploidy classes. Van Noorden et al.[11] rightly remarked that heterogeneity of the parenchymal cell population should be taken into account with regard not only to the metabolic zonation but also to the ploidy classes.

The liver of the adult is a slowly self-replacing tissue with a low level of DNA synthesis and mitotic activity. Carriere[4] described a mitotic index of 0.03% with varying standard error in adult male rats. According to Brodsky and Uryvaeva,[12] DNA synthesis is hardly detectable, and [³H]thymidine administration to mice for several days results in labeling of less than 1% of the hepatocytes. It was reported that the labeled cells tend to have a periportal distribution, but because mitoses are so few in the normal adult liver, it must be assumed that normal growth and reparative growth are randomly distributed.

Partial hepatectomy or toxic injury causes proliferation of the remaining cells; however, it is not clear whether forced liver regeneration corresponds to normal regeneration. Since regeneration after operation or toxic damage leads to persistent elevation in polyploidy, experimentally induced proliferation only faintly resembles the normal condition. The observation, however, that 24 hr after partial hepatectomy DNA synthesis was found by means of autoradiographic techniques to be concentrated in the periportal area (later extending toward the terminal hepatic venule and becoming randomly distributed[13]) suggests that the periportal zone is the regenerative area of liver parenchyma.

2.4. Ultrastructure

In general, the liver parenchymal cells exhibit a submicroscopic organization similar to that of other eukaryotic cells (Fig. 4).

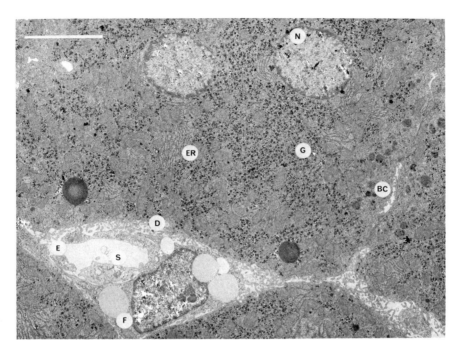

Figure 4.   Electron micrograph of a rat liver cell. (N) Nucleus of a parenchymal cell; (G) glycogen field; (ER) endoplasmic reticulum; (BC) bile canaliculus; (S) sinusoid; (D) space of Disse; (E) endothelial cell; (F) fat-storing cell. Scale bar: 5 μm. Original by Dr. L. Landmann.

The cytoplasm consists of two major components: solid structure and the cytosol. The cytosol contains soluble proteins, RNA, and enzymes that comprise about 25% of the total cell protein.[14] Of the numerous submicroscopic structures present (for quantitative data, see Table II), only those that have been especially studied in hepatocytes or that play a particular role in the function of these cells will be described. However, it must be stressed that intracellular structures can vary in both size and number in hepatocytes lining the sinusoids.

2.4.1. Mitochondria

The mitochondria of the liver cell exhibit the typical two-membrane structure. They vary in size and shape and make up about 20% of the cytoplasmic volume. In the rat liver, the mitochondria are on average shorter and larger at the beginning of the sinusoid and become progressively longer and thinner toward its end. The mean volume of mitochondria in the periportal cells is more than double that of perivenous mitochondria.[15]

Table II.   Ultrastructural Composition of Rat Liver Parenchymal Cells Calculated per Average Cell (Nucleus)[a]

Composition	Peripheral	Midzonal	Central
Volume (μm^3)			
Total cytoplasm[b]	5,100	5,100	5,100
Mitochondria	995	1,046	765
Peroxisomes	87	92	87
Lysosomes	10	10	20
Lipid	5	10	10
Glycogen	1,050	1,100	867
Other	2,953	2,842	3,351
Membrane area (μm^2)			
Agranular endoplasmic reticulum[c]	17,000	10,600	28,800
Granular endoplasmic reticulum[c]	30,400	29,200	22,600
Mitochondrial envelope	7,470	7,790	8,300
Mitochondrial cristae[d]	39,600	32,800	31,400
Number			
Mitochondria	1,160	1,480	1,530
Peroxisomes	490	560	490

[a] Data from Wiener et al.[61]

[b] Cytoplasmic volume was measured per nucleus because of the significant number of large binucleate parenchymal cells and is approximately equivalent to that of an average mononucleate cell.

[c] These figures, which were obtained by multiplying the measured membrane area per unit volume by the average volume per cell, have been further increased by 50% to correct for the effect of oblique sectioning on the observability of membrane profiles.

[d] These numbers are based on higher-magnification measurements of intramitochondrial structure reported elsewhere.

2.4.2. Lysosomes

Hepatic lysosomes are cytoplasmic particles surrounded by a membrane that is usually tripartite. They contain a variety of hydrolases, but are most often characterized by their content of acid phosphatase. The primary lysosomes (coated vesicles) contain acid hydrolases that are not involved in intracellular digestion. When this primary lysosome merges with a phagosome, digestion starts and the lysosome becomes a secondary lysosome and usually shows a variety of inclusions. Remains of undigested material are described as residual bodies. Lysosomes that are involved in the degradation of endogenous material are called autophagic; others that degrade exogenous material are heterophagic. In hepatocytes, the lysosomes take part in a number of different autophagic processes.[16]

The primary lysosomes originate from the Golgi apparatus or, more precisely, the GERL, a complex related to the inner aspect of the Golgi stack, containing a specialized region of smooth endoplasmic reticulum that forms the lysosomes.[17] According to Loud,[15] the distribution pattern of lysosomes suggests a trend toward greater numbers in the perivenous hepatocytes.

2.4.3. Peroxisomes

Peroxisomes are especially numerous and large in hepatocytes, where they have a mean diameter of 0.6 μm. These spherical or ellipsoid particles consist of a unit membrane, a fine granular matrix, and sometimes a dense, paracrystalline core that consists of urate oxidase in rat hepatocytes. Human hepatic peroxisomes lack both urate oxidase and cores.[18] The peroxisomes originate from the endoplasmic reticulum, which also appears to equip these particles with a group of oxidases for a variety of substrates. These enzymes produce hydrogen peroxide, which is decomposed by the leading enzyme of peroxisomes: catalase. The volume density of peroxisomes does not differ with the position of hepatocytes along the sinusoid, but the number of peroxisomes per cell increases toward the terminal hepatic venule.[15]

2.4.4. Endoplasmic Reticulum

The endoplasmic reticulum builds up an extensive network of tubules, vesicles, and lamellae. The lumina of the rough endoplasmic reticulum (RER) are 20–30 nm in diameter; those of the smooth endoplasmic reticulum (SER) 30–60 nm. Quantitative data indicate that SER is significantly more abundant in perivenous hepatocytes than at the beginning of the sinusoid; the RER is distributed without significant variations.[15]

2.4.5. Cytoskeletal Structures

These structures account for the regulation of cell shape and mobility and for the movement of structures within the cell. The actomyosin system consists of microfilaments that measure 4–7 nm in diameter. It forms a three-dimensional network and is mainly concentrated in the outer regions of the hepatocytes and especially around the bile canaliculi, where it plays an important role in secretion. Tubular structures with diameters between 6 and 11 nm make up a system of filaments of intermediate sizes that maintains cell shape and stability as well as divides the cell into compartments and controls the movement of organelles.[19] Finally, microtubules with an outer diameter of 20–26 nm traverse the cytoplasm of hepatocytes for long distances. These are also responsible for cell shape and the movement of organelles, particularly during mitotic division.

The submicroscopic organization of liver cells also displays regularity with regard to the intracellular distribution of the organelles. For example, if the cytoplasm of a liver cell is divided into zones concentric to the middle of the nucleus and beginning at the nuclear envelope, the quantitative analysis of ER and mitochondria shows the following distribution pattern: In the regions associated with the sinusoidal and the biliary pole, ER and mitochondria reach a maximum concentration in the zone nearest the nucleus. The mitochondria show a further maximum concentration at the periphery of the biliary canalicular pole. In cases of forced glycogen accumulation after fructose feeding, the main glycogen content is found in the intermediate zone of the cytoplasm, producing a relative concentration of ER and mitochondria around the nucleus and, in the case of the mitochondria, a less pronounced maximum at the cell periphery.[20]

2.5. Sinusoidal Cells

Aside from the fibrocytes and cells of the bile ductules, the sinusoidal cells form by far the greatest part by volume of the nonepithelial hepatocytes. On the basis of recent results, especially electron-microscopic observation, sinusoidal cells of the liver can be classified as follows: endothelial cells, Kupffer cells, fat-storing cells, and pit cells. They are self-proliferating cell types. They differ in morphology, enzyme content, capacity for endocytosis, and responses to different experimental conditions.

According to the morphometric data of Blouin,[21] the endothelial cells contribute 44.4%, Kupffer cells of 33.3%, fat-storing cells 10–25%, and the pit cells 5% to the volume of the nonhepatocytes.

2.5.1. Endothelial Cells

Endothelial cells are evenly distributed in the liver parenchyma; they are streamlined in shape and bulge only slightly into the sinusoidal lumen. Seen under the electron microscope, these cells have flat processes with typical fenestrations, occurring in groups to form the "sieve plates." According to Wisse et al.,[22] the endothelial lining in the perivenous zone shows a higher porosity than elsewhere. This finding, together with the longer perimeter of the sinusoids in this area by which blood flow rate might decrease, suggests that exchange processes between the blood and the parenchymal cells become easier at the distal end of the sinusoid. Gumucio and Miller,[23] however, postulated on the basis of their measurements a greater probability for solute–sinusoidal wall interaction in the periportal area. Endothelial cells are capable of endocytosis, but only to a degree, which distinguishes them fundamentally from the Kupffer cells; endothelial cells are unable to endocytose particles with a diameter of more than 100 nm and therefore have, in comparison with Kupffer cells, a much lower capacity for endocytosis. They are regarded as a self-proliferating cell class.[24,25]

2.5.2. Kupffer Cells

Kupffer cells are macrophages with a phagocytotic capacity for rather large particles (0.1–0.8 μm). They are highly variable in shape, most of the total surface being exposed to the sinusoidal bloodstream. Kupffer cells are part of the endothelial lining, but because of their high mobility, they can reach into the space of Disse or even become detached. These macrophages are not equally distributed throughout the liver parenchyma, but are situated predominantly in the periportal area. The surface of a Kupffer cell is equipped with a fuzzy coat that consists of proteins. The perikaryon is rich in cytoplasm with characteristic organelles, and typically includes tubelike structures that are thought to serve as a pool of spare cell membrane available for phagocytosis. The most apparent characteristic is the abundance of lysosomes, and these underline the digestive capacity of this cell type. Because of their high phagocytotic potency, Kupffer cells can be specifically labeled under experimental conditions. Kupffer cells are characterized histochemically by a high endogenous peroxidase activity and by high activities of glucose-6-phosphate dehydrogenase.[24,25]

2.5.3. Fat-Storing Cells

Fat-storing cells were first described by Ito and Nemoto.[26] They are characterized by their intracytoplasmic fat droplets and their ability to store vitamin A, which therefore serves as a marker for these cells. They occupy fixed positions evenly distributed along the sinusoidal wall. Typically, fat-storing cells are situated exclusively in the space of Disse, and they are often compressed into the recesses between hepatocytes. In normal rats, fat-storing cells contain an average of 25.3% by volume of fat droplets. Depending on their location and on the amount of fat stored, the perikarya can bulge into the sinusoidal lumen. Often, the fat-storing cells in the perivenous area show very few fat droplets, and have therefore been called "leere Fettspeicherzellen" (empty-fat-storing cells).[26]

Fat-storing cells probably have several functions. They are known to be sites of fat metabolism, since fat synthesis and the presence of fat droplets have been observed.[27] Moreover, fat-storing cells may have a mechanical function insofar as they support the sinusoidal wall. There is even some evidence of their ability to produce fibrous tissue, since, in areas of damaged liver parenchyma, local accumulations of fat-storing cells and fibroblasts have been observed. Fat-storing cells have been interpreted as resting fibroblasts that may be responsible for "intralobular" fibrogenesis.[24,28]

2.5.4. Pit Cells

Pit cells comprise a new sinusoidal cell class, the origin and function of which remain hypothetical. They are considered to have no preferential location in the liver parenchyma. Because of their characteristic granules, they have been named "pit cells."[29] Since the granules resemble those in endocrine cells, an endocrine function is feasible. Kaneda and Wake,[30] however, consider pit cells to be derived from the peripheral blood and to be closely related to lymphocytes.

2.6. Architecture of Liver Parenchyma

Histological sections reveal the relatively simple architecture of the mammalian liver parenchyma, which is composed of epithelial cells, blood vessels, bile ductules, and, depending on the species, a more or less prominent connective tissue. This lack of specific histological characteristics has led to difficulties in describing and defining a structural and functional liver unit. Even now, controversial opinions on these matters crop up in the literature and continue a discussion that reaches back to the beginning of light microscopy. Three main concepts are accepted (Fig. 5), although there are many discrepancies that will be discussed later.

2.6.1. Liver Lobule

These structural units were first described by Wepfer[31] and Malpighi[32] as small clumps of liver tissue adhering to minute blood vessels. The precise definition of the liver lobule was given by Kiernan[33] after his extensive studies on

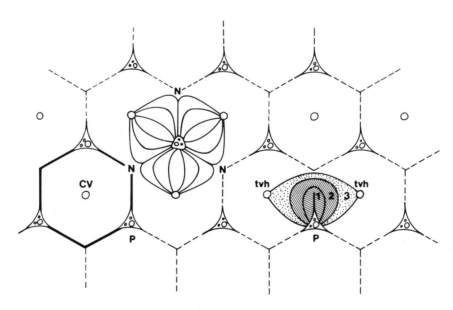

Figure 5.   Schematic drawing of the three main liver units. *Left:* Hexagonal liver lobule, surrounded by Glisson's portal triads (P) and drained by the central vein (CV). *Middle:* Portal unit, the center of which is formed by the triad. The lines point to the more or less bent sinusoids; the periphery of the portal unit is marked by central veins or by nodal points (N). *Right:* Liver acinus, the center of which is formed by the terminal afferent vessels and the periphery of which is drained by terminal hepatic venules (tvh). There are three different acinar zones: the periportal zone (1), the intermediate zone (2), and the perivenous zone (3).

the histology of pig liver. He stated that the liver lobule is a polygonal area of parenchyma with a boundary of connective tissue. The corners of the polygon are occupied by portal spaces containing a triad of structures: a branch of the portal vein, a branch of the hepatic artery, and a bile ductule. These vessels are surrounded by connective tissue, which accompanies the terminal arterial and venous branches running between the lobules to supply the sinusoids. The sinusoids lead the blood in the direction of the so-called central vein, which is situated in the center of the lobule ("central vein unit") and drains the whole of it.

Although this definition has been accepted by almost all writers of textbooks of histology since the time of Kiernan, there are three important arguments against it. In the first place, the fibrous septa that easily allow the lobules to be recognized are a peculiarity of the pig liver (and of certain rare species as well), but are absent in man and in most laboratory animals, in which the single lobule can be detected only with some difficulty. The second argument against the concept of the liver lobule is derived from the disparity between this description of a structural unit and a corresponding functional unit. Since the liver is not only a digestive organ, which acts on and is connected with the intestinal blood-stream, but is equally a secretory gland, the essential function of bile secretion is ignored both morphologically and conceptually. Therefore, soon after Kiernan's publication, alternative concepts were suggested that described liver units as bile lobules. The third argument against the central vein unit was the histochemical discovery that the periphery of the lobule is not uniform.

2.6.2. Portal Unit

Mall[34] presented a concept of the structural unit of the liver parenchyma that met the arguments against the lobule. He pointed out that in all other glands, the duct is the center of the structural unit. In his view, everything radiates from the portal space: arterial and portal blood vessels, bile ducts, lymphatics, nerves, and connective tissue. This portal space is therefore defined as the center of the portal unit. The sinusoids themselves are the first collecting vessels, because of their own anastomosing system, but there are differences in their length and direction. The shortest course between the portal and the hepatic veins is taken by perfectly straight sinusoids, and as the region away from the straight course is approached, the general direction of the sinusoids becomes more and more bent. It is obvious that the deflected sinusoids from several adjoining lobules come together at certain points. These nodal points and the adjacent intralobular ("central") veins mark the outline of each portal unit.

The concept of the portal unit is superior, in the view of many hepatologists, to that of the central vein unit, though both share the disadvantage of being difficult to recognize. Another striking argument against this concept is that the portal channels—the center of the portal unit—are preterminal vessels that, being *pre*terminal, function only to a limited extent as distribution vessels to the sinusoids.

2.6.3. Liver Acinus

Taking into account pathohistological findings and the knowledge of the microcirculation, Rappaport *et al.*[35] described a subdivision of the hexagonal liver lobule into a structural and functional unit, namely, the liver acinus. This concept was further elaborated in the following years.[36] According to Rappaport, the acinus is a clump of parenchyma oriented around the terminal afferent (portal and arterial) vessels. Together with the bile ductules, these vessels form the axis of the acinus, from which it is supplied by blood. In the periphery of the acinus lies the terminal hepatic venule (the former "central vein"), which drains the periphery of several adjacent acini. Since the quality of the blood passing through the sinusoids is altered by exchanges with the hepatocytes, three different zones have been postulated: the periportal zone (1) around the axis, which is supplied by blood with high oxygen content, the intermediate zone (2), and the perivenous zone (3), which receives blood that has already exchanged gases and metabolites with cells in zones 1 and 2. The intermediate zone is regarded as a transitional stretch of tissue.

Although liver acini are discernible only with special techniques (e.g., by injection of the afferent vessels), the concept of the liver acinus has become more widely accepted because of several major advantages that it possesses. When the axis, which includes the terminal afferent blood vessels and the first bile ductules, is regarded as the center of the unit, both the ingestive and the secretory functions of liver parenchyma are taken into account. Further, the functional aspect is regarded as the more important for the definition of the unit, and it therefore serves as a basis for the interpretation of the heterotopy of liver functions.[37] This functional heterogeneity of liver cells led to the concept of metabolic zonation.[38]

2.6.4. General Conclusions

The concept of the liver lobule, which used to be generally accepted as the anatomical and pathological unit for diagnostic purposes, has given way to a more modern concept that allows function and structure to be integrated. The liver acinus, rather than the portal unit, prevails as the basis for the interpretation of the functional aspects in the field of microcirculation and histochemistry. All the units that have been described above share the disadvantage that they require schematization to become definable and understandable. Although the real situation is more or less reflected, it is never totally represented (Fig. 6).

Although it is true that the hexagonal or polygonal lobules can be recognized in certain parts of a liver section, it is nearly impossible to divide up a whole

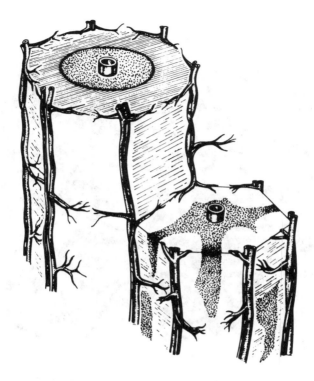

Figure 6.   Schematic drawing of the functional units of the liver. *Left:* In the liver lobule, a peripheral and a pericentral functional area are discernible, which are oriented concentrically around the central vein. *Right:* In the liver acinus, the arrangement of metabolic zones depends on their proximity to the terminal afferent vessels. Therefore, the (stippled) perivenous zone is irregularly shaped.

section into such units. It has therefore been necessary to describe larger units such as the collecting lobule (Sammelläppchen). Comparable difficulties obviously appear with respect to the acinus, the berrylike shape of which is hardly evident. The zones described above can be demonstrated histochemically by enzyme activity; however, these seldom correspond to the idealized concept.

Other proposals for the hepatic unit have not led to a solution of these difficulties. The meticulous studies on the angioarchitecure of the liver by Matsumoto *et al.*[39] resulted in a subdivision of the liver lobule ("secondary lobule") into six to eight "primary lobules" with sickle zones in the periportal area; however, these primary lobules do not present a clearly visible outline in normally stained histological sections. Other authors, such as Bloch[40] and later Teutsch,[41] have tried to overcome the difficulties of recognition by regarding the sinusoid, together with the space of Disse and the abutting hepatocytes, as the functional unit. This has the result, however, that either each lining hepatocyte belongs to two units or the unit includes only one half of the cell.

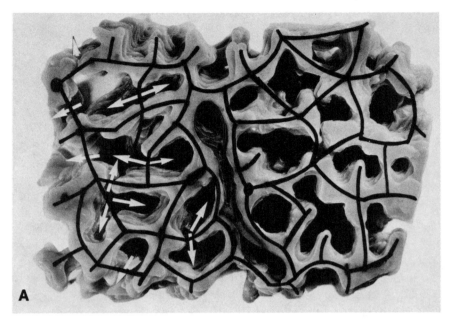

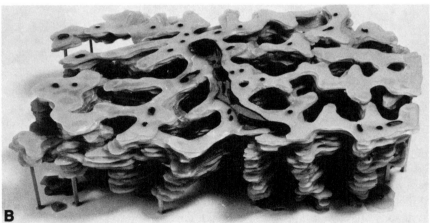

Figure 7.   Microreconstruction of a human liver after an endocrine shock caused by a pheochro-mocytoma. The perivenous areas are reconstucted. (A) The dark lines indicate the borders of the liver lobules. The white arrows demonstrate the continuity of the perivenous zones. The whole parenchyma proves to be an irregular interdigitating system. (B) Side aspect of the microreconstruc-tion.

Examination of a microreconstruction of liver parenchyma with periportal or perivenous zonal necrosis (Fig. 7) makes it clear that the periportal and perivenous areas together build up a continuum that is oriented around the terminal afferent and efferent branches of the hepatic blood vessels. As a whole, the liver parenchyma can be described as an irregular interdigitating system of regions related to these terminal vessels. The specific relationship of liver cells to certain metabolic conditions that are found at different positions along the sinusoid can be established only in areas where sinusoids are seen histologically as arising from the terminal afferent vessels and ending in the terminal hepatic venule.

3. INNERVATION OF THE LIVER

3.1. Macroscopic Aspects

The mammalian liver is richly supplied by afferent and efferent nerves of the autonomic nervous system from two communicating plexuses surrounding the portal vein and the hepatic artery.

The smaller anterior hepatic plexus is situated in the hepatoduodenal ligament and is chiefly associated wih the hepatic artery. It is composed of parasympathetic fibers from the vagus nerve: direct hepatic branches of the anterior (left) vagal trunk, branches from the main nerves of the lesser curvature of the stomach, and bundles of fibers arising predominantly from the posterior (right) vagal trunk via the celiac plexus. Sympathetic nerves come from the celiac plexus, which is itself composed of celiac ganglia and fibers from the splanchnic nerves. The nerves of the anterior hepatic plexus supply the liver, the bile ducts, and the gallbladder.

The larger posterior hepatic plexus is situated behind the portal vein and is mainly associated with it. The parasympathetic fibers predominantly stem from the posterior (right) vagal trunk; the sympathetic fibers come out of the celiac plexus. The nerves enter the liver in association with the blood vessels and bile duct.[42–44]

3.2. Microscopic Aspects

Various methods have been used for the study of intrinsic hepatic nerves. Many histological staining techniques based on silver impregnation, which often leads to difficulty in distinguishing between nerve fibers and reticular fibers, have been used to study the liver. The more modern techniques used in this field include histochemical procedures, such as the demonstration of specific enzyme activity (acetylcholinesterase, monoamine oxidase), autoradiographic techniques, and catecholamine fluorescence. A further approach is made possible by the use of the electron microscope, sometimes after surgical or chemical degeneration.

The data on liver innervation that have been published in the last 20 years are extremely contradictory owing to the different techniques employed, and are further complicated by apparent species differences.[45] Nevertheless, physiological and biochemical results point out that intrinsic nerves play an essential role in the regulation of blood flow and liver metabolism. Hepatic afferent nerves are connected to chemoreceptors, osmoreceptors, and baroreceptors;[46] they are also involved in the regulation of short-term feeding behavior.[47] Efferent nerves are responsible for the vasomotor regulation of the liver blood flow. Other efferent nerves terminating on the hepatocytes can exert control over the metabolic function of the liver.[46,48]

Afferent and efferent fibers are present in both the adrenergic (sympathetic) nerves and the cholinergic (parasympathetic) nerves. These nerves originate from or terminate in nuclei of the central nervous system. Shimazu[48] was able to localize centers of autonomic innervation by electrostimulation. Stimulation of the ventromedial hypothalamic nucleus, for instance, causes glycogenolysis, the impulses being conveyed via the splanchnic nerves, whereas electrical stimulation of the lateral hypothalamic nucleus of the vagus promotes glycogenesis. By applying horseradish peroxidase to the hepatic branch of the vagus in rats, Rogers and Hermann[49] were able to elucidate a predominate pattern of afferent terminations within the left subnucleus gelatinosus, the medial division of the left nucleus solitarius, and the left lateral edge of the area postrema. Efferent nuclei were concentrated in the left dorsal motor nucleus of the vagus and in some neurons in the right one, as well as in the left anterior nucleus ambiguus.

The morphological findings on hepatic innervation can be summarized as follows:

A positive acetylcholinesterase reaction, which might with reservations be interpreted as a parasympathetic signal, was found in nerve bundles in the connective tissue of the adventitia of the portal vein, of the hepatic artery, and of the hepatic veins.[50,51] In addition to the external plexus, de Luca et al.[52] described an inner plexus at the level of the transitional zone between adventitia and media and in the outer layers of the media. Cholinergic innervation can be traced as far as the portal spaces[53,54] and to the lamina of hepatic cells that abut the portal area.

The detection of monoaminergic (noradrenergic) fibers by fluorescence techniques reveals a remarkably rich innervation of the hepatic artery and especially of the portal vein.[50] It was demonstrated in all branches of these afferent vessels.[54] Electron-microscopic investigations demonstrated nerve fibers in all three layers of the portal vein. Between the muscle layers of the media, there are axons in close connection with the smooth muscle cells, and terminals have also been found in the intima.[55] Fine varicose monoaminergic fibers run parallel to the axis of the preterminal and terminal portal vessels. Many fewer monoaminergic fibers are present in the walls of the hepatic veins. Noradrenergic innervation of the bile ducts appears to be sparse.

While the results described above apply to a greater or lesser extent to most of the mammalian species that have so far been investigated, the direct connection of hepatocytes to nerve fibers depends on the species examined. Forssmann and Ito[56] and Metz and Forssmann[57] pointed to the important interspecies variations of hepatocellular innervation, which have also been confirmed by others.

In general, cholinergic nerve fibers have been found only in connection with the cells of the outer limiting plate of the parenchyma. Acetylcholinesterase-positive nerves enter the periportal area only in guinea pigs.[50]

A marked species variation concerns the density of adrenergic innervation of the liver parenchyma. Human liver and liver of the rhesus monkey, baboon, cynomolgus monkey, and guinea pig show a high density of parenchymal adrenergic fibers. An intermediate group is formed by the rabbit, cat, pig, cow, and horse. Species with little or no parenchymal innervation are said to include the rat and the mouse,[58] although an intralobular nerve supply has been described in rats by Skaaring and Bierring[53] and in mice by Yamada.[59]

Because the hepatic cells in the tree shrew are extensively innervated but have few gap junctions, and in the mouse and rat few hepatocytes have a nerve supply but possess many gap junctions, Forssmann and Ito[56] suggested that a lack of innervation could possibly be compensated for by direct intercellular communicative junctions.

3.3. Electron-Microscopic Aspects

The morphology of intraparenchymatous nerves has been studied in various species by use of the electron microscope.[54,56,57,60] The results in man, monkey, *Tupaia belangeri,* and guinea pig (and to some extent in the rat) indicate that bundles of autonomic fibers, most of them surrounded by satellite cells and a basal lamina, lie in the portal spaces. The nerves contain empty and dense core vesicles of different sizes. From here, small fascicles branch off and enter the spaces of Disse, thus taking a radial course in the direction of the terminal hepatic venule (Fig. 8). These fibers are associated in groups and are either partially surrounded by satellite cells or unmyelinated. The axons have intervaricose segments of 400–500 nm that contain numerous neurotubules. These intervaricose segments are often localized within deep grooves or notches of the liver cells, partly enclosed by the hepatocyte membrane on the side of the space of Disse. The varicose expansions exhibit a diameter of 650–1300 nm and are normally in close contact with the hepatocyte. Single axons with prominent varicosities and without Schwann cells also make contact with endothelial cells, fat-storing cells, or Kupffer cells. The varicosities contain clusters of mitochondria and of transmitter vesicles of three types: (1) large, dense core vesicles, 80 nm in diameter; (2) smaller dense core vesicles, 40 nm in diameter; and (3) clear

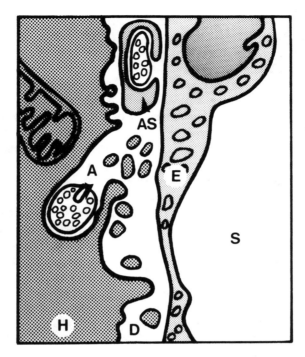

Figure 8. Schematic drawing of guinea pig innervation. Axon, surrounded by a satellite cell (AS), in the space of Disse (D). Another axon (A) is in contact with a hepatocyte (H). (E) Endothelial cell; (S) sinusoidal lumen. After Metz and Forssmann.[57]

vesicles, 40 nm in diameter. Synaptic membrane specializations are absent from these neuroeffector junctions. The interspace between the axon and the hepatocyte membrane is formed by a small cleft of about 20 nm.

4. SUMMARY

Liver development starts from the entodermal epithelium of the intestine and from the mesenchymal cells of the septum transversum. In each liver parenchymal cell, the double function of the whole organ is perceptible; thus, the liver cell both is part of a gland secreting the bile into a canalicular system and has surfaces oriented to the sinusoidal bloodstream for the exchange of metabolites. The "muralium hepatis" is interspersed with sinusoidal capillaries that are surrounded by characteristic cells: the endothelial cells, which are modified reticulum cells, the phagocytotic Kupffer cells, the fat-storing cells, and the pit cells.

Even today, it is difficult to describe a specific structural unit of liver parenchyma. Of the more frequently discussed concepts, the liver lobule, the portal unit, and the liver acinus are described. The liver lobule might serve as a suitable basis for the description of pathohistological diagnosis. The liver acinus, however, is more apt for the demonstration of liver function, and therefore for the distribution patterns of enzyme activities that indicate metabolic zonation. It is suggested that defining a liver unit requires a schematization that does not totally reflect the real situation, but that might be described as an irregularly interdigitating system of metabolically differing zones.

An important prerequisite for the regulation of the metabolic functions of the liver parenchyma is its autonomic innervation. Contradictory data in the literature point out that fibers of the sympathetic and parasympathetic nervous system arrive at and come from the liver. Both systems supply the afferent blood vessels and the bile ducts. The innervation of liver parenchymal cells is species-dependent; while adrenergic innervation has been found in many species, a cholinergic innervation of the liver epithelium remains questionable.

REFERENCES

1. Daoust, R., 1958, The cell population of liver tissue and the cytological reference bases, *Am. Inst. Biol. Sci. Publ.* **4:**3–10.
2. Elias, H., 1955, Liver morphology, *Biol. Rev.* **30:**263–310.
3. Jacobj, W., 1925, Über das rhythmische Wachstum der Zellen durch Verdoppelung ihres Volumens, *Roux Arch.* **106:**124–192.
4. Carriere, R., 1969, The growth of liver parenchymal nuclei and its endocrine regulation, *Int. Rev. Cytol.* **25:**201–277.
5. Amano, M., 1967, Metabolism of RNA in the liver cells of the rat. I. Isolation and chemical composition of nucleus, nucleolus, chromatin, nuclear sap and cytoplasm, *Exp. Cell Res.* **46:**169–179.
6. Münzer, F. T., 1923, Über die Zweikernigkeit der Leberzellen, *Arch. Mikrosk. Anat.* **98:**249–282.
7. Alfert, M., and Geschwind, J. J., 1958, Development of polysomaty in the rat liver, *Exp. Cell Res.* **15:**230–232.
8. Nadal, D., and Zajdela, F., 1966, Polyploïdie somatique dans le foie de rat. I. Le rôle des cellules binuclées dans la génèse des cellules polyploïdes, *Exp. Cell Res.* **42:**99–116.
9. James, J., Tas, J., Bosch, K. S., de Meere, A. J. P., and Schuyt, H. C., 1979, Growth patterns of rat hepatocytes during postnatal development, *Eur. J. Cell Biol.* **19:**222–226.
10. Geller, S., 1965, Intralobular distribution of polyploid cells in rat liver, *Anat. Rec.* **151:**352–353.
11. Van Noorden, C. J. F., Bhattacharya, R. D., and Fronik, G., 1984, Glucose-6-phosphate dehydrogenase activity in individual rat hepatocytes of different ploidy classes. II. Day time dependent variations, *Chronobiologia* (in press).
12. Brodsky, W. Y., and Uryvaeva, J. V., 1977, Cell polyploidy: Its relation to tissue growth and function, *Int. Rev. Cytol.* **50:**275–332.
13. Bucher, N. L. R., 1963, Regeneration of mammalian liver, *Int. Rev. Cytol.* **15:**245–300.
14. Denk, H., and Franke, W. W., 1982, Cytoskeletal filaments, in: *The Liver: Biology and Pathobiology* (J. M. Arias, H. Popper, D. Schachter, and D. A. Shafritz, eds.), Raven Press, New York.
15. Loud, A. V., 1968, A quantitative stereological description of the ultrastructure of normal rat liver parenchymal cells, *J. Cell Biol.* **37:**27–46.

16. Novikoff, A. B., and Shin, W. Y., 1978, Endoplasmic reticulum and autophagy in rat hepatocytes, *Proc. Natl. Acad. Sci. U.S.A.* **75**:5039–5042.
17. Novikoff, A. B., and Novikoff, P. M., 1977, Cytochemical contributions to differentiating GERL from the Golgi apparatus, *Histochem. J.* **9**:525–551.
18. Hruban, Z., and Rechcigl, M., 1969, *Microbodies and Related Particles*, Academic Press, New York.
19. Jahn, W., 1980, The cytoskeleton of rat liver parenchymal cells, *Naturwissenschaften* **67**:568.
20. Riede, U. N., and Sasse, D., 1981, Quantitative topography of organelles in the liver: A combined histochemical and morphometric analysis, *Cell Tissue Res.* **221**:209–220.
21. Blouin, A., 1977, Morphometry of liver sinusoidal cells, in: *Kupffer Cells and Other Liver Sinusoidal Cells* (E. Wisse and D. L. Knook, eds.), pp. 61–71, Elsevier/North-Holland, Amsterdam.
22. Wisse, E., DeZanger, R., and Jacobs, R., 1982, Lobular gradients in endothelial fenestrae and sinusoidal diameter favour centrolobular exchange processes: A scanning EM study, in: *Sinusoidal Liver Cells* (D. L. Knook and E. Wisse, eds.), pp. 61–67, Elsevier, Amsterdam.
23. Gumucio, J. J., and Miller, D. L., 1982, Liver cell heterogeneity, in: *The Liver: Biology and Pathobiology* (J. M. Arias, H. Popper, D. Schachter, and D. A. Shafritz, eds.), Raven Press, New York.
24. Wisse, E., 1977, Ultrastructure and function of Kupffer cells and other sinusoidal cells in the liver, in: *Kupffer Cells and Other Liver Sinusoidal Cells* (E. Wisse and D. L. Knook, eds.), pp. 33–60, Elsevier/North-Holland, Amsterdam.
25. Hosemann, W., Teutsch, H. F., and Sasse, D., 1979, Identification of G6PDH active sinusoidal cells as Kupffer cells in the rat liver, *Cell Tissue Res.* **196**:237–247.
26. Ito, T., and Nemoto, M., 1952, Über die Kupfferschen Sternzellen und die "Fettspeicherungszellen" ("fat storing cells") in der Blutkapillarenwand der menschlichen Leber, *Okajimas Folia Anat. Jpn.* **24**:243–258.
27. Bronfenmajer, S., Schaffner, F., and Popper, H., 1966, Fat storing cells (lipocytes) in human liver, *Arch. Pathol.* **82**:447–453.
28. MacGee, J. O. D., and Patrick, R. S., 1972, The role of perisinusoidal cells in hepatic fibrogenesis: An electron microscopic study of acute carbon tetrachloride liver injury, *Lab. Invest.* **26**:429–440.
29. Wisse, E., Noordende, J. M., Van't Meulen, J., and Van der Daems, W. T. H., 1976, The pit cell: Description of a new type of cell occurring in rat liver sinusoids and peripheral blood, *Cell Tissue Res.* **173**:423–435.
30. Kaneda, K., and Wake, K., 1983, Distribution and morphological characteristics of the pit cells in the liver of the rat. *Cell Tissue Res.* **233**:485–505.
31. Wepfer, H. E., 1664, *De dubiis anatomicis, epistula ad Jacob. Hen. Paulum,* Nürnberg.
32. Malpighi, M., 1666, *De viscerum structura exercitatio anatomica,* London.
33. Kiernan, F., 1833, The anatomy and physiology of the liver, *Philos. Trans. R. Soc. London,* pp. 711–770.
34. Mall, F. P., 1906, A study of the structural unit of the liver, *Am. J. Anat.* **5**:227–308.
35. Rappaport, A. M., Borowy, Z. J., Longheed, W. M., and Lotto, W. N., 1954, Subdivision of hexagonal liver lobules into a structural and functional unit: Role in hepatic physiology and pathology, *Anat. Rec.* **119**:11–34.
36. Rappaport, A. M., 1976, The microcirculatory acinar concept of normal and pathological hepatic structure, *Beitr. Pathol.* **157**:215–243.
37. Zeiger, K., 1952, Zur funktionellen Anatomie der Leber, *Dtsch. Z. Verdau. Stoffwechselkr. Sonderbd.* 22–31.
38. Jungermann, K., and Sasse, D., 1978, Heterogeneity of liver parenchymal cells, *Trends Biochem. Sci.* **3**:198–202.
39. Matsumoto, T., Komori, R., Magara, T., Ui, T., Kawakami, M., Tokuda, T., Takasaki, S.,

Hayashi, H., Jo, K., Hano, H., Fujino, H., and Tanaka, H., 1979, A study on the normal structure of the human liver, with special reference to its angioarchitecture, *Jikeikai Med. J.* **26**:1–40.

40. Bloch, E. H., 1970, The determination of hepatic arterioles and the functional unit of the liver as determined by microscopy of the living organ, *Ann. N. Y. Acad. Sci.* **170**:78–87.

41. Teutsch, H. F., 1981, Chemomorphology of liver parenchyma, *Prog. Histochem. Cytochem.* **14**(3).

42. Riegele, L., 1928, Über das feinere Verhalten der Nerven in der Leber von Mensch und Säugetier, *Z. Mikrosk.-Anat. Forsch.* **14**:73–98.

43. Alexander, W. F., 1940, The innervation of the biliary system, *J. Comp. Neurol.* **72**:357–370.

44. Stelmasiak, M., and Kurylcio, L., 1971, Nerwy watroby i drog zolciowych, *Folia Morphol. (Warsaw)* **30**:169–182.

45. Lautt, W. W., 1980, Hepatic nerves: A review of their functions and effects, *Can. J. Physiol. Pharmacol.* **58**:105–123.

46. De Wulf, H., and Carton, H., 1981, Neural control of glycogen metabolism, in: *Short-Term Regulation of Liver Metabolism* (L. Hue and G. Van de Werve eds.), Elsevier/North-Holland, Amsterdam.

47. Russek, M., 1971, Hepatic receptors and the neurophysiological mechanisms controlling feeding behavior, in: *Neuroscience Research* (S. Ehrenpreis, ed.), pp. 213–282, Academic Press, New York.

48. Shimazu, T., 1981, Central nervous system regulation of liver and adipose tissue metabolism, *Diabetologia* **20**(Suppl.)343–356.

49. Rogers, R. C., and Hermann, G. E., 1983, Central connections of the hepatic branch of the vagus nerve: A horseradish peroxidase histochemical study, *J. Auton. Nerv. Syst.* **7**:165–174.

50. Ungvary, G., 1977, *Functional Morphology of the Hepatic Vascular System*, Adadémiai Kiadó, Budapest.

51. Tonelli, F., Amenta, F., Cavalotti, C., and Ferrante, F., 1981, Cholinergic nerves in the human liver, *Histochem. J.* **13**:419–424.

52. De Luca, C., Cantagalli, A., De Angelis, E., and Amenta, F., 1982, Cholinergic nerves in the rat portal vein, *Experientia* **38**:397–398.

53. Skaaring, P., and Bierring, F., 1977, Further evidence for the existence of intralobular nerves in the rat liver, *Cell Tissue Res.* **177**:287–290.

54. Reilly, F. D., McCuskey, A. P., and McCuskey, R. S., 1978, Intrahepatic distribution of nerves in the rat, *Anat. Rec.* **191**:55–67.

55. Ungváry, G., and Varga, B., 1971, Intralobular redistribution of tissue circulation in the canine liver. II. Effect of the stimulation on certain peripheral nerves, *Acta Physiol. Acad. Sci. Hung.* **40**:347–357.

56. Forssmann, W. G., and Ito, S., 1977, Hepatocyte innervation in primates, *J. Cell Biol.* **74**:299–313.

57. Metz, W., and Forssmann, W. G., 1980, Innervation of the liver in guinea pig and rat, *Anat. Embryol.* **160**:239–252.

58. Moghimzadeh, E., Nobin, A., and Rosengren, E., 1982, Adrenergic nerves and receptors in the liver, *Brain Res. Bull.* **9**:709–714.

59. Yamada, E., 1965, Some observations on the nerve terminal on the liver parenchymal cell of the mouse as revealed by electron microscopy, *Okajimas Folia Anat. Jpn.* **40**:663–677.

60. Nobin, A., Baumgarten, H. G., Falck, F., Jngemansson, S., Moghimzadeh, E., and Rosengren, E., 1978, Organization of the sympathetic innervation in liver tissue from monkey and man, *Cell Tissue Res.* **195**:371–380.

61. Wiener, J., Loud, A. V., Kimberg, D., and Spiro, D., 1968, A quantitative description of cortisone induced alteration in the ultrastructure of rat liver parenchymal cells, *J. Cell Biol.* **37**:47–62.

Chapter 2

Hepatic Hemodynamics and Microcirculation

P. G. Withrington and P. D. I. Richardson

1. INTRODUCTION

In this chapter, we aim to give an overview of normal values for hepatic hemodynamic variables (Section 2), followed by a brief résumé of some techniques used experimentally (Section 3). This is in turn followed by details of the control and pharmacological responses of the hepatic arterial (Section 4) and portal venous (Section 5) resistance vessels, their interrelationship (Section 6), and the hepatic capacitance and exchange vessels (Section 7). The relationship between liver circulation and liver function is reviewed briefly (Section 8). A summary (Section 9) concludes the chapter.

Glossary. Following are definitions of some technical terms used in this chapter:

Resistance. This is used exactly as in Ohm's law. The vascular resistance of a tissue or organ (i.e., liver) is defined as the mean pressure gradient (i.e., hepatic arterial minus hepatic venous pressure *or* hepatic portal minus hepatic venous pressure) divided by the simultaneously measured mean blood flow.

P. G. WITHRINGTON • Department of Pharmacology, The Medical College of St. Bartholomew's Hospital, London EC1M 6BQ, England.   P. D. I. RICHARDSON • Medical Department, Astra Pharmaceuticals Ltd., Home Park Estate, Kings Langley, Hertfordshire WD4 8DH, England.

Conductance. This is the reciprocal of the vascular resistance, i.e., concomitant mean flow/pressure gradient.

Vasoconstriction. An active increase in vascular resistance of a tissue caused by reduction in the caliber of the primary resistance sites, i.e., the arterioles or capillary sphincters.

It is important to realize that vasodilatation and vasoconstriction are terms used to describe active changes in vascular resistance rather than any passive changes brought about by alterations in the perfusion pressure gradient.

Capacitance. The available volume of the intravascular space of a tissue or organ. Changes in vascular capacity are usually associated with alterations, either active or passive, in tone of the venous smooth muscle.

Compliance. An estimate of the change of the capacity of a vascular bed usually obtained by elevating the venous pressure of a tissue or organ while measuring its volume, i.e., dV/dP.

Tachyphylaxis. The phenomenon whereby in a series of injections of the same dose of a drug or hormone into a vascular bed the vascular responses become smaller with subsequent administration.

2. HEPATIC VASCULAR RESISTANCE: CONTROL VALUES

Under "physiological conditions" of normal arterial and venous pressures, the principal determinant of hepatic arterial blood flow (HABF) is hepatic arterial vascular resistance (HAVR).

In the anesthetized dog, a species for which much information is available, mean hepatic arterial pressure (i.e., systemic BP) is about 100–110 mm Hg, hepatic venous (i.e., inferior vena caval) pressure is 1 or 2 mm Hg, and HABF is about 50 ml min^{-1} 100 g^{-1} expressed in terms of liver weight. Liver weight is about 2–4% of total body weight. This gives an HAVR of 1.5–3.0 mm Hg ml^{-1} min 100 g.

In contrast, hepatic portal venous blood flow (HPVF) is not determined primarily by intrahepatic portal vascular resistance, but by the blood flow through the intestine and spleen, the venous drainage of which, together with that from the pancreas and omentum, constitutes the portal venous blood supply. Portal blood flow depends ultimately on vascular resistances of the intestine[1] and spleen,[2] which are reviewed elsewhere. Intrahepatic vascular resistance to portal blood flow is low; in the dog, portal flow is about 75–90 ml min^{-1} 100 g^{-1} and portal venous pressure 5–10 mm Hg, giving a calculated intrahepatic portal vascular resistance of 0.02–0.10 mm Hg ml^{-1} min 100 g—about 1/30th that of the arterial tract.

Lists of values for pressure, flow, and vascular resistance are available elsewhere,[3] and a discussion of the interrelationship between the hepatic arterial and portal vascular systems is presented in Section 6.

3. TECHNIQUES

Clinically, accurate measurement of total liver blood flow is possible,[4-6] but the techniques necessarily impose two restrictions: The measurements are discontinuous, and they do not differentiate between hepatic arterial and portal venous blood flows. The techniques are also more or less invasive and are in use in only a limited number of centers.

For this reason, much reliance has to be placed on the results of animal experimentation. If we assume that the fundamental point of most animal experimentation is to elucidate more of the function and pathology of the human liver, major problems arise.

Much experimental work can be grouped into two categories. The first category comprises "biochemical" experiments using either cellular liver preparations or livers perfused with physiological solutions through the portal vein alone. Often there is no measurement of vascular variables, and the portal bed is exposed to unphysiological pressures associated with either high or low perfusion fluid flows. Moreover, with perfusion through the portal vein alone, oxygen supply is appreciably reduced below normal, when at least 50% would be supplied by the hepatic artery.

The second category is that of "perfusion" experiments typified by the early work of Burton-Opitz[7] and the more recent work of Greenway and Lautt[8-10] and Richardson and Withrington.[3,11] In these experiments, the livers of anesthetized animals were perfused *in situ* via both the hepatic artery and the portal vein, and intravascular pressures, blood flows, oxygen uptake, and liver volume were the principal variables measured. In most but not all[12] of these experiments, it was impossible to estimate the functional integrity of the liver in terms of its metabolic activity or potential for activity. It is conceivable that such experimental preparations, which may involve several hours of major surgery, cannulation of blood vessels, manipulation of the liver itself, and hemodilution, could cause changes in liver function that make subsequent observations atypical.

Nevertheless, major contributions to our understanding of the liver circulation have been made using these techniques. Physical access to the liver and its blood vessels is inherently difficult, and accurate noninvasive methods that would give continuous blood flow data do not seem likely to emerge in the near future.

The development of microvascular techniques in other organs has led to their use in the liver. Microsphere techniques have been used to study blood-flow distribution in the various lobes of the liver[13]; though valuable information has been obtained using microspheres, the measurements are intrinsically isolated rather than continuous. Transillumination techniques have been applied successfully to the margins of the liver[14,15] and have yielded important information about the physiological and pharmacological responses of the hepatic microvessels and sinusoids. The single problem with this approach is that the vessels at the extreme edges of the liver that are amenable to transillumination may not be representative in anatomy, physiology, or pharmacology of the bulk of vessels deeper in the organ.

4. HEPATIC ARTERIAL RESISTANCE

4.1. Intrinsic Regulation

The hepatic arterial vascular bed exhibits intrinsic regulatory mechanisms, though their quantitative contribution to the physiological control of hepatic arterial blood flow (HABF) is undoubtedly small.

Some studies have revealed hepatic arterial autoregulation, i.e., a decreased hepatic arterial resistance at low arterial pressure, and vice versa, effects that tend to maintain a constant HABF.[16,17] In other experiments that cannot be differentiated technically, no sign of hepatic arterial autoregulation could be found[18]; the controversy over the existence of autoregulation should not cloud the main conclusion of all experiments—that hepatic arterial autoregulation is weak or nonexistent and is not quantitatively an important control of HABF. In the small intestine,[19] autoregulation is more evident in the fed than in the fasted state, and it has been suggested that a comparable situation may occur between the metabolically active compared to the "quiescent" liver[20]; however, the relationship between HABF and hepatic metabolic activity is controversial,[21] and at present it seems improbable that differences in metabolic activity explain the discrepancies among different series of investigations of the presence or absence of hepatic arterial autoregulation.

Elevation of hepatic venous pressure increases hepatic arterial vascular resistance (HAVR),[17] and although the response is modest, this is unequivocal evidence[1] of an intrinsic myogenic response of the hepatic arterial resistance sites to increased transmural pressure.

Further evidence of intrinsic regulation of the hepatic arterial vasculature comes from the response of postocclusion reactive hyperemia[16,17]; such responses are indicative of intrinsic control, and are probably explained by a local buildup of vasodilator "metabolites" during the period of arterial occlusion—a metabolic as opposed to a myogenic[1,3] response—since the response is dependent on the magnitude and duration of the hepatic arterial flow restriction.

4.2. Blood Gases

Weak intrinsic control of blood flow is consistent with weak vascular responses to alterations in systemic arterial pO_2 and pCO_2. Reduction of arterial pO_2 to about 36–44 mm Hg failed to alter hepatic arterial resistance in the cat[22] and the dog.[23] Extreme hypoxia (pO_2 = 25 mm Hg) caused an increased HAVR.[24]

Hypercapnia (pCO_2 = 65 mm Hg) increases, and hypocapnia (pCO_2 = 24 mm Hg) decreases, canine HABF,[23] though the changes are small.

4.3. Osmolarity

Increases in arterial osmolarity increase regional blood flow in many organs, but the principal interest with respect to hepatic circulation concerns increases in portal venous plasma osmolarity such as would occur consequent on absorption from the intestines. Increased portal osmolarity increases HABF in the cat[25] and dog[26]; even moderate increments in portal osmolarity (30–35 mosmoles/liter), which are associated with trivial increases in systemic arterial osmolarity (0–5 mosmoles/liter), and which are about the same as postprandial changes in plasma osmolarity,[27] reduce hepatic arterial resistance by about 10%.[26] We believe that changes in portal venous osmolarity may be an important physiological control of HABF, and consequently oxygen delivery to the liver, at times of increased demand such as during absorption and metabolic stimulation.

4.4. Nervous Control

The principal nervous regulation of hepatic arterial resistance, and consequently blood flow, is by the hepatic periarterial sympathetic nerves. Experimentally, electrical stimulation of the peripheral (hepatic) end of this nerve bundle increases hepatic arterial resistance and reduces HABF in a frequency-dependent manner.[27–30]

In the cat[31,32] but not the dog,[29] maintained hepatic arterial nerve stimulation fails to evoke a maintained vasoconstriction, and the blood flow slowly returns toward control values—autoregulatory escape. Hepatic nerve stimulation does not cause redistribution of blood flow within the liver; microsphere studies[13] suggest an equivalent vasoconstriction in all lobes and areas of the liver when the hepatic nerves are stimulated. However, other reports using different techniques suggest that these observations are not uniform in all species.

The experimental observations are clear, but their physiological relevance requires critical assessment, for, *a priori*, one would expect a vital organ such as the liver to be spared extreme vasoconstriction during generalized sympathetic stimulation, when the portal blood flow would certainly be compromised due to intestinal[1] and splenic[2] vasoconstriction.

Carneiro and Donald[28] stimulated the sympathetic supply to the liver indirectly via the baroreceptor reflex and, by reducing the carotid sinus blood pressure to 40 mm Hg, maximally increased HAVR by about 45%. This is the same increase as that produced by direct hepatic periarterial stimulation at 1–2 Hz[30] and probably indicates the limit on changes in HAVR under physiological conditions. At constant arterial pressure, a 45% increase in vascular resistance is equivalent to about a 30% reduction in blood flow.

4.5. Gastrointestinal and Pancreatic Hormones

The synthetic gastrin analogues, pentagastrin,[33,34] secretin,[34,35] cholecystokinin-pancreozymin (CCK-PZ),[34] and glucagon[34,35] all cause hepatic arterial vasodilatation when injected or infused into the hepatic artery; the effect of glucagon is particularly protracted.[34,35]

Although pharmacologically interesting, these effects probably do not illustrate a physiological vasoregulatory role of any one of these hormones, since the quantities administered in these experiments were in excess of those likely to be encountered physiologically or even pathologically. Consideration of the potential systemic roles of individual gastrointestinal hormones may be misleading, however, since they are naturally released sequentially (e.g., gastrin, secretin), concomitantly (secretin, CCK-PZ) or locally (e.g., vasoactive intestinal peptide), and until some information is available on the effects of hormones administered in a way and at a concentration that closely resemble their natural release, it is premature to pass judgment on their possible role as hepatic arterial vasoregulators.

Glucagon has proved of particular interest, for not only is it a weak hepatic arterial vasodilator, but it also inhibits hepatic arterial vasoconstriction due to hepatic nerve stimulation,[29] noradrenaline, angiotensin, and vasopressin.[36]

The concept that glucagon, released physiologically into the portal vein, may "protect" the hepatic arterial blood supply from vasoconstrictor influences receives support from the observation that infusing glucagon into the portal vein to produce concentrations about the same as those that occur physiologically inhibits hepatic arterial constriction due to intraarterial noradrenaline[37] or hepatic nerve stimulation.[30]

Because this property is not common to other vasodilator peptide hormones, is exhibited by low portal venous blood levels of glucagon, and appears to be antagonistic to vasoconstriction of any origin, it is possible that in states of stress, hypoglycemia, and shock, elevated portal venous glucagon concentrations help to maintain constant liver perfusion and oxygen supply by alleviating the vasoconstriction that would otherwise occur due to sympathetic nervous activation, circulating catecholamines, angiotensin, and vasopressin.

4.6. Catecholamines and Related Drugs

The effects of the α and β adrenoceptor stimulants can be explained in terms of the hepatic arterial resistance sites containing α-receptors, which when stimulated cause vasoconstriction, and β_2-receptors, which mediate vasodilatation.

Consistent with this, the pure α-stimulant phenylephrine causes hepatic arterial vasoconstriction,[38] whereas isoprenaline[16,35,38,39] and the β_2-stimulant salbutamol[38] evoke vasodilatation. Adrenaline (and, to a lesser extent, noradrenaline) causes vasoconstriction followed by vasodilatation when injected into the hepatic artery[38]; by infusion, low doses cause vasodilatation and high doses vasoconstriction.[37] These effects are explicable because the mixed α- and β-agonist causes vasodilatation by β-receptor stimulation (hence the dilator component is blocked by propranolol[38]) and vasoconstriction by α-receptor stimulation.

Dopamine at low doses causes hepatic arterial vasodilatation by activating specific dopamine receptors; at high doses, vasoconstriction due to α-receptor activation occurs.[40]

Physiologically, the responses to adrenaline are of greatest interest: Low (and therefore "physiological") concentrations cause vasodilatation and would increase hepatic arterial blood flow if the arterial pressure remained constant. It is questionable whether hepatic arterial vasoconstriction ever occurs due to "pathophysiological" release of adrenaline, and in any case the role of the sympathetic innervation is probably of greater importance in mediating hepatic arterial vasoconstriction. We are not aware of any studies of the possible interrelationship between elevated adrenaline levels and hepatic nerve stimulation.

4.7. Autacoids and Systemic Peptide Hormones

4.7.1. Autacoids

4.7.1a. Bradykinin. Bradykinin is the most potent hepatic arterial dilator yet studied with an ED_{50} of under 3×10^{-13} M. Released from the gastrointestinal tract pathologically, its potency makes it a candidate for increasing liver perfusion under pathological conditions.[41]

4.7.1b. Histamine. Histamine is a hepatic arterial vasodilator,[35,42] but is among the less potent group of dilators, making any natural vasoregulatory role improbable. The dilatation is mediated principally via H_1 receptors, the role (if any) of H_2 receptors being minor.[41]

4.7.1c. Serotonin (5-HT). 5-HT causes weak hepatic arterial vasoconstriction,[41,42] though there is sometimes a weak initial vasodilatation. The effects are so weak that it is improbable that serotonin alone has any hepatic arterial regulatory role.

4.7.1d. Prostaglandins. Prostaglandins E_1 and E_2 cause hepatic arterial vasodilatation,[34,43] as do A_1, A_2, and B_1.[44]

4.7.1e. Comment. The autacoids, with the clear exception of bradykinin, are probably not sufficiently potent to regulate HABF singly. What has not been adequately investigated is the possibility that these substances may regulate HABF when released concomitantly as a group, under which circumstances they could act synergistically.

4.7.2. Systemic Peptide Hormones

4.7.2a. Angiotensin. Angiotensin is a potent hepatic arterial vasoconstrictor,[36] though the response is not sustained during intraarterial infusions or after repeated intraarterial injections—tachyphylaxis is exhibited (Richardson and Withrington, unpublished data).

4.7.2b. Vasopressin. Vasopressin also causes hepatic arterial vasoconstriction,[45] and the responses are, in contrast to those of angiotensin, sustained.

4.7.2c. Comment. The possible roles of angiotensin and vasopressin in controlling HABF have not been investigated fully. From experimental studies,[11] it seems improbable that they exert a physiological role, but when plasma concentrations are elevated pathologically, it is possible that either or both may act as hepatic arterial vasoconstrictors.

4.8. Summary

The maintenance of HABF and therefore oxygen supply to the liver is essential for metabolism, detoxification, and other vital hepatic functions. It is consequently understandable that most of the control systems are directed toward maintaining a constant or enhanced HABF, rather than dramatic alterations. Consistent with this are (1) a relatively weak response to sympathetic nerve activation, (2) a dilator response to "physiological" concentrations of adrenaline, (3) the antagonism by glucagon of hepatic arterial vasoconstrictor responses, and (4) tachyphylaxis in the constrictor responses to angiotensin. The potential physiological dilator roles of the gastrointestinal hormones and pathological dilator roles of bradykinin, histamine, and prostaglandins all require further investigation. The efficiency of these extrinsic mechanisms in maintaining a constant HABF, coupled with the intimate relationship between hepatic arterial and portal venous blood flows (see Section 6), apparently obviates the need for profound intrinsic regulation of the hepatic arterial vasculature.

5. PORTAL VENOUS RESISTANCE

It is important to emphasize again (cf. Section 2) that portal venous blood pressure and flow are determined by two principal factors, the intrahepatic resistance to portal inflow [hepatic portal vascular resistance (HPVR)] and the mesenteric and splenic vascular resistances. Here we shall be dealing predominantly with modifications of the intrahepatic portal inflow resistance, which may occur at both pre- and postsinusoidal sites. However, significant alterations in portal hemodynamics may occur *in vivo* by changes in the mesenteric and splenic resistances concomitant with, but also in the absence of, alterations in portal inflow resistance. The changes in portal inflow resistance induced by any experimental procedure may be in the same direction or in the direction opposite to any changes in the vascular resistance of the splenic and mesenteric beds. These factors must be considered when predicting the effects on either the portal pressure or the flow of any imposed stimulus.

In a low-pressure system such as the portal vein, significant changes in portal resistance to flow may occur as the result of physical alterations in the distensibility of the vessel wall. Alterations in portal vein compliance due to drugs and other mechanisms may prove to be an important factor to consider, since reflex alterations in portal vein stiffness have been reported to have substantial functional implications.[46]

5.1. Intrinsic Regulation

The portal intrahepatic vascular circuit appears to be a passive channel in that it lacks intrinsic myogenic mechanisms to control and maintain portal pressure in response to wide alterations in portal inflow. Experimental work in many species[18,47–49] reports a linear pressure–flow relationship. Autoregulation of the intrahepatic portal inflow might be considered to be superfluous, since both mesenteric and splenic circuits demonstrate well-defined autoregulation.

5.2. Blood Gases

Local changes in portal venous pH, pCO_2, and pO_2, unaccompanied by systemic alterations,[50] reveal that a decrease in portal pH increases portal vascular resistance such that a fall in portal pH of 0.1 unit increases HPVR by 9%. Increases in portal pH have the opposite effect, but induce smaller changes. An increase in portal pCO_2 causes an increase in vascular inflow resistance, and portal pressure and consequently a fall in portal inflow. An increase in portal O_2 content causes a decrease in portal vascular resistance with an increase in portal inflow. The mesenteric circulation responds very actively to changes in systemic pCO_2, pO_2, and pH, so that the portal flow will be modified indirectly by any such systemic changes. Thus, hypercapnia in the dog[23] caused substantial increases (43%) in portal flow as the result of mesenteric vasodilatation.

5.3. Osmolarity

In the dog, graded intraportal infusions of mannitol increased portal plasma osmolarity by 170 mosmoles/liter, and although there were significant increases in hepatic arterial blood flow (HABF), there were no accompanying changes in portal inflow resistance. When the hepatic arterial vasodilatation was almost maximal, there was a small concomitant increase in HPVR.[26] Almost certainly this increase in HPVR was a result of the elevated HABF and derived from the reciprocal relationship between the two inflow circuits (see Section 6.1). When the intraportal osmolarity was elevated experimentally sufficient to also raise systemic osmolarity, there was an increase in mesenteric outflow into the portal vein indicative of the sensitivity of the mesenteric resistance sites to elevated systemic osmolarity. Elevated portal osmolarity, therefore, may increase portal blood flow, not as a result of a direct mechanism effecting the portal inflow resistance, but indirectly through mesenteric vasodilatation with consequent increased drainage into the portal system.

5.4. Nervous Control

In the cat, stimulation of the hepatic periarterial nerves causes graded increases in portal pressure at constant inflow volume.[32] The absolute changes in HPVR were small compared with the increases in mesenteric resistance, and the authors suggested that the portal system acts as a constant-flow conduit. In the dog,[13,30] periarterial nerve stimulation evokes graded increases in HPVR, with the threshold frequency (1–2 Hz) being higher than for the arterial responses. In both species, the portal responses are maintained throughout the period of nerve stimulation. The definitive study of the reflex changes in portal vascular inflow resistance[28] has shown that graded alteration in carotid sinus pressure (CSP) produces graded changes in HPVR and that an inverse relationship exists between CSP and HPVR. When the baroreceptor drive is minimal (CSP = 40 mm Hg), the HPVR increases by 22%, and when the baroreceptor drive exerts maximal inhibition (CSP = 240 mm Hg), the HPVR decreases by 18% from controls. These changes are small compared with the potential range of alteration in HPVR that can be induced by stimulation of the periarterial nerves and suggest that physiological control of the portal inflow resistance by baroreceptors is slight.

5.5. Gastrointestinal and Pancreatic Hormones

Gastrin, secretin, cholecystokinin-pancreozymin (CCK-PZ), vasoactive intestinal peptide (VIP), and glucagon all induce profound hepatic arterial vasodilatation (see Section 4.5). In contrast, they are without any direct vascular action on the portal inflow resistance sites.[33,51,52]

When injected or infused intraportally or intravenously or injected into the hepatic artery, they may evoke a slight increase in portal inflow resistance at the very highest doses when hepatic arterial vasodilatation is almost maximal. This increase in portal resistance is almost certainly an indirect response to the increase in arterial blood flow as part of the reciprocal relationship between the two inflow circuits described in Section 6.1. However, once again, these peptide substances may increase portal inflow because of the potent vasodilator activity that they possess on the mesenteric bed in the whole animal.[3] The primary influence on portal flow under conditions when the systemic levels of these substances are elevated is not hepatic portal inflow resistance, but the lowered vascular resistance of those vascular territories that drain into the portal tract.

5.6. Catecholamines and Related Drugs

5.6.1. α-Adrenoceptor Agonists

Injections of phenylephrine, adrenaline, and noradrenaline into either the hepatic portal vein or the hepatic artery produce only increases in portal vascular resistance, indicating portal vasoconstriction. On a molar basis, adrenaline is the most potent, followed by noradrenaline and then phenylephrine. These vasoconstrictor responses of the portal vascular bed are antagonized competitively by α-adrenoceptor blocking drugs, but are unaltered by the administration of β-blocking drugs, such as propranolol.[53]

5.6.2. β-Adrenoceptor Agonists

Intraportal or intraarterial injections of the nonselective β-adrenoceptor agonist isoprenaline do not alter the intrahepatic portal inflow resistance.[18]

These results imply that the portal inflow resistance sites have a distribution of α-adrenoceptors that when activated cause portal vasoconstriction. In the cat and dog, there appear to be no β-adrenoceptors present in the portal inflow circuit, and so β-agonists and β-antagonists would not be predicted to alter portal inflow resistance directly. Of course, because of the high β-adrenoceptor density in the mesenteric[1] and splenic[2] circulations, β-adrenoceptor agonists and antagonists would alter portal vein blood flow and pressure by changing drainage from these tissues into the portal vein.

5.6.3. Dopamine

Intraportal injections of dopamine cause hepatic portal vasoconstriction without any vasodilator component.[40] The vasoconstrictor response is attenuated by haloperidol (a dopamine antagonist) and also by phentolamine (an α-adrenoceptor antagonist). The nonspecificity of blockade with haloperidol suggested that the portal vasoconstriction produced by dopamine is not associated with activation of specific dopamine receptors in the portal bed, but results from dopamine activation of α-adrenoceptors.

5.7. Autacoids and Systemic Peptide Hormones

5.7.1. Histamine

Intraportal administration of histamine increases the calculated portal inflow resistance.[41,42] In addition to constricting portal inflow resistance sites, it also directly contracts the hepatic veins in the dog, causing an "outflow block."[8] Intraarterial histamine also increases HPVR, there being little quantitative difference between the increases in HPVR induced by the same dose of histamine whether it is given intraportally or intraarterially,[42] suggesting that its principal site of action is beyond the point of mixing of the two inflow streams, i.e., postsinusoidal. The increase in HPVR to histamine is blocked by doses of the H_1 antagonist mepyramine, but not by the H_2 antagonist metiamide,[41] indicating that the portal vasoconstrictor response is predominantly due to interaction with an H_1-receptor population.

5.7.2. Angiotensin

Intraportal or intraarterial injections or infusions of angiotensin increase portal inflow vascular resistance.[54–56] There is a pronounced tachyphylaxis to the portal response, since if a series of portal injections of the same dose are administered within a short interval, then the portal vascular response to successive doses is markedly diminished. Unless sufficient time intervals are allowed between doses, the dose–response relationship of the portal resistance site to angiotensin appears to be bell-shaped rather than sigmoid.

5.7.3. Vasopressin

Intraportal, intraarterial, and intravenous vasopressin have all been shown to reduce the hepatic portal inflow resistance,[45,54] and vasopressin is the only substance so far investigated that directly lowers the intrahepatic portal vascular resistance. Since vasopressin also causes a marked intestinal vasoconstriction with a fall in venous drainage into the portal vein, the peptide would cause a profound decline in portal blood flow and portal pressure. Concomitant with the fall in portal flow, there is a marked hepatic arterial vasoconstriction; the overall effect of vasopressin is a substantial fall in total liver blood flow. In addition, the hepatic arterial vasoconstriction would cause, through the reciprocal relationship between the two inflow circuits, a further reduction in portal inflow resistance and portal pressure.

5.7.4. Bradykinin

Intraportal injections or infusions of bradykinin[41,56] are without direct effect on the intrahepatic portal inflow resistance. Elevated systemic arterial levels due to experimental administration or to high portal levels accompanying gastrointestinal pathology may significantly increase portal blood flow by a direct vasodilator action on the mesenteric[1] and splenic[2] arterial resistance sites and so increase venous drainage from these structures into the portal vein.

5.7.5. Prostaglandins

Prostaglandins B_1, B_2, and E_2 are without direct action on the hepatic portal inflow resistance, while PGA_1 and A_2 both increase the portal vascular resistance, PGA_2 being the more potent.[44]

5.7.6. 5-Hydroxytryptamine

Any hepatic portal vascular responses to 5-HT are weak and variable. Intraportal 5-HT causes small reductions in HPVR at low doses (below 100 μg), while higher doses (up to 1.0 mg) either have no direct effect or cause a mild portal vasoconstriction.[41,42] It is probable that these very small responses of the intrahepatic portal resistance sites to 5-HT are an indirect consequence of primary changes in the hepatic arterial resistance and blood flow induced by 5-HT administration.

5.8. Summary

The hepatic portal vein is a unique vascular channel. It receives a large flow of partially oxygenated blood draining the spleen and gastrointestinal tract. The principal determinants of portal hemodynamics and portal pressure are (1) the outflow volume of blood draining the spleen and gastronintestinal tract, determined by the vascular resistances of these organs, and (2) the inflow resistance of the portal vein tract within the liver. The intrahepatic portal resistance is low and the sites contain only α-adrenoceptors, so that both sympathetic nerve stimulation and circulating adrenaline cause only an increase in intrahepatic portal vascular resistance. However, the response of the portal resistance sites to many circulating substances is unusual (see Table I), since intraportal histamine causes portal vasoconstriction while vasopressin causes a fall in portal resistance. A wide variety of substances, active at most other vascular sites, produced either

Table I. Vascular Effects of Nerve Stimulation and of Various Drugs, Hormones, and Experimental Procedures on the Hepatic Arterial and Portal Inflow Circuits [a]

Stimulus	Hepatic arterial response	Hepatic portal response
Nerve stimulation		
Sympathetic	Vasoconstriction	Vasoconstriction
Parasympathetic	?	?
Catecholamines		
α-Agonists		
(e.g., phenylephrine)	Vasoconstriction	Vasoconstriction
β-Agonists		
(e.g., isoprenaline)	Vasodilatation	No effect
Mixed agonists		
(e.g., adrenaline)	Biphasic—vasodilatation, then vasoconstriction	Vasoconstriction only
Dopamine	Biphasic—vasodilatation, then vasoconstriction	Vasoconstriction only
Simple amines		
Histamine	Vasodilatation	Marked vasoconstriction
5-Hydroxytryptamine	Biphasic—vasodilatation, then vasoconstriction	Weak vasoconstriction
Peptides		
Angiotensin	Vasoconstriction with tachyphylaxis	Vasoconstriction with tachyphylaxis
Vasopressin	Vasoconstriction	Vasodilatation
Bradykinin	Vasodilatation	No effect
Vasoactive intestinal peptide	Vasodilatation	No effect
Substance P	Vasodilatation	No effect
CCK-PZ	Vasodilatation	No effect
Secretin	Vasodilatation	No effect
Glucagon	Prolonged vasodilatation	No effect
Pentagastrin	Vasodilatation	No effect
Prostaglandins	Vasodilatation	No effect or weak vasoconstriction
Hyperosmolarity (local)	Vasodilatation	No effect
Hypercapnia (local)	Vasodilatation	Vasoconstriction
Hypoxia (local)	Weak vasodilatation	Vasoconstriction (?)

[a] The information in this table is derived mainly from the anesthetized dog. The drug and hormone responses refer to direct injections into the appropriate circuit.

normally (VIP, glucagon, secretin, CCK-PZ) or in pathological conditions (bradykinin, prostaglandins, 5-HT) either are without any direct vascular action on the portal outflow resistance or have a very low potency. In addition, changes of portal osmolarity or gas tensions have little direct action on the portal vasculature. The two principal influences on the intrahepatic portal inflow resistance are the concomitant HABF and pressure (the reciprocal relationship between the two circuits) and the portal inflow volume and pressure themselves, which determine the intrinsic resistance to blood flow from the portal vein into the liver.

6. INTERRELATIONSHIP BETWEEN THE HEPATIC ARTERY AND THE PORTAL VEIN

6.1. Mutual Pressure–Flow Curves

One of the earliest experimental observations[7] was that there exists a physical interrelationship between the hepatic artery and the portal vein such that a reduction in blood flow in one of the circuits leads to a fall in inflow resistance and an increase in blood flow in the other circuit. This effect, termed reciprocity, has been thought of as a mechanism unique to the liver vasculature whereby a compensation occurs when one of the inflow circuits is compromised to ensure that an almost constant total liver blood flow is maintained.

Quantitative studies by several groups in which perfusion of both the arterial and portal circuits in the dog have been established under controlled conditions of pressure and flow[17,18,57,58] have shown that experimental increases in hepatic arterial blood pressure and flow (HABF) are associated with linear increases in hepatic portal vascular resistance, while increases in portal flow and pressure cause linear increases in hepatic arterial vascular resistance (see Fig. 1). Total occlusion of one inflow, either hepatic arterial or portal, causes a fall in the calculated inflow resistance of the remaining circuit of approximately 20% irrespective of whether this is the arterial or the portal supply. It became apparent that although such vascular interactions occur, they are quantitatively small and probably inadequate to fully compensate for a compromised blood flow in one of the circuits. Although an increased generalized sympathetic drive will cause hepatic arterial vasoconstriction and therefore a reduction in portal inflow resistance, the concomitant reduction in venous drainage from the gastrointestinal tract due to the increased sympathetic tone would substantially lower portal blood flow to the liver despite the decline in portal inflow resistance.

More recently, the concept has been reinvestigated in the dog using slightly different perfusion techniques[59] and the suggestion made that rather than the maintenance of an almost constant total liver blood flow, these intrinsic interrelating mechanisms are designed to keep oxygen delivery to the liver cells constant. A relevant observation to consider here is that hepatic arterial occlusion not only increases hepatic portal blood flow by lowering portal inflow resistance, but also increases arteriovenous shunting through the intestine and other beds draining into the portal circuit. Such an effect increases the oxygen content of the portal vein blood and further increases the efficiency of any compensatory mechanism.[60]

6.2. "Transhepatic" Drug Effects

It has been observed by several authors[18,61] using perfusion techniques in which both hepatic inflow circuits were perfused simultaneously that the injection

A

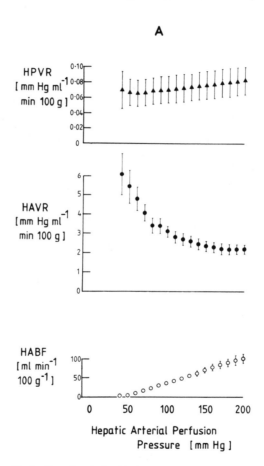

Figure 1. Reciprocal hydrodynamic relationship between the hepatic artery and the hepatic portal vein in the dog. The figure illustrates observations made in experiments in which both the hepatic artery and the hepatic portal vein were perfused with blood of the appropriate composition under controlled conditions of pressure and flow. (A) The abscissa represents the hepatic arterial perfusion pressure, which is altered experimentally, and illustrates the consequences to the hepatic arterial and portal perfusion circuits. As the perfusion pressure is increased, once an opening threshold pressure has been reached (around 50 mm Hg), the hepatic arterial blood flow (HABF) rises while the calculated hepatic arterial vascular resistance (HAVR) falls. In contrast, the topmost graph reveals that the inflow resistance of the *portal* circuit increases in response to the elevated hepatic *arterial*

or infusion of vasoactive substances into one of the circuits is accompanied by substantial vascular changes in both inflow circuits, not just the one directly receiving the injection.

In a series of publications,[18,42,45] it has been reported that intraarterial injections of noradrenaline, angiotensin, and vasopressin all cause hepatic arterial vasoconstriction and that, in addition, noradrenaline and angiotensin cause portal vasoconstriction while vasopressin causes portal vasodilatation. In contrast, in-

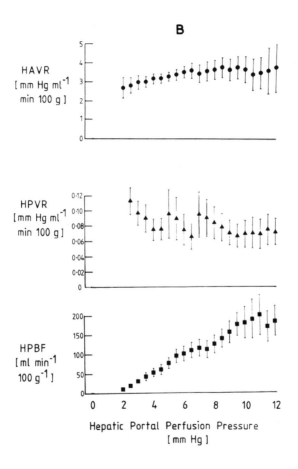

pressure. Hepatic portal vasoconstriction is the consequence of increased hepatic arterial pressure and flow. (B) The abscissa represents experimental alterations in portal perfusion pressure (i.e., HPVP-IVCP) and shows that as this variable is increased, there is a concomitant increase in portal blood flow (HPBF) with a small fall in portal inflow resistance (HPVR). The uppermost graph reveals that as the portal pressure and flow are elevated, the hepatic arterial vascular resistance (HAVR) increases, indicating hepatic *arterial vasoconstriction*. The reader should consult the original reference[18] for further details of perfusion techniques and measurements. The figure is reprinted, slightly modified, with permission of the editors of the *Journal of Physiology, London.*

traarterial histamine causes hepatic arterial vasodilatation concomitant with portal vasoconstriction. Intraportal injections of angiotensin, noradrenaline, and histamine cause portal vasoconstriction, but while angiotensin and noradrenaline evoke accompanying arterial vasoconstriction, histamine causes concomitant hepatic arterial vasodilatation. In contrast, intraportal vasopressin reduces portal inflow resistance but increases hepatic arterial inflow resistance. All the vascular effects on the second inflow circuit are the appropriate changes expected from the primary actions of these substances on that circuit and do not arise as passive reciprocal changes in the second inflow circuit as an indirect consequence of primary vascular changes in the circuit receiving the direct injection. Indeed, several vasoactive substances such as isoprenaline, bradykinin, PGE_2, or vasoactive intestinal peptide that are without any direct vascular action on the portal inflow circuit may, when administered intraportally, cause significant increases in HABF without any accompanying systemic responses indicative of entry into the systemic circulation (see Fig. 2).

An analysis of the latencies from the time of injection to the appearance of the hepatic arterial and portal responses after either arterial or portal injection revealed that the hepatic arterial and portal responses occurred simultaneously irrespective of the circuit that received the direct injection. The vascular responses in both the arterial and the portal inflow circuits occurred after a significantly shorter delay than any accompanying systemic changes such as BP, HR, and superior mesenteric vascular responses. These results suggest strongly that the vascular response of the hepatic inflow circuit not directly receiving the injection is not the result of recirculation and reentry into the liver from the systemic circuit but is the result of access to resistance sites of both the arterial and the portal circuits within the liver irrespective of the route of administration, either intraarterial or intraportal.

The physiological significance of such "transhepatic effects" is considerable, since it implies that vasoactive substances released by the gastrointestinal tract or ingested after oral administration may enter the liver in the portal inflow and without necessarily entering the systemic circulation influence the supply of arterial, oxygenated blood to the hepatic parenchyma. Such a potential route is especially functionally significant for vasoactive substances that are released from the gut with short half-lives of survival within the blood or that are destroyed during passage through the cardiopulmonary circuit.

7. CAPACITANCE AND EXCHANGE

7.1. Regulation of Liver Volume

In most species, the liver is an important blood reservoir, although in the dog, its role in this respect is exceeded by that of the spleen.[62] Most estimates

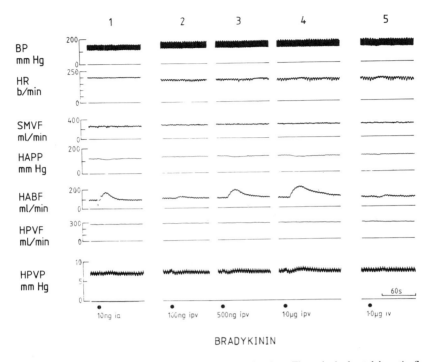

BRADYKININ

Figure 2. Record of a liver perfusion experiment in the dog. The principal total hepatic flow determinants, i.e., hepatic arterial blood flow (HABF), superior mesenteric venous flow (SMVF), hepatic arterial perfusion pressure (HAPP), hepatic portal venous flow (HPVF), and hepatic portal venous pressure (HPVP), are all continuously measured and recorded. In addition, systemic arterial blood pressure (BP) and heart rate (HR) are recorded. The record shows in a series of panels (1–5) the hepatic vascular effects of the potent vasodilator peptide bradykinin when injected intraarterially [i.e., into the hepatic artery (ia)], intraportally (ipv), and intravenously [(iv) into the inferior vena cava (ivc) at the level of the diaphragm]. In (1), bradykinin is injected directly into the hepatic artery and evokes a marked increase in HABF without any other cardiovascular changes. Bradykinin is rapidly inactivated by passage through the cardiopulmonary circuit and therefore does not enter the systemic circuit in concentrations that would cause vasodilatation of any other peripheral vascular beds and a consequent fall in BP. In (2), (3), and (4), bradykinin is injected directly into the portal inflow circuit in increasing doses. No change is seen on the portal inflow pressure, indicating that bradykinin has no direct action on portal inflow resistance. However, as the dose of bradykinin is raised, marked increases in HABF occur in the absence of any systemic changes in BP, HR, and SMVF. If bradykinin were entering the systemic circulation and producing the hepatic arterial vasodilatation observed in the series of ipv injections by recirculation, concomitant alterations in BP, HR, and SMVF would be expected. In (5), the largest dose of bradykinin (1.0 μg) that was administered by ipv injection is here administered iv at the level of the diaphragm. There are small resultant changes in BP, HR, and HABF indicative of some survival of the administered dose into the systemic circulation to provoke small cardiovascular changes. A comparison of the effects between (4) and (5) makes it apparent that for the same dose of bradykinin, the vascular effect on the hepatic arterial circuit is much greater for the intraportal injection than that administered into the ivc. This is explained by the proposition that vasoactive substances entering the liver in the portal circuit have access within the liver to those sites that control hepatic arterial resistance to inflow.

of liver blood volume are about 20–25 ml/100 g liver weight,[63] and the three most important factors that influence liver blood content are the hepatic venous pressure, the hepatic arterial and portal blood inflows, and the activity of the hepatic sympathetic innervation.

It is well established that the liver decreases in size when either the hepatic or the splanchnic nerves are stimulated, and quantitative aspects of this control system have been studied in both the cat and the dog.[13,28,64] The maximum expulsion of hepatic stored blood occurs at rates of whole sympathetic nerve stimulation of 4–8 Hz in both species and represents about 50% of the hepatic blood in the cat and even more in the dog. About 80% of this maximum removal of stored blood from the liver by nerve stimulation is achieved within 20 sec, although a much longer period is required for recovery to control hepatic volume.

An important physiological aspect of this nervous control of hepatic volume and mobilization of stored blood is the extent of any involvement in cardiovascular reflexes. While in the cat, occlusion of the common carotids, eliciting reflexes of both baro- and chemoreceptor origin, does not produce a consistent change in liver volume,[9] in the dog, the liver capacity is very sensitive to changes in reflex activity. Carotid sinus hypotension results in a reduction in hepatic blood volume of 16%, while carotid sinus hypertension increases liver volume by 20%. Combined withdrawal of both carotid baroreceptor and cardiopulmonary afferent drive results in a decrease in liver blood content of 42%.[28] An abrupt increase in carotid sinus pressure from 40 to 240 mm Hg representing maximal and minimal reflex activation of the hepatic sympathetic innervation leads to a rapid increase in liver volume that is 80% complete within 25 sec.

The liver, therefore, can act as an important blood reservoir from which a significant shift of blood can occur rapidly and in a precise and controlled manner as determined by the activity of the sympathetic innervation.

As would be predicted from the effects of sympathetic stimulation, hemorrhage reduces liver volume[28] in a graded manner related to the severity of the hemorrhage and the fall in systemic BP. However, experiments in conscious dogs[65] suggest that the mobilization of the hepatic blood reservoir does not occur in all situations of stress. The severity of the stress is undoubtedly an important consideration, since adrenal medullary catecholamines, adrenaline and noradrenaline, both decrease liver volume.[66] In addition, the vasoconstrictor peptides angiotensin and vasopressin, both of which circulate in higher concentrations in stress, reduce hepatic volume in the cat,[66] although to different extents.

Histamine is without significant effect on liver volume in the cat,[66] but has a potent and unique action in the dog,[8] leading to hepatic enlargement and congestion.

A number of potent vasodilator drugs seem to have little action on the hepatic capacitance vessels and liver volume.[67]

An important experimental consideration in studies of liver volume is knowledge of the concomitant hepatic venous pressure and whether this pressure is maintained constant during any experimental procedures. There is a substantial compliance of the hepatic capacitance vessels,[68] about 10 times that of the systemic circulation, and minor alterations in hepatic venous pressure may cause large alterations in liver volume. The extent to which liver volume is affected by changes in hepatic arterial and portal inflow volumes confirms the earlier suggestion[69] that the liver acts as a passive reservoir either to add to the circulating blood volume or to remove blood from the circulation when deviations from normal venous pressures and inflows occur. These additions and removals occur without the active participation of the innervation, but arise as a consequence of the compliance of the hepatic capacitance system.

7.2. Exchange in the Hepatic Microcirculation

In the cat, elevation of the hepatic venous pressure leads to a biphasic increase in liver volume.[64] The initial phase is associated with passive distension of the capacitance vessels and provides an estimate of their compliance[9] (1.3–3.4 ml mm Hg^{-1} · 100 g^{-1}). The succeeding second phase in liver volume increase is due predominantly to the trans-sinusoidal filtration of fluid into the interstitial space, and its rate gives an important numerical value in the study of hepatic microcirculation. Basically, the net fluid movement is determined by two principal factors, the net filtering pressure across the sinusoidal wall determined by the balance between hydrostatic and osmotic gradients and the "capillary filtration coefficient" (CFC), a measure of hydraulic conductance that depends on both permeability and surface area available for exchange. In the series of experiments of the type described above, the CFC was calculated, after certain assumptions, to be approximately 0.3 ml min^{-1} mm Hg^{-1} 100 g^{-1}.

Further numerical values of the "Starling equilibrium" have been evaluated in the liver of the dog.[70] By determining the protein concentration of hepatic prenodal lymph, Laine et al.[70] revealed that, uniquely, when the hepatic venous pressure was elevated, the lymph protein composition did not decrease. Therefore, the sinusoid endothelium does not offer an effective barrier to protein movement that would be expected to become apparent especially at high rates of lymph flow when the venous pressure was elevated. The osmotic reflexion coefficient, a sensitive index of the restrictive properties of vessel exchange barriers, was calculated to be close to zero; i.e., in the liver sinusoid, no effective barrier exists to the movement of protein. The consequence of this phenomenon is that fluid movement across the hepatic sinusoid would appear to be determined by a single factor, the hydrostatic pressure gradient. This assumes that the sinusoidal permeability cannot be increased further and that any particular procedure does not effectively reduce permeability. Determinations of the distribution of pressures through out the hepatic vasculature have been made using implanted capsules subsequently used to measure tissue pressure.[70] The control sinusoidal pressure was estimated to lie between 5.8 and 7.0 mm Hg, with approximately 90% of any change in inferior vena caval pressure being transmitted through to the sinusoid. An important measurement was that the interstitial hydrostatic pressure was around 5.8 mm Hg indicating the very small hydrostatic gradient that normally exists across the sinusoid walls. This indicates that a slender margin exists for filtration from the vascular to the extravascular space. Substantial alterations in filtration and formation of interstitial fluid, lymph, and ascitic fluid must be possible by trivial changes in extravascular pressure secondary to changes in capsular tone or intraabdominal pressure. These types of experiments lead to minimal values of CFC calculated by two groups[70,71] to be around 0.085 ml min^{-1} mm Hg^{-1} 100 g^{-1}.

However, few experimental factors seem to alter hepatic fluid filtration, and an unusual feature of this equilibrium in the cat liver[64] is that it is unaffected by sympathetic nerve stimulation or by intraarterial injections of adrenaline, isoprenaline, or histamine.[66]

Although the hepatic sinusoidal lining contains a spectrum of pore sizes that are apparently sufficiently large to allow free movement of plasma proteins by diffusion and convection, nevertheless they offer a barrier to the outward movement of RBCs. Elevations in hepatic venous pressure (HVP) therefore lead to increases in hepatic venous hematocrit.[68] When HVP is elevated initially, the hepatic venous hemoglobin increases due to filtration of plasma unaccompanied by RBCs into the hepatic extravascular compartment. The venous hemoglobin then falls to a plateau maintained above control levels for the duration of HVP elevation. This is due to the maintained increase in sinusoidal pressure resulting in increased filtration into the interstitial space, lymphatics, and peritoneal cavity as ascites. When the HVP is lowered to control, then blood is displaced from the liver and reabsorption of plasma from the extravascular space of Disse also leads to a fall in hepatic venous hematocrit.

8. RELATIONSHIP OF LIVER CIRCULATION TO LIVER FUNCTION

8.1. Postprandial Hyperemia

Total liver blood flow increases after eating,[72,73] and there is evidence, at least in the sheep,[73] of an increased hepatic arterial, as well as the well-established increase in intestinal, blood flow. The mechanism of this hepatic arterial postprandial hyperemia is unknown, and it has not been confirmed in other species[72] or in man.

8.2. Metabolic Stimulation

It has been accepted that hepatic arterial blood flow (HABF) is likely to increase at times of increased hepatic metabolic activity. The thesis is attractive in that one might expect an increased activity to be dependent on an increased oxygen supply to the hepatocytes and in turn on an increased arterial blood flow. There is experimental support for this view: Metabolic stimulation in the isolated sheep liver increases O_2 consumption and HABF.[74] In the dog, amino acid infusions increase HABF,[75] and in man, enzyme induction increases HABF.[76]

Most of these observations are susceptible to alternative interpretations—for instance, that the hyperemia associated with amino acids is a pharmacological response to the amino acids rather than a response to metabolic stimulation *per se*. Lautt[21] has shown that alterations in hepatic oxygen demand during metabolic stimulation changes hepatic oxygen extraction and to some extent changes portal blood flow; changes in hepatic arterial blood flow are largely secondary ("transhepatic") to the altered portal flow (see Section 6).

It is unwise to be dogmatic about the relationship between HABF and metabolic activity. Only recently has it been appreciated that the extraction of oxygen varies widely in many organs, including the liver, to meet changing demands. It is evidently incorrect to expect proportionate changes in metabolic activity and HABF, and systemic changes (e.g., hypoxia, hemodilution) that alter intestinal and therefore portal blood flow undoubtedly evoke "intrahepatic" changes in HABF. What is not established is whether changes in metabolism that are localized to the liver evoke increases in HABF flow as well as increases in oxygen extraction.[21]

9. SUMMARY

Liver blood flow comprises two intimately linked supplies—the portal venous and the hepatic arterial inflow. The portal inflow is determined by vascular resistance in the intestine and spleen, while the arterial supply is determined by intrahepatic resistance and vessel tone. Hepatic arterial blood flow alters reciprocally with portal flow in an attempt to maintain a constant total liver blood flow, but this reciprocity is only partially effective. Intrinsic vasoregulation is weak,[3] but recent work suggests an intrinsic control of hepatic oxygen extraction[21] that may be more important than the regulation of blood flow. Extrinsic controls are directed toward the maintenance of a high, constant, blood flow with weak vasoconstrictor influences, more prevalent vasodilator influences, and the important "transhepatic" responses whereby material present in portal venous blood modulates hepatic arterial blood flow.

REFERENCES

1. Granger, D. N., Richardson, P. D. I., Kvietys, P. R., and Mortillaro, N. A., 1980, Intestinal blood flow, *Gastroenterology*, **78**:837–863.

2. Davies, B. N., and Withrington, P. G., 1973, The actions of drugs on the smooth muscle of the capsule and blood vessels of the spleen, *Pharmacol. Rev.* **25**:373–413.

3. Richardson, P. D. I., and Withrington, P. G., 1981, Liver blood flow I, *Gastroenterology,* **81**:159–173.

4. Feely, J., and Wood, A. J. J., 1983, Effects of inhibitors of prostaglandin synthesis on hepatic drug clearance, *Br. J. Clin. Pharmacol.* **15**:109–111.

5. Feely, J., Wilkinson, G. R., and Wood, A. J. J., 1981, Reduction of liver blood flow and propranolol metabolism by cimetidine, *N. Engl. J. Med.* **304**:692–695.

6. Grainger, S. L., Keeling, P. W. N., Brown, I. M. H., Marigold, H. J., and Thompson, R. P. H., 1983, Clearance and non-invasive determination of the hepatic extraction of indocyanine green in baboons and man, *Clin. Sci.* **64**:207–212.

7. Burton-Opitz, R., 1911, The vascularity of the liver. II. The influence of the portal blood flow upon the flow in the hepatic artery, *Q. J. Exp. Physiol.* **4**:93–102.

8. Greenway, C. V., and Oshiro, G., 1973, Effects of histamine on hepatic volume (outflow block) in anaesthetized dogs, *Br. J. Pharmacol.* **47**:282–290.

9. Lautt, W. W., and Greenway, C. V., 1976, Hepatic venous compliance and role of liver as a blood reservoir, *Am. J. Physiol.* **231**:292–295.

10. Lautt, W. W., 1977, Effect of stimulation of hepatic nerves on hepatic O_2 uptake and blood flow, *Am. J. Physiol.* **232**:H652–656.

11. Richardson, P. D. I., and Withrington, P. G., 1981, Liver blood flow II, *Gastroenterology,* **81**:356–375.

12. Lautt, W. W., 1980, Control of hepatic arterial blood flow: Independence from liver metabolic activity, *Am. J. Physiol.* **239**:H559–564.

13. Greenway, C. V., and Oshiro, G., 1972, Comparison of the effects of hepatic nerve stimulation on arterial flow, distribution of arterial and portal flows and the blood content of the livers of anaesthetized cats and dogs, *J. Physiol. (London)* **227**:487–501.

14. Koo, A., and Liang, I. Y. S., 1979, Stimulation and blockade of cholinergic receptors in terminal liver microcirculation in rats, *Am. J. Physiol.* **236**:E728–732.

15. Koo, A., and Liang, I. Y. S., 1979, Microvascular filling pattern in rat liver sinusoids during vagal stimulation, *J. Physiol. (London)* **295**:191–199.

16. Hanson, K. M., 1973, Dilator responses of the canine hepatic vasculature, *Angiologica* **10**:15–23.

17. Hanson, K. M., and Johnson, P. C., 1966, Local control of hepatic arterial and portal venous flow in the dog, *Am. J. Physiol.* **211**:712–720.

18. Richardson, P. D. I., and Withrington, P. G., 1978, Pressure–flow relationships and the effects of noradrenaline and isoprenaline on the simultaneously-perfused hepatic arterial and portal venous vascular beds of the dog, *J. Physiol. (London)* **282**:451–470.

19. Norris, C. P., Barnes, G. E., Smith, E. E., and Granger, H. J., 1979, Autoregulation of superior mesenteric blood flow in fasted and fed dogs, *Am. J. Physiol.* **237**:H174–177.

20. Richardson, P. D. I., and Withrington, P. G., 1982, Physiological regulation of the hepatic circulation, *Annu. Rev. Physiol.* **44**:57–69.

21. Lautt, W. W., 1983, Relationship between hepatic blood flow and overall metabolism: The hepatic arterial buffer response, *Fed. Proc. Fed. Am. Soc. Exp. Biol.* **42**:1662–1666.

22. Larsen, J. A., Krarup, N., and Munck, A., 1976, Liver hemodynamics and liver function in cats during graded hypoxic hypoxemia, *Acta Physiol. Scand.* **98**:257–262.

23. Scholtholt, J., and Shiraishi, T., 1970, The reaction of liver and intestinal blood flow to a general hypoxia, hypocapnia and hypercapnia in the anaesthetized dog, *Pfluegers Arch.* **318**:185–201.

24. Hughes, R. L., Mathie, R. T., Campbell, D., and W. Fitch, 1979, Systemic hypoxia and hyperoxia and liver blood flow and oxygen consumption in the greyhound, *Pfluegers Arch.* **381**:151–157.

25. Lautt, W. W., MacLachlan, T. L., and Brown, L. C., 1977, The effect of hypertonic infusions on hepatic blood flows and liver volume in the cat, *Can. J. Physiol. Pharmacol.* **55**:1339–1344.

26. Richardson, P. D. I., and Withrington, P. G., 1980, Effects of intraportal infusions of hypertonic solutions on hepatic haemodynamics in the dog, *J. Physiol. (London)* **301**:82–83P.

27. Carr, D. H., and Titchen, D. A., 1978, Postprandial changes in parotid salivary secretion and plasma osmolarity and the effects of intravenous infusions of saline solutions, *Q. J. Exp. Physiol.* **63**:1–21.

28. Carneiro, J. J., and Donald, D. E., 1977, Change in liver blood flow and blood content in dogs during direct and reflex alteration of hepatic sympathetic nerve activity, *Circ. Res.* **40**:150–158.

29. Richardson, P. D. I., and Withrington, P. G., 1977, Glucagon inhibition of hepatic arterial responses to hepatic nerve stimulation, *Am. J. Physiol.* **233**:H647–654.

30. Richardson, P. D. I., and Withrington, P. G., 1978, The effects of intraportal infusions of glucagon on the responses of the simultaneously-perfused hepatic arterial and portal venous vascular beds of the dog to periarterial nerve stimulation, *J. Physiol. (London)* **284**:102–103P.

31. Lautt, W. W., 1977, The effect of stimulation of hepatic nerves on hepatic oxygen uptake and blood flow, *Am. J. Physiol.* **232**:H652–656.

32. Greenway, C. V., Lawson, A. E., and Mellander, S., 1967, The effects of stimulation of the hepatic nerves, infusion of noradrenaline and occlusion of the carotid arteries on liver blood flow in the anaesthetised cat, *J. Physiol. (London)* **192**:21–41.

33. Post, J. A., and Hanson, K. M., 1975, Hepatic vascular and biliary responses to infusion of gastrointestinal hormones and bile salts, *Digestion* **12**:65–77.

34. Richardson, P. D. I., and Withrington, P. G., 1977, The effects of glucagon, secretin, pancreozymin and pentagastrin on the hepatic arterial vascular bed of the dog, *Br. J. Pharmacol.* **59**:148–156.

35. Richardson, P. D. I., and Withrington, P. G., 1976, The vasodilator actions of isoprenaline, histamine, prostaglandin E_2, glucagon and secretin on the hepatic arterial vascular bed of the dog, *Br. J. Pharmacol.* **57**:581–588.

36. Richardson, P. D. I., and Withrington, P. G., 1976, The inhibition by glucagon of the vasoconstrictor actions of noradrenaline, angiotensin and vasopressin on the hepatic arterial vascular bed of the dog, *Br. J. Pharmacol.* **57**:93–102.

37. Richardson, P. D. I., and Withrington, P. G., 1979, Responses of the hepatic arterial and portal venous vascular beds of the dog to intra-arterial infusions of noradrenaline and adrenaline: Inhibition of hepatic arterial vasoconstrictor responses by intraportal infusions of glucagon, *Br. J. Pharmacol.* **66**:82P.

38. Richardson, P. D. I., and Withrington, P. G., 1977, The role of beta-adrenoceptors in the responses of the hepatic arterial vascular bed of the dog to phenylephrine, isoprenaline, noradrenaline and adrenaline, *Br. J. Pharmacol.* **60**:239–49.

39. Greenway, C. V., and Lawson, A. E., 1969, Beta adrenergic receptors in the hepatic arterial bed of the anesthetized cat, *Can. J. Physiol. Pharmacol.* **47**:415–419.

40. Richardson, P. D. I., and Withrington, P. G., 1978, Responses to the canine hepatic arterial and portal venous vascular beds to dopamine, *Eur. J. Pharmacol.* **48**:337–349.

41. Richardson, P. D. I., and Withrington, P. G., 1977, A comparison of the effects of bradykinin, 5-hydroxytryptamine and histamine on the hepatic arterial and portal venous vascular beds of the dog: Histamine H_1 and H_2 receptors, *Br. J. Pharmacol.* **60**:123–133.

42. Richardson, P. D. I., and Withrington, P. G., 1978, Responses of the simultaneously-perfused hepatic arterial and portal venous vascular beds of the dog to histamine and 5-hydroxytryptamine, *Br. J. Pharmacol.* **64**:581–588.

43. Geumei, A., Bashour, F. A., Swamy, B. V., and Nafrawi, A. F., 1973, Prostaglandin E_1: Its effects on heptic circulation in dogs, *Pharmacology* **9**:336–347.

44. Hanson, K. M., and Post, J. A., 1976, Splanchnic vascular responses to the infusion of prostaglandins A_1, A_2 and B_1, *Pharmacology* **14**:166–181.

45. Richardson, P. D. I., and Withrington, P. G., 1978, Effects of intra-arterial and intraportal injections of vasopressin on the hepatic arterial and portal venous vascular beds of the dog, *Circ. Res.* **43**:496–503.

46. Auden, R. M., and Donald, D. E., 1975, Reflex responses of the isolated, *in situ,* portal vein of the dog, *J. Surg. Res.* **18**:35–42.

47. Price, J. B., McFate, P. A., and Shaw, R. F., 1964, Dynamics of blood flow through the normal canine liver, *Surgery* **56**:1109–1120.

48. Brauer, R. W., Leong, G. F., and McElroy, R. F., 1956, Haemodynamics of the vascular tree of the isolated rat liver preparation, *Am. J. Physiol.* **185**:537–542.

49. Drapnas, T., Zemel, R., and Vang, J. O., 1966, Haemodynamics of the isolated perfused pig liver, *Ann. Surg.* **164**:522–537.

50. Gelman, S., and Ernst, E. A., 1977, Role of pH, PCO_2 and oxygen content of portal blood in hepatic circulatory autoregulation, *Am. J. Physiol.* **233**:E255–E262.

51. Ross, G., 1970, Cardiovascular effects of secretin, *Am. J. Physiol.* **218**:1166–1170.

52. Richardson, P. D. I., and Withrington, P. G., 1978, The effects of intraportal infusions of glucagon on the hepatic arterial and portal venous vascular beds of the dog: Inhibition of hepatic arterial vasoconstrictor responses to noradrenaline, *Pfluegers Arch. (Eur. J. Physiol).* **378**:135–150.

53. Richardson, P. D. I., and Withrington, P. G., 1977, Alpha and beta adrenoceptors in the hepatic portal venous vascular bed of the dog, *Br. J. Pharmacol.* **60**:283–284P.

54. Richardson, P. D. I., and Withrington, P. G., 1977, The effects of intraportal injections of noradrenaline, adrenaline, vasopressin and angiotensin on the hepatic portal venous vascular bed of the dog: Marked tachyphylaxis to angiotensin, *Br. J. Pharmacol.* **59**:293–301.

55. Kelly, K. A., and Nyhus, L. M., 1966, Angiotensin and the liver, *Am. J. Physiol.* **210**:305–311.

56. Scholtholt, J., and Shiraishi, T., 1968, The action of acetylcholine, bradykinin and angiotensin on the liver blood flow of the anaesthetized dog and on the pressure in the ligated ductus choledochus, *Pfluegers Arch.* **300**:189–201.

57. Green, H. D., Hall, L. S., Sexton, J., and Deal, C. P., 1959, Autonomic vasomotor responses in the canine hepatic arterial and venous beds, *Am. J. Physiol.* **196**:196–202.

58. Sato, T., Shirataka, M., Ikeda, N., and Grodins, F. S., 1977, Steady-state systems analysis of hepatic hemodynamics in the isolated perfused canine liver, *Am. J. Physiol.* **233**:R188–197.

59. Mathie, R. T., and Blumgart, L. H., 1983, The hepatic haemodynamic response to acute portal venous blood flow reductions in the dog, *Pfluegers Arch.* **399**:223–227.

60. Lindell, B., and Aronsen, K. F., 1977, Changes in cardiac output distribution after liver dearterialization in the rat, *Acta. Chir. Scand.* **143**:207–213.

61. Hirsch, L. J., Ayabe, T., and Glick, G., 1976, Direct effects of various catecholamines on liver circulation in dogs, *Am. J. Physiol.* **230**:1394–1399.

62. Carneiro, J. J., and Donald, D. E., 1977, Blood reservoir function of dog spleen, liver and intestine, *Am. J. Physiol.* **232**:H67–H72.

63. Greenway, C. V., and Stark, R. D., 1971, Hepatic vascular bed, *Physiol. Rev.* **51**:23–65.

64. Greenway, C. V., Stark, R. D., and Lautt, W. W., 1969, Capacitance responses and fluid exchange in the cat liver during stimulation of the hepatic nerves. *Circ. Res.* **25**:277–284.

65. Guntheroth, W. G., and Mullins, G. H., 1963, Liver and spleen as venous reservoirs, *Am. J. Physiol.* **204**:35–41.

66. Greenway, C. V., and Lautt, W. W., 1972, Effects of adrenaline, isoprenaline and histamine on trans-sinusoidal fluid filtration in the cat liver, *Br. J. Pharmacol.* **44**:185–191.

67. Greenway, C. V., 1979, Effects of sodium nitroprusside, isosorbide dinitrate, phentolamine and prazosin on hepatic venous responses to sympathetic nerve stimulation in the cat, *J. Pharmacol. Exp. Ther.* **209**:56–61.

68. Bennett, T. D., and Rothe, C. F., 1981, Hepatic capacitance responses to changes in flow and hepatic venous pressure in dogs, *Am. J. Physiol.* **240**:H18–H28.

69. Lautt, W. W., 1977, Hepatic vasculature: A conceptual review, *Gastroenterology,* **73**:1163–1169.

70. Laine, G. A., Hall, J. T., Laine, S. H., and Grainger, H. J., 1979, Trans-sinusoidal fluid dynamics in canine liver during venous hypertension, *Circ. Res.* **45**:317–323.

71. Granger, D. N., Miller, T., Allen, R., Parker, R. E., Parker, J. C., and Taylor, A. E., 1979, Permselectivity of cat liver blood–lymph barrier to endogenous macromolecules, *Gastroenterology,* **77**:103–109.

72. Hopkinson, B. R., and Schenk, W. G., 1968, The electromagnetic measurement of liver blood flow and cardiac output in conscious dogs during feeding and exercise, *Surgery* **63**:970–975.

73. Katz, M. L., and Bergman, E. N., 1969, Simultaneous measurements of hepatic and portal venous blood flow in the sheep and dog, *Am. J. Physiol.* **216**:946–952.

74. Linzell, J. L., Setchell, B. P., and Lindsay, D. B., 1971, The isolated perfused liver of the sheep: An assessment of its metabolic synthetic and excretory functions, *Q. J. Exp. Physiol.* **56**:53–71.

75. Scholtholt, J., 1970, Das Verhalten der Durchblutung der Leber bei Steigerung des Sauerstoffverbrauches der Leber, *Pfluegers Arch.* **318**:202–216.

76. Ohnhaus, E. E., Coninx, S., Ramos, M. R., and Noelpp, U., 1976, Liver blood flow and enzyme induction in man, *Br. J. Clin. Pharmacol.* **3**:352–353P (abstract).

II

Methods

Chapter 3

Histology and Histochemistry

Dieter Sasse

1. INTRODUCTION

Obviously, it is not possible to present in this chapter a comprehensive survey of all aspects and details of qualitative and quantitative histological and histochemical techniques that in the past have been the subject of almost encyclopedic volumes.[1–10] The methods selected for description herein include the most frequently used techniques of tissue pretreatment, histological staining, quantitative histology, and qualitative and quantitative histochemistry appropriate for the elucidation of the structure and the histochemical distribution patterns of liver parenchyma.

While the histological staining methods are largely standardized, the histochemical techniques are often modified from laboratory to laboratory. The reason for developing such modifications is to improve either the preservation of the histological structure or the precise localization and stainability of the reaction product. This latter object, however, is largely dependent on the individual point of view, so that histochemical methods are sometimes regarded as unspecific, and it is considered that the results of "staining histochemistry" can be assessed only with reservations. In those cases, however, where the results of qualitative histochemical techniques have already been compared directly with

DIETER SASSE • Institute of Anatomy, University of Basel, CH-4056 Basel, Switzerland.

the results of microquantitative methods (periodic acid–Schiff reaction, enzyme distribution patterns of glucose-6-phosphate dehydrogenase, 6-phosphogluconate dehydrogenase, and malic enzyme), it has been found that an excellent correspondence exists in liver parenchyma between the subjective assessment and the values measured.

Only those techniques and methods that have proved reliable in our laboratory are described.

2. HISTOLOGY

2.1. Tissue Pretreatment

2.1.1. Fixation

The aim of fixation is to achieve a permanent preservation of cells and tissues that will allow investigation of their structure and, as far as possible, of their chemical composition. To obtain results that reflect the situation during life, the process of fixation has to begin either by perfusion of the living organ or immediately after the removal of the tissue, in order to limit postmortem alterations. It is important to take into consideration early the influences that the fixative will have on the physical properties and the stainability of the tissue.

Chemical fixation is still widely used as a prerequisite for the microscopic study of tissue selections. Fixation leads principally to a linkage of molecules, and necessarily results in an alteration of the morphology and the chemistry of the tissue. Wolman[11] stated that a good morphological fixation is one in which the changes that occur in the structures take place below the resolving power of the optical system, whereas a good histochemical fixation is a good morphological fixation in which the chemical groups studied can still be recognized by the appropriate reagents. In this section, some fixation methods that lead to an adequate preservation of structure and allow subsequent histochemical demonstration techniques will be briefly described.

2.1.1a. Formaldehyde and Glutaraldehyde. Formaldehyde is more suitable for the fixation of a number of enzymes and the preservation of their activity; glutaraldehyde is an excellent fixative for structures. The tissue proteins undergo different complex reactions with both aldehydes, in many cases forming cross-links between protein end-groups. Moreover, aldehydes react with thiols and with lipophilic groups, leading to the appearance of more hydrophilic groups. Because of the slow penetration of aldehydes, the edges of the tissue block should not exceed 0.5 cm.

Aqueous solutions of 4% phosphate-buffered (pH 7.2–7.4) formaldehyde and of 2–3% cacodylate-buffered (pH 7.2–7.4) glutaraldehyde are recommended.

The fixation temperature should be fairly low (4°C), and the fixation time depends largely on the density of the tissue, although 2–5 hr is usually sufficient. After fixation, the tissue has to be washed in running tap water or, more carefully, in Holt's mixture[12] (30 g sucrose and 1 g gum acacia being mixed and then distilled water added to make up 100 ml). The washing procedure should last as long as the fixation time. The tissue can then be frozen and cut at −20°C in a cryostat, or it can be dehydrated with acetone and xylene and transferred to paraffin. Permeation with paraffin should be completed after 5 hr (see Section 2.1.4).

2.1.1b. Carnoy's Fixative. This mixture yields excellent morphological preservation together with good stainability of the nucleic acids. The fixative consists of 60 ml ethyl alcohol, 30 ml chloroform, and 10 ml glacial acetic acid. A variation of Carnoy's fluid is the fixative Methacarn,[13] in which methanol is substituted for ethyl alcohol. Fixation in these mixtures should be continued at 0–4°C for 12–24 hr. Final dehydration is achieved in 100% ethyl alcohol or 100% methyl alcohol.

2.1.1c. Gendre's Fixative. This mixture is also recommended for good morphological preservation and when the subsequent histochemical demonstration of glycogen and other polysaccharides is required.[14] The mixture consists of 85 parts of saturated picric acid in 96% ethyl alcohol, 10 parts of 40% formaldehyde, and 5 parts of glacial acetic acid. Best results are achieved when fixation is carried out at 0–4°C for 12–24 hr. Final dehydration is achieved by 100% ethyl alcohol.

2.1.2. Freeze–Substitution

This histological technique was introduced by Simpson[15] and Lison.[16] Its rationale is to replace the water in tissues frozen well below the melting point with liquid dehydrating agents. Depending on the substituent used, tissue preservation is achieved by either dehydration or fixation.

One prerequisite for a good result is the quenching of very small tissue blocks (3 mm in diameter) at a low temperature (−190°C), e.g., in isopentane–liquid nitrogen. The tissue is then immersed in a substituent at a temperature below the eutectic point.[17] There have been divergent opinions on the best media to use and on the optimal temperature and duration of the procedure. In the meantime, programmed thermostats by which freeze–substitution temperatures can be regulated have become available. With these devices, either maintenance of temperature or rewarming of the substituting bath at the rate or time desired is possible. Our experiments[18] with small blocks of liver, trachea, neonatal kidneys, and uterine segments, quenched in isopentane (−190°C) and then transferred to absolute acetone, absolute ethanol, or Rossman's fluid (similar to Gendre's fluid)—each at −62°C—showed that the best results could be attained by progressive rewarming of the substituent up to 20°C for a period of 2–4 days.

2.1.3. Freeze–Drying

There is no doubt that under optimal conditions, freeze–drying leads to the best results for both the morphology and the chemical composition of the tissue. However, it must be stated that despite repeated recommendations of this method, freeze–drying is still seldom used by histologists. This might be due not only to the cost of the technique, but also to the disappointing results that may unexpectedly occur. Very often, the tissue is damaged by the formation of ice crystals during the procedure or by incomplete drying of the tissue.

In the field of histochemistry, freeze–drying (or lyophilization) is used as a pretreatment for tissue sections in which substances or enzyme activity are later to be demonstrated by qualitative histochemical means or that are to be microdissected for quantitative analysis by techniques introduced by Lowry and his colleagues (see Chapter 5).

The following procedure can be recommended for the lyophilization of tissue sections[19]: Small blocks of tissue are rapidly frozen in isopentane cooled with liquid nitrogen ($-190°C$). These can then be stored in airtight tubes at $-70°C$ until use. When required, 10-μm sections of the unfixed material are cut at $-20°C$ in a cryostat and then placed in individual compartments in a precooled sample holder.[20] The sample holder is placed in a lyophilization tube and transferred to a cryostat, and the tubes are connected to a vacuum gauge equipped with a foreline adsorption trap. Alternate sections can be taken for conventional slide histochemical procedures. The sections are dried from the frozen state for 12–24 hr at a vacuum equivalent to 6.7×10^{-1} Pa. These lyophilized sections may again be stored at $-70°C$ under vacuum or warmed up to room temperature under vacuum by connecting the lyophilization tube to the vacuum pump for 60 min.

2.1.4. Embedding and Sectioning

Fixed material that may not be cut in a frozen state must be embedded, and this is mostly done in paraffin. Before the tissue can be infiltrated by melted paraffin wax, it must be dehydrated, usually by taking it through a series of aqueous solutions of increasing alcoholic concentration until absolute alcohol is reached. For histochemical purposes, however, when it is intended to demonstrate the activity of enzymes able to withstand 2–3 hr of formaldehyde fixation (alkaline phosphatase, peptidases, esterases of the endoplasmic reticulum and of lysosomes, as well as acid phosphatase or β-glucuronidase), a more cautious method of dehydration is recommended.[9] Tissue, after having been washed in Holt's mixture, is transferred at first into a 50% aqueous solution of acetone (45 min, 4°C) and then into 100% acetone for 12–24 hr. The acetone should be changed at least three times; during the final immersion, the tissue is allowed to reach room temperature. The tissue is then transferred to xylene (3 × 10 min) and immersed in low-melting-point paraffin (56°C), which should be kept liquid for at least 45 min. The tissue, embedded in paraffin blocks, is cut on a suitable microtome into sections of 5–10 μm.

The most usual method of sectioning unfixed tissue for histochemical purposes employs a cryostat. Particularly recommended are cryostats with two separate cooling systems that allow different temperatures for the frozen tissue block and the cryostat chamber. The temperature of the tissue should be lower for fat-rich tissue (-30°C) and higher for water-rich tissues (-15 to -20°C). The temperature of the cryostat chamber is kept at -20°C. It has been found that tissue sections of good quality and of approximately similar thickness can be obtained by using a microtome equipped with a continuously running motor. The appropriate thickness of the cryostat sections depends on the subsequent technique; 10-μm sections are generally used. The sections are conveniently thawed on cover glasses before proceeding to the next step.

Before staining procedures can be carried out on paraffin sections, the sections must be transferred to xylene for 1–3 min and then taken through the series absolute alcohol, 90% alcohol, and 70% alcohol (1 min each), and then put into distilled water.

After staining, the sections can be mounted directly in a hydrophilic mounting medium (glycerine jelly: 15 g gelatin in 100 ml distilled water, warm, add 100 g glycerol, filtrate, and add a drop of phenol). For permanent preparations, the sections must be dehydrated through a series of increasing alcohol to xylene and mounted in a suitable medium (e.g., DePeX).

2.1.5. Quantitative Methods in Histology

The subjective visual impression that is obtained by looking at planar histological and electron-microscopic sections can be described in objective terms by using morphometric methods. The quantitative methods to be used for the evaluation of the structure parameters depend on the problems to be solved.[21] If volumes and surfaces are to be measured, the simple manual or the optomanual methods are recommended. In these cases, grids of various sizes are placed either in the eyepiece or on the surface of the electron photomicrograph. According to Haug,[22] the network density should be at a level where each structure in the measurement field registers between 1 and 15 hits. With manual methods, the values are registered on check sheets or simple counters; optomanual procedures require electric counters with many registers.

If, in addition to volume and surface measurements, particle-size determinations are also required, semiautomatic methods are preferable. In this case, the boundaries of the structures are outlined on a table with a tracer. Magnetostrictive systems are most commonly available. Either the electron photomicrograph is placed directly on the plate or light-microscopic specimens are reflected onto the plate by a microscope equipped with a drawing apparatus. The results of the semiautomatic analysis are stored and analyzed by a computer.

Fully automatic measurements are carried out with a television tube; the analyzing beam counts changes of contrast across a predetermined threshold and calculates the results directly by means of a computer.

The various quantities that can be measured are represented as letters, where the subscript letter represents the denominator or overall quantity (e.g., total volume, total number of points). The following letters are commonly used in biology[22,23]:

A = planar surface (partial or overall surface)
I = intersection (grid line cut off at the boundary of a structure)
L = length of a grid line, or structure length, or length of a structure boundary
N = number of particles
P = number of grid points (= "hits," when they fall within the required structure)
Q = transection (protrusions of lengthwise structures through the grid area)
S = surface of structure (flat or arched)
T = thickness of section
d = interval distance of the grid
k = size of the smallest recognizable particle
r = mean radius of a structure

On the basis of the morphometric data, the methods of stereology allow conclusions to be drawn about the measurements in three dimensions. According to Weibel,[5] "stereology is a body of mathematical methods—relating three-dimensional parameters defining the structure to two-dimensional measurements obtainable on sections of the structure." Stereological methods are essential mainly to solve the question: "How is the size of a certain profile related to the size of the object of interest?"

The results of these methods are substantially influenced by the techniques of preparation, by structural inhomogeneities, and by the thickness of the section. Stereological procedures permit the determination of volumes, surfaces, length and number of particles, and several other values in tissue sections, so that the terms volume density, surface density, length density, curvature density, and numerical density describe these quantitative properties of the structure in relation to the structure space.

To evaluate the components of liver parenchyma, the hierarchical model of liver structure in Fig. 1 was described.[5] The various stages are defined as follows:

Stage I: Light microscopy, magnification × 200
Reference volume: total liver tissue
Stage II: Electron microscopy, final magnification × 6,200
Reference volume: liver parenchyma
Stage III: Electron microscopy, final magnification × 19,000
Reference volume: hepatocyte cytoplasm
Stage IV: Electron microscopy, final magnification × 96,000
Reference volume: hepatocyte cytoplasm

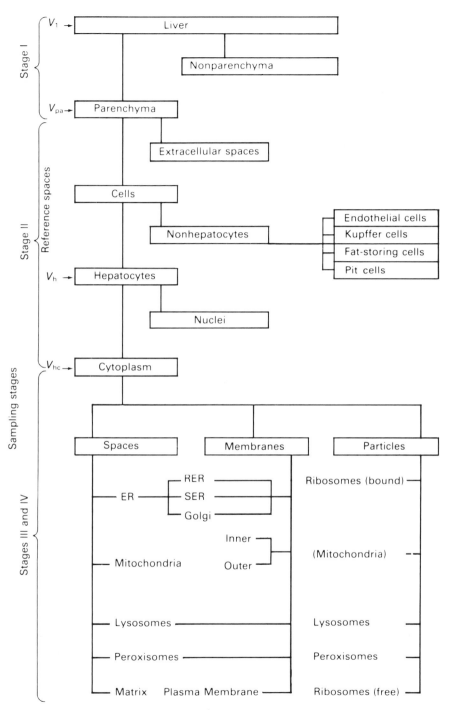

Figure 1. Hierarchical model of liver structure. After Weibel.[5]

2.2. Routine Staining Methods

Hematoxylin–eosin staining is the standard method for making the cell nuclei and the cytoplasmic structures visible. Instead of the classic procedure, it is easier to use Mayer's hemalum for routine staining and to omit counterstaining with eosin or erythrosin, which often leads to a greasy appearance of the cytoplasm.

Hemalum staining alone leads to an excellent and clear presentation of the dark-blue-stained nuclei as well as of the cytoplasmic structures.

2.2.1. Mayer's Hemalum[1]

Solutions: In 1000 ml distilled water, dissolve:

Hematoxylin	1.0 g
Sodium iodate	0.2 g
Potassium alum	50.0 g

Shake the mixture for some hours until it turns blue-violet. Then add:

Chloral hydrate	50.0 g
Citric acid crystals	1.0 g
The solution then turns a red-violet color.	

Staining procedure: Fixed sections in water or unfixed sections are immersed in the solution for 4–6 min. The sections are then washed thoroughly in tap water for 10 min before being dehydrated through the alcohols and xylene and mounted.

2.2.2. Trichrome Stain after van Gieson[24]

Good results are obtained with this trichrome stain, a combination of hematoxylin, picric acid, and acid fuchsin. With this method, the nuclei are stained brownish black, the collagen tissue red, and the muscle yellow. Other components, such as colloid, hyalin, or mucin, are recognized by their differing color intensities.

Solutions

a. Celestine blue B	0.5 g
Ferrous ammonium sulfate	5.0 g
Glycerol	14.0 ml
Distilled water	100.0 ml

Ferrous ammonium sulfate is dissolved in distilled water, and the celestine blue is added and the mixture gently heated. After cooling and filtration, glycerol is added. The solution is stable for at least 6 months at 4°C.

b. Mayer's hemalum (see above)	
c. Saturated solution of picric acid in distilled water	90 ml
1% Acid fuchsin in distilled water	10 ml

Both solutions (c) are mixed and boiled for 3 min. This combination is stable and can be stored as a stock solution at 4°C.

Staining procedure: Fixed and deparaffinated in water are immersed in solution (a) (celestine blue) for 5 min and then washed in tap water for several minutes. They are then stained for 5 min in solution (b) (Mayer's hemalum), washed once more in tap water for 5 min, and finally stained in solution (c) (picric acid–fuchsin). After this, the sections are rapidly washed in distilled water again and then dehydrated through the alcohols and xylene and mounted.

2.2.3. Azan[1]

This method is rather complicated, although it yields the best results in precise color localization and stability. Azan staining can be regarded as one of the sharpest and most brilliant of the classic histological procedures. Collagen and reticular connective tissue are stained blue, nuclei and chromatin red, and muscle tissue orange-red. Intracellular granules stain yellow, red, or blue depending on their chemical composition.

Solutions

a. Azocarmine G	0.1 g
Distilled water	100.0 ml

The solution is rapidly heated to 100° C, allowed to cool, and filtered. To 100 ml of filtered solution, add:

Glacial acetic acid	1.0 ml
b. Aniline	1.0 ml
90% Ethanol	1000.0 ml
c. Glacial acetic acid	1.0 ml
96% Ethanol	100.0 ml
d. Phosphotungstic acid	5.0 g
Distilled water	100.0 ml
e. Aniline blue	0.5
Orange G	2.0 g
Distilled water	100.0 ml
Glacial acetic acid	8.0 ml

The solution (e) is boiled for minutes and then filtered. Before use, it is diluted 1 : 2 with distilled water.

Staining procedure: Fixed and deparaffinized sections in water are stained in solution (a) (azocarmine) at 60°C for 45–60 min and then washed in distilled water. Differentiation takes place in solution (b) (aniline–ethanol) under microscopic control until only the nuclei remain pink and is then halted by transfer of the sections into solution (c) (acetic ethanol). After some minutes, the sections are put into solution (d) (phosphotungstic acid) and allowed to remain for 2 hr. After being rinsed with distilled water, they are stained in solution (e) (aniline blue) for 1–3 hr. The sections are then passed very rapidly through distilled water and differentiated in 96% ethanol before being further dehydrated through the alcohols and xylene and mounted.

2.3. Special Staining Methods

2.3.1. Bile Canaliculi[1]

With this procedure, bile canaliculi are impregnated and rendered brownish black (Fig. 2).

Fresh, unfixed blocks of liver, smaller than 1 cm³, are immersed 3 times for 24 hr in fresh portions of the following solution:

4 Parts of an aqueous solution of 3% potassium dichromate

1 Part of an aqueous solution of 1% osmium tetroxide

The tissue blocks are then transferred to an aqueous solution of 0.75% silver nitrate for 24–48 hr. The specimens are then washed in distilled water for 0.5–1 hr and fixed in the course of dehydration through alcohols of increasing concentration. They may later be taken through xylene into paraffin, or they can be cut in a cryostat.

2.3.2. Reticulin Fibers[1,24] (Gomori, 1937)

Reticulin fibers are impregnated by silver nitrate and appear black, nuclei gray, and collagen fibers grayish red (Fig. 3). Best results are obtained with Carnoy- (Methacarn-)fixed liver tissue.

Solutions

    a.   Aqueous solution of 1% potassium permanganate
    b.   Aqueous solution of 2% potassium metabisulfite
    c.   Aqueous solution of 2% ferrrous ammonium sulfate
    d.   Aqueous solution of 10% neutral formaldehyde
    e.   Aqueous solution of 0.2% gold chloride
    f.   Aqueous solution of 2.5% sodium thiosulfate
    g.   Ammoniacal solution of silver nitrate:
        Mix: Aqueous solution of 10% silver nitrate 10 ml
             Aqueous solution of 10% potassium hydroxide 2 ml

To this mixture, add ammonia solution (about 25%) drop by drop. The mixture has to be shaken continuously during the procedure to avoid precipitation. Then, again, 10% silver nitrate is added until the first precipitations occur. Finally, an equal volume of distilled water is added and the solution is filtered.

Staining procedure: Sections out of water are oxidized in solution (a) (po-

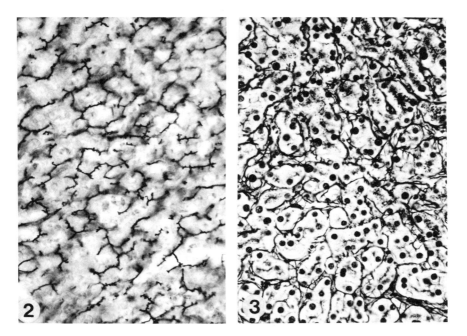

Figure 2. Bile canaliculi, human liver. Silver impregnation.

Figure 3. Reticulin fibers, human liver. Silver impregnation.

tassium permanganate) for 2 min. Sections are then briefly washed in distilled water and transferred to solution (b) (potassium metabisulfite) for 1 min. Again wash sections in distilled water. Then immerse sections in solution (c) (ferrous ammonium sulfate) for 1 min. Wash thoroughly in tap water and distilled water. Impregnate sections with solution (g) (ammoniacal silver nitrate). Wash for a short time with distilled water. Hold the slide at an angle while pouring solution (d) (neutral formaldehyde) over it. It must then be laid on a slide rack placed immediately above the surface of the formaldehyde solution. Wash the section for 3 min with tap water and stain in solution (e) (gold chloride) for 5–10 min, before further washing in distilled water and treating with solution (b) (potassium metabisulfite) for 1 min. Again wash the section in distilled water and immerse in solution (f) (sodium thiosulfate) for 2 min before a further final wash in distilled water, dehydration through the alcohols, and mounting.

2.3.3.   Kupffer Cells and Fat-Storing Cells[1,25,26]

Both these cell types can be marked by intravital staining. The staining procedures may be carried out for one cell type only or for both.[25] The following description includes the volumes necessary for rat tissue.

Solutions

A (for Kupffer cells)
    a. Saturated aqueous solution of sodium bicarbonate   100 ml
    b. Carmine   2.5 g
Boil the solution for 10 min and then filter
B (for fat-storing cells)
    Solution of vitamin A acetate (1,000,000 IU/g)   1 g
    dissolved in peanut oil   5 ml

Staining procedure: For the demonstration of Kupffer cells, 1 ml carmine solution is injected intravenously into the rat (200–300 g body weight), and the procedure is repeated after 1 hr. At 90 min after the last injection, the animal is killed and the liver removed.

For the demonstration of fat-storing cells, 330,000 IU/kg body weight of vitamin A solution is injected subcutaneously on 4 consecutive days. The total dosage of vitamin A is 1,320,000 IU/kg. At 14 days after the last injection, the animal is killed and the liver removed.

For the simultaneous demonstration of Kupffer cells and fat-storing cells, vitamin A as described in (B) should be injected; after 14 days, carmine [see (A) above] is administered.

For the visualization of Kupffer cells, unfixed cryostat sections can be used directly or after counterstaining with Mayer's hemalum. The UV fluorescence of fat-storing cells can be seen in unfixed cryostat sections without any further treatment.

3. HISTOCHEMISTRY

3.1. Substances

3.1.1. Glycogen

The most sensitive method for the demonstration of glycogen is the periodic acid–Schiff (PAS) reaction[27,28] (Fig. 4). Since this reaction demonstrates not only the 1,2-glycol groups of glycogen but also those of glycoproteins and other compounds, a parallel section is necessary for prior incubation in α-amylase. On comparing the two adjacent sections, glycogen can be seen as a red color in those sites where no staining is visible in the control (Figs. 5 and 6).

Solutions

    a. Aqueous solution of 0.5% periodic acid
    b. Schiff's reagent:
        Dissolve 5 g pararosaniline in 150 ml 1 N HCl

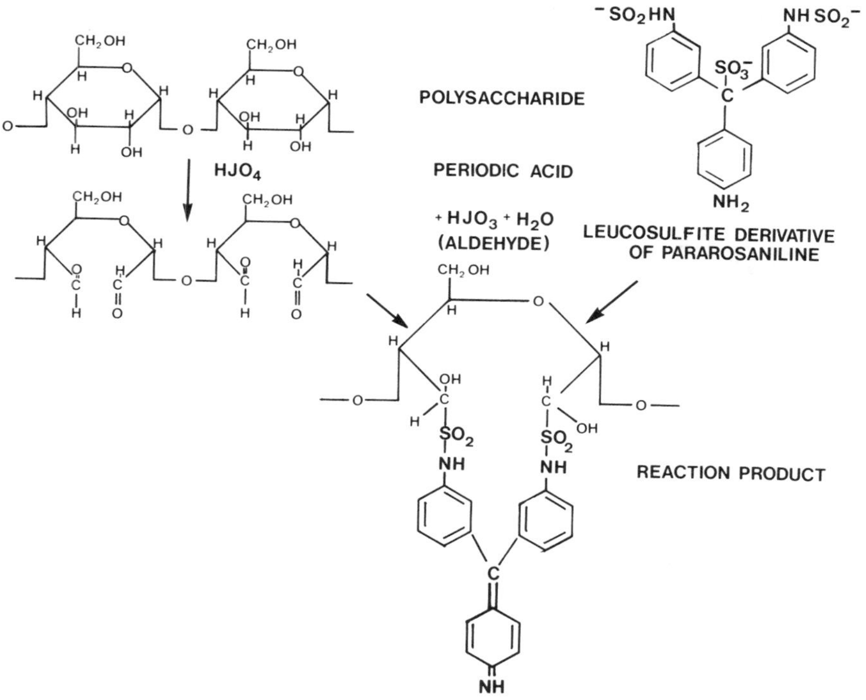

POLYSACCHARIDE

PERIODIC ACID

$+ HJO_3 + H_2O$
(ALDEHYDE)

LEUCOSULFITE DERIVATIVE
OF PARAROSANILINE

REACTION PRODUCT

Figure 4. Periodic acid–Schiff (PAS) reaction.

Add:
5 g Potassium disulfite dissolved in
850 ml Double-distilled water

The red solution turns yellow within 24 hr. The solution is then shaken with 3 g activated charcoal and filtered twice.

c. Aqueous solution of:

10% Potassium metabisulfite	30	ml
1.0 N HCl	30	ml
in double-distilled water	600	ml

Staining procedure: Gendre-fixed sections in water or unfixed cryostat sections without further pretreatment are immersed in solution (a) (periodic acid) for 10 min, and then washed in tap water for 10 min and rinsed twice for 2 min in distilled water. They are then placed in solution (b) (Schiff's reagent) for 30 min. Thereafter, the sections are treated with freshly prepared solution (c) (potassium metabisulfite) (3 × 2 min) and then washed in tap water for 5 min.

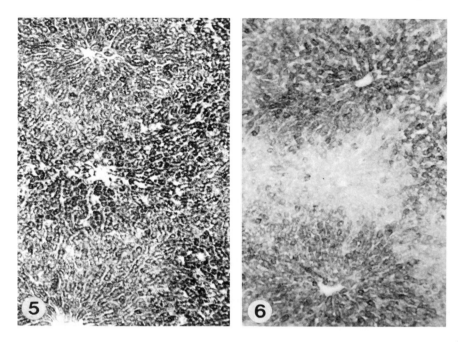

Figure 5. Liver glycogen in a fed rat. PAS reaction. Note the glycogen content in all hepatocytes, mainly in the periportal zone.

Figure 6. Liver glycogen in rat after 8 hr of starving. PAS reaction. Note that the glycogen content is restricted to the perivenous zones.

After immersion in distilled water, the sections are dehydrated through alcohol and xylene and finally mounted.

Control: Before the PAS reaction, Gendre-fixed sections in water or unfixed cryostat sections are immersed in:

Aqueous solution of α-amylase   (2800 IU/g) 1 g
in double-distilled water   100 ml

for 2 hr at room temperature. They are then rinsed twice in distilled water and thereafter treated as for the PAS reaction.

3.1.2. Fat

Staining of lipids is possible by dyes the solubility of which in fat exceeds their solubility in the solvent. For the demonstration of the neutral fat content of liver cells, staining with Oil Red 0 was found to be quite sensitive.[29] The stained lipid droplets appear bright red (Fig. 7).

Solutions

a. Aqueous solution of 60% isopropanol
b. Oil Red solution: 0.5 g
    To prepare stock solution, dissolve, Oil
       Red 0
    in 99% isopropanol   100 ml
    Before use, add 4 ml distilled water to
       6 ml of the stock solution. After 24
       hr, the solution is filtered and used
       immediately.

Staining procedure: Formaldehyde-fixed sections in water or unfixed cryostat sections are immersed in solution (a) (60% isopropanol) for 5 min, stained
in solution (b) (Oil Red O) for 10 min, and, if necessary, differentiated rapidly
again in solution (a). They are then rinsed in distilled water. Counterstaining
with Mayer's hemalum for 3–5 min is recommended. The sections should then
be washed in tap water for 10 min and mounted directly in glycerine jelly.

3.1.3. Nucleic Acids

A simultaneous demonstration of RNA and DNA is obtained with gallocyanin–chrome alum staining. Gallocyanin is a stable metal–dye complex that
binds to nucleic acids by mordanting mechanisms. The metal is bound coordinately both to groups on the tissue and to groups on the dye. It has been described
as a sensitive method that also allows cytophotometric quantification.[30] Both
RNA- and DNA-containing cell structures are dark blue (Fig. 8).

Solutions

Chrome alum	5.0	g
Gallocyanin	0.15	g
Double-distilled water	100.0	ml

Boil the solution for 5 min. After cooling to room temperature, filter and pour
double-distilled water through the filter to obtain a final volume of 100 ml. The
solution is stable for 4 weeks.

Staining procedure: Carnoy- or Methacarn-fixed sections in water are stained
at room temperature for 48 hr, washed in tap water for 10 min, and dehydrated
through the alcohols and xylene before mounting.

Control: For the demonstration of exclusively RNA- or DNA-containing
structures, Carnoy- or Methacarn-fixed sections are taken out of water and immersed in:

40 ml   Aqueous solution of of 10 mg (2000 IU/mg) deoxyribonuclease or 10 mg (50 IU/mg)
            ribonuclease

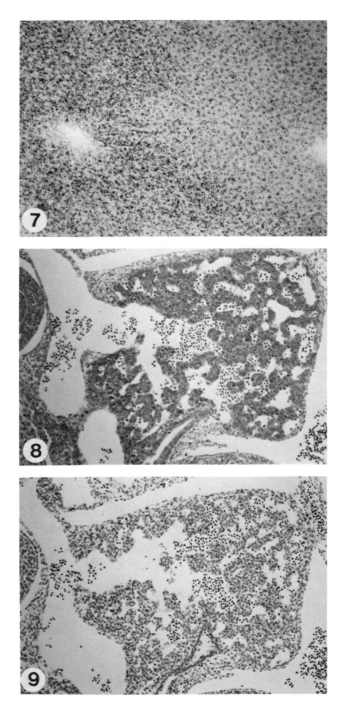

for 2 hr at room temperature, washed with tap water for 20 min, and stained with gallocyanin–chrome alum (Fig. 9).

3.1.4. Iron[31]

Fe^{2+} and Fe^{3+} can be demonstrated by the Turnbull Blue reaction. Iron-containing structures are stained blue.

Solutions

  a.   Aqueous solution of 10% ammonium sulfide
  b.   Equal parts of an aqueous solution of potassium ferricyanide (III) 20% and HCl 10%

Staining procedure: Formaldehyde-fixed sections in water or unfixed cryostat sections are immersed in solution (a) (ammonium sulfide) for 15 min, then rinsed three times for 2 min with distilled water before being immersed in freshly prepared solution (b) (potassium ferricyanide) for 15 min. The sections are then rinsed with distilled water, dehydrated through the alcohols and xylene, and mounted.

3.2. Enzymes

Enzyme histochemical techniques allow the localization of enzyme activity in the tissue. For this purpose, methods are principally used that correspond to the biochemical determination. For *in situ* demonstration, however, some additional difficulties have to be taken into consideration. The enzyme content and activity in a 10-μm tissue section are usually very low and must be preserved as far as possible in the section during the procedure, and the histochemical reactions do not take place under the optimal *in vitro* conditions of a biochemical assay. Furthermore, a histochemical method should not alter the histological structure. Finally, as the result of the reaction, the product has to be visible under the microscope, and this requires the formation of a pigment. This pigment must be insoluble and must be precipitated exactly at the site of the enzyme activity in the cell.

There are four principal approaches for the histochemical detection of enzyme activity: metal-salt trapping methods, coupling methods, tetrazolium meth-

---

Figure 7.   Lipid content of rat liver, starved 2 days and refed for 3 days with a carbohydrate-rich diet. Oil Red 0. Lipid droplets are accumulated mainly in the periportal zone.

Figure 8.   Prenatal liver, golden hamster (15 days, 8 hr of development). Simultaneous demonstration of RNA and DNA with gallocyanin–chrome alum.

Figure 9.   Same animal as in Fig. 8, parallel section preincubated with ribonuclease. Demonstration of DNA with gallocyanin–chrome alum.

ods, and the demonstration of product. Examples appropriate to liver metabolism are presented in Sections 3.2.2–3.2.5.

3.2.1. Microscopic Photometry of Enzyme Activity

The demonstration of enzymes with qualitative histochemical methods allows the differentiation of sites of relatively high or low activity, and therewith the recognition of distribution patterns on the basis of staining intensities. To attain a higher grade of objectivity, the staining results are often listed in categories (0, ±, +, + +, + + +), an approach for which the term "semiquantitative" is as common as it is euphemistic. Despite the usually good reproducibility of qualitative histochemical methods, it is not possible to compare such subjective estimations with the genuinely quantitative results that can be attained by the biochemical methods of controlled fragmentation of tissue and cells or by the ultramicrochemical analysis (Lowry technique) of one or more cells. Therefore, increasingly successful attempts have been made in recent decades to obtain a quantification of the histochemical reaction product *in situ* at the light-microscopic level by the use of microscope photometers. The addition of equipment to microscopes with programmed computers serves to automate the measuring procedures and to collect data from a greater number of points.[32]

According to Pette and Wimmer,[33] the method of microscopic photometry has to fulfil the following requirements:

1. Availability of a specific and stoichiometric reaction suitable for direct photometric measurement of the reaction rate.
2. Process of measuring reaction at stable conditions and stability of the photometrically determined reaction product.
3. Proportionality between reaction rate and local enzyme concentration.

Numerous investigations have been carried out on the problem of the specificity of enzyme histochemical procedures. The measurement of enzyme activity in model systems is very suitable for solving this question. The requirements for the quantitative measurement of final reaction products were investigated by van Duijn[32] and co-workers, who studied the problems of quantitative determinations of phosphatases and questions connected with the kinetics of the capture reaction and the diffusion of the reaction in model experiments, using polyacrylamide films. The photometric evaluation of metal-salt trapping, however, represents an end-point measurement. Deductions about enzyme activity are more reliable when it is possible to confirm that the underlying reaction rate is linear with time.

These questions were studied by Pette and co-workers,[34–36] who directed their efforts toward enzyme reactions that can be coupled to the reduction of tetrazolium salts (glutamate dehydrogenase, lactate dehydrogenase, malate dehydrogenase, isocitrate dehydrogenase, glucose-6-phosphate dehydrogenase, NADH tetrazolium reductase). By the incorporation of enzyme preparations into different matrix systems, they were able to simulate the situation of an enzyme in a cell and to assess whether the conditions of Lambert–Beer's law were fulfilled.

Further important prerequisites for the microphotometric measurement of enzyme activity have been worked out. The introduction of the gel film technique and the use of viscous media in which it is possible to record the specifically catalyzed reaction at initial rate conditions minimize artifacts due to light-scattering and distribution error. The media contain the complete reaction mixture, which is placed on the tissue section mounted on the microscope stage.

To improve the reliability of the microphotometric determinations, measurements were taken within the same section from different preselected measuring fields of equal size. Thus, a direct comparison of microphotometrically determined enzyme reaction rates is possible, because the area of the measuring field, thickness of the section, temperature, and reaction medium are identical. The use of a microscope stage that can be moved by two stepping motors along rectangular coordinates guided by a special computer program allows measurements of numerous different preselected measuring positions. The continuous recording of extinction changes at initial rates provides an equally continuous control of the reaction kinetics and also offers the possibility of evaluating maximum initial reaction rates.

By these methods, it is now possible to obtain detailed objective information on heterogeneous distribution patterns of enzyme activity in structurally complex organs such as the liver.[37]

3.2.2. Metal-Salt Trapping

3.2.2a. Glucose-6-phosphatase (E.C.3.1.3.9) (Modified, Maly and Sasse, 1983)[38]

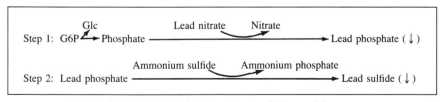

Reaction scheme for demonstrating G6Pase activity

Unfixed cryostat sections, 10 μm, placed on coverslips are used.

Incubation medium		*Final concentration*
2.5 ml	a. 200 mM tris maleate buffer, pH 6.5	50 mM
2.0 ml	b. 100 mM G6P in double-distilled water	20 mM
4.5 ml	c. Double-distilled water	
1.0 ml	d. 46 mM Pb(NO$_3$)$_2$ in double-distilled water	4.6 mM

Stock solutions (storable at $-70°$C) are prepared from solutions (a–c) in 9-ml portions, and these are warmed to room temperature. Then 1.0 ml solution (d) (storable at 4°C) is added, with continuous stirring. Incubation temperature: 25°C; incubation time: 10 min.

It is essential to shake the medium during incubation. This may be done by hand or on an eccentrically rotating mixer with about 35 movements/min at an angle of inclination of 10°. After incubation, the tissue sections, placed on coverslips, are rinsed in distilled water for 1 min and immersed in a 1 : 100 aqueous solution of 27% ammonium sulfide for 2 min. Thereafter, the sections are again rinsed in distilled water and finally mounted in glycerine jelly. The reaction product is brown-black (Fig. 10).

3.2.3. Coupling Methods

3.2.3a. Alkaline Phosphatase (E.C. 3.1.3.1) (Modified, Lojda et al., 1979)[9]

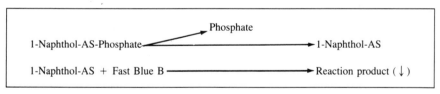

Reaction scheme for demonstrating alkaline phosphatase activity

Either 10-μm unfixed or formaldehyde-fixed cryostat sections or formaldehyde-fixed paraffin sections in water may be used. They are placed on coverslips.

Incubation medium

Naphthol-AS-phosphate (or naphthol-AS-MX-, naphthol-AS-D-, naphthol-AS-BI-, or naphthol-AS-TR-phosphate)	10–25 mg
Dissolved in *N,N*-dimethylformamide	0.5 ml

| 200 mM Tris-HCl buffer, pH 8.2–9.2 | 50 ml |
| Fast blue BB (or fast blue RR, B, or fast red TR) | 50 mg |

These reagents must be mixed thoroughly and filtered. Incubation temperature: 37°C; incubation time: 15 min. After incubation, the sections should be rinsed with distilled water and immersed for several hours in a 4% formaldehyde solution. Counterstaining with Mayer's hemalum is possible. The sections are then washed with tap water and distilled water and mounted in glycerine jelly. The reaction product is stained according to the nature of the azo dye used.

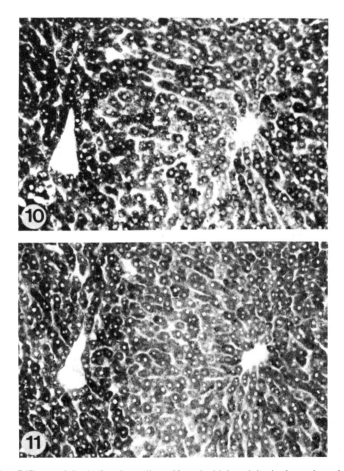

Figure 10. G6Pase activity in female rat liver. Note the high activity in the periportal zone.

Figure 11. SDH activity in female rat liver. Parallel section to Figure 10. Note the high activity in the periportal zone.

3.2.3b. β-Glucuronidase (E.C. 3.2.1.31) (Hayashi et al., 1964)[39]

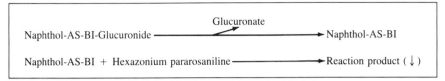

Reaction scheme for demonstrating β-glucuronidase activity

Formaldehyde or glutaraldehyde-fixed cryostat sections, 10 μm, placed on coverslips, are washed for 5 min in tap water and rinsed for a short time in distilled water. The medium should be freshly prepared just prior to the incubation.

Incubation medium

Naphthol AS-BI-D-glucuronide	4.0 mg
Dissolved in *N,N*-dimethylformamide	0.25 ml
Buffered hexazonium-*p*-rosaniline (from 19.4 to 18.2 ml 200 mM sodium acetate buffer and 0.6–1.8 ml hexazonium-*p*-rosaniline, pH 5.0, adjusted with NaOH)	20 ml

These reagents should be mixed thoroughly and filtered. Incubation temperature: 37°C; incubation time: 30–60 min. After incubation, the sections are rinsed with distilled water and immersed for several hours in a 4% formaldehyde solution. Counterstaining with Mayer's hemalum is possible. The sections are then washed with tap water and distilled water and mounted in glycerine jelly. The reaction product is red.

3.2.4. Tetrazolium Methods

3.2.4a. Succinate Dehydrogenase (E.C. 1.3.99.1) (Modified)

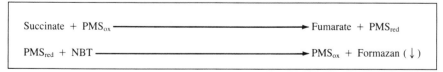

Reaction scheme for demonstrating SDH activity

Unfixed cryostat sections, 10 μm, placed on coverslips are air-dried (5 min, 37°C) and then covered with the incubation medium; incubation should be carried out in the dark.

Incubation medium   *Final concentration*

4.5 ml	41 mg Nitroblue tetrazolium (NBT) in 4.5 ml double-distilled water	5.0 mM
2.5 ml	Phosphate buffer, pH 7.5, 200 mM	50.0 mM
1 ml	50 mg $MgCl_2 \times 6H_2O$ in 5 ml double-distilled water	5.0 mM
1 ml	338 mg Succinate disodium salt in 5.0 ml double-distilled water	50.0 mM
0.6 ml	Double-distilled water (or buffer for pH adjustment)	

This medium can be stored at $-70°C$. Before use, warm up to room temperature and add:

0.2 ml	65 mg NaN_3 in 2.0 ml double-distilled water	10.0 mM
0.2 ml	10 mg Phenazine methosulfate (PMS) in 2.0 ml double-distilled water	0.32 mM

Incubation temperature: 37°C; incubation time: 10 min. After incubation, the sections are washed in 0.9% NaCl solution (1 min, 37°C), postfixed in 4% formaldehyde, 2% $CaCl_2$, 7.5% polyvinylpyrrolidone (20 min, 0°C), rinsed in double-distilled water (2 × 5 min), and mounted in glycerine jelly. The reaction product is blue-violet (Fig. 11).

The histochemical demonstration of the activity of the soluble enzymes LDH, G6PDH, 6PGDH, and of malic enzyme is complicated because enzyme diffusion has to be inhibited during incubation. Two different approaches have been most commonly used to minimize this artifact: interposition of a semipermeable membrane between section and medium and increase of the viscosity of the incubation medium by the addition of polyvinyl alcohol [(PVA), 20%].[40,41] Extensive studies in our laboratory have shown that the addition of PVA permits an accurate demonstration of cytoplasmic enzyme activity in the liver parenchyma.

3.2.4b. Lactate Dehydrogenase (E.C. 1.1.1.27) (Modified)

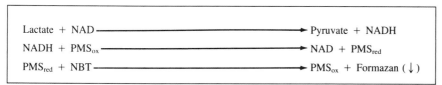

Reaction scheme for demonstrating LDH activity

Cryostat sections, 10 μm, are placed on coverslips and air-dried (5 min, 37°C). Lipids can be removed with 100% chloroform (5 min, 0°C). Then the sections are again air-dried (3 min, 37°C). The sections are covered with the medium described below. Incubation should be carried out in the dark.

Incubation medium		*Final concentration*
1.1 ml	45 mg NBT in 1.1 ml double-distilled water	5.0 mM
1.3 ml	Tris-HCl buffer, pH 7.4, 200 mM	50.0 mM
1.0 ml	50 mg $MgCl_2$ × $6H_2O$ in 5.0 ml double-distilled water	5.0 mM
1.0 ml	240 mg Lactic acid, lithium salt in 5.0 ml	100.0 mM
0.2 ml	70.5 mg NAD-monolithium salt × $2H_2O$ in 2 ml	1.0 mM
5.0 ml	20 g PVA (05/140) in 50.0 ml Tris-HCl-buffer, 50 mM, pH 7.4 (dissolved at 95°C by stirring; pH adjusted to 7.4)	20% (wt./vol.)

This medium can be stored at −70°C. Before use, warm up to room temperature and add:

		Final concentration
0.2 ml	65 mg NaN_3 in 2.0 ml double-distilled water	10.0 mM
0.2 ml	10 mg PMS in 2.0 ml double-distilled water	0.32 mM

Incubation temperature: 37°C; incubation time: 5–10 min. After incubation, the sections are washed in 0.9% NaCl solution (1 min, 37°C), postfixed in 4% formaldehyde, 2% $CaCl_2$, 7.5% polyvinylpyrrolidone (20 min, 0°C), rinsed in double-distilled water (2 × 5 min), and mounted in glycerine jelly. The reaction product is blue-violet.

3.2.4c. Glucose-6-phosphate Dehydrogenase (E.C. 1.1.1.49), 6-Phosphogluconate Dehydrogenase (E.C. 1.1.1.43), and Malic Enzyme (E.C. 1.1.1.40) (Rieder et al.,1978)[42]

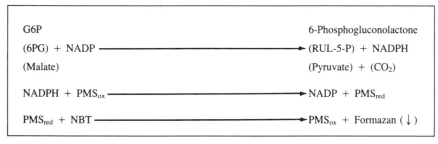

Reaction scheme for demonstrating the activity of G6PDH, 6PGDH, and malic enzyme.

Cryostat sections, 10 μm, are placed on coverslips and air-dried (5 min, 37°C). Lipids can be removed with 100% acetone (5 min, 0°C), 100% chloroform

(10 min, $-20°C$), 100% acetone (1 min, 0°C), and air-drying (3 min, 37°C).[43,44] The sections are covered with the medium described below. Incubation should be carried out in the dark.

Incubation medium		*Final concentration*	
1.1 ml	45 mg NBT in 1.1 ml double-distilled water	5.0	mM
1.3 ml	Tris-HCl buffer, pH 7.4	50.0	mM
1.0 ml	50 mg $MgCl_2 \times 6H_2O$ in 5.0 ml double-distilled water		
1.0 ml	152 mg Di-Na-glucose-6-phosphate (G6P) in 5.0 ml double-distilled water or, instead of G6P:	5.0	mM
(1.0 ml)	189 mg Tri-Na-6-phosphogluconate (6PG) in 5.0 ml double-distilled water	10.0	mM
(1.0 ml)	78mg Na-L-malate in 5.0 ml double-distilled water (pH adjusted to 7.4)	10.0	mM
0.2 ml	63 mg Di-Na-NADP in 2.0 ml double-distilled water		
5.0 ml	20 g PVA (05/140) in 50.0 ml Tris-HCl-buffer, 50.0 mM, pH 7.4 (dissolved at 95°C by stirring; pH adjusted to 7.4)	10.0	mM
		0.8	mM

This medium can be stored at $-70°C$. Before use, warm up to room temperature and add:

0.2 ml	65 mg NaN_3 in 2.0 ml double-distilled water	10.0	mM
0.2 ml	10 mg PMS in 2.0 ml double-distilled water	0.32	mM

Incubation temperature: 37°C; incubation time: 10–15 min. After incubation, the sections are washed in 0.9% NaCl solution (1 min, 37°C), postfixed in 4% formaldehyde, 2% $CaCl_2$, 7.5% polyvinylpyrrolidone (20 min, 0°C), rinsed in double-distilled water (2 × 5 min), and mounted in glycerine jelly. The reaction product is blue-violet (Figs. 12–15).

3.2.5. Product Demonstration

3.2.5a. Phosphorylase (E.C. 2.4.1.1) (Modified)

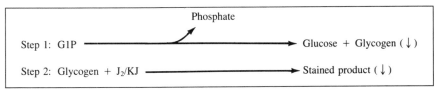

Reaction scheme for demonstrating phosphorylase activity

Unfixed cryostat sections, 20 μm, placed on coverslips are air-dried (5 min, 37°C) and incubated in the following medium:

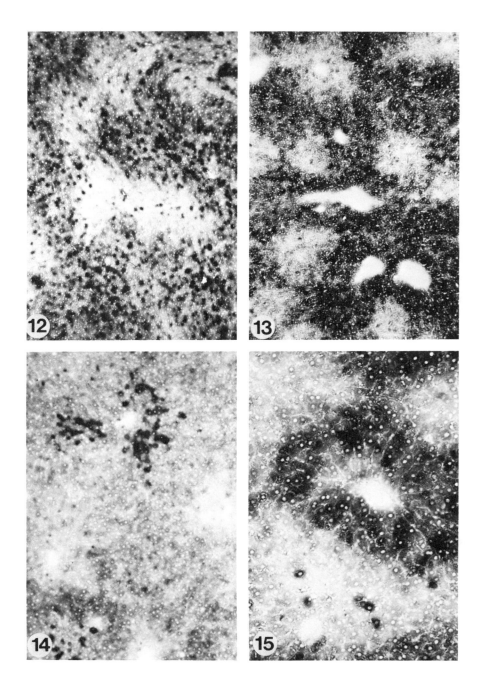

Incubation medium	*Final concentration*
Polyvinylpyrrolidone (K 30) dissolved in	900 mg
Acetate buffer, 100 mM, pH 5.6	10 ml
Absolute ethanol	2 ml
Glucose-1-phosphate (G1P) disodium salt × $4H_2O$	100 mg
EDTA, disodium salt	37 mg
Sodium fluoride	180 mg

pH 6.8, adjusted with NaOH

Incubation temperature: 37°C; incubation time: 1 hr. After incubation, the sections are washed in 0.9% NaCl solution (1 min, 37°C) and in 300 mM aqueous solution of sucrose (3 min). The newly formed glycogen is stained with Lugol's solution, diluted 1 : 10. Sections are mounted in glycerine jelly to which a drop of Lugol's solution has been added. The reaction product is brown-violet (Fig. 16).

The sections must be photographed immediately because the staining is unstable.

4. SUMMARY

Histological and histochemical methods are essential for the recognition of the structural and chemomorphological organization of liver parenchyma. A basic requirement for these microscopic studies is the adequate preservation of the tissue. Fixation with aldehydes and with the mixtures of Gendre and Carnoy (Methacarn) have proved suitable, particularly for the liver, for various subsequent staining procedures. For some problems, the techniques of freeze–substitution and freeze–drying are also advantageous. With quantitative methods, structural features can be evaluated. A short survey has been concerned with morphometric and stereological procedures.

Of the numerous histological techniques, staining with Mayer's hemalum, van Gieson's trichrome stain, and Heidenhain's azan stain have been described, all of which give excellent histological results. Special staining procedures have been mentioned that demonstrate typical elements of liver parenchyma: the silver

---

Figure 12. G6PDH activity in male rat liver. Note the activity in the epithelial liver cells and the high activity in the Kupffer cells, mainly in the periportal zone.

Figure 13. G6PDH activity in female rat liver. Note the high activity in the epithelial liver cells of the perivenous zone. Highly reactive Kupffer cells are located mainly in the periportal zone.

Figure 14. Malic enzyme activity in male rat liver. There is high activity only in scattered hepatocytes of the periportal zone.

Figure 15. Malic enzyme activity in female rat liver. There is high activity in the perivenous zone and in scattered hepatocytes of the periportal zone.

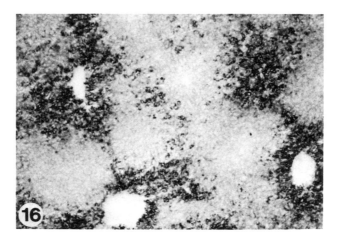

Figure 16. Phosphorylase activity in male rat liver. There is high activity in the periportal zone.

impregnation methods for the demonstration of bile canaliculi and reticulin fibers and the intravital marking of Kupffer cells and fat-storing cells.

Reliable histochemical methods for the demonstration of glycogen, intracellular fat droplets, nucleic acids, and iron have been described. As examples of functions relevant to liver metabolism, enzyme histochemical procedures have been briefly characterized and the possibilities of their quantification by microscopic photometry outlined. Methods have been described for the demonstration of the following enzyme activities: metal-salt trapping (glucose-6-phosphatase), coupling methods (alkaline phosphatase, β-glucuronidase), tetrazolium methods (succinate dehydrogenase, lactate dehydrogenase, glucose-6-phosphate dehydrogenase, 6-phosphogluconate dehydrogenase, and malic enzyme), and the product demonstration of phosphorylase activity.

REFERENCES

1. Romeis, B., 1968, *Mikroskopische Technik,* Oldenbourg Verlag, Munich and Vienna.
2. Gabe, M., 1976, *Histological Techniques,* Masson, Paris; Springer, Berlin.
3. McManus, J. F. A., and Mowry, R. A., 1960, *Staining Methods, Histologic and Histochemical,* Hoeber, New York.
4. Underwood, E. E., 1970, *Quantitative Stereology,* Addison-Wesley, Reading, Massachusetts, Menlo Park, California, and London; Don Mills, Ontario.
5. Weibel, E. R., 1979, *Stereological Methods,* Vol. I, *Practical Methods for Biological Morphometry,* Academic Press, London, New York, Toronto, Sydney, and San Francisco.
6. Oberholzer, M., 1983, *Morphometrie in der klinischen Pathologie: Allgemeine Grundlagen,* Springer-Verlag, Berlin, Heidelberg, New York, and Tokyo.
7. Thompson, S.W., 1966, *Selected Histochemical and Histopathological Methods,* Charles C Thomas, Springfield, Illinois.

8. Pearse, A. G. E., 1972, 1980, *Histochemistry: Theoretical and Applied*, 2 vols., Churchill Livingstone, Edinburgh, London, and New York.

9. Lojda, Z., Gossrau, R., and Schiebler, T. H., 1979, *Enzyme Histochemistry*, Springer-Verlag, Berlin, Heidelberg, and New York.

10. Horobin, R. W., 1982, *Histochemistry*, Gustav Fischer Verlag, Stuttgart and New York; Butterworths, London.

11. Wolman, M., 1955, Problems of fixation in cytology, histology, and histochemistry, *Int. Rev. Cytol.* **4**:79–102.

12. Holt, S., Hobbiger, E. L., and Pawan, G. L. S., 1960, Preservation of integrity of rat tissues for cytochemical staining purposes, *J. Biophys. Biochem. Cytol.* **7**:383–386.

13. Puchtler, H., Waldrop, F. S., Meloan, S. N., Terry, M. S., and Conner, H. M., 1970, Methacarn (methanol-Carnoy) fixation: Practical and theoretical considerations, *Histochemie* **21**:97–116.

14. Sasse, D., and Graumann, W., 1965, Untersuchungen zum cytochemischen Glykogennachweis. V. Chemische Fixation mit weiteren alkoholischen und dioxinhaltigen Pikrinsäuregemischen, *Acta Histochem.* **20**:25–38.

15. Simpson, W. L., 1941, An experimental analysis of the Altmann technic of freeze–drying, *Anat. Rec.* **80**:173–189.

16. Lison, L., 1949, Sur la fixation histochimique du glycogène, *C. R. Soc. Biol.* **143**:115–116.

17. Bell, L. G. E., 1952, The application of freezing and drying techniques in cytology, *Int. Rev. Cytol.* **1**:35–63.

18. Sasse, D., and Matthaei, C., 1977, Improvement of freeze–substitution by programmed rewarming, *Stain Technol.* **52**:299–300.

19. Teutsch, H. F., 1981, Chemomorphology of liver parenchyma: Qualitative histochemical distribution patterns and quantitative sinusoidal profiles of G6Pase, G6PDH and malic enzyme activity and of glycogen content, *Prog. Histochem. Cytochem.* **14**(3):1–92.

20. Lowry, O. H., and Passonneau, J. V., 1972, *A Flexible System of Enzymatic Analysis*, Academic Press, New York, San Francisco, and London.

21. Weibel, E. R., and Elias, H., 1967, *Quantitative Methods in Morphology*, Springer-Verlag, Berlin, Heidelberg, and New York.

22. Haug, H., 1980, The significance of quantitative stereologic experimental procedures in pathology, *Pathol. Res. Pract.* **166**:144–164.

23. Weibel, E. R., 1974, Selection of the best method in stereology, *J. Microsc.* **100**:261–269.

24. Smith, A., and Bruton, J., 1977, *A Colour Atlas of Histological Staining Techniques*, Wolfe, London.

25. Hosemann, W., Teutsch, H. F., and Sasse D., 1979, Identification of G6PDH-active sinusoidal cells as Kupffer cells in the rat liver, *Cell Tissue Res.* **196**:237–247.

26. Wake, K., 1974, Development of vitamin-A-rich lipid droplets in multivesicular bodies of rat liver stellate cells, *J. Cell Biol.* **63**:683–691.

27. McManus, J. F. A., 1948, Histological and histochemical uses of periodic acid, *Stain Technol.* **23**:99–108.

28. Graumann, W., 1953, Zur Standardisierung des Schiffschen Reagens, *Z. Wiss. Mikrosk.* **61**:225–226.

29. Lillie, R. D., 1944, Various oil soluble dyes as fat stains in the supersaturated isopropanol technic, *Stain Technol.* **19**:55–58.

30. Sandritter, W., Kiefer, G., and Rick, W., 1963, Über die Stöchiometrie von Gallocyaninchromalaun mit Desoxyribonucleinsäure, *Histochemie* **3**:315–340.

31. Arnold, M., 1968, *Histochemie: Einführung in Grundlagen und Prinzipien der Methoden*, Springer-Verlag, Berlin, Heidelberg, and New York.

32. Van Duijn, P., 1976, Prospects for microscopic cytochemistry. *Histochem. J.* **8**:653–676.

33. Pette, D., and Wimmer, M., 1979, Kinetic microphotometric activity determination in enzyme containing gels and model studies with tissue sections, *Histochemistry* **64**:11–22.

34. Nolte, J., and Pette, D., 1972, Microphotometric determination of enzyme activity in single cells in cryostat sections, *J. Histochem. Cytochem.* **20:**567–576.

35. Pette, D., Wasmund, H., and Wimmer, M., 1979, Principle and method of kinetic microphotometric enzyme activity determination *in situ, Histochemistry* **64:**1–10.

36. Pette, D., and Wimmer, M., 1980, Microphotometric determination of enzyme activities in cryostat sections by the gel film technique, *Trends Enzyme Histochem. Cytochem.: Ciba Found. Symp.* **73:**121–134.

37. Wimmer, M., and Pette, D., 1979, Microphotometric studies on intraacinar enzyme distribution in rat liver, *Histochemistry* **64:**22–33.

38. Maly, I. P., and Sasse, D., 1983, A technical note on the histochemical demonstration of G6Pase activity, *Histochemistry* **78:**409–411.

39. Hayashi, M., Nakajima, Y., and Fishman, W. H., 1964, The cytologic demonstration of beta-glucuronidase employing naphthol AS-BI-glucuronide and hexazonium pararosaniline: A preliminary report, *J. Histochem. Cytochem.* **12:**293–297.

40. Altmann, F. P., and Chayen, J., 1965, Retention of nitrogenous material in unfixed sections during incubation for histochemical demonstration of enzymes, *Nature (London)* **207:**1205–1206.

41. Altman, F. P., 1971, The use of a new grade of polyvinyl alcohol for stabilising tissue sections during histochemical incubations, *Histochemie* **28:**236–242.

42. Rieder, H., Teutsch, H. F., and Sasse, D., 1978, NADP-dependent dehydrogenases in rat liver parenchyma. I. Methodological studies on the qualitative histochemistry of G6PDH, 6PGDH, malic enzyme and ICDH, *Histochemistry* **56:**283–298.

43. Jacobsen, N. O., 1969, The histochemical localization of lactic dehydrogenase isoenzymes in the rat nephron by means of an improved polyvinyl alcohol method, *Histochemie* **20:**250–265.

44. Mellgren, S. I., 1971, The distribution of lactate dehydrogenase (lactate tetrazolium reductase) in the hippocampal region of the rat: A reinvestigation with the polyvinyl alcohol method, *Z. Zellforsch.* **120:**187–203.

Chapter 4

Immunohistochemistry

Jeffrey Baron, Jeffrey M. Voigt, Thomas T. Kawabata,
and Jan A. Redick

1. INTRODUCTION

Knowledge of the precise intratissue and intracellular localizations and distributions of enzymes and other biological molecules is often a prerequisite for understanding the metabolic and regulatory functions of these substances. Such information is also frequently required for defining the biological functions of specific cells and for elucidating the underlying biochemical bases for any differences in metabolic capabilities that may exist among morphologically different cell types as well as among morphologically similar cells. Unfortunately, the acquisition of this information is frequently hindered by a number of factors that include, but are not necessarily limited to, the presence of low tissue and/or cellular levels and/or activities of enzymes and other biological molecules and the fact that mammalian tissues are not composed of a single, homogeneous population of cells. In this respect, although the liver is commonly considered to be a fairly homogeneous tissue, it must be appreciated that significant differences in biochemical and physiological characteristics and functions have frequently been detected among hepatic parenchymal cells, or hepatocytes. A

JEFFREY BARON, JEFFREY M. VOIGT, THOMAS T. KAWABATA, and JAN A. REDICK • The Toxicology Center, Department of Pharmacology, The University of Iowa College of Medicine, Iowa City, Iowa 52242.

number of these differences are considered in greater detail in Sections III and IV of this volume.

In many instances, information regarding the intratissue and intracellular localizations and distributions of enzymes and other biological molecules can be obtained only through the application of exquisitely sensitive and specific immunohistochemical and immunocytochemical staining techniques that allow for the visualization of antigens within tissues and cells, respectively. These techniques allow for the investigation of antigens that are present within limited regions of tissues and cells and/or at levels that may be below the limits of detection of more conventional biochemical and biophysical methodologies.

In 1942, Coons et al.[1] provided the first description of an immunohistochemical staining technique and its application for demonstrating the presence of a specific antigen within tissues. Since the publication of that initial report, the combined use of immunological and histological procedures has evolved into one of the most widely employed and powerful research and diagnostic methods available and, as such, has proven to be an invaluable technique in all fields of biology, as well as in diagnostic pathology.

The utilization of immunohistochemical staining techniques for investigating the localizations and distributions and hence the intercellular compartmentations of biological molecules within complex tissues is associated with some obvious advantages. The most notable of these relate to the extreme sensitivity of the methods, the ability to determine the *in situ* localizations and distributions of biological molecules, and the ability to simultaneously examine an antigen within all the different cell types that are present in a given tissue. Not unexpectedly, however, immunohistochemical techniques also possess some disadvantages. For instance, they do not provide information regarding the enzymatic activities and/or other biological functions of antigens at their intratissue sites of localization. Moreover, the procedures that are required for the preparation of tissues for immunohistochemical investigations may result in the loss of the antigen from the tissue and/or in alterations in antigenic determinants and thereby give rise to artifacts in staining. In addition, nonspecific background staining in tissue sections can hinder, if not prevent, the proper interpretation of experimental findings, while both false-positive and false-negative results can frequently be obtained. Furthermore, homogeneous preparations of antigens are essential for the production of the specific antibodies needed for use in these techniques. Although these and other difficulties associated with the application of immunohistochemical staining procedures for studies on the intratissue localizations and distributions of antigens may appear to be insurmountable, such problems can often be resolved. However, it is imperative that the investigator be aware of the caveats associated with the utilization of immunohistochemical staining techniques and take the necessary precautions to ensure that artifacts in immunohistochemical staining do not occur or, at the very least, are minimized. It is also essential that the concentrations of all reagents used in any immunohisto-chemical staining procedure, as well as the staining protocol itself, be optimized for each antigen, tissue, and experimental manipulation so that the resulting immunohistochemical staining will be limited solely by the antigen.

The very marked increase in the utilization of immunohistochemical and immunocytochemical technologies for basic and clincial research, as well as for diagnostic pathology, has resulted during the past two decades in the development of numerous modifications in staining procedures. These modifications, in turn, have led to significant improvements in accuracy, reproducibility, and sensitivity. This chapter concentrates on the application of immunohistochemical methods for the study of antigens within tissues at the light-microscopic level. There will be no attempt to describe immunocytochemical methods that are employed for investigating antigens at the electron-microscopic level or to provide a compre-hensive review of all the many different immunohistochemical staining tech-niques now available. Descriptions of immunocytochemical staining techniques and additional information regarding immunohistochemical staining methods can be found in a number of excellent monographs and books that deal specifically with these methods and their principles.[2–12] Information relating to routine his-tological procedures, such as tissue sectioning, are described in detail in most standard references dealing with histological methodology. The intent of this chapter, rather, is to illustrate how immunohistochemical staining techniques can be utilized for investigations on the intratissue (i.e., intercellular) compart-mentations of biological molecules. To accomplish this, attention will be pri-marily focused on those immunohistochemical procedures that have been suc-cessfully employed by this laboratory during the past several years to investigate the localizations and distributions of several xenobiotic-metabolizing enzymes within the liver[13–25] and certain extrahepatic tissues.[26–31]

2. TISSUE PREPARATION

2.1. General Considerations

To successfully localize an antigen immunohistochemically, a number of requirements must initially be satisfied. Many of these requirements relate di-rectly to the preparation of the tissue employed for the immunohistochemical study. Of primary importance to immunohistochemical analyses is that the mol-ecule under study must be retained in the tissue, its antigenicity must be pre-served, and its movement (i.e., diffusion) within the tissue must be prevented throughout all procedures involved in the preparation of the tissue. At the same time, the more critical morphological and cytological characteristics of the tissue must also be preserved. Thus, optimal conditions must be employed for tissue preparation. Unfortunately, although some general guidelines are available, conditions necessary for the proper preparation of tissues are largely dependent on both the antigen and the tissue under investigation and, consequently, must usually be empirically selected in a process that is both quite time-consuming and tedious. Even so, when new studies are initiated, a variety of methods for tissue preparation must be evaluated in order to prevent or greatly minimize the possibility of artifacts in immunohistochemical staining and, further, to ensure that reproducible results are obtained.

2.2. Fixation Procedures

In many instances, immunohistochemical studies are conducted using fixed and embedded tissue specimens. For these analyses, as indicated above, fixation must preserve the tissue's morphological and cytological characteristics (i.e., osmotic damage and shrinkage must be minimized during fixation) while allowing for the retention of tissue constituents and their antigenicities. Fixation is also often necessary to prevent diffusion of antigens within the tissue itself. These requirements, however, are frequently not satisfied by only a single fixative. There are a number of fixatives that provide excellent retention of antigens and their antigenicities without causing marked morphological and/or cytological distortions detectable with light microscopy. These fixatives range from the more powerful cross-linking agents, such as aldehydes, to the weaker denaturing agents, such as alcohols. Fixation can be accomplished either by perfusion of the tissue or organ *in situ* or by immersion of freshly obtained tissue blocks or pieces in the fixative solution. When tissues are perfused with a fixative solution, care must be exercised to ensure that perfusion pressure does not result in gross morphological alterations such as separation of the cords of parenchymal cells in the liver.

Aldehydes react with amino acids to form cross-links between proteins and thereby provide both excellent structural preservation and a high degree of retention of diffusible proteins. For these reasons, formaldehyde, glutaraldehyde, and other aldehydes are widely used as fixatives for both light- and electron-microscopic analyses. Unfortunately, the formation of cross-links can cause modifications in antigentic determinants and/or result in the denaturation of antigen molecules. Thus, the antigenicities of many proteins and enzymes are often altered and may be completely lost when aldehydes are employed as fixatives. For those substances that cannot withstand exposure to aldehyde-containing fixatives, a weaker bifunctional cross-linking agent, such as dimethyl-suberimidate, [32–34] can often be of considerable use. However, while the weaker cross-linking agents do preserve the antigenic determinants of most antigens, and are therefore useful for many immunohistochemical studies,[26–28] we have found that most of the weaker cross-linking fixatives, including dimethylsuberimidate, do not provide sufficient preservation of the morphological features of many tissues, including the liver, to allow for the proper interpretation of immunohistochemical findings. The notable exception to this is p-benzoquinone.

p-Benzoquinone is a relatively weak, bifunctional cross-linking agent that is capable of reacting with amino acids, proteins, amines, thiols, and imidazoles.[34–39] In addition to providing excellent preservation of the morphological features of tissues, p-benzoquinone preserves antigenic determinants which are often either altered or destroyed by the more powerful cross-linking agents. This chemical has been successfully used by us as a fixative for immunohistochemical investigations of the intrahepatic localizations and distributions of several membrane-bound and cytosolic xenobiotic-metabolizing enzymes[13–25,40,41]; results of these immunohistochemical studies are described in detail in Chapter 13. Since p-benzoquinone is both light- and oxygen-sensitive, precautions must be exercised in its use. Moreover, the commercially obtained chemical should be purified prior to use. Recrystallization from petroleum ether yields long, bright yellow crystals that provide much more uniform fixation and hence greater reproducibility in immunohistochemical staining. The following procedure is routinely employed in this laboratory for the fixation of animal and human liver with p-benzoquinone: After the liver has been excised, it is cut into blocks or slices, approximately 1–2 mm thick. The use of thin blocks and slices promotes rapid and even penetration of the fixative into the tissue. The liver blocks or slices are immersed and agitated in a solution containing 0.35–0.5% (wt./vol.) p-benzoquinone and 0.02 M $CaCl_2$ in 0.2 M sodium cacodylate buffer, pH 7.4, for 3 hr. This solution should be replaced with freshly prepared fixative every 20 min during the initial 2 hr, and an additional change of fixative solution should be made during the 3rd hour. The entire fixation procedure is conducted at 4°C in the dark to avoid excessive oxidation of p-benzoquinone.

As an alternative to cross-linking agents, solutions consisting of 95–99% (vol./vol.) ethanol and 1% (vol./vol.) acetic acid can also be employed for the fixation of tissues such as the liver. This fixative causes the aggregation or precipitation of cellular proteins and provides excellent retention of antigenicity. However, fixation of tissues with ethanol–acetic acid solutions may result in the loss of soluble antigens during the fixation process and/or in the diffusion of antigens within the fixed tissue. Moreover, morphological and cytological properties may not be well preserved, since shrinkage and distortion frequently occur as a consequence of the rapid dehydration that results when tissues are placed into alcoholic solutions.

As indicated above, tissue fixation, especially when one of the stronger cross-linking agents is employed, can frequently result in decreased or absolute loss of a molecule's antigenicity. However, the exposure of sections prepared from fixed tissues to trypsin,[9,42–45] protease,[45,46] pronase,[47] or pepsin[44] appears to result in degradation of many of the protein cross-links, including those involving antigenic determinants. Thus, these enzymes can be employed to unmask antigenic sites after tissues have been fixed. The incubation of sections prepared from fixed tissues in a 10% (wt./vol.) sucrose solution has also been suggested to be an effective means for restoring lost antigenicity.[9] It must be appreciated, however, that prolonged exposure to high concentrations of proteolytic enzymes can also result in the digestion of tissue sections; furthermore, exposure of tissue sections to proteolytic enzymes and/or sucrose may not result in the complete restoration of a molecule's antigenicity once the tissue has undergone fixation. Since any loss in a molecule's antigenicity could result in false-negative immunohistochemical findings, it is essential that immunohistochemical staining for a new antigen or tissue be evaluated by using a number of different fixatives as well as unfixed, frozen sections (see Section 2.4). Only in this manner can fixation-induced artifacts in immunohistochemical staining be identified and circumvented.

2.3. Embedding Procedures

Once a tissue has been fixed, it must be embedded in a solid medium that both supports the tissue and provides sufficient rigidity to allow for the preparation of thin sections that are not damaged during sectioning. Paraffin is used most commonly and is the most convenient medium. Sections between 4 and 12 μm in thickness can readily be cut from paraffin-embedded tissues, and the paraffin can be easily and completely removed from tissue sections by immersing slides with attached sections in xylene. To ensure that the paraffin completely infiltrates the tissue, the fixed tissue must first be dehydrated and cleared (i.e., the dehydrating agent removed and the tissue rendered translucent) by immersion in nonpolar organic solvents. Although there are a number of effective dehydrating and clearing agents, procedures utilized in our laboratory for embedding fixed liver specimens will be given as an example. Initially, fixed liver specimens are dehydrated by immersion in 70% (vol./vol.) ethanol for 2 hr. The ethanol should be changed three or four times during this period. This step can be omitted if the liver specimens have been fixed using an ethanol–acetic acid solution. Complete dehydration is then achieved by immersing the liver specimens in ethylene glycol monoethyl ether (cellosolve) for 4 hr, with four or five changes of fresh solvent during that period of time. These steps are conducted at 4°C with continuous agitation. The dehydrated liver specimens are then cleared by immersion and agitation in Histosol® (National Diagnostics, Somerville, New Jersey) at 24°C for 1 hr; the clearing agent should be changed two or three times during this period. Once the liver specimens have been dehydrated and cleared, they are embedded using paraffin with a melting point between 54 and 58°C. The liver specimens are initially immersed in freshly melted paraffin for 30 min. For complete paraffin infiltration, the immersed specimens are then transferred to a vacuum oven for 3 hr, with three changes of fresh paraffin being made during this period of time. The tissue specimens are then removed from the paraffin and placed in plastic embedding molds that have been filled with freshly melted paraffin. Once the paraffin has solidified, the embedded tissue specimens are refrigerated. We have found that immunohistochemical staining for xenobiotic-metabolizing enzymes remains unaltered over prolonged periods of time (e.g., years) when the fixed, paraffin-embedded tissue specimens are stored at 0–4°C.

2.4. Unfixed, Frozen Sections

Extremely labile antigens cannot withstand exposure to even the weakest of fixatives and must therefore be immunohistochemically investigated using unfixed, frozen tissue sections. It must be noted, however, that soluble antigens can readily diffuse within or be entirely lost from unfixed sections during immunohistochemical staining protocols and, further, that morphological and cytological features are frequently not preserved very well in such sections. In addition, it is often difficult to obtain serial sections when tissues have not been fixed. To circumvent at least some of these problems, sections prepared from unfixed, frozen tissues can be lightly fixed by brief exposure to a relatively weak fixative such as acetone or ethanol.

The rate at which tissues are frozen is a critical determinant of the morphological and cytological characteristics of unfixed, frozen sections, since ice crystals will form from any water present within intracellular and/or extracellular spaces, with larger crystals being produced when the freezing process is slow. The formation of ice crystals can result in tissue tearing, tissue and cell shrinkage due to osmotic changes, membrane disruption, and redistribution of intracellular organelles and soluble molecules. It has been suggested that ice-crystal formation can be reduced by the prior infusion of 0.6–1.0 M sucrose into the tissue.[48] For freezing, relatively thin tissue specimens (i.e., blocks or slices 1–2 mm thick) are mounted on cork stubs using a polyethylene glycerol-based embedding medium such as Tissue Tek O.C.T. compound and are frozen by immersion in either an isopentane–dry ice bath or liquid nitrogen. The frozen specimens are then transferred to a cryostat (usually maintained at − 18 to − 20°C) for equilibration prior to sectioning. For immunohistochemical analyses, cryostat sections, 8–12 μm thick and usually cut at − 20°C, are mounted on clean glass coverslips that have been coated with an adhesive such as chrome alum–gelatin or Histostik® (Accurate Chemical and Scientific Corp., Westbury, N.Y.) and are allowed to air-dry for approximately 2 hr prior to their use in immunohistochemical staining procedures. In contrast to sections from fixed, embedded tissues, which are stable when stored for prolonged periods of time, unfixed, frozen sections must frequently be used shortly after preparation, since storage may result in their dehydration and/or in the diffusion or loss of small or soluble antigens. As noted above, the brief exposure of unfixed, frozen tissue sections to a fixative may prevent the loss of many, but unfortunately not of all antigens.

3. IMMUNOENZYMATIC TECHNIQUES

3.1. General Considerations

The initial immunohistochemical staining procedure introduced in 1942 by Coons *et al.*[1] involved the use of an antibody that had been conjugated with a fluorochrome, fluorescein isothiocyanate. As discussed in greater detail in Section 4, immunofluorescence staining procedures still enjoy widespread use. Unfortunately, their routine application is associated with a number of difficulties and limitations. Primarily because of these disadvantages, fluorescence immunohistochemical techniques have been replaced, in many instances, by immunoenzymatic procedures in which enzyme-conjugated, rather than fluorochrome-conjugated, antibodies are employed. It is important to note that immunoenzymatic techniques appear to be at least as sensitive as the corresponding immunofluorescence methods.[3,4,7,10,49–52]

The wide acceptance gained by immunoenzymatic methodologies is due, in large measure, to the many advantages they offer: (1) immunoenzymatic staining can usually be readily visualized by means of conventional light-microscopic techniques; (2) most of the "stains" that are employed in immunoenzymatic procedures are stable, so that immunoenzymatically stained sections can usually be kept indefinitely for future retrieval and analysis; (3) in most instances, fixed, embedded tissue specimens can be utilized, and this facilitates the preparation of serial sections and allows for the preservation of morphological and cytological details, which in turn permits both the precise histological localization of the antigen and the proper interpretation of immunohistochemical findings; (4) immunoenzymatically stained sections can be counterstained to delineate the morphological and cytological features of the tissue; and (5) retrospective investigations can be easily conducted by preparing sections from previously fixed and embedded tissue specimens.

Immunoenzymatic staining techniques were introduced in 1967 when Nakane and Pierce[53,54] and Avrameas[55,56] independently demonstrated that an active enzyme such as horseradish peroxidase could be conjugated with a specific antibody and that the resulting conjugate could then be utilized for immunohistochemically investigating the *in situ* localizations of antigens. It must be appreciated that immunoenzymatic staining is absolutely dependent on the ability of the antibody-conjugated enzyme to catalyze the formation of a colored reaction product that will precipitate at the site of the antigen–antibody complex and that can then be visualized under the light microscope.

A number of different enzymes, including glucose oxidase,[56,57] alkaline phosphatase,[56] and acid phosphatase,[54] have been conjugated with antibodies and used as enzyme labels for immunoenzymatic staining procedures. However, the vast majority of immunoenzymatic procedures involve the use of horseradish peroxidase conjugates.[3–6,8–12,49,50,53–75] The principal reasons for this are that horseradish peroxidase is a relatively small protein that does not interfere with the interaction between an antibody and its antigen in tissue sections, it is a stable enzyme, and it is commercially available in highly purified forms. Moreover, horseradish peroxidase catalyzes the oxidation of a wide variety of electron donors (chromogen substrates) to yield colored reaction products that can be easily visualized under the light microscope.

3,3'-Diaminobenzidine tetrahydrochloride is the chromogen substrate that is most frequently utilized in immunoperoxidase procedures. In 1966, Graham and Karnovsky[58] demonstrated that in the presence of hydrogen peroxide, horseradish peroxidase catalyzes the oxidative polymerization of 3,3'-diaminobenzidine to form an insoluble brown reaction product. The subsequent chelation of this reaction product with osmium tetroxide results in the formation of osmium black, thereby enhancing the brown color and increasing the stability of the 3,3'-diaminobenzidine reaction product (i.e., osmication prevents any fading of the colored product that may occur over long periods of time).[59] More recently, a number of procedures have been described for intensifying the 3,3'-diaminobenzidine reaction product. These procedures involve the addition of imidazole[60] or heavy metals[61] to solutions of 3,3'-diaminobenzidine and the use of a thioglycolic acid solution together with a silver-nitrate-containing developer after 3,3'-diaminobenzidine has been oxidized.[62] The inclusion of metallic ions in 3,3'-diaminobenzidine solutions has also been reported to result in the modification of the color of the final 3,3-diaminobenzidine reaction product.[63]

The primary disadvantage associated with the use of 3,3'-diaminobenzidine as a chromogen substrate for horseradish peroxidase in immunoperoxidase procedures is that it is carcinogenic and thus must be used with extreme care. Although it remains the most widely employed chromogen substrate, 3,3'-diaminobenzidine can be replaced by a number of other chemicals, including: *p*-phenylenediamine dihydrochloride and pyrocatechol (the Hanker–Yates reagent),[64] 3-amino-9-ethylcarbazole,[65] and 4-chloro-1-naphthol.[66] Unfortunately, the reaction products which are formed during the horseradish peroxidase-catalyzed oxidations of 3-amino-9-ethylcarbazole and 4-chloro-1-naphthol are soluble in alcohols and other organic solvents. Thus, tissue sections must be mounted in aqueous media when either of these two chemicals is used as the chromogen substrate in immunoperoxidase staining procedures.

Despite the many advantages offered by immunoperoxidase staining techniques for immunohistochemical investigations on the intratissue localizations and distributions of antigens, their usefulness is hindered by several factors. Of greatest concern is the presence of endogenous peroxidase activity in the tissue being studied. High levels of endogenous peroxidase activity can give rise to and/or accentuate any nonspecific background staining in tissue sections. This can result in the appearance of false-positive staining and interfere markedly with the visualization and interpretation of the specific immunohistochemical staining for an antigen. To circumvent problems associated with the presence of endogenous peroxidase activity, it is customary to irreversibly inhibit the endogenous enzyme's activity prior to performing immunohistochemical staining. A number of procedures are available for inhibiting endogenous peroxidase activity in tissue sections. The most commonly employed method involves pretreatment of tissue sections with a methanolic hydrogen peroxide solution.[67,68] Although effective, this method causes some degree of damage to unfixed, cryostat sections, which often contain large numbers of blood cells. To avoid this problem, unfixed as well as fixed tissue sections can be exposed to phenylhydrazine, another inhibitor of peroxidase activity.[69] In our experience, phenylhydrazine has been found to be superior to methanolic hydrogen peroxide for blocking the endogenous peroxidase activity in both unfixed, frozen and fixed, paraffin-embedded sections that have been prepared from liver and other tissues.[28,30]

The presence of nonspecific background staining in tissue sections can present significant difficulties when immunoperoxidase techniques are employed, since such staining often has the appearance of a uniform dark background on which the specific immunohistochemical staining for an antigen is superimposed. Although both the presence and the degree of nonspecific background staining may vary for reason(s) not completely understood, it must be appreciated that antibodies can adhere nonspecifically to highly charged connective tissue elements and collagen, as do most proteins.[9,11] Exposure of tissue sections to innocuous proteins such as albumin or those present in preimmune or nonimmune sera prior to exposure to antibodies appears to be the most effective means for reducing or eliminating nonspecific background staining. Although nonspecific background staining can also be reduced by decreasing antibody concentrations, the use of high dilutions of antibodies can result in decreased or total loss of specific immunohistochemical staining for an antigen.

To identify and overcome problems associated with nonspecific background staining in tissue sections, as well as other difficulties that may arise during the application of immunoenzymatic procedures, it is essential that the specificity of immunohistochemical staining be routinely verified through the use of appropriate controls.[3–12,70–77] The principal source of nonspecific background staining appears to be the nonspecific binding of antibodies to tissue components, although nonimmunological reagents employed in staining protocols may also interact nonspecifically with tissue components.

One test for antibody specificity that is frequently employed in conjunction with immunoperoxidase and other types of immunohistochemical staining procedures involves the removal of the primary antibody (i.e., the antibody that has been raised against the antigen under study) by adsorption with the purified antigen. Theoretically, any staining observed in a tissue section exposed to an adsorbed primary antibody should be due to nonspecific background staining. However, if contaminants were present in the original preparation of the antigen used to elicit the production of the antibody, as well as in the preparation used for adsorption, antibodies directed against these contaminants would also be removed by adsorption, and thus, nonspecific staining could, and probably would, be mistakenly identified as representing immunohistochemical staining for the specific antigen.

A number of other tests for antibody specificity are also commonly utilized. For example, the primary antibody can be replaced with an identical dilution of preimmune or nonimmune serum (or another appropriate preparation, such as an IgG fraction) that has been obtained from the same animal or species, respectively, as was the primary antibody. The preimmune or nonimmune preparation should contain all the components found in the preparation of the primary antibody except, of course, the specific antibody. Also, the primary antibody can be either omitted or replaced with buffer. Alternatively, the primary antibody can be replaced with an antibody raised in the same species as was the primary antibody but directed against an antigen absent from the tissue under investigation. Great care must be taken to ensure that this antigen is indeed absent from the tissue being studied. When these controls are employed, any staining detected in tissue sections would be attributed to the nonspecific binding of other reagents, immunological as well as nonimmunological, that were used in the immunohistochemical staining procedure.

Many of the immunoenzymatic procedures described below involve the use of two or more different antibodies. In these cases, tests for the specificities of all antibodies employed in the immunohistochemical staining procedure should be routinely conducted. Whenever possible, other sensitive and specific techniques, such as immunoblotting,[78] should also be utilized to demonstrate the specificity of each antibody used in an immunohistochemical staining procedure.

From the foregoing, it should be obvious that the routine use of appropriate controls are absolutely essential for the validation and proper interpretation of results obtained when immunoenzymatic and other immunohistochemical staining techniques are utilized. The actual controls used will depend, in large measure, on the immunohistochemical staining procedure employed.

As indicated above, the most commonly employed immunoenzymatic staining techniques involve the use of horseradish peroxidase as the enzyme label. Four of the most widely used of these techniques are the direct and indirect peroxidase methods,[3,4,9,11,53,54,56,66,70,71,76] the unlabeled antibody peroxidase–antiperoxidase technique,[3,4,9,11,45,47,49,52,70,71,73,75–77] and the avidin–biotin–peroxidase method.[9,11,50,75]

3.2. Direct and Indirect Peroxidase Methods

The direct peroxidase, or enzyme-labeled, technique is the simplest immunoperoxidase staining procedure that can be utilized for immunohistochemical studies. This method is analogous to the fluorescence immunohistochemical staining technique described in 1942 by Coons *et al.*[1] Horseradish peroxidase is directly conjugated with the primary antibody which has been raised against the antigen under study.[3,4,53–56,66] A purified antibody, rather than whole antiserum, is usually required for the preparation of enzyme conjugate.

Although direct peroxidase staining involves a fairly straightforward and rapid procedure, it does possess some disadvantages. The most important of these is that a different horseradish peroxidase-conjugated primary antibody is required for each antigen to be studied. Also, the direct method appears to be the least sensitive of all the immunoperoxidase techniques which are available.[66]

The following controls are needed to verify the specificity of immunohistochemical staining that is produced when the direct peroxidase staining technique is employed: (1) removal of the primary antibody by adsorption with the purified antigen and (2) replacement of the horseradish peroxidase-conjugated antibody with buffer, with horseradish peroxidase-conjugated IgG that has been prepared from preimmune or nonimmune serum, and/or with a horseradish peroxidase conjugate of an antibody that does not react with any antigen present in the tissue being studied.

The indirect peroxidase staining technique offers greater sensitivity than the direct peroxidase method and involves the use of two different antibodies: The primary antibody which has been produced in one species (e.g. rabbit) and a second antibody which has been produced in a different species (e.g. sheep) and which is directed against antibodues (e.g. IgGs) of the first species.The second antibody is conjugated with horseradish peroxidase and is used to label the primary antibody that is bound to the specific antigen in the tissue section. It should be apparent that the indirect peroxidase method is a much more versatile technique than the direct method, since a single horseradish peroxidase-conjugated secondary antibody can be utilized for immunohistochemical investigations of a variety of antigens. Moreover, many different horseradish peroxidase-conjugated second antibodies are available from numerous commercial sources. Suitable controls for this immunohistochemical staining procedure include: adsorption of the primary antibody with the purified antigen against which it is directed; substitution of an equivalent dilution of preimmune or nonimmune serum, or other appropriate preimmune or nonimmune preparation, for the primary antibody; and omission of the horseradish peroxidase-conjugated second antibody.

One of the major disadvantages associated with both direct and indirect peroxidase staining techniques relates to the conjugation of antibodies with horseradish peroxidase. Although a number of procedures have been described for conjugating antibodies with enzymes,[3,4,53–56] all these methods involve the formation of a covalent linkage between the enzyme and the antibody molecule. Because of this, the conjugation process may give rise to alterations in the activity of the conjugated enzyme and/or modifications in the antibody molecule that in turn may result in alterations in subsequent antigen–antibody interactions. Thus, the mere conjugation of an antibody with an enzyme can markedly decrease or totally abolish immunohistochemical staining for the antigen. Furthermore, the conjugation reaction is frequently incomplete and residual unconjugated antibody may compete for antigenic sites in tissue sections. These difficulties have been largely circumvented and sensitivity has been greatly improved through the development and application of two other immunoperoxidase techniques: the unlabeled antibody peroxidase–antiperoxidase method and the avidin-biotin-peroxidase method.

3.3.   Unlabeled Antibody Peroxidase–Antiperoxidase Method

The unlabeled antibody peroxidase–antiperoxidase method, or the unlabeled antibody enzyme technique, was introduced in 1970 by Sternberger et al.[49] This immunoperoxidase method circumvents many of the aforementioned disadvantages associated with the use of enzyme-conjugated primary and secondary antibodies in both the direct and the indirect peroxidase techniques (i.e., the possible alteration or denaturation of antibodies and inactivation of enzymes, as well as the presence of residual unconjugated antibody and free enzyme). In addition, the unlabeled antibody peroxidase–antiperoxidase method offers significantly enhanced sensitivity for antigen detection.[3,4,49,51,52] For these reasons, this technique has become the most widely utilized immunoperoxidase method for routine immunohistochemical studies.

The unlabeled antibody peroxidase–antiperoxidase method involves the sequential exposure of tissue sections to three different antibodies: the primary antibody, which has been raised in species A (e.g., rabbit) against the antigen being investigated; a second antibody, which has been raised in species B (e.g., sheep) and is directed against IgG molecules of species A; and a soluble antigen–antibody complex consisting of species A anti-horseradish peroxidase and horseradish peroxidase. The second antibody acts as a link, or bridge, between the primary antibody, which is bound to the antigen in the tissue section, and the soluble peroxidase–antiperoxidase complex, so that the active horseradish peroxidase is localized at the site of the antigen in the tissue section. Since the peroxidase–antiperoxidase complex consists of 3 molecules of horseradish peroxidase and 2 antiperoxidase molecules,[64] the use of this complex results in a greater amount of active enzyme at the site of the antigen. Thus, as indicated above, this method provides greater sensitivity for antigen detection than either the direct or the indirect immunoperoxidase method. Because of this greater sensitivity, more dilute preparations of primary antibodies can usually be employed than would be possible with the direct or the indirect peroxidase method, and this in turn frequently minimizes nonspecific background staining in tissue sections. Moreover, since the horseradish peroxidase is a component of an antigen–antibody complex, rather than being conjugated with an antibody, there is little if any loss of enzyme activity. One potential disadvantage associated with this technique is that in order to attain maximum sensitivity in immuno-histochemical staining, the anti-horseradish peroxidase and the primary antibody directed against the antigen being studied usually must be raised in the same species, and the required anti-horseradish peroxidase may not be commercially available. In certain instances, however, there may be a sufficient degree of cross-reactivity between immunoglobulins from different species to allow for the use of heterologous antibodies.[79]

To illustrate how unlabeled antibody peroxidase–antiperoxidase staining can be accomplished, the procedure employed routinely in this laboratory to inves-tigate the intrahepatic localizations of microsomal and cytosolic xenobiotic-me-tabolizing enzymes is described in detail below. It must be stressed that when utilizing any immunohistochemical staining technique, the procedures involved in the prepration of tissues and the reagents used in the staining protocol must be optimized to ensure the proper interpretation of experimental findings.

1. Fixed, paraffin-embedded liver sections, 4–7 μm thick, are deparaf-finized in xylene and then rehydrated through a series of graded meth-anols.

2. After washing with five changes of distilled water, the tissue sections are exposed for 40 min at 24°C to aqueous 10% (vol./vol.) dimethyl-sulfoxide. This as been found to markedly enhance the uniform pen-etration of antibodies into tissue sections and to result in more repro-ducible staining.

3. The sections are washed with water and then with three changes of 0.05 M Tris-HC1 buffer, pH 7.75, containing 0.154 M NaCl [Tris-bufferred saline (TBS)].

4. To block endogenous peroxidase activity, the sections are exposed for 1 hr at 37°C to 0.01–0.05% (wt./vol.) phenylhydrazine in TBS.

5. The tissue sections are washed for 10 min at 24°C with three changes of TBS and are placed in humidified incubation chambers (e.g., petri dishes lined with moist filter paper).

6. To reduce nonspecific antibody binding, the sections are precoated for 10 min at 24°C with 10% nonimmune serum (or IgG) in TBS. The precoat serum should be obtained from the same species as was the second antibody. If nonspecific background staining presents major problems for the detection and interpretation of specific staining, all immunochemical reagents used subsequently can be prepared in the diluted precoat serum (or IgG) rather than in TBS.

7. The sections are drained, without washing, of excess precoat serum (or IgG) are are exposed for 2 hr at 37°C to appropriate dilutions of the primary antibody (this may be whole antiserum, an IgG preparation, affinity-purified antibody, Fab or Fab′ fragments, or a monoclonal antibody).

8. The sections are washed for 10 min at 24°C with three changes of TBS. It is important that slides with sections that have been exposed to different antibodies be washed separately (i.e., in separate Coplin jars) to avoid cross-contamination.

9. The sections are then exposed for 30 min at 24°C to appropriate dilutions of the second antibody, which is directed against the IgG of the species in which the primary antibody was raised. As previously indicated, this antibody acts as a link between the primary antibody and the soluble peroxidase–antiperoxidase complex.

10. The sections are washed for 10 min with three changes of TBS.

11. The sections are exposed for 30 min at 24°C to appropriate dilutions of the soluble horseradish peroxidase–antiperoxidase complex.

12. The sections are washed for 10 min with three changes of 50 mM Tris-HCl buffer, pH 7.75.

13. The sections are then incubated in the dark for 20–30 min at 24°C with 0.015% (wt./vol.) 3,3'-diaminobenzidine tetrahydrochloride and 0.005% H_2O_2 in 50 mM Tris-HCl buffer, pH 7.75.

14. The peroxidase reaction is terminated by washing the sections with three changes of distilled water.

15. The sections are then briefly exposed to aqueous 0.2% (wt./vol.) OsO_4 to intensify and stabilize the immunoperoxidase stain.

16. The sections are washed with three changes of distilled water.

17. Finally, the sections are dehydrated through graded methanols to xylene, mounted in a nonaqueous medium such as Permount® (Fisher Scientific Co., Chicago, IL), and examined by transmitted-light microscopy without further staining.

To ensure that the endogenous peroxidase activity in the tissue sections has been blocked, after exposure to phenylhydrazine, the sections are immediately placed in 3,3'-diaminobenzidine and H_2O_2, and the remainder of the protocol is carried out. Two additional method controls are also used for this immuno-histochemical staining protocol. In one, the second antibody is omitted and replaced with buffer, or, preferably, with preimmune or nonimmune serum (or IgG preparation, etc.) obtained from the same animal or species as was the second antibody. In the other, the peroxidase–antiperoxidase complex is omitted and replaced with buffer. To demonstrate the specificity of immunohistochemical staining produced using the unlabeled antibody peroxidase–antiperoxidase staining technique, the primary antibody should be replaced with either preimmune or nonimmune serum (or IgG preparation, etc.) or an adsorbed antibody preparation.

3.4. Avidin–Biotin–Peroxidase Method

One of the most recently developed immunoperoxidase techniques involves the use of an avidin–biotin–peroxidase complex.[9,11,50,75] Avidin, a glycoprotein found in egg white, has a very great affinity for biotin; in addition, each avidin molecule is capable of interacting with 4 biotin molecules.[80] Because of these features, the avidin–biotin–peroxidase method provides a very high degree of sensitivity for the immunohistochemical detection of antigens in tissues.[9,11,50,75] However, since biotin is present in many mammalian tissues,[81] nonspecific background staining in tissue sections is a potential problem. On the other hand, nonspecific background staining due to the presence of biotin can be greatly reduced or eliminated by pretreating tissue sections with avidin. The unoccupied biotin binding sites on the bound avidin molecules are then blocked by the subsequent exposure or the tissue section to excess unlabeled biotin.[82]

The protocol routinely employed for utilizating the avidin–biotin–peroxidase staining technique is essentially identical to that described above for the unlabeled antibody peroxidase–antiperoxidase method, with two exceptions: (1) The second antibody is biotinylated and (2) an avidin–biotin–peroxidase complex is used in place of the peroxidase–antiperoxidase complex. In addition, significantly less primary antibody is required for producing satisfactory immunohistochemical staining with the avidin–biotin–peroxidase method than with the unlabeled antibody peroxidase–antiperoxidase procedure. As would be expected, similar method and specificity controls are utilized for both the avidin–biotin–peroxidase and the unlabeled antibody peroxidase–antiperoxidase techniques.

4. IMMUNOFLUORESCENCE TECHNIQUES

4.1. General Considerations

Since its introduction in 1942,[1] immunofluorescence has proven to be an invaluable technique in both research and diagnostic settings.[2–8,10,12] Fluorescence immunohistochemical methodologies are as specific as immunoenzymatic methods, but are generally less time-consuming. However, they frequently provide significantly less sensitivity for antigen detection than do many of the more recently introduced immunoenzymatic techniques, especially the unlabeled antibody peroxidase–antiperoxidase and avidin–biotin–peroxidase methods.[3,4,70,72,76] The application of immunofluorescence technology is also associated, unfortunately, with a number of more serious disadvantages: Specialized microscopic techniques are required for the examination of fluorescently stained tissue sections; unfixed tissue specimens must be used in many instances; morphological detail often cannot be accurately or thoroughly assessed, especially when unfixed tissue specimens are studied; the immunofluorescent stain is not stable; and finally, tissue autofluorescence can hinder the visualization of specific immunohistochemical staining and thereby interfere with the proper interpretation of experimental findings.

For immunofluorescence analyses, either primary or secondary antibodies are conjugated with fluorochromes, and the antigen under study is visualized with a light microscope equipped for fluorescence. Incident-light, or epi-illumination, fluorescence microscopy is usually preferred for examining immunofluorescently stained tissue sections, rather than more traditional transmitted-light fluorescence microscopy; epi-illumination provides excitation light with an especially high intensity, and the emitted fluorescence is usually not significantly affected by the thickness of the tissue section being examined.

A variety of fluorochromes are available for antibody conjugation. Fluorescein isothiocyanate (FITC), which produces a bright, apple-green fluorescence, and tetramethylrhodamine isothiocyanate (TRITC), which gives rise to an orange-red fluorescence, are the fluorochromes of choice for most immunofluorescence studies.[2–8,10,12,83,84] These compounds exhibit excellent fluorescence efficiencies, can be quite easily conjugated with antibodies, and in many instances are more stable than other fluorochromes. One disadvantage inherent in the use of these and other fluorescent dyes is their tendency to fade on illumination with high-intensity light.[85,86] This is especially true for FITC. However, fluorescence fading can be signficantly retarded by including p-phenylenediamine,[87,88] 1,4-diazobicyclo-(2,2,2)-octane (DABCO),[86,89] or n-propyl gallate[90] in the mounting medium.

4.2. Direct Immunofluorescence

The direct immunofluorescence method, which was initially developed by Coons *et al.*,[1] involves the use of a primary antibody conjugated with a fluorochrome. Thus, this immunohistochemical staining technique is analogous to the direct immunoenzymatic procedure described above and, as such, suffers from the same limitations as that method; i.e., large amounts of primary antibodies are required, a different conjugated primary antibody is needed for each antigen studied, the sensitivity for antigen detection is rather low, and, of greatest importance, conjugation of the fluorochrome directly to the immunoglobulin molecule may cause the antigen binding site to be modified in such a manner that the specific interaction between the antibody and its antigen is decreased or totally abolished. On the other hand, the direct immunofluorescence method is rapid, the staining procedure is simple and straightforward, and the technique can be quite useful for studying a single antigen in a large number of tissue specimens. As for all types of immunohistochemical staining procedures, appropriate controls must be employed. For direct immunofluorescence staining, suitable controls would include the substitution of preimmune or nonimmune serum, or other appropriate preimmune or nonimmune preparation, for the primary antibody, as well as removal of the primary antibody–fluorochrome conjugates by adsorption with the purified antigen.

4.3. Indirect Immunofluorescence

The indirect fluorescent antibody method enjoys much more widespread use than the direct immunofluorescence technique. Except for the use of a fluorochrome-conjugated second antibody, indirect immunofluorescence is comparable to the indirect immunoenzymatic procedure that was previously described. Thus, the indirect immunofluorescence technique possesses many of the same advantages and limitations as the indirect immunoenzymatic method. In addition, similar methods and specificity controls must be used to ensure that any staining detected in a tissue section is the result of a specific interaction between the primary antibody and its antigen.

Indirect immunofluoresent antibody staining has been employed with considerable success by this laboratory to investigate the intrahepatic localizations and distributions of a number of membrane-bound and cytoplasmic enzymes participating in the activation and detoxication of a multitude of xenobiotics and endogenous substances.[17–22,24,25] The procedure employed routinely for these investigations using fixed, paraffin-embedded liver specimens is described in detail below. It must again be stressed that the concentrations of all reagents used in the staining protocol must be optimized for each antigen and tissue to ensure the proper interpretation of results.

1. Fixed, paraffin-embedded liver sections, 4–7 μm thick, are deparaffinized in xylene and then rehydrated through a series of graded methanols.
2. After washing with five changes of distilled water, the tissue sections are exposed for 40 min at 24°C to aqueous 10% (vol./vol.) dimethylsulfoxide.
3. The tissue sections are washed with five changes of distilled water and then placed in 50 mM Tris-HCl buffer, pH 7.75, containing 0.154 M NaCl [Tris-buffered saline (TBS)]. After a 10-min period, the following steps are carried out in moist chambers (e.g., petri dishes lined with moist filter paper).
4. To reduce nonspecific antibody binding, the sections are precoated for 10 min at 24°C with 10% nonimmune serum (or IgG) in TBS. The precoat serum should be obtained from the same species as was the fluorochrome-conjugated second antibody. If there is a considerable degree of nonspecific background staining, all immunochemical reagents used subsequently can be prepared in the diluted precoat serum (or IgG) rather than in TBS.
5. The sections are drained, without washing, of excess precoat serum (or IgG) and are exposed overnight at 4°C to appropriate dilutions of the primary antibody (this may be whole antiserum, an IgG preparation, affinity-purified antibody, Fab or Fab' fragments, or a monoclonal antibody).

6. The sections are washed for 10 min at 24°C with three changes of TBS.
7. The sections are then exposed for 1 hr at 37°C to appropriate dilutions of FITC conjugates of the second antibody (usually an IgG preparation) that is directed against the IgG of the species in which the primary antibody was produced.
8. The sections are washed for 10 min with three changes of TBS.
9. Finally, since the FITC molecule fluoresces maximally at alkaline pH,[91,92] the sections are mounted with 90% (vol./vol.) glycerol containing 20 mM sodium phosphate buffer, pH 8.2, and 15.4 mM NaCl. To retard fluorescence fading, DABCO is included in the mounting medium at a concentration of 25 mg/ml.

The fluorescently stained tissue sections are then examined by means of incident-light fluorescence microscopy in which the excitation light is directed onto the tissue section through the microscope objective. In incident-light fluorescence microscopy, the full aperture of the microscope objective is utilized for excitation. Thus, the highest possible fluorescence intensity is obtained, since there is no loss of excitation light due to either light scattering or absorption by the specimen. Such losses occur when transmitted-light fluorescence microscopy is utilized. A dichroic beam-splitting mirror allows the appropriate wavelengths of the emitted fluorescence to pass through to the eyepiece to form the image while filtering out light at the excitation wavelengths. The excitation light can be provided by either a mercury or a xenon lamp and should encompass a fairly narrow wavelength range to minimize both tissue autofluorescence and nonspecific background staining. We have found that the following conditions allow for the optimum examination of immunofluorescence staining when the second antibody has been conjugated with FITC, a fluorochrome that exhibits an excitation maximum at 490 nm and an emission maximum at 525 nm: Excitation light is provided by a 150-watt xenon lamp; the tissue section is irradiated using an E. Leitz Ploemopak 2.1 fluorescence illuminator; and a K2 filter block is employed to provide the appropriate excitation and emission wavelengths (i.e., excitation at 470–490 nm and emission above 515 nm). Other commercially available fluorescence illuminators and filter combinations can also be utilized. Since the fluorescence will eventually fade, the stained sections must be photographed to provide a permanent record of the experimental findings.

To verify the specificity of indirect fluorescent antibody staining, the primary antibody can be replaced with preimmune or nonimmune serum (or IgG preparation, etc.) or an adsorbed antibody preparation. Additionally, to evaluate the presence and degree of nonspecific background staining and/or tissue autofluorescence, the fluorochrome-conjugated second antibody can be omitted or replaced with either unconjugated second antibody or an appropriate preimmune or nonimmune preparation.

5. DUAL-LABELING TECHNIQUES

5.1. General Considerations

In certain instances, information is needed regarding the localizations and distributions of two or more antigens within a given tissue such as the liver. This type of information can sometimes be obtained by utilizing any of the previously described methods to immunohistochemically localize each of the antigens under study in adjacent serial sections. However, the procedures employed for the routine histological preparation of tissues frequently do not allow for the preparation of serial sections sufficiently thin to facilitate the immunohistochemical localizations of multiple antigens within the same cell. To circumvent this problem, a number of dual-label immunohistochemical staining techniques have been developed with which the localizations of two or more antigens can be simultaneously investigated within a single tissue section.[3,4,66,93–100]

5.2. Dual Immunoenzymatic Labeling Methods

In general, these procedures, which lead to the formation of reaction products possessing contrasting colors, are rather time-consuming. However, one method that can be completed in less than 4 hr has been described for the simultaneous immunoenzymatic demonstration of two antigens.[95] In most dual-label immunoenzymatic procedures, one antigen is examined by means of an immunoperoxidase staining method, while another enzyme, such as alkaline phosphatase[95] or glucose oxidase,[98] is utilized to study the second antigen. Alternatively, two immunoperoxidase staining procedures can be utilized, providing that the different chromogen substrates used (e.g., 3,3'-diaminobenzidine and 3-amino-9-ethylcarbazole) yield reaction products with different colors.[3,4,66,99]

In the more commonly employed dual-label immunoenzymatic techniques in which two antigens are simultaneously investigated, the tissue section is sequentially exposed to the primary antibodies, preferably produced in different species, which are directed against the two antigens being studied.[66,98,99] The two antigens can then be immunohistochemically localized using, again sequentially, the indirect immunoenzymatic procedure, the unlabeled antibody peroxidase–antiperoxidase method, and/or the avidin–biotin–peroxidase technique. Although the application of dual-label immunoenzymatic methods allows for the simultaneous study of two different antigens within the same tissue section, considerable care must be exercised to ensure that the concentrations of all reagents used, as well as the immunohistochemical staining protocols themselves, have been optimized to preclude any possible quenching of one colored reaction product by the other.[100] Moreover, it is imperative that the procedure used to immunohistochemically stain the tissue section for one antigen not interfere with the method used to stain the section for the second antigen.

5.3. Dual Immunofluorescence Labeling Methods

Methods in which antibodies conjugated with fluorochromes that fluoresce at different wavelengths (i.e., with different colors) and that allow for the simultaneous immunofluorescence investigation of two antigens within a single tissue section have been available for nearly two decades.[12,83,92,101–106] As previously indicated, the fluorochromes most commonly utilized in these immunohistochemical procedures are fluorescein isothiocyanate (FITC) and tetramethylrhodamine isothiocyanate (TRITC), although other compounds such as lissamine rhodamine sulfonyl chloride (RB200SC)[101] have also been employed. Due to the contrasting colors of the fluorochromes (e.g., the fluorescence emitted by FITC is bright green, whereas TRITC emits an orange-red fluorescence), the simultaneous localizations of two antigens within different cells can easily be accomplished. Dual immunofluorescence labeling techniques are quite useful for identifying and studying one antigen that is present at low levels in the presence of much higher levels of a second antigen, especially when the two antigens are present within the same cell. However, dual immunofluorescence staining within a given cell may give rise to an intermediate color which might interfere with the proper interpretation of the experimental findings. To circumvent this problem, specific filters which provide light at the appropriate excitation wavelengths and permit the transmission of emitted fluorescence at the appropriate wavelengths, are required for visualizing and photographing immunofluorescence staining due to each of the fluorochromes utilized.

Dual-label immunofluorescence procedures can involve direct and/or indirect immunofluorescence techniques; that is, fluorochromes can be conjugated with either primary antibodies[101] or second antibodies.[107] Indirect immunofluorescence methods are applicable only when there is no possibility of cross-reactivity between the two primary antibodies (which must be obtained from different species) and the fluorochrome-conjugated second antibodies. Regardless of which method or combination of methods is used, fluorochrome-conjugated antibodies can be applied either sequentially or simultaneously.[102] Following completion of the immunofluorescence staining protocols, sections are mounted in buffered glycerol at a pH that allows for maximal fluorescence of both fluorochromes.[91,92] To obtain a permanent record of results when dual-label immunofluorescence procedures are employed, the fluorescently stained sections should be photographed using double-exposure techniques in conjunction with conditions that allow for the optimal fluorescence of each fluorochrome.

5.4. Combined Immunoenzymatic and Immunofluorescence Labeling Methods

Combinations of immunoenzymatic, especially immunoperoxidase, and immunofluorescence staining techniques have also been successfully employed for simultaneously localizing two different antigens within the same tissue sections.[108-111] The use of combined immunoenzymatic and immunofluorescence techniques is especially effective in those situations in which other dual-label immunohistochemical methodologies yield unclear results, for instance, when color mixing of fluorochromes within a single cell results in fluorescence of an intermediate color. To obtain satisfactory results when a combination of immunoenzymatic and immunofluorescence staining techniques is employed, it is essential that the procedures for tissue fixation and embedding be selected with consideracare, as many of these procedures, while appropriate for immunoenzymatic studies, may give rise to unwanted nonspecific tissue autofluorescence.

In most procedures involving combinations of immunoenzymatic and immunofluorescence procedures that have been described, one antigen is initially localized by means of indirect immunofluorescence, and the second antigen is then localized employing an immunoenzymatic method. It must be noted, however, that immunofluorescence staining can be quenched in the presence of osmium black and other reaction products that are formed as a result of immunoenzymatic staining.[110] To partially overcome such technical problems, the enzymatic reaction should be conducted under suboptimal conditions, since the intensity of emitted fluorescence will increase as the intensity of immunoenzymatic staining decreases.[110] After completion of the two immunohistochemical staining protocols, the tissue section is mounted in buffered glycerol and examined by incident-light fluorescence microscopy to visualize immunofluorescence staining. Routine transmitted-light microscopy is then employed to visualize immunoenzymatic staining in the tissue section. As for all immunofluorescence staining procedures, the sections must be photographed to obtain permanent records of the experimental findings.

6. QUANTITATIVE IMMUNOHISTOCHEMICAL TECHNIQUES

6.1. General Considerations

Immunohistochemical findings are routinely evaluated by means of both visual inspection and subjective grading of staining intensity within and among different cells in tissue sections. In many instances, however, more accurate determminations of immunohistochemical staining intensities are required, especially for investigations of the intratissue distributions of specific antigens. To accomplish this, microdensitometric and microfluorometric techniques can be employed to quantitate immunoenzymatic and immunofluorescence staining intensities, respectively.

The validity of quantitative immunohistochemistry, like that of quantitative histochemistry and cytochemistry, is based on the ability to accurately measure a chemical substance within a cell. However, the products of immunoenzymatic and immunofluorescence staining are often not homogeneously distributed throughout cells. Primarily because of differences in the physical characteristics of immunoenzymatic and immunofluorescence stains (i.e., immunoenzymatic staining usually occurs in the form of discrete particles, whereas immunofluoresence staining is commonly of a much more diffuse or uniform nature), heterogeneity in the intracellular distribution of immunohistochemical stains presents a much more serious problem for microdensitometric analyses of immunoenzymatic staining than for microfluorometric analyses of immunofluorescence staining.

In addition to concerns relating to the heterogeneous intracellular distribution of immunohistochemical staining, the accuracy of quantitative immunohistochemistry requires that the following criteria be satisfied: (1) the procedures employed for the preparation of the tissues used for quantitative immunohistochemical analyses must not result in any loss or diffusion of the antigen under study or in any modification in its antigenicity; (2) the Beer–Lambert law must apply; i.e., there must be a linear relationship between the concentration of the absorbing or fluorescing material and the respective microdensitometric or microfluorometric measurements; (3) the immunohistochemical stain must not diffuse within the tissue section or be soluble in the mounting medium; and (4) the immunohistochemical staining protocol utilized must be optimized so that the intensity of immunoenzymatic or immunofluorescence staining is limited solely by the level of the antigen. In the case of microdensitometric analyses of immunoenzymatic staining, the accuracy of mesurement is also dependent on the thickness of the tissue section, since transmitted-light microscopic techniques are employed. Finally, the apparatus used for microdensitometric or microfluorometric analysis should be standardized to ensure that any observed variations in the intensities of immunohistochemical staining are due to differences in the level of the antigen and not to measurement error.[84]

6.2. Microdensitometry

Microdensitometry is based on the principles of optical absorption spectrophotometry and is therefore markedly affected by the heterogeneous intracellular distribution of the light-absorbing material. To circumvent such "distributional errors," scanning and integrating microdensitometry must be utilized.[112–121] In this technique, the diameter of the light beam that is transmitted through the tissue specimen should approximate the size of the smallest heterogeneously distributed immunoenzymatic reaction product (e.g., osmium black), and microdensitometric measurements should be obtained from a great many areas or spots within the cell. The absorbance of every "spot" is then integrated to yield a mean absorbance value for the cell. This relative mean absorbance value can then be converted into an absolute mean absorbance value through the use of neutral-density filters possessing known, absolute absorbance. If the molar absorptivity of the final reaction product is known, the absolute mean absorbance value can then be used to determine the concentration of the chromophore within that specific cell. Since both the molar absorptivity and the optical absorption band maximum of the chromophore may vary depending on whether the chromophore is in solution or in a solid matrix,[122] the optical absorption characteristics of the chromophore must be determined in tissue sections.

Although microdensitometry has not been applied widely to quantitative immunohistochemistry, scanning and integrating microdensitometry have been utilized to investigate and determine the distribution of immunoperoxidase staining for NADPH-cytochrome P-450 reductase across the lobule in rat liver.[25] For these analyses, the unlabeled antibody peroxidase–antiperoxidase technique was employed, and measurements of the absorption of osmium black, the product formed by the osmication of oxidized 3,3'-diaminobenzidine, were obtained at 430 nm (osmium black exhibits a relatively broad optical absorption band having a maximum at this wavelength) from numerous small areas, 0.5 μm in diameter, in the optical plane of the tissue section, within hepatocytes across the liver lobule. Measurements were obtained from within corresponding cells in serial sections that had been exposed to sheep antiserum, to NADPH-cytochrome P-450 reductase, and to nonimmune sheep serum. The absorption values calculated for cells exposed to nonimmune serum represent the amount of light absorption at 430 nm due to both light scattering and nonspecific background staining. To calculate the absorbance due to specific immunohistochemical staining, i.e., to determine the intensities with which hepatocytes were specifically stained by the antibody to the cytochrome P-450 reductase, the mean microdensitometric values obtained from within hepatocytes exposed to nonimmune serum were subtracted from the values obtained from within corresponding cells in serial sections exposed to the antireductase serum. Since the unlabeled antibody peroxidase–antiperoxidase staining protocol was optimized so that the intensity of immunoperoxidase staining was limited only by the amount of antigen, the microdensitometric determinations of immunoperoxidase staining thus directly reflect the intracellular levels of NADPH-cytochrome P-450 reductase. In this manner, the intralobular distribution of an antigen can be accurately and reproducibly investigated.[25] The results of these microdensitometric analyses are shown in Fig. 2 in Chapter 13.

6.3. Microfluorometry

Microfluorometry offers a number of advantages over microdensitometry for quantitative immunohistochemical analyses. Since immunofluorescence staining is much more diffusely and homogeneously distributed within cells than are particulate, immunoenzymatic stains, microfluorometry is associated with significantly less distributional error than that seen with microdensitometry. In addition, immunofluorescence staining of thick or opaque tissue sections can be readily and accurately investigated by means of incident-light fluorescence microscopy. Microfluorometry does, however, possess some limitations. For instance, immunofluorescence fading can interfere with and at times prevent accurate microfluorometric analysis of tissue sections. Moreover, although microfluorometers can be standardized with uranyl glass filters,[84] microfluorometric measurements usually cannot be equated with the absolute concentration of the fluorochrome. Thus, such determinations are only semiquantitative. Despite these limitations, microfluorometry is theoretically more precise than microdensitometry.[123] In addition, Smith *et al.*[25] demonstrated that there is significantly less (i.e., one third to one half as much) variability in microfluorometric determinations of immunofluorescence staining than in microdensitometric determinations of immunoperoxidase staining for the same antigen. Nevertheless, the two methods do yield comparable results.

This laboratory has utilized microflurometric techniques extensively for semiquantitative analyses of the intensities of immunofluorescence staining for several different xenobiotic-metabolizing enzymes within centrilobular, midzonal, and periportal hepatocytes.[17–22,24,25] The results of these analyses are summarized in Chapter 13. For these investigations, tissue sections were stained for each of the antigens using the indirect immunofluorescence technique described earlier and fluorescein isothiocyanate (FITC)–conjugated second antibodies. Immediately after completion of the immunofluorescence staining procedure, microfluorometric measurements were obtained as follows: The immunofluorescently stained liver sections were examined by means of incident-light fluorescence microscopy using a modified E. Leitz MPV-1 microscope photometer system[17–22,24,25,27–29,124] (other commercially available microscope photometer systems can also be used), a 150-watt Osram xenon lamp, and a Leitz Ploemopak 2.1 fluorescence illuminator containing a K2 filter block that possesses the appropriate filters for the excitation and fluorecence emission of FITC. Fluorescence emitted at 525 nm (the fluorescence emission maximum for FITC) from within small areas (excluding nuclei) in cells was detected by an end-on photomultiplier tube. The signal from the photomultiplier tube was then amplified by a photometer, the output of which (i.e., voltage corresponding to transmittance) was fed into a computer that stored and statistically analyzed the data. The intensity of emitted fluorescence should be linearly related to the concentration of FITC conjugated with the second antibody, which is bound to the antigen, and hence to the concentration of the antigen under study. However, because absorbance is a linear function of sample concentration, whereas transmittance is a logarithmic function, the transmittance values of the emitted fluorescence are converted into absorbance values. Furthermore, since the absorbance at 525 nm decreases as the intensity of emitted fluorescence at this wavelength increases, the absorbance values are subtracted from 1, and the data are exposed in terms of $1 -$ absorbance ($\times 100$). In this manner, a positive, linear relationship is obtained between the intensities of immunofluorescence staining and the microfluorometric measurements that directly reflect the intracellular levels of the antigen.

Any emitted fluorescence due to nonspecific background staining and/or nonspecific tissue autofluorescence must be accounted for to calculate the intensity of specific immunofluorescence staining. To accomplish this, microfluorometric measurements are obtained from within cells in serial sections that have been exposed to the appropriate preimmune or nonimmune serum, or other preimmune or nonimmune preparation (e.g., IgG). These measurements are then subtracted from those obtained from within corresponding cells in serial sections exposed to the specific antibody. The resulting values represent the relative extents of binding of the specific antibody and are directly proportional to intracellular levels of the antigen, and thus can be used to determine the intratissue distribution of the antigen.

7. SUMMARY

Many enzymes and other biological molecules that participate in various metabolic processes are heterogeneously distributed in tissues such as the liver. While it is obvious that the levels and/or enzymatic activities of these substances frequently differ among morphologically dissimilar cell types, such differences can and do exist among morphologically similar cells, including hepatic parenchymal cells. The combined application of histological and immunological methodologies provides a very sensitive and specific means for investigating such intratissue and intercellular compartmentation *in situ*. The investigator has the option of utilizing these powerful methods as the sole means for conducting these investigations or of employing them in conjunction with one or more of the other techniques (e.g., histochemical and microbiochemical methods) that are considered in the other chapters in this section of the book.

During the past two to three decades, numerous immunoenzymatic and immunofluorescence staining procedures have been developed that permit biological molecules and other antigens to be visualized at the light-microscopic level within complex tissues. Moreover, the introduction of microdensitometric and microfluorometric techniques allows for quantitative analyses of immunohistochemical staining intensity and, thereby, the intratissue distributions of antigens.

REFERENCES

1. Coons, A. H., Creech, H. J., Jones, R. N., and Berliner, E., 1942, The demonstration of pneumococcal antigen in tissues by the use of a fluorescent antibody, *J. Immunol.* **45:**159–170.
2. Goldman, M., 1968, *Fluorescent Antibody Methods,* Academic Press, New York.
3. Sternberger, L. A., 1974, *Immunocytochemistry,* Prentice-Hall, Englewood Cliffs, New Jersey.
4. Sternberger, L. A., 1979, *Immunocytochemistry,* 2nd ed., John Wiley, New York.
5. Bullock, G. R., and Petrusz, P. (eds.), 1982, *Techniques in Immunocytochemistry,* Vol. 1, Academic Press, London.
6. Bullock, G. R., and Petrusz, P. (eds.), 1983, *Techniques in Immunocytochemistry,* Vol. 2, Academic Press, London.

7. Wick, G., Traill, K. N., and Schauenstein, K. (eds.), 1982, *Immunofluorescence Technology: Selected Theoretical and Clinical Aspects*, Elsevier, Amsterdam.
8. Cuello, A. C. (ed.), 1983, *Immunohistochemistry*, John Wiley, Chichester.
9. Wordinger, R. J., Miller, G. W., and Nicodemus, D. S., 1983, *Manual of Immunoperoxidase Techniques*, American Society of Clinical Pathologists Press, Chicago.
10. Beutner, E. H., Nisengard, R. J., and Albini, B. (eds.), 1983, *Defined Immunofluorescence and Related Cytochemical Methods, Ann. N. Y. Acad. Sci.* **420.**
11. Bourne, J. A., 1983, *Handbook of Immunoperoxidase Staining Methods*, DAKO Corp., Santa Barbara.
12. Polak, J. M., and Van Noorden, S. (eds.), 1983, *Immunocytochemistry: Practical Applications in Pathology and Biology*, John Wright, Bristol.
13. Baron, J., Redick, J. A., Greenspan, P., and Taira, Y., 1978, Immunohistochemical localization of NADPH-cytochrome *c* reductase in rat liver, *Life Sci.* **22:**1097–1102.
14. Kapke, G. F., Redick, J. A., and Baron, J., 1978, Immunohistochemical demonstration of an adrenal ferredoxin-like iron-sulfur protein in rat hepatic mitochondria, *J. Biol. Chem.* **253:**8604–8608.
15. Baron, J., Redick, J. A., and Guengerich, F. P., 1978, Immunohistochemical localizations of cytochromes P-450 in rat liver, *Life Sci.* **23:**2627–2632.
16. Baron, J., Redick, J. A., and Guengerich, F. P., 1980, Immunohistochemical localization of epoxide hydratase in rat liver, *Life Sci.* **26:**489–493.
17. Taira, Y., Redick, J. A., and Baron, J., 1980, An immunohistochemical study on the localization and distribution of NADPH-cytochrome *c* (P-450) reductase in rat liver, *Mol. Pharmacol.* **17:**374–381.
18. Taira, Y., Greenspan, P., Kapke, G. F., Redick, J. A., and Baron, J., 1980, Effects of phenobarbital, pregnenolone-16α-carbonitrile, and 3-methylcholanthrene pretreatments on the distribution of NADPH-cytochrome *c* (P-450) reductase within the liver lobule, *Mol. Pharmacol.* **18:**304–312.
19. Redick, J. A., Kawabata, T. T., Guengerich, F. P., Krieter, P. A., Shires, T. K., and Baron, J., 1980, Distributions of monooxygenase components and epoxide hydratase within livers of untreated male rats, *Life Sci.* **27:**2465–2470.
20. Baron, J., Redick, J. A., and Guengerich, F. P., 1981, An immunohistochemical study on the localizations and distributions of phenobarbital- and 3-methylcholanthrene-inducible cytochromes P-450 within livers of untreated rats, *J. Biol. Chem.* **256:**5931–5937.
21. Kawabata, T. T., Guengerich, F. P., and Baron, J., 1981, An immunohistochemical study on the localization and distribution of epoxide hydrolase within livers of untreated rats, *Mol. Pharmacol.* **20:**709–714.
22. Baron, J., Redick, J. A., and Guengerich, F. P., 1982, Effects of 3-methylcholanthrene, β-naphthoflavone, and phenobarbital on the 3-methylcholanthrene-inducible isozyme of cytochrome P-450 within centrilobular, midzonal, and periportal hepatocytes, *J. Biol. Chem.* **257:**953–957.
23. Redick, J. A., Jakoby, W. B., and Baron, J., 1982, Immunohistochemical localization of glutathione *S*-transferases in livers of untreated rats, *J. Biol. Chem.* **257:**15,200–15,203.
24. Kawabata, T. T., Guengerich, F. P., and Baron, J., 1983, Effects of phenobarbital, *trans*-stilbene oxide, and 3-methylcholanthrene on epoxide hydrolase within centrilobular, midzonal, and periportal regions of rat liver, *J. Biol. Chem.* **258:**7767–7773.
25. Smith, M. T., Redick, J. A., and Baron, J., 1983, Quantitative immunohistochemistry: A comparison of microdensitometric analysis of unlabeled antibody peroxidase–antiperoxidase staining and of microfluorometric analysis of indirect fluorescent antibody staining for NADPH-cytochrome *c* (P-450) reductase in rat liver, *J. Histochem. Cytochem.* **31:**1183–1189.
26. Redick, J. A., Kapke, G. F., Van Orden, L. S., III, and Baron, J., 1977, Immunohistochemical localization of adrenal ferredoxin in bovine adrenal cortex, *Life Sci.* **20:**1139–1148.
27. Baron, J., Redick, J. A., Kapke, G. F., and Van Orden, L. S., III, 1978, Immunohistochemical

localization of adrenal ferredoxin and distribution of adrenal ferredoxin and cytochrome P-450 in the rat adrenal, *Biochim. Biophys. Acta* **540**:443–454.

28. Taira, Y., Redick, J. A., Greenspan, P., and Baron, J., 1979, Immunohistochemical studies on electron transport proteins associated with cytochromes P-450 in steroidogenic tissues. II. Microsomal NADPH-cytochrome *c* reductase in the rat adrenal, *Biochim. Biophys. Acta* **583**:148–158.

29. Kawabata, T. T., Wick, D. G., Guengerich, F. P., and Baron, J., 1984, Immunohistochemical localization of carcinogen-metabolizing enzymes within the rat and hamster exocrine pancreas, *Cancer Res.* **44**:215–223.

30. Ishii-Ohba, H., Guengerich, F. P., and Baron, J., 1985, Localization of epoxide-metabolizing enzymes in rat testis, *Biochim. Biophys. Acta* **802**:326–334.

31. Baron, J., Kawabata, T. T., Redick, J. A., Knapp, S. A., Wick, D. G., Wallace, R. B., Jakoby, W. B., and Guengerich, F. P., 1983, Localization of carcinogen-metabolizing enzymes in human and animal tissues, in: *Extrahepatic Drug Metabolism and Chemical Carcinogenesis (J. Rydstrom, J. Montelius, and M. Bengtsson, eds.), pp. 73–88. Elsevier/North-Holland, Amsterdam.*

32. Yamamoto, N., and Yasuda, K., 1977, Use of a water soluble carbodiimide as a fixing agent, *Acta Histochem. Cytochem.* **10**:14–37.

33. Hand, A. R., and Hassell, J. R., 1976, Tissue fixation with diimidoesters as an alternative to formaldehyde. II. Cytochemical and biochemical studies of rat liver fixed with dimethylsuberimidate, *J. Histochem. Cytochem.* **24**:1000–1011.

34. Pearse, A. G. E., and Polak, J. M., 1975, Bifunctional reagents as vapour- and liquid-phase fixatives for immunohistochemistry, *Histochem. J.* **7**:179–186.

35. Morrison, M., Steele, W., and Danner, D. J., 1969, The reaction of benzoquinone with amines and proteins, *Arch. Biochem. Biophys.* **134**:515–523.

36. Lorenz, K., 1976, On the nature of protein benzoquinone complexes, *Experientia* **32**:1502–1503.

37. Brandt, J., Anderson, L. O., and Porath, J., 1975, Covalent attachment of proteins to polysaccharide carriers by means of benzoquinone, *Biochim. Biophys. Acta* **386**:196–202.

38. Mason, H. S., and Peterson, E. W., 1965, Melanoproteins. I. Reactions between enzyme-generated quinones and amino acids, *Biochim. Biophys. Acta* **111**:134–146.

39. Leterrier, F., Balny, C. and Douzou, P., 1967, Formation de complexes entre la *p*-benzosemiquinone et l'imidazole et ses derives, *Biochim. Biophys. Acta* **154**:444–479.

40. Bentley, P., Waechter, F., Oesch, F., and Staubli, W., 1979, Immunochemical localization of epoxide hydratase in rat liver: Effects of 2-acetylaminofluorene, *Biochem. Biophys. Res. Commun.* **91**:1101–1108.

41. Wolf, C. R., Moll, E., Friedberg, T., Oesch, F., Buchmann, A., Kuhlmann, W. D., and Kunz, H. W., 1984, Characterization, localization and regulation of a novel phenobarbital-inducible form of cytochrome P-450, compared with three further P-450-isoenzymes, NADPH P-450 reductase, glutathione transferases and microsomal epoxide hydrolase, *Carcinogenesis* **5**:993–1001.

42. Huang, S., Minassian, H., and More, J. D., 1976, Application of immunofluorescent staining in paraffin sections improved by trypsin digestion, *Lab. Invest.* **35**:383–396.

43. Curran, R. C., and Gregory, J., 1977, The unmasking of antigens in paraffin sections of tissues by trypsin, *Experientia* **33**:1400–1401.

44. Brozman, M., 1978, Immunohistochemical analysis of formaldehyde and trypsin- or pepsin-treated material, *Acta Histochem.* **63**:251–260.

45. Mepham, B. L., Frater, W., and Mitchell, B. S., 1979, The use of proteolytic enzymes to improve immunoglobulin staining by the PAP technique, *Histochem. J.* **11**:345–357.

46. Radaszkiewicz, T., Dragosics, B., Abdelfattahgad, M., and Denk, H., 1979, Effect of protease pretreatment on immunologic demonstrations of hepatitis B-surface antigen in conventional paraffin-embedded liver biopsy material, *J. Immunol. Methods* **29**:27–33.

47. Denk, H., Radaszkiewicz, T., and Weirich, E., 1977, Pronase pretreatment of tissue sections

enhances sensitivity of the unlabeled antibody–enzyme (PAP) technique, *J. Immunol. Methods* **15**:163–167.

48. Tokuyasu, K. T., 1973, A technique for ultramicrotomy of cell suspensions and tissues, *J. Cell Biol.* **57**:551–565.

49. Sternberger, L. A., Hardy, P. H., Cuculis, J. J., and Meyer, H. G., 1970, The unlabeled antibody enzyme method of immunohistochemistry. Preparation and properties of soluble antigen–antibody complex (horseradish peroxidase–antihorseradish peroxidase) and its use in identification of spirochetes, *J. Histochem. Cytochem.* **18**:315–333.

50. Hsu, S. M., Raine, L., and Fanger, H., 1981, Use of avidin–biotin–peroxidase complex (ABC) in immunoperoxidase techniques: A comparison between ABC and unlabeled antibody (PAP) procedures, *J. Histochem. Cytochem.* **29**:577–580.

51. Bergroth, V., Reitamo, S., Konttinen, Y. T., and Lalla, M., 1980, Sensitivity and nonspecific staining of varius immunoperoxidase techniques, *Histochemistry* **68**:17–22.

52. Burns, J., 1975, Background staining and sensitivity of the unlabeled antibody–enzyme (PAP) method. Comparison with the peroxidase labeled sandwich method using formalin fixed paraffin embedded material, *Histochemistry* **43**:291–294.

53. Nakane, P. K., and Pierce, G. B., 1966, Enzyme labeled antibodies: Preparation and application for the localization of antigens, *J. Histochem. Cytochem.* **14**:929–931.

54. Nakane, P. K., and Pierce, G. B., 1967, Enzyme-labeled antibodies for the light- and electronmicroscopic localization of tissue antigens, *J. Cell Biol.* **33**:307–318.

55. Avrameas, S., and Uriel, J., 1966, Methode de marquage d'antigenes et d'anticorps avec des enzymes et son application en immunodiffision, *C. R. Acad. Sci.* **262**:2543–2545.

56. Avrameas, S., 1967, Coupling of enzymes to proteins with glutaraldehyde. Use of conjugates for the detection of antigens and antibodies, *Immunochemistry* **6**:43–52.

57. Clark, C. A., Downs, E. C., and Primus, F. J., 1982, An unlabeled antibody method using glucose oxidase–antiglucose oxidase complexes (GAG): A sensitive alternative to immunoperoxidase for the detection of tissue antigens, *J. Histochem. Cytochem.* **30**:27–34.

58. Graham, R. C., and Karnovsky, M. J., 1966, The early stages of absorption of injected horseradish peroxidase in the proximal tubules of mouse kidney: Ultrastructural cytochemistry by a new technique, *J. Histochem. Cytochem.* **12**:291–302.

59. Seligman, A. M., Karnovsky, M. J., Wasserkrug, H. L., and Hanker, J. S., 1968, Nondroplet untrastructural demonstration of cytochrome oxidase with a polymerizing osmophilic reagent, diaminodenzidine (DAB), *J. Cell Biol.* **38**:1–14.

60. Straus, W., 1982, Imidazole increases the sensitivity of the cytochemical reaction of peroxidase with diaminobenzidine at a neutral pH, *J. Histochem. Cytochem.* **30**:491–493.

61. Adams, J. C., 1981, Heavy metal intensification of DAB-based HRP reaction product, *J. Histochem. Cytochem.* **29**:775–777.

62. Gallyas, F., Gorcs, T., and Merchenthaler, I., 1982, High-grade intensification of the end-product of the diaminobenzidine reaction for peroxidase histochemistry, *J. Histochem. Cytochem.* **30**:183–184.

63. Hsu, S.-M., and Soban, E., 1982, Color modification of diaminobenzidine (DAB) precipitation by metallic ions and its application for double immunohistochemistry, *J. Histochem. Cytochem.* **30**:1079–1082.

64. Hanker, J. S., Yates, P. E., Metz, C. B., and Rustioni, A., 1977, A new, specific, sensitive, and non-carcinogenic reagent for the demonstration of horseradish peroxidase, *Histochem. J.* **9**:789–792.

65. Graham, R. C., Ludholm, U., and Karnovsky, M. J., 1965, Cytochemical demonstration of peroxidase activity with 3-amino-9-ethylcarbazole, *J. Histochem. Cytochem.* **13**:150–152.

66. Nakane, P. K., 1968, Simultaneous localization of multiple tissue antigens using the peroxidase-labeled antibody method: A study in the pituitary glands of the rat, *J. Histochem. Cytochem.* **16**:557–560.

67. Straus, W., 1971, Inhibition of peroxidase by methanol and by methanol-nitroferricyanide for use in immunoperoxidase procedures, *J. Histochem. Cytochem.* **19:**682–688.

68. Streefkerk, J. G., 1972, Inhibition of erythrocyte pseudoperoxidase activity by treatment with hydrogen peroxide following methanol, *J. Histochem. Cytochem.* **20:**829–831.

69. Straus, W., 1972, Phenylhydrazine as an inhibitor of horseradish peroxidase for use in immunoperoxidase procedures, *J. Histochem. Cytochem.* **20:**949–951.

70. Taylor, C. R., 1978, Immunoperoxidase techniques: Practical and theoretical aspects, *Arch. Pathol. Lab. Med.* **102:**113–121.

71. Heyderman, E., 1979, Immunoperoxidase techniques in histopathology: Application, methods, and controls, *J. Clin. Pathol.* **32:**971–978.

72. DeLellis, R. A., Sternberger, L. A., Mann, R. B., Banks, P. M., and Nakane, P. K., 1979, Immunoperoxidase technics in diagnostic pathology. Report of a workshop sponsored by the National Cancer Institute, *Am. J. Clin. Pathol.* **71:**483–488.

73. Bosman, F.T., and Nieuwenhuijzen Kruseman, A. C., 1979, Clinical applications of the enzyme labeled antibody method. Immunoperoxidase methods in diagnostic pathology, *J. Histochem. Cytochem.* **27:**1140–1147.

74. MacIver, A. G., and Mepham, B. L., 1982, Immunoperoxidase techniques in human renal biopsy, *Histopathology* **6:**249–267.

75. Lewis, R. E., Johnson, W. W., and Cruse, J. M., 1983, Pitfalls and caveats in the methodology for immunoperoxidase staining in surgical pathologic diagnosis, *Surv. Synth. Pathol. Res.* **1:**134–152.

76. Bosman, F. T., 1983, Some recent developments in immunocytochemistry, *Histochem. J.* **15:**189–200.

77. Espinoza, C. G., Pillarisetti, S. G., and Azar, H. A., 1983, Selected applications of immunoperoxidase techniques in surgical pathology, *Ann. Clin. Lab. Sci.* **13:**240–248.

78. Towbin, H., Stachelin, T., and Gordon, J., 1976, Electrophoretic transfer of proteins from polyacrylamide gels to nitrocellulose sheets: Procedures and some applications, *Proc. Natl. Acad. Sci. U.S.A.* **76:**4350–4354.

79. Erlandsen, S. L., Parsons, J. A., Burke, J. P., Redick, J. A., Van Orden, D. E., and Van Orden, L. S., III, 1975, A modification of the unlabeled antibody enzyme method using heterologous antisera for the light microscopic and ultrastructural localization of insulin, glucagon and growth hormone, *J. Histochem. Cytochem.* **23:**666–677.

80. Bayer, E., Skutelsky, E., and Wilchek, M., 1979, The avidin–biotin method in affinity cytochemistry, *Methods Enzymol.* **62:**308–316.

81. Dakshinamurti, K., and Mistry, S. P., 1963, Tissue and intracellular distribution of biotin-$C^{14}OOH$ in rats and chicks, *J. Biol. Chem.* **238:**297–301.

82. Wood, G. S., and Warnke, R., 1981, Suppression of endogenous avidin binding activity in tissues and its relevance to biotin–avidin detection systems, *J. Histochem. Cytochem.* **29:**1196–1204.

83. Nairn, R. C., 1976, *Fluorescent Protein Tracing*, 4th ed., Churchill Livingstone, New York.

84. Ploem, J. S., 1970, Standards for fluorescence microscopy, in: *Standardization in Immunofluorescence* (E. J. Holbrow, ed.), pp. 137–153, Blackwell, London.

85. Storz, H., 1982, Investigations of fading of immunofluorescence objects, *Acta Histochem.* **71:**2–9.

86. Johnson, G. D., Davidson, R. S., McNamme, K. C., Russell, G., Goodwin, D., and Holborow, E. T., 1982, Fading of fluorescence during microscopy: A study of the phenomenon and its remedy, *J. Immunol. Methods* **55:**231–242.

87. Huff, J. C., Weston, W. L., and Wanda, K. D., 1982, Enhancement of specific immunofluorescent findings with use of a para-phenylenediamine mounting buffer, *J. Invest. Dermatol.* **78:**449–450.

88. Platt, J. L., and Michael, A. F., 1983, Retardation of fading and enhancement of intensity of immunofluorescence of *p*-phenylenediamine, *J. Histochem. Cytochem.* **31:**840–842.

89. Langanger, G., De Mey, J., and Adam, H., 1983, 1,4-Diazobicyclo-(2,2,2)-octane (DABCO) is retarding fading of immunofluorescence preparations, *Mikroskopie* **40**:237–241.

90. Giloh, H., and Sedat, J. W., 1982, Fluorescence microscopy: Reduced photobleaching of rhodamine and fluorescein protein conjugates by *n*-propyl gallate, *Science* **217**:1252–1255.

91. Nairn, R. C., Herzog, F., Ward, H. A., and DeBoer, W. G. R. M., 1969, Microphotometry in immunofluorescence, *Clin. Exp. Immunol.* **4**:697–705.

92. Hiramoto, R., Bernecky, J., Jurand, J., and Hamlin, M., 1964, The effect of hydrogen ion concentration on fluorescent labeled antibodies, *J. Histochem. Cytochem.* **12**:271–274.

93. Halliday, D., Davey, F. R., Call, F., and Marucci, A. A., 1977, Identification of intracellular immunoglobulin in extramedullary myeloma, *Arch. Pathol. Lab. Med.* **101**:522–525.

94. Mason, D. Y., and Sammons, R. E., 1979, The labeled antigen method of immunoenzyme staining, *J. Histochem. Cytochem.* **27**:832–840.

95. Falini, B., de Solas, I., Halverson, C., Parker, J. W., and Taylor, C. R., 1982, Double labeled-antigen method for demonstration of intracellular antigens in paraffin-embedded tissues, *J. Histochem. Cytochem.* **30**:21–26.

96. El Etreby, M. F., and Fath el Bab, M. R., 1977, The utility of antisera to canine growth hormone and canine prolactin for immunocytochemical staining of dog pituitary gland, *Histochemistry* **53**:1–15.

97. Erlandsen, S. L., Hegre, O. D., Parsons, J. A., McEvoy, R. C., and Elde, R. P., 1976, Pancreatic islet cell hormones: Distribution of cell types in the islet and evidence for the presence of somatostatin and gastrin within the D cell, *J. Histochem. Cytochem.* **24**:883–897.

98. Campbell, G. T., and Bhatnagar, A. S., 1976, Simultaneous visualization by light microscopy of two pituitary hormones in a single tissue section using a combination of indirect immunohistochemical methods, *J. Histochem. Cytochem.* **24**:448–452.

99. Sternberger, L. A., and Joseph, S. A., 1979, The unlabeled antibody method: Contrasting color staining of paired pituitary hormones without antibody removal, *J. Histochem. Cytochem.* **27**:1424–1436.

100. Valnes, K., and Brandtzaeg, P., 1982, Comparison of paired immunofluorescence and paired immunoenzyme staining methods based on primary antisera from the same species, *J. Histochem. Cytochem.* **30**:518–524.

101. Korsrud, F. R., and Brandtzaeg, P., 1982, Characterization of epithelial elements in human major salivary glands by functional markers: Localization of amylase, lactoferrin, lysozyme, secretory component, and secretory immunoglobulins by paired immunofluorescence staining, *J. Histochem. Cytochem.* **30**:657–666.

102. Enestrom, S., 1982, Immunofluorescent staining of epon embedded kidney sections through simultaneous use of two different fluorochrome-conjugated antisera, *Stain Technol.* **57**:31–38.

103. Hiramoto, R., and Hamlin, M., 1965, Detection of two antibodies in single plasma cells by the paired fluorescence technique, *J. Immunol.* **95**:214–224.

104. Scott, D. G., 1960, Immuno-histochemical studies of connective tissue: The use of contrasting fluorescent protein tracers in the comparison of two antisera, *Immunology* **3**:226–236.

105. Shiino, M., and Rennels, E. G., 1966, Cellular localization of prolactin and growth hormone in the anterior pituitary glands of the rat and rabbit, *Tex. Rep. Biol. Med.* **24**:659–673.

106. Silverstein, A. M., 1957, Contrasting fluorescent labels for two antibodies, *J. Histochem. Cytochem.* **5**:94–95.

107. Beutner, E. H., Holborow, E. J., and Johnson, G. D., 1956, A new fluorescent antibody method: Mixed antiglobulin immunofluorescence or labelled antigen indirect immunofluorescence staining, *Nature (London)* **208**:353–355.

108. Notani, G. W., Parsons, J. A., and Erlandsen, S. L., 1979, Versatility of *Staphylococcus aureus* protein A in immunocytochemistry. Use in unlabeled antibody enzyme system and fluorescent methods, *J. Histochem. Cytochem.* **27**:1438–1444.

109. Valnes, K., and Brandtzaeg, P., 1981, Unlabeled antibody peroxidase–antiperoxidase method combined with direct immunofluorescence, *J. Histochem. Cytochem.* **29**:703–711.

110. Lechago, J., Sun, N. C. J., and Weinstein, W. M., 1979, Simultaneous visualization of two antigens in the same tissue section by combining immunoperoxidase with immunofluorescence techniques, *J. Histochem. Cytochem.* **27:**1221–1225.
111. Brozman, M., Chorvath, D., and Jakubovsky, J., 1977, Immunohistochemical staining using coupled immunofluorescence and immunocomplex technique, *Acta Histochem.* **59:**61–69.
112. Deeley, E. S., 1955, An integrating microdensitometer for biological cells, *J. Sci. Instrum.* **32:**263–267.
113. Isaka, K., 1972, *Introduction to Microspectrophotometry,* Olympus Optical Co., Tokyo.
114. Altman, F. P., 1975, Quantitation in histochemistry: A review of some commercially available microdensitometers, *Histochem. J.* **7:**375–395.
115. Chayen, J., 1978, The cytochemical approach to hormone assay, *Int. Rev. Cytol.* **53:**333–396.
116. Chayen, J., 1978, Microdensitometry, in: *Biochemical Mechanisms of Liver Injury* (T. F. Slater, ed.), pp. 257–291, Academic Press, New York.
117. Grove, G. L., Lavker, R. M., and Kligman, A. M., 1978, Use of microspectrophotometry in dermatological investigations, *J. Soc. Cosmet. Chem.* **29:**537–544.
118. Bahr, G. F., 1979, Frontiers of quantitative cytochemistry. A review of recent developments and potentials, *Anal. Quant. Cytol.* **1:**1–19.
119. Cabrini, R. L., 1981, Practical applications of the microphotometric quantification of histoenzyme reactions, *Histochem. J.* **13:**241–250.
120. Duijndam, W. A. L., Smeulders, A. W. M., Van Duijn, P., and Verweij, A. C., 1980, Optical errors in scanning stage absorbance cytophotometry. I. Procedures for correcting apparent integrated absorbance values for distributional, glare, and diffraction errors, *J. Histochem. Cytochem.* **28:**388–394.
121. Duijndam, W. A. L., Van Duijn, P., and Riddersma, S. H. 1980, Optical errors in scanning stage absorbance cytophotometry. II. Application of correction factors for residual distributional error, glare, and diffraction error in practical cytophotometry, *J. Histochem. Cytochem.* **28:**395–400.
122. Baker, J. R., 1958, *Principles of Biological Microtechnique,* Methuen, London.
123. Lowry, O. H., and Passonneau, J., 1972, *A Flexible System of Enzymatic Analysis,* Academic Press, New York.
124. Van Orden, L. S., III, 1970, Quantitative histochemistry of biogenic amines. A simple microspectrofluorometer, *Biochem. Pharmacol.* **19:**1105–1117.

Chapter 5

Quantitative Histochemical Measurements within Sublobular Zones of the Liver Lobule

Frederick C. Kauffman and Franz M. Matschinsky

1. INTRODUCTION

It is well established that parenchymal cells in different zones of the hepatic lobule differ in function, biochemical properties, and susceptibility to hepatotoxins.[1-3] The experimental approaches that have been used most extensively over the years to describe the biochemical heterogeneity of the liver lobule are classic microscopic histochemistry and quantitative histochemistry. The object of this chapter is to describe the latter approach and illustrate its application to analyses of selected substrates and enzyme activites in microdissected samples from specific zones of the liver lobule. Methods of high specificity and sensitivity are required for such analyses because the number of cells that can be obtained conveniently from specific zones of the liver lobule range in number from about 100 to 500 depending on the age and species of animal studied. The average mass of a rat liver cell is estimated to be on the order of 1×10^{-9} g. Thus, an intermediate such as ATP, which is estimated to be about 5 mmoles/kg wet weight liver, would be about 5×10^{-15} mole/cell or about $0.5-2.5 \times 10^{-12}$

FREDERICK C. KAUFFMAN • Department of Pharmacology and Experimental Therapeutics, University of Maryland School of Medicine, Baltimore, Maryland 21201. FRANZ M. MATSCHINSKY • Department of Biochemistry and Biophysics, Diabetes Research Center, University of Pennsylvania, Philadelphia, Pennsylvania 19104.

mole/microdissected sample. Although this amount of substrate is below the range detected by conventional biochemical analytical techniques, this level of substrate can be measured conveniently via pyridine-nucleotide-dependent enzymatic cycling assays[4,5] and some bioluminescence assays.[6,7] Each of these types of analyses can be applied to specimens obtained by quantitative histochemical sampling procedures.

Quantitative histochemical methods have been in use for more than 50 years. Holter and Linderstrom-Lang[8] introduced these methods to measure pepsin and perform histology on adjacent frozen sections of the intestine and demonstrated unequivocally that the enzyme was localized in chief cells. Further development of this approach to analyze biochemical intermediates in adjacent tissue sections that differ in cellular composition was accomplished by Anfinsen et al.,[9] who demonstrated that histological analyses and determination of specific enzymes in layers of the retina could be accomplished in the same sections if these were dried at $-20°C$ over P_2O_5 prior to assessment of their cellularity using a mild staining procedure. The early technique was advanced further by the introduction of a quartz-fiber microbalance,[10] which was applied to determining acetylcholinesterase and NAD in microdissected samples of bovine retina.[11,12] Since these early studies, the techniques of histochemistry have been greatly refined, principally by O. H. Lowry and his colleagues, who have applied the techniques to the analysis of a wide array of substrates and enzymes in many tissues. The historical development of this approach has been described in several excellent reviews,[13,14] and the practical aspects of the technique are discussed in some detail in the book *A Flexible System of Enzymatic Analysis.*[5] A summary of these techniques and a discussion of their application to the analysis of sublobular zones of the liver is presented below.

2. PREPARATION OF TISSUE SAMPLES FOR ANALYSES

2.1. Sampling and Sectioning of Tissues

Samples of liver for analyses may be frozen by either immersing a small biopsy of the tissue in a freezing medium[15,16] or pressing an aluminum mallet chilled to liquid nitrogen temperature against the surface of the liver.[17,18] Rapid freezing is necessary to minimize ice-crystal formation and to maintain concentrations of labile substrates, which may change rapidly during brief periods of anoxic ischemia. The history of the tissue prior to freezing is less critical for the determination of most enzyme activities; however, exceptions exist. For example, maximal conversion of phosphorylase *b* to phosphorylase *a* in response to changes in cytosolic calcium in hepatic parenchymal cells occurs over a period of 10 sec.[19] Because heat conduction is slow in tissues, rapidly freezing areas more than a few millimeters below the surface of the liver is difficult. Samples weighing less than a gram are best frozen by immersion and rapid stirring in Freon 12 ($CC1_2F_2$) brought to its freezing point ($-150°C$) by a surrounding bath of liquid nitrogen. Freezing in this medium is faster than in liquid nitrogen at its boiling point ($-196°C$) because the formation of an insulating layer of gas is avoided. Samples weighing more than a gram can be frozen in liquid nitrogen brought from its boiling point to its freezing point ($-210°C$) by rapid evaporation under vacuum.[5] Use of liquid nitrogen brought to its freezing point prevents the formation of gas, and the colder temperature enhances freezing at depths greater than 3–4 mm.[20]

Frozen samples should be stored at temperatures below $-40°C$ to avoid ice-crystal growth and loss of labile enzyme activities and substrates that occur at the temperature ($-20°C$) of conventional freezers. Although detailed tests of labile constituents in frozen liver have not been made, detailed studies of the stability of several metabolites in samples of mouse brain indicate that 20% of ATP is lost over 24 hr at $-20°C$ and 20% of glucose-6-phosphate is lost after only 1 hr at $-20°C$. Other substrates that are known to decline significantly in mouse brain kept only a few hours at $-20°C$ include AMP, fructose-1,6-diphosphate, 3-phosphoglycerate, and glucose. In contrast, none of these substrates decreased in tissues kept at $-35°C$ over 1 week.[5] The same considerations apply to many enzyme activities in frozen tissues that may be lost after only a brief period of time at $-20°C$ but are maintained indefinitely at temperatures below $-40°C$.

Frozen samples are allowed to warm to -15 to $-20°C$ for a brief period of time before cutting and mounting blocks for sectioning in a cryostat. Blocks of tissue are mounted in a paste of mounting medium maintained at its freezing temperature on wooden or aluminum dowels. Freezing of the mounted tissue is accomplished by immediately immersing the mounting assembly in heptane or hexane maintained at dry-ice temperature. Mounted tissues are allowed to equilibrate to -20 to $-25°C$ in a cryostat before being sectioned. Normally, 20 μm serial sections of liver, obtained using a conventional cryostat microtome, are transferred to a suitable holder. The holder and tissue sections are placed in a special drying tube that can be evacuated. Great care is taken not to allow the holder and tube to warm above the temperature of the cryostat before transferring the drying assembly to a constant-temperature box maintained at -35 to $-40°C$.

2.2. Drying and Storage of Samples

Sections are lyophilized at this temperature to maintain histological structures and avoid ice-crystal formation. At a vacuum equivalent to about 0.01 mm Hg, essentially all the water can be removed from the tissues in 6–8 hr. Once water has been removed from tissue sections by this method, most labile enzymes and substrates can be stored indefinitely *in vacuo* at $-20°C$. Metabolites and enzymes are also quite stable in sections maintained at room temperature for the brief periods of time necessary for microdissection and weighing.

2.3. Identification of Sublobular Zones and Histological Control

Microdissection and weighing of samples are carried out in a room in which temperature can be maintained at or below 25°C and humidity held below 50%. Since tissue sections and dissected samples are very light, it is necessary to reduce air currents by surrounding the dissection bench with lightweight curtains. Handling of lyophilized tissue sections is performed after they have been allowed to equilibrate to room temperature *in vacuo* to avoid condensation of atmospheric moisture. When sections are lyophilized as above to minimize ice-crystal formation and shrinkage, it is possible to recognize structural details such as portal triads, central veins, and bile canaliculi in unstained sections.[18] Histological staining of adjacent serial sections can be used as an aid to identify specific structures and facilitate dissection. Histochemical staining for specific enzymes concentrated in periportal or pericentral zones of the liver can also be employed. For example, histochemical staining for glucose-6-phosphate dehydrogenase can be used to localize pericentral hepatocytes,[21] and staining for succinate dehydrogenase can be used to identify periportal hepatocytes.[22] Permanent dissecting maps of sections analyzed can be made using a camera lucida. Maps of staining patterns of specific markers for periportal and pericentral hepatocytes can be superimposed on adjacent freeze–dried sections to facilitate dissection of samples from specific sublobular zones.[16]

2.4. Dissection and Weighing of Samples

Identified structures are dissected freehand using knives constructed from fragments of razor blades fixed to flexible fiber shafts. Samples as small as 10–20 μm in diameter can be isolated using these tools and a conventional dissecting microscope. The dissected samples can be picked up and transferred with a short piece of hair mounted to a pencil-shaped glass or plastic holder. The size of dissected samples can be measured in several ways, but the most satisfactory method is to determine the dry weight of the sample using a quartz-fiber "fishpole" balance. This balance is a simple device consisting of a fine quartz fiber mounted horizontally within the barrel of a syringe.[5,23] A detailed description of methods employed in constructing quartz-fiber balances is given in the book by Lowry and Passonneau.[5] Samples to be weighed are placed on the free end of the quartz fiber, and the resulting displacement is measured using a micrometer ocular in a low-power stereoscopic microscope. This simple balance is considerably more useful in weighing microdissected samples because it can be contained in a very small chamber where air currents are minimal. Samples as small as 0.01 μg can be weighed accurately to within 1 or 2%. Microdissected samples of sublobular zones of the liver weighing 0.1–0.3 μg are easily handled by the procedures described above.

3. ANALYTICAL PROCEDURES

3.1. General Considerations

3.1.1. Enzymatic Cycling

A variety of methods exist that can be applied to measuring biochemical intermediates in microdissected samples of the liver lobule; however, the use of fluorometry of pyridine nucleotides in combination with amplification provided by enzymatic cycling has proven to be an exceptionally useful approach. Over the years, a very large array of compounds that are capable of being coupled enzymatically to the oxidation or reduction of diphosphopyridine nucleotide or triphosphopyridine nucleotide have been measured either spectrophotometrically or fluorometrically. The reduced forms of these pyridine nucleotides differ from the oxidized forms in their near-ultraviolet absorption properties and consequently can be either measured at 340 nm using a spectrophotometer or determined by their capacity to fluoresce at 420 nm when excited at 340 nm. The first use of pyridine nucleotides in a biochemical assay took place in Warburg's laboratory in 1935 when Negelein and Haas[24] determined glucose-6-phosphate dehydrogenase activity by the increase in absorption produced by NADPH. Pyridine nucleotide fluorescence was first employed to measure metabolites[25] and enzyme activities[26] in the mid-1950s. Since these early applications, the use of pyridine nucleotides in coupled enzymatic reactions has become a mainstay of modern analytical biochemistry.

Several properties of pyridine nucleotides, in addition to their absorption and fluorescence characteristics, contribute to their great utility in biochemical assays. Among these are their differential stability in acid and base[27] and the capacity of the oxidized species to form highly fluorescent products when heated in strong alkali.[28] Reduced forms of the pyridine nucleotide can be measured accurately at concentrations ranging between 10^{-5} and 2×10^{-4} M by conventional spectrophotometry and at concentrations down to 10^{-7} M by fluorometry. When treated with acid, the reduced forms are rapidly destroyed and the oxidized forms are unaffected. In contrast, the oxidized form is destroyed and the reduced form is maintained when treated with alkali. Thus, at the completion of a reaction, excess oxidized or reduced pyridine nucleotide remaining in the assay mixture can be destroyed and the form generated during the course of the reaction can be measured by one of the following procedures. If great amplification is not required, the product of the reaction can be treated with strong alkali to form a fluorescent product that can be accurately measured down to 10^{-8} M. If an oxidized pyridine nucleotide is formed, this is converted to the oxidized form by treatment with H_2O_2 before generating the fluorescent product with strong alkali.[4,5] A much greater amplification of pyridine nucleotides formed during the course of reactions can be achieved by "enzymatic cycling" in which the oxidized or reduced product serves as catalytic intermediate in a two-enzyme system.

The principles involved in determining metabolic intermediates or enzymes via pyridine-nucleotide-coupled enzymatic assays can be best illustrated by a specific example. For example, five intermediates or two enzyme activities may be measured by the following two reactions:

$$\text{Glucose} + \text{ATP} \xrightarrow[\text{(hexokinase)}]{\text{Mg}^{2+}} \text{Glucose-6-P} + \text{ADP} \tag{1}$$

$$\text{Glucose-6-P} + \text{NADP}^+ \xrightarrow[\substack{\text{(glucose-6-phosphate} \\ \text{dehydrogenase)}}]{} \text{6-Phosphogluconate} \\ + \text{NADPH} + \text{H}^+ \tag{2}$$

Based on the presence of the other components in nonlimiting amounts, either glucose, ATP, Mg^{2+}, or hexokinase can be measured via reaction 1. Reaction 2, which is the "indicator reaction," can be applied to the measurement of either glucose-6-phosphate, $NADP^+$, or glucose-6-phosphate dehydrogenase. Substrates in the range of 10^{-10} to 10^{-11} mole can be measured in a volume of 1 ml based on native fluorescence of NADPH. Tenfold greater sensitivity can be achieved via measurement of alkali-induced fluorescence after destruction of the remaining $NADP^+$ in the reaction mixture. $NADP^+$ is destroyed by adjusting the pH of the reaction mixture to pH 12 and heating at 80°C for 15–20 min.[5] NADPH ranging down to 1×10^{-15} mole can be measured readily by "enzymatic cycling" via the following scheme[4,5]:

In the presence of high activities of the two enzymes and excess glucose-6-phosphate, α-ketoglutarate, and NH_4^+, NADP is continuously oxidized and reduced in a cyclic fashion. The cycling rate is directly proportional to the content of $NADP^+$ or NADPH added to the reaction mixture and may be as high as

20,000 cycles/hour. The source of glucose-6-phosphate dehydrogenase is an important determinant of cycling rates. The crystalline enzyme from baker's yeast causes destruction of NADPH, and this leads to a sharp decline in cycling rates with time.[29] This difficulty can be solved by using glucose-6-phosphate dehydrogenase from *Leuconostoc mesenteroides,* which does not destroy NADPH and has kinetic properties that are very favorable for high cycling activity. Enzyme cycling reagents containing this enzyme are capable of amplifying 100,000-fold in 4 hr at 38°C or 350,000-fold in 3 days at 15°C.[29] At the end of a predetermined time, the cycling reaction is stopped by boiling, and 6-phosphogluconate formed is measured using 6-phosphogluconate dehydrogenase and NADP$^+$. NADPH formed in this last reaction is either measured directly or measured after treatment with H_2O_2 and strong alkali. If greater sensitivity is required, excess NADP$^+$ used in the last reaction is destroyed with alkali, and the cycling step is repeated to measure NADPH generated from 6-phosphogluconate. Repetition of the cycling step provides enormous amplification of the initial product (e.g., 4×10^8 -fold if each cycling step was for 1 hr), allowing less than 10^{-18} mole to be determined. This degree of amplification is more than necessary for most of the intermediates and enzymes of interest in microdissected samples of the liver lobule.

The cycling system commonly used to amplify NAD$^+$ or NADH involves the use of alcohol, oxaloacetate, alcohol dehydrogenase, and malate dehydrogenase according to the following scheme[30]:

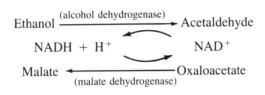

Malate formed in this cycling system is determined with either NAD$^+$ or NADP$^+$ using either malate dehydrogenase or malic enzyme, respectively.

The concept of enzymatic cycling is not new, and a number of analyses have been developed using this principle. The earliest application was probably by Warburg *et al.*[31] who measured nicotinamide adenine dinucleotide phosphate by O_2 consumed during alternate oxidation and reduction of the nucleotide via "old yellow enzyme" and glucose-6-phosphate dehydrogenase. More recent applications of this technique include cycling methods to measure glutamate of α-ketoglutarate,[5] adenine nucleotides,[32] and guanine nucleotides.[33]

3.1.2. Bioluminescence Assays

The development of modern instruments that permit measurement of emitted light with great precision and the commercial availability of substrates and enzymes for light-emitting systems has led to the development of a wide variety of bioluminescent assays for biologically important molecules. For the most part, these assays involve the use of luciferase systems isolated from either fireflies or bioluminescent bacteria. Light emitted by the firefly system in the presence of excess luciferin and magnesium is directly proportional to ATP either added directly or generated via coupled enzymatic reactions. The bacterial systems can be employed to measure the appearance or disappearance of reduced pyridine nucleotides, NADH and NADPH. The emerging use of these systems as powerful analytical tools is underscored by the devotion of an entire volume of *Methods in Enzymology*[34] to this subject and the continuing appearance of a large number of original research reports involving the application of bioluminescence assay systems. Some of the more widely used assays are summarized below along with selected recent developments to illustrate the great utility of this approach.

The firefly luciferin–luciferase system has been widely used as an analytical system to measure ATP or other substrates that can be linked to ATP formation via coupled enzymatic reactions.[6,7,35,36] The major advantages of this analytical system are that it is specific for ATP, can be performed with relatively simple equipment, and requires fewer steps than the enzymatic cycling technique. It was not long after McElroy[37] demonstrated that light emitted from crude extracts of firefly lanterns was proportional to added ATP that this phenomenon was employed in an assay system. Strehler and Totter[35] described conditions under which as little as 2 pmoles ATP could be determined using the luciferin–luciferase system and a quantum counting photomultiplier. Since these early studies, the commercial availability of purified luciferase and synthetic luciferin has stimulated the development of many assays based on bioluminescence generated via this system. Combination of this analytical system with quantitative histochemical sampling procedures described above has led to the convenient measurement of ATP, ADP, total adenylates, and phosphocreatine in the range of 0.1–80 pmoles.[7,38] Measurement of total adenylates in lyophilized samples (1–3 μg) of mouse cerebellum by the luciferin–luciferase method and enzymatic cycling of NADPH generated via hexokinase and glucose-6-phosphate dehydrogenase gave essentially the same results.[7]

The principle of using luciferin–luciferase to measure picomole amounts of adenine nucleotides and phosphocreatine is based on detecting the relatively steady level of bioluminescence generated in the presence of ATP. A variety of instruments equipped with photomultipliers have been employed to monitor light emitted during the course of the reaction, including photometers, filter fluorometers,[7] and liquid scintillation counters.[36] ATP in tissue extracts is measured directly by adding sample to luciferin–luciferase reagent and monitoring light emitted. If assays are carried out using crude luciferase preparations, measurements of ATP may be complicated by contaminating amounts of myokinase. This problem can be averted by including P[1],P[5]-di(adenosine-5′)pentaphosphate, a specific inhibitor of myokinase,[39] in the reaction mixture. This inhibitor may also be added to reagents used to convert phosphocreatine to ATP via creatine kinase prior to addition to luciferin–luciferase reagents. ADP is measured via addition of phosphoenolpyruvate and pyruvate kinase to the initial detector reagent, which is usually contained in a volume of 10μl or less. Total adenylates are determined by adding myokinase to the reaction mixture used to measure ADP.

Sensitivity of the assays for adenylate phosphates and phosphocreatine can be increased by adding additional luciferin to the indicator reaction mixture.[7,36] Since the light emitted via the luciferin–luciferase assay declines slightly with time,[40] it is advisable to read samples and standards at the same time interval after addition to the indicator reaction. More constant light emission may be obtained by reducing the concentration of luciferse in the reaction mixture.[7]

Bacterial luciferases involve the shunting of electrons from reduced substrates to oxygen via flavin. Light emission occurs when a reduced FMN species complexes with bacterial luciferase and reacts with a long-chain aldehyde to produce FMN, acid, water, and light.[41,42] Bacterial luciferases used in analytical systems have been obtained from *Beneckea harvei, Photobacterium fisheri, and P. phosphoreum.* Several examples of the use of these luciferases to measure biochemical substrates are presented below. Glucose-6-phosphate and 6-phosphogluconate have been measured employing a bacterial luciferase system specific for NADPH.[43] While this assay system is useful to measure picomole amounts of glucose-6-phosphate and 6-phosphogluconate, difficulties encountered with high blanks due to phosphorescence and relatively slow onset of bioluminescence generated via the indicator luciferase have limited wide use of this analytical system.

A sensitive bioluminescent assay for free fatty acids in biological samples has been developed recently based on the activation of free fatty acids by acyl-CoA synthetase.[44] Pyrophosphate formed via this reaction is linked to NADH formation and the bacterial luciferase system from *Vibrio harvei.* Although a complex series of coupled enzymatic reactions are employed in this assay involving acyl-CoA synthetase, pyrophosphate fructose-6-phosphate phosphotransferase, aldolase, and glyceraldehyde phosphate dehydrogenase, the generation of light in this reaction was linearly proportional to fatty acids ranging from 1 to 30 nmoles. An NADH-linked bioluminescent assay has also been reported recently for determining glycerol. This assay is a kinetic assay based on determining rates of NADH formation via glycerol dehydrogenase.[45]

A recent advance in bioluminescent assays employing NAD(P)H:FMN oxidoreductase and a bacterial luciferase involves the use of coupled enzymes immobilized on an insoluble matrix.[42] The advantages of such preparations are that they are more stable and more efficient than soluble systems. Through the use of appropriate enzymes, bioluminescent assays have been developed for D-glucose, L-lactate, 6-phosphogluconate, L-malate, L-alanine, L-glutamate, NAD, and NADP. In general, 10–100 pmoles of substrate can be readily determined using these systems, which seem to have greater sensitivity with NADP as a cofactor.

3.1.3. Radiochemical Assays

The combination of sensitive radiochemical or radioimmunoassays with quantitative histochemical sampling procedures offers another experimental approach to defining the biochemical microheterogeneity of the liver lobule. This approach has not yet been applied to any large extent in studies of the liver. A few examples of this approach are presented in the hope that they will stimulate an expansion of the application of radiochemical technologies to studies of the cellular heterogeneity of the liver. Use of conventional counting techniques such as liquid scintillation to assay the content of specific intermediates in sublobular zones of the liver will likely be limited to those that are present in abundant amounts and labeled with isotopes of the highest specific activity. An example of the use of direct counting techniques in combination with quantitative histochemical sampling procedures is illustrated by a study employing [^{14}C]glucose to determine the turnover of protein in discrete areas of rat brain.[46] Labeled glucose was injected serially over a $5\frac{1}{2}$-hr period to label pools of amino acids in equilibrium with protein. Measurements of the specific activity of free glutamate and glutamate residues in proteins were used to calculate the turnover of protein in whole brain and specific histological areas of the cerebellum, cortex, and hippocampus. The apparent mean half-life for proteins in whole brain was 85 hr. Analyses of histologically distinct regions indicated that rates of protein turnover were highest in areas rich in cell bodies, which were 2- to 4-fold greater than those observed in areas rich in fiber tracts and dendrites. Approaches similar to this could be taken to study the turnover of total and possibly specific proteins in discrete regions of the liver.

A novel radiometric microassay was recently introduced for measuring the intralobular distribution of glucose phosphorylation in the liver and for determining glucokinase in pancreatic islet tissue.[47] The assay is based on the liberation of T_2O from glucose 2-T-glucose-6-phosphate, which is the product of the phosphorylation reaction using 2-T-glucose and ATP as substrates. The liberation of T_2O is accomplished with the help of hexosephosphate-isomerase, and the product T_2O is separated from the primary substrate 2-T-glucose by a diffusion step. This radiometric assay has one important advantage over the more widely employed fluorometric microassay.[48] In the presence of 3–10 mM glucose-6-phosphate, the assay registers primarily the high-K_m enzyme glucokinase. This is because glucose-6-phosphate inhibits hexokinase without affecting glucokinase. Therefore, it is possible to study glucokinase in situations in which hexokinase contributes in a major way to glucose phosphorylation, which is the case in pancreatic islet tissue, and also when determining the K_m of glucokinase for glucose. The sensitivity of this radiometric assay of glucose phosphorylation enzymes can be greatly enhanced by working with an oil-well method.[49] Using this approach, glucokinase was quantitated in as little as 50 ng of pancreatic freeze–dried islet tissue and 10 ng of freeze–dried liver tissue.

Radioimmunoassays have been employed in combination with microdissection techniques to measure a number of biochemical intermediates. One of the more widely used applications of this approach involves the measurement of cyclic nucleotides. Radioimmunoassays of cyclic AMP and cyclic GMP have been developed by generating antibodies to 2'-O-succinyl derivatives of these nucleotides complexed to proteins.[50] Immunoassay curves based on the displacement of ^{125}I-labeled 2'-O-succinyl cyclic AMP permit femtomole quantities of cyclic AMP to be measured conveniently. Use of such assays to determine cyclic nucleotides in microdissected samples from lyophilized tissue sections is illustrated by the study of Rubin and Ferrendelli,[51] who examined the influence of various drugs on cyclic AMP and cyclic GMP in various cellular layers of the mouse cerebellum.

3.1.4. Gas–Liquid Chromatography Mass Spectrometry and Atomic Absorption

New advances are being made in quantitative histochemistry using gas–liquid chromatography (GLC) mass spectrometry analysis of various low–molecular-weight substances and by applying atomic absorption and x-ray probes for the analysis of Na, K, Mg, and Ca contents of tissues. GLC mass spectrometry in the selected ion-monitoring mode was used to carry out detailed quantitative histochemical studies of myoinositol distribution in brain tissue.[52] The sensitivity of this method reaches the low femtomole range. To complement the GLC mass spectrometric method for myoinositol, a pyridine-nucleotide-dependent enzymatic fluorometric oil-well method was developed and was applied to measurements of myoinositol in various types of tissues. The oil-well method for myoinositol has a sensitivity of about one tenth that of the mass spectrometric technique.[53] The microprocedure has been used to quantitate myoinositol in discrete layers of the rabbit retina. The measurements showed that diabetes caused a fall of myoinositol in all layers including the retinal pigment epithelium. This drop of myoinositol could be causally related to the development of diabetic retinopathy.[54] Using a carbon rod attachment to the atomic absorption spectrometer and computer controlled stepwise combustion of solid samples, it has become feasible to quantitate the Na and K contents of bits of freeze–dried tissue weighing just a few nanograms. For the analysis of the less abundant Ca and Mg, a fraction of $1\mu g$ of freeze–dried tissue is needed.[55] Using this approach, measurements have been made in retinal and cerebellar microscopic layers as well as in samples from distinct intralobular locations of the liver parenchyma. These measurements can be complemented by elemental analysis of cellular substructures. Electron-probe microanalysis applied to ultrathin freeze–dried tissue sections has allowed measurements of Na, K, Ca, and Mg, and of other elements in ultramicroscopic substructures of the cell, e.g., mitochrondria and sarcoplasmic reticulum.[56,57] It is believed that the application of these sophisticated techniques will be of great advantage for studies of the cellular heterogeneity of the hepatic parenchyma.

3.2. Examples of Quantitative Histochemical Measurements in Liver

A few samples of measurements of selected enzymes and substrates in specific zones of the liver are presented to illustrate the utility of the quantitative histochemical approach. The reader interested in comprehensive surveys of biochemical measurements made in sublobular zones is referred to two excellent reviews that have appeared recently.[1,58]

3.2.1. Enzyme Measurements

An early application of the techniques described above involved the measurement of pyridine-nucleotide-dependent enzymes in regenerating and degenerating areas of the rat liver lobule.[15] Measurements of these enzymes are among the easiest because oxidized pyridine nucleotides are produced during the course of these reactions and can be measured fluorometrically either directly or via alkali-induced fluorescence. Microchemical techniques were used in combination with microdissection of lyophilized sections to measure total protein, total hemoglobin, total lipid, and nine enzymes in four zones of the liver lobule of animals exposed to carbon tetrachloride.[15,59] Enzyme measurements were made using samples ranging between 0.2 and 0.8 µg. Regenerative processes dominated the portal midzone area of the injured lobule, while degenerative processes were localized largely in the central area. Degenerating areas were characterized by increases in glucose-6-phosphate dehydrogenase and by decreases in lactate dehydrogenase, isocitrate dehydrogenase, glutamic dehydrogenase, and β-hydroxybutyrate dehydrogenase. Lactate dehydrogenase was elevated in the regenerating area of the liver, while the other pyridine-nucleotide-linked dehydrogenases remained unchanged. These data were interpreted to indicate that many specialized functions are maintained in regenerating areas and that lactate may serve as a special substrate for gluconeogenesis and energy production via the tricarboxylic acid cycle in regenerating hepatocytes. Another example of changes in a pyridine-nucleotide-dependent enzyme that changes in response to a physiological stimulus is illustrated by hepatic glucose-6-phosphate dehydrogenase, which can be induced 10-fold by realimentation of fasted animals.[60] Quantitative measurements of this activity can be made with 0.1 µg dry weight samples added directly to 1 ml of complete reagent and following the rate of NADPH generated using a simple filter fluorometer.[21] Using this approach, Welsh [21] found that the induction of glucose-6-phosphate dehydrogenase that occurs with realimentation is greater in centrilobular than in periportal hepatocytes.

The intralobular distribution of glucokinase in the liver was studied by fluorometric and radiometric assays.[47,48] An activity gradient rising from the periportal to the perivenous regions was observed similarly with both methods. With the radiometric methods, it was possible to determine the K_m for glucose with tissue samples as small as 10–20 ng. The radiometric microassay was sufficiently reliable for demonstrating the sigmoidal glucose dependency of the phosphorylation reaction. The application of these techniques promises to be useful in studies of hepatic glucose metabolism in starvation, diabetes, alcoholic liver injury, and possibly other situations.

Highly fluorescent methylumbelliferyl-conjugated substrates and 7-hydroxycoumarin have been employed to measure β-glucuronidase and glucuronosyltransferase in sublobular zones of the liver.[61] UDP-glucuronosyltransferase was measured quantitatively in microdissected samples of periportal and pericentral hepatocytes from normal and phenobarbital- and 3-methylcholanthrene-treated rats using 7-hydroxycoumarin as substrate. Glucuronosyltransferase activities were consistently higher in pericentral than in periportal regions of livers from all groups. Treatment with phenobarbital increased activities about 2-fold in both areas, and 3-methylcholanthrene elevated activities 8- to 9-fold in the two zones. By pooling samples dissected from the two areas, kinetic studies of this activity in periportal and pericentral hepatocytes could be performed. The K_m for the aglycone, 7-hydroxycoumarin, was unaffected by the various treatments; however, the K_m of the enzyme for UDP-glucuronic acid differed in the two zones of the liver lobule and was increased after treatment with 3-methylcholanthrene. β-Glucuronidase, which may influence net glucuronide production by the liver,[62] has been assayed in sublobular zones of the liver lobule using methylumbelliferyl glucuronide as a substrate and found not to differ in the two areas. Although other hydrolytic enzymes could be determined conveniently in periportal and pericentral zones using either methylumbelliferyl- or *p*-nitrophenyl-conjugated substrates, only alkaline phosphatase[15] appears to have been studied.

UDP-glucuronosyltransferase in microdissected samples of periportal and pericentral regions of the liver lobule has also been determined by measuring the disappearance of the fluorescent substrate, 1-naphthol.[63] Results obtained using this quantitative assay and immunohistochemical localization indicated that the 3-methylcholanthrene-inducible form of glucuronosyltransferase is concentrated in centrilobular hepatocytes.

3.2.2. Substrate Analyses

Although a considerable number of quantitative histochemical measurements of enzyme activities have been made in microdissected samples of the liver lobule, measurements of various substrates are limited. To date, substrates that have been determined employing either enzymatic cycling or bioluminescent techniques include adenine nucleotides,[16] pyridine nucleotides,[16,18] inorganic phosphate,[16] glucose-6-phosphate,[64] α-glycerophosphate, and dihydroxyacetone phosphate.[16] Further understanding of the functional implications of the bio-chemical heterogeneity of the hepatic lobule will require that additional deter-minations of substrates be made under a variety of physiological conditions.

A recent study exploring the influence of the translobular gradient of oxygen and nutrients on the oxidation–reduction in periportal and pericentral hepatocytes involved measurement of α-glycerophosphate and dihydroxyacetone to calculate free $NAD^+/NADH$ ratios.[16] Samples of lyophilized tissue weighing between 0.01 and 0.1 μg were analyzed using the "oil-well" technique of enzymatic cycling. Newly developed assays were employed for α-glycerophosphate in the range of 2–10×10^{-14} mole and dihydroxyacetone ranging between 0.5 and 2.5×10^{-14} mole. Measurements of these intermediates along with ATP, ADP, and inorganic phosphate in normal rat livers and in livers exposed to brief periods of ischemia indicated that the oxidation–reduction and phosphate potentials are uniform throughout the entire liver lobule of fed rats.

Measurements of $NADP^+$ and NADPH have been made in isolated perfused livers during the course of mixed-function oxidation of 7-ethoxycoumarin.[18] Rapid freezing of the liver surface during perfusion was achieved by gently pressing an aluminum mallet chilled in liquid nitrogen against the left lateral lobe of the liver. Small blocks of tissue were prepared from this area of the liver and processed for quantitative histochemical measurements of the pyridine nu-cleotides. During mixed-function oxidation of 7-ethoxycoumarin, the oxida-tion–reduction state of NADP(H) was similar in both regions of the liver lobule. Infusion of xylitol decreased $NADP^+/NADPH$ ratios and stimulated rates of drug metabolism in both zones, suggesting that under certain conditions, the supply of reduced cofactor can be an important rate determinant of mixed-function oxidation in both zones.

4. ADVANTAGES AND LIMITATIONS OF THE QUANTITATIVE HISTOCHEMICAL APPROACH

The major advantage of the quantitative histochemical approach is that it permits quantitative biological measurements to be made in well-defined histo-logical zones of heterogeneous tissues. By combining microdissection techniques with powerful analytical schemes such as enzymatic cycling and bioluminescent assays, a wide variety of biologically important substrates and enzymes can be determined in lyophilized sections. Concentrations of most substrates and enzyme activities are maintained at levels at which they exist in the intact organ by quick freezing. Samples as small as 5–10μm in diameter can be isolated and cofactors, metabolites, and enzyme activities in amounts lower than 10^{-15} mole can be measured by pyridine-nucleotide-linked enzymatic cycling procedures. Where sensitivity is not a great factor, a variety of other analytical techniques are available for quantitative biochemical measurements in discrete histological zones.

As with other analytical schemes, limitations exist. The methods described above do not distinguish between bound and free metabolites in tissues, and they do not provide information on the distribution of various enzymes and substrates in subcellular compartments. Another problem is the failure of some enzyme systems to survive the freeze–drying process. This is particularly a problem in studies related to hepatic drug metabolism because the P-450-dependent mixed-function oxidase activity is lost during lyophilization. Another limitation of this analytical scheme is that the level of resolution is not as great as that achieved via high-resolution staining and radioautographic techniques. Quantitative histochemical measurements necessarily depend on invasive sampling procedures; therefore, it is difficult if not impossible to study the behavior of specific enzyme systems as a function of time in sublobular zones of the intact organ. These deficiencies, however, should not detract from the great usefulness of the quantitative histochemical approach. When this approach is combined with other approaches such as the use of noninvasive microlight guides, miniature oxygen electrodes, immunohistochemical staining procedures, and x-ray diffraction studies, a more comprehensive understanding of the physiological importance of metabolic zonation in the liver will be achieved.

REFERENCES

1. Gumucio, J. J., and Miller, D. L., 1981, Functional implications of liver cell heterogeneity, *Gastroenterology* **80**:393–403.
2. Jungermann, K. K., and Katz, N., 1985, Metabolism of carbohydrate, in: *Regulation of Hepatic Metabolism: Intra- and Intercellular Compartmentation* (R. G. Thurman, F. C. Kauffman, and K. Jungermann, eds.), Chapter 9, Plenum Press, New York.
3. Jungermann, K., and Sasse, D., 1978, Heterogeneity of liver parenchymal cell, *Trends Biochem Sci.* **3**:198–202.
4. Lowry, O. H., Passonneau, J. V., Schulz, D. W., and Rock, M. K., 1961, The measurement of pyridine nucleotides by enzymatic cycling, *J. Biol. Chem.* **236**:2746–2755.
5. Lowry, O. H., and Passonneau, J. V., 1972, *A Flexible System of Enzymatic Analysis*, Academic Press, New York.
6. Lundin, A., Rickardsson, A., and Thore, A., 1976, Continuous monitoring of ATP-converting reactions by purified firefly luciferase, *Anal. Biochem.* **75**:611–620.
7. Lust, W. D., Feussner, G. K., Barbehenn, E. K., and Passonneau, J. V., 1981, The enzymatic measurement of adenine nucleotides and P-creatine in picomole amounts, *Anal. Biochem.* **110**:258–266.
8. Holter, H., and Linderstrom-Lang, K., 1935, The distribution of pepsin in the gastric mucosa of pigs, *C. R. Lab. Carlsberg Ser. Chim.* **20**:1–32.
9. Anfinsen, C. B., Lowry, O. H., and Hastings, A. B., 1942, The application of the freeze–drying technique to retinal histochemistry, *J. Cell. Comp. Physiol.* **20**:231–237.
10. Lowry, O. H., 1944, A simple quartz torsion balance, *J. Biol. Chem.* **152**:293–294.
11. Anfinsen, C. B., 1944, The distribution of cholinesterase in the bovine retina, *J. Biol. Chem.* **152**:267–278.
12. Anfinsen, C. B., 1944, The distribution of diphosphopyridine nucleotide in the bovine retina, *J. Biol. Chem.* **152**:274–284.

13. Lowry, O. H., 1975, Quantitative histochemistry, in: *The Nervous System,* Vol. 1, (D. B. Tower, ed.), pp. 523–533, Raven Press, New York.
14. Lowry, O. H., 1973, An unlimited microanalytical system, *Acc. Chem. Res.* **6:**289–293.
15. Morrison, G. R., Brock, F. E., Karl, I. E., and Shank, R. E., 1965, Quantitative analysis of regenerating and degenerating areas within the lobule of carbon tetrachloride-injured liver, *Arch. Biochem. Biophys.* **111:**448–460.
16. Ghosh, A. K., Finegold, D., White, W., Zawalich, K., and Matschinsky, F. M., 1982, Quantitative histochemical resolution of oxidation–reduction and phosphate potentials within the simple hepatic acinus, *J. Biol. Chem.* **257:**5476–5481.
17. Wollenberger, A., Ristau, O., and Schoffa, G., 1960, A simple technique for extremely rapid freezing of large pieces of tissue, *Pflügers Arch.* **270:**399–412.
18. Belinsky, S. A., Kauffman, F. C., Ji, S., Lemasters, J. J., and Thurman, R. G., 1983, Stimulation of mixed-function oxidation of 7-ethoxycoumarin in periportal and pericentral regions of the perfused rat liver by xylitol, *Eur. J. Biochem.* **137:**1–6.
19. Charest, R., Blackmore, P. F., Berthon, B., and Exton, J. H., 1983, Changes in free cytosolic Ca^{2+} in hepatocytes following α_1-adrenergic stimulation: Studies on Quin-2 loaded hepatocytes, *J. Biol. Chem.* **258:**8769–8773.
20. Ferrendelli, J. A., Gay, M. H., Sedgwick, W. G., and Chang, M. M., 1972, Quick freezing of the mouse central nervous system: Comparison of regional cooling rates and metabolite levels when using liquid nitrogen or Freon-12, *J. Neurochem.* **19:**979–987.
21. Welsh, F. A., 1972, Changes in distribution of enzymes within the liver lobule during adaptive increases, *J. Histochem. Cytochem.* **20:**107–111.
22. Loud, A. V., 1968, Quantitative stereological description of the ultrastructure of normal rat liver parenchymal cells, *J. Cell Biol.* **37:**27–46.
23. Lowry, O. H., 1953, The quantitative histochemistry of the brain: Histological sampling, *J. Histochem. Cytochem.* **1:**420–428.
24. Negelein, E., and Haas, E., 1935, Uber die Wirkungsweise des Zwischenferment, *Biochem. Z.* **282:**206–220.
25. Greengard, D., 1956, Determination of intermediary metabolites by enzymatic fluorimetry, *Nature (London)* **178:**632–634.
26. Lowry, O. H., Roberts, N. R., and Chang, M. L. W., 1956, The analysis of single cells, *J. Biol. Chem.* **222:**97–107.
27. Lowry, O. H., Passonneau, J. V., and Rock, M. K., 1961, The stability of pyridine nucleotides, *J. Biol. Chem.* **236:**2756–2757.
28. Kaplan, N. O., Colowick, S. P., and Barnes, C. C., 1951, Effect of alkali on diphosphopyridine nucleotide, *J. Biol. Chem.* **191:**461–472.
29. Chi, M. M. Y., Lowry, C. V., and Lowry, O. H., 1978, An improved enzymatic cycle for nicotinamide-adenine dinucleotide phosphate, *Anal. Biochem.* **89:**119–129.
30. Kato, T., Berger, S. J., Carter, J. A., and Lowry, O. H., 1973, An enzymatic cycling method for nicotinamide-adenine dinucleotide with malic and alcohol dehydrogenases, *Anal. Biochem.* **53:**86–97.
31. Warburg, O., Christian, W., and Griese, A., 1935, Wasserstoffübertragendes C0-ferment; Seine Zusammensetzung und Wirkungsweise, *Biochem. Z.* **282:**157–205.
32. Breckenridge, B. M., 1964, The measurement of cyclic adenylate in tissues, *Proc. Natl. Acad. Sci. U.S.A.* **52:**1580–1586.
33. Goldberg, N. D., Larner, J., Sasko, H., and O'Toole, A. G., 1969, Enzymatic analysis of cyclic 3′,5′-AMP in mammalian tissues and urine, *Anal. Biochem.* **28:**523–544.
34. DeLuca, M. A., 1978, *Bioluminescence and Chemiluminescence,* Academic Press, New York, San Francisco, and London.
35. Strehler, B. L., and Totter, J. R., 1952, Firefly luminescence in the study of energy transfer mechanisms. I. Substrate and enzyme determination, *Arch Biochem. Biophys.* **40:**28–41.

36. Kimmich, G. A., Randles, J., and Brand, J. S., 1975, Assay of picomole amounts of ATP, ADP and AMP using the luciferase enzyme system, *Anal. Biochem.* **69:**187–206.

37. McElroy, W. D., 1947, The energy source for bioluminescence in an isolated system, *Proc. Natl. Acad. Sci. U.S.A.* **33:**342–345.

38. Sinicropi, D. V., Dombrowski, A., Montgomery, C. W., Evans, R. K., and Kauffman, F. C., 1980, Maintenance of the adult rat superior cervical ganglion *in vitro:* Comparison of organ and explant culture systems, *J. Neurochem.* **34:**1280–1287.

39. Lienhard, G. E., and Secemski, I. I., 1973, P^1,P^5-Di(adenosine-5')pentaphosphate, a potent multisubstrate inhibitor of adenylate kinase, *J. Biol. Chem.* **248:**1121–1123.

40. Matthews, J. C., and Cormier, M. J., 1978, Rapid microassay for the calcium-dependent protein modulator of cyclic nucleotide phosphodiesterase, *Methods Enzymol.* **57:**107–112.

41. Hastings, J. W., 1978, A sensitive kinetic assay for glycerol using bacterial bioluminescence, *Anal. Biochem.* **139:**510–515.

42. Wienhausen, G., and DeLuca, M. A., 1982, Bioluminescent assays of picomole levels of various metabolites using immobilized enzymes, *Anal. Biochem.* **127:**380–388.

43. Palmisano, J., and Schwartz, J. H., 1982, Microassays for glucose-6-phosphate and 6-phosphogluconate based on bioluminescent techniques, *Anal. Biochem.* **126:**409–413.

44. Kather, H., and Wieland, E., 1984, Bioluminescent determination of free fatty acids, *Anal. Biochem.* **140:**349–353.

45. Lavi, J. T., 1984, A sensitive kinetic assay for glycerol using bacterial bioluminescence, *Anal. Biochem.* **139:**510–515.

46. Austin, L., Lowry, O. H., Brown, J. G., and Carter, J. C., 1972, The turnover of protein in discrete areas of rat brain, *Biochem. J.* **126:**351–359.

47. Bedoya, F., Meglasson, M., Wilson, J., and Matschinsky, F., 1985, Radiometric oil well assay for glucokinase in microscopic structures, *Anal. Biochem.* **144:**504–513.

48. Trus, M., and Matschinsky, F. M., 1980, Hexokinase and glucokinase distribution in the liver lobule, *J. Histochem. Cytochem.* **28:**579–591.

49. Matschinsky, F. M., Passonneau, J. V., and Lowry, O. H., 1968, Quantitative histochemical analysis of glycolytic intermediates and cofactors with an oil well technique, *J. Histochem. Cytochem.* **16:**29–39.

50. Steiner, A. L., 1974, Assay of cyclic nucleotides by radioimmunoassay methods, *Methods Enzymol.* **38:**96–105.

51. Rubin, E. H., and Ferrendelli, J. A., 1977, Distribution and regulation of cyclic nucleotide levels in cerebellum, *in vivo*, *J. Neurochem.* **29:**43–51.

52. Godfrey, D. A., Hallcher, L. M., Laird, M. M., Matschinsky, F. M., and Sherman, W. H., 1982, Distribution of myoinositol in the cat cochlear nucleus, *J. Neurochem.* **38:**939–947.

53. MacGregor, L. C., and Matschinsky, F. M., 1984, An enzymatic fluorimetric assay for myoinositol, *Anal. Biochem.* **141:**382–389.

54. MacGregor, L., and Matschinsky, F. M., 1985, In preparation.

55. Sussman, I., MacGregor, L., and Matschinsky, F. M., 1985, In preparation.

56. Somlyo, A. P., Somlyo, A. V., and Shuman, H., 1979, Electron probe analysis of vascular smooth muscle: Composition of mitochondria, nuclei and cytoplasm, *J. Cell Biol.* **81:**316–335.

57. Somlyo, A. V., Gonzalez-Serratos, H. Shuman, H., McClellan, G., and Somlyo, A. P., 1980, Calcium release and ionic changes in the sarcoplasmic reticulum of tetanized muscle: An electron probe study, *J. Cell Biol.* **90:**577–594.

58. Jungermann, K., and Katz, N., 1982, Functional hepatocellular heterogeneity, *Hepatology* **2:**385–395.

59. Shank, R. E., Morrison, G., Cheng, C. H., Karl, I., and Schwartz, R., 1959, Cell heterogeneity within the hepatic lobule (quantitative histochemistry), *J. Histochem. Cytochem.* **7:**237–239.

60. McDonald, B. E., and Johnson, B. C., 1965, Metabolic response to realimentation following chronic starvation in the adult male rat, *J. Nutr.* **87:**161–167.

61. Tsukuda, T., Thurman, R. G., and Kauffman, F. C., 1983, Effect of inducing agents on the distribution and kinetic properties of UPD-glucuronosyl transferase in periportal and pericentral zones of the liver, *Fed. Proc. Fed. Am. Soc. Exp. Biol.* **42:**912.

62. Sokolove, P. M., Wilcox, M. A., Thurman, R. G., and Kauffman, F. C., 1984, Stimulation of hepatic microsomal β-glucuronidase by calcium, *Biochem. Biophys. Res. Commun.* **121:**987–993.

63. Ullrich, D., Fischer, G., Katz, N., and Bock, K. W., 1984, Intralobular distribution of UDP-glucuronosyltransferase in livers from untreated, 3-methylcholanthrene- and phenobarbital-treated rats, *Chem.-Biol. Interact.* **48:**181–190.

64. Jungermann, K., Heilbronn, R., Katz, N., and Sasse, D., 1982, The glucose/glucose-6-phosphate cycle in the periportal and perivenous zone of rat liver, *Eur. J. Biochem.* **123:**429–436.

Chapter 6

Separation of Functionally Different Liver Cell Types

Kai O. Lindros, Gunnar Bengtsson, Mikko Salaspuro, and
Hannu Väänänen

1. INTRODUCTION

It is becoming increasingly evident that the mammalian liver is more heterogeneous than was previously thought.[1,2] Among the functionally different
cell types identified, the hepatocytes (parenchymal cells) contribute more than
90% to the total volume occupied by liver cells.[3,4] The nonhepatocytes or nonparenchymal cells are much smaller than the hepatocytes and constitute about
40% of the cells by number. They consist of sinusoidal cells, i.e., Kupffer cells,
endothelial cells, fat-storing cells, and pit cells (for reviews, see van Berkel[4]
and Zahlten et al[5]) and of cells from the vascular trees.[6] Our present knowledge
of hepatic cell heterogeneity is based mainly on microscopy combined with
morphometry, histochemistry, autoradiography, and immunofluorescence. Although many functional characteristics of various cell types have been revealed
with these techniques, they exclude studies on metabolic dynamics. Regulation
of synthetic and catabolic pathways and functional coordination among the different cell types are best studied by means of isolated intact cells. Basic functions

KAI O. LINDROS, GUNNAR BENGTSSON, MIKKO SALASPURO, and HANNU VÄÄNÄNEN • Research Laboratories of the Finnish State Alcohol Company, Alko, Ltd., SF-00101 Helsinki 10, Finland.   Dr.
Bengtsson's present address is National Institute of Forensic Toxicology, N-0372 Oslo, Norway.

of the liver—e.g., the uptake and metabolism of xenobiotics, the maintenance of blood glucose homeostasis, the regulation of plasma protein synthesis, the production of lipoproteins, and the development of pathological states such as fibrosis—are all better understood through studies of separated cell types. It is therefore not unexpected that the existence of enzymatic techniques for dispersion of tissue into isolated intact cells has provoked the development of techniques for the subsequent isolation of various cell types.

Hepatic cells can also be subdivided on the basis of their original location within the acinus. Since the morphological differences among cells from different acinar zones are far from distinct, their separation must be verified biochemically, on the basis of the metabolic heterogeneity within the acinus. Convincing evidence for biochemical differences between the periportal (afferent) and perivenous (efferent) part of the acinus has been provided by microbiochemical enzyme activity analysis of subacinar samples obtained by microdissection (for reviews, see Jungermann and Katz[2] and Jungermann and Sasse[7]). Separation of intact cells according to their acinar locations is, however, more difficult than the separation of different cell types. Many previous attempts have failed, and not until recently has successful separation of hepatocytes from the different acinar zones been reported.

This review will outline current methods for dispersion of liver tissue into intact cells and the subsequent separation of the various functionally different cell types. Since separation of nonhepatocytes has been treated in several recent reviews,[4,5,8,9] this section will be brief, emphasizing only the most recent developments. Separation of hepatocytes into subclasses and the relationship to their acinar origin will be discussed in more detail, in view of the potential importance of this approach for studies on the metabolic heterogeneity in the liver acinus.

2. DISPERSION OF LIVER TISSUE INTO ISOLATED CELLS

To study the specific biochemical and physiological functions of cell types, isolated intact cells are needed so that they can be further characterized and cultured. Mechanical and chemical methods used in the past were crude and ineffective. The increased knowledge of the molecular basis for cell-to-cell adhesion has, however, immensely increased our possibilities for obtaining reasonably pure, intact cells from various tissues including liver.[10,11]

2.1. Mechanical and Chemical Methods

Methods used in general for the separation of cells from various tissues are applicable to the liver as well and have recently been reviewed by Waymouth.[11]

In the past, liver tissue was disrupted mechanically by mincing, slicing, pipetting, shaking with glass beads, homogenization with a loosely fitted pestle[12,13] or sieving through a coarse screen. The softness of liver tissue makes its mechanical disintegration easy, but the yield of isolated cells from these treatments is modest; more important, the vast majority of the cells are damaged, thus severely restricting their further use. These crude methods have now been succeeded by more sophisticated techniques.[9,11]

Although the exact nature of the forces that attach adjacent cells is still unclear, the role of the divalent cations Ca^{2+} and Mg^{2+} was recognized as early as 1900.[14] By removal of Ca^{2+} from the medium and/or the use of a chelator such as citrate, EDTA, or EGTA, the yield of isolated cells increased drastically due to the loosening of adhesive forces,[15] but the treatment still caused irreversible damage to most of the cells. Recently, however, Berry et al.[16] reported that a reasonably good yield of intact hepatocytes could be obtained by prolonged perfusion of the liver with Ca^{2+}-free medium supplemented with 2 mM EDTA followed by centrifugation through Percoll. Since the enzymatic digestion described below may affect receptor and other membrane functions,[13] this method may be useful. On the other hand the prolonged absence of calcium may have other irreversible effects on both hepatocytes and nonparenchymal cells.

2.2. Enzymatic Methods

Disintegration of tissue with trypsin or other proteolytic enzymes has been widely used for many years.[11] The crude trypsin preparations actually contain a number of different enzymes, such as chymotrypsin, elastase, collagenase, RNase, and amylase. The unspecific action of these preparations limits their use for preparation of intact isolated liver cells. Better results may be obtained with specific purified single enzymes. For the purpose of isolating liver cells, the collagenases are best because they hydrolyze the collagens of the extracellular connective tissue but do not affect the plasma membrane. In 1967–1968, Howard et al.[17,18] used a mixture of collagenase and hyaluronidase to release hepatocytes from liver slices. In 1969, Berry and Friend[19] were able to increase the yield of intact cells dramatically by perfusing the enzyme solution through the liver. The method based on this principle is now used routinely with some modifications in many laboratories. Seglen[9,20] demonstrated that the Ca^{2+}-free preperfusion need not contain a chelator, hyaluronidase can be omitted, and 4–5 mM Ca^{2+} should be added to the collagenase medium. Using this procedure, preferentially followed by incubation in oxygenated albumin–supplemented medium, a large yield of metabolically intact cells with normal morphology can be obtained. The suspension obtained contains hepatocytes and various types of sinusoidal cells. Depending on the purpose of the study, a specific type of cells can be further separated from the mixture by the methods described below.

3. SEPARATION OF HEPATOCYTES AND NONHEPATOCYTES

The collagenase perfusion method (see Section 2.2) gives a suspension of liver cells, and in addition, a whitish material constituting the vascular trees is obtained after sieving. From these two fractions, various liver cell types may be prepared (Fig.1), and of the "nonparenchymal" liver cells, sinusoidal cells and vascular nonhepatocytes are separated. If the method utilizes pieces of liver without a sieving step, all kinds of nonhepatocytes may be released.

3.1. Centrifugation Methods

Hepatocytes can be purified from a crude suspension of collagenase-released liver cells by repeated gentle differential centrifugation in fresh incubation medium, e.g., for 1, 0.5, and 0.5 min, respectively, at about $40 \times g$. Normally, 3–4 g of packed cells with a purity of 98% and a viability of 90–95% is produced from a 10-g rat liver. Sinusoidal cells can be prepared from the supernatants by differential centrifugation.[21] Higher yields of sinusoidal cells are obtained if the liver is disrupted at 0–5°C and if the centrifugations are done without preincubation of the cells. This prevents Kupffer cells from sticking to vessel walls or cell debris. Isopycnic centrifugation in metrizamide[22,23] or Percoll[24,25] has been used for separation of hepatocytes and nonhepatocytes.

3.2. Enzymatic Methods

By these methods, nonhepatocytes are prepared by selective destruction of hepatocytes with pronase, a mixture of proteolytic enzymes from *Streptomyces griseus,* or with enterotoxin from *Clostridium perfringens.* Using diced liver tissue, it is possible to prepare nonhepatocytes by incubation for 90 min with pronase.[26] A modification of this method includes perfusion with pronase solution before dicing and incubation.[27,28] Collagenase-released liver cells can also be used as a starting material for incubation with pronase[29] or enterotoxin.[30]

4. SEPARATION OF VARIOUS TYPES OF NONHEPATOCYTES

Methods for preparation of sinusoidal liver cells have been discussed at two international symposia, the First and the Second Kupffer Cell Symposia in Holland. Readers interested in this subject are referred to the proceedings[31,32] as well as to a comprehensive report from the second symposium.[33]

There is no method available yet for separation of all types of liver cells in high purity and yield from the same liver. With existing methods, the optimum conditions for preparation of one cell type include losses of other types. The scheme in Fig. 1 is theoretical but useful for discussion. If a preparation of

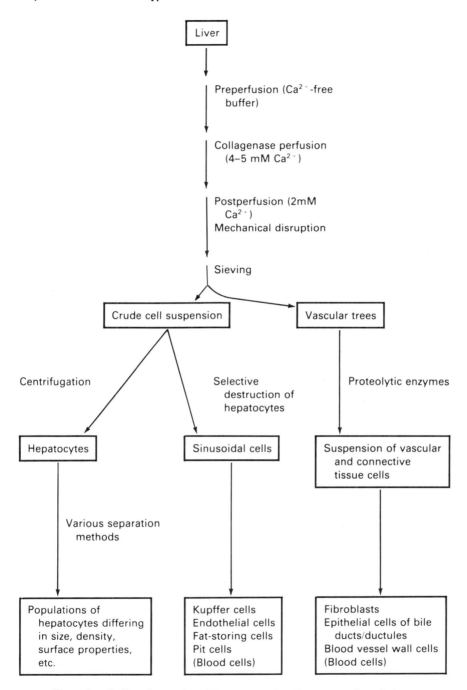

Figure 1. Outline of separation of hepatocyte and nonhepatocyte subpopulations.

mostly sinusoidal nonhepatocytes is desired, collagenase-released liver cells can be used for subsequent selective destruction of hepatocytes with pronase[29] or enterotoxin.[30] If, on the other hand, vascular nonhepatocytes are desired, the tissue retained after sieving should be treated with pronase. The degree of separation of sinusoidal and vascular nonhepatocytes by these methods is unclear. For example, the activity of various lysosomal enzymes, among them cathepsin D, which is enriched in Kupffer cells, was the same in both types of preparations.[34] Also, bile ductule cells were found in a typical sinusoidal cell preparation.[35]

4.1. Kupffer Cells and Endothelial Cells

Old methods depending on the specific loading of Kupffer cells with colloidal iron and other techniques will not be reviewed here. The modern methods include enzymatic digestion of the liver to release cells followed by removal of the hepatocytes (see Sections 3.1 and 3.2). Kupffer cells and endothelial cells can be separated from a suspension of sinusoidal cells by specific adherence of the Kupffer cells to glass[36] or by means of centrifugal elutriation.[37–40] An alternative method for preparation of endothelial cells consists of perfusion with pronase and with collagenase plus pronase, incubation of the resulting pastelike substance with collagenase plus pronase, and purification on a metrizamide cushion.[41] An interesting possibility is the separation of periportal and perivenous Kupffer cells by elutriation.[42]

It is important to choose the conditions for enzymatic digestion to avoid loss of specific surface receptors. For example, lipoprotein receptors are destroyed by pronase, but not by collagenase. Also, attachment of the separated cells to a substratum during culture may differ.[30,36]

4.2. Fat-Storing Cells and Pit Cells

Fat-storing cells contaminate preparations of Kupffer cells and endothelial cells separated by elutriation.[30,43] An approximately 70% pure preparation of fat-storing cells can be obtained by centrifugation of a suspension of sinusoidal cells (released by pronase plus collagenase) in a discontinuous metrizamide gradient followed by elutriation of a low-density cell population.[44]

Sleyster *et al.*[43] found pit cells in a certain population of elutriated sinusoidal liver cells, but to our knowledge no method has yet been developed for isolation of this cell type.

4.3. Cells from the Vascular Trees

Various blood cells are almost always found in preparations of nonhepatocytes, even though the liver is normally preperfused with a physiological solution to rinse out these cells. On the other hand, cells making up the walls of blood vessels and bile ductules are normally not observed. However, in one study, by centrifugation of nonhepatocytes released by collagenase plus hyaluronidase in metrizamide gradients, a band containing a mixture of bile ductule cells and Kupffer cells was obtained.[35] Biliary epithelial cells have also been enriched by centrifugal elutriation.[45]

5. SEPARATION OF PERIPORTAL AND PERIVENOUS HEPATOCYTES

5.1. Background

The accumulating awareness of the implications of acinar heterogeneity has focused interest on methods to separate cells from the periportal and the perivenous area. In principle, such attempts should be based either on their different location or, if a "total" cell suspension is first prepared, on zone differences between cells with respect to their morphological or surface properties.

To verify the origin of the separated cells, reliable markers indicating the identity of the cells are needed. Acinar gradients of a number of enzyme activities have been obtained by analysis of microdissected subacinar speciments.[7] The enzymes with the most pronounced activity differences have been used as markers for the acinar origin of isolated cell populations. A few studies have attempted prelabeling of cells in a specific acinar zone with fluorescent or radioactive compounds as a means of identifying released cells. Fluorescein diacetate, acridine orange, and rhodamine B are reported to bind predominantly to cells in the periportal area, while perivenous cells exhibited stronger fluorescence after perfusion with fluorescein isothiocyanate.[46,47] In addition, several attempts have been made to produce or strengthen intraacinar heterogeneity by suitable pretreatment of the donor animals to specifically change the content of smooth endoplasmic reticulum, glycogen, or neutral fat in one zone. [48-51]

5.2. Separation Based on Physicochemical Differences

Various sedimentation techniques separate cells according to size or density. Phase partitioning and receptor binding techniques are based on differences in cell surface properties. Free-flow electrophoresis separates cells according to their average charge. These techniques have been used in attempts to separate hepatocyte populations[9,52-55]

The average diameter of rat hepatocytes from various acinar zones is almost the same,[56] at least in rats younger than 6 months.[57] Ultrastructural differences have, however, been found. Perivenous cells contain more but smaller mitochondria and a larger proportion of smooth endoplasmic reticulum.[56-59] These differences should influence cell density, making isopycnic density-gradient centrifugation useful for separation of periportal and perivenous cells. The density is, however, much more influenced by the cell content of neutral fat and, to some extent, by the content of glycogen. The acinar distribution of fat and glycogen is commonly uneven and easily changed diurnally and with the nutritional state. The influence of fat and glycogen on the density distribution must therefore be carefully avoided, e.g., by depleting fat and glycogen stores as completely as possible before cell isolation.

5.2.1. Density-Gradient Centrifugation

Most of the procedures aimed at separating various hepatocyte populations after collagenase dissociation of the liver are based on differences in cell density, which is determined by the composition of the cell. As noted above, ultrastructural differences between periportal and perivenous hepatocytes exist, but they are not great enough to suggest that separate bands of isolated hepatocytes should be found in linear density gradients. Instead, a single-band distribution is expected.[9] With properly used density-gradient separation of cells, a high resolution of density is achieved.[60] Multiple bands have been observed in several studies.[48,61-63] These probably represent various degrees of cell damage caused by excessive centrifugal force or by using an unphysiological density-gradient medium.[64] Cell damage during centrifugation could also occur because the cells were not preincubated under physiological conditions and thus were not able to recover from the stress of collagenase perfusion and mechanical separation. Stepwise changes in the cellular contents of glycogen or neutral fat as a basis of multiple bands in normal livers seem unlikely. For instance, a 3-fold difference in lipid content between cells of high and low density did not result in separate bands.[65] Only under experimental conditions causing marked fat accumulation in some cells have separate bands been observed.[66] On the other hand, it must be stressed that hepatocytes derived from nonstarved rats have a rapid glycogen breakdown and that female rats accumulate lipid in the liver on starvation. Both these factors could change the distribution of cells within a single band. Therefore, the best liver donors are starved male rats.

A method giving a bell-shaped density distribution curve (Fig. 2A) and a separation of periportal and perivenous hepatocytes will be described here. For more details, see Bengtsson et al.[67]

Isolated hepatocytes are incubated 25 min at 37°C in a buffered salt solution containing 2% defatted bovine serum albumin before they are rapidly (within 7 min) mixed evenly into a linear, isoosmotic gradient of metrizamide. The gradient ($1.07-1.12$ g/cm^3) itself is formed in the same step. This procedure minimizes the danger of hypoxia and clumping of cells that occur when cells are added onto a layer at the top of a preformed gradient. Also, the "wall effect", i.e., the collision of peripheral cells with the wall of the centrifuge tube, is reduced. The risk of hypoxia is further reduced by keeping the temperature at 12°C during the

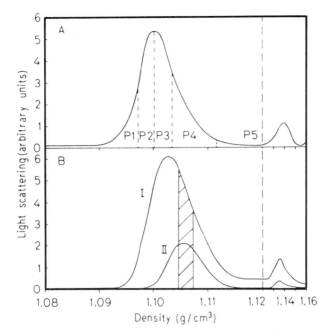

Figure 2. Distribution of hepatocytes in metrizamide gradients (A) and rebanding (B). (A) Enzymatically isolated hepatocytes from starved rats were separated according to density in linear metrizamide gradients with a bottom cushion (centrifugation for 5 min at 130*g*). Cell populations P1–P5 (dashed-line limits) were recovered and analyzed for biochemical parameters. The graph is the average of light-scattering records from ten experiments. The area under the curve is proportional to the recovered wet weight of cells derived from the cellocrit measurements, and unity on the ordinate indicates the average cell concentration in the gradient. The figure is drawn to anotheer scale above 1.12 g/cm^3 (dashed line) to correspond to the actual volume of the bottom cushion in relation to the gradient. (B) Isolated hepatocytes (350 mg wet weight of packed pellet) were centrifuged in a linear metrizamide gradient and recovered in 47 fractions (distribution curve I). A density population (diagonally hatched area) was washed and centrifuged in a second gradient (distribution curve II). (From Bengtsson et al.[67])

entire separation procedure. The gradient is centrifuged in a swing-out rotor for 5 min at 130 × *g*, allowing in addition 2 min for acceleration and 3 min for spontaneous deceleration. About 40 fractions are collected by upward fractionation through a conical lid. The cell concentration is continuously monitored in the effluent by light scattering. The gradient fractions may be combined into density populations of cells, which are subsequently washed free of gradient solution by centrifugation in incubation medium. The main band of hepatocytes is enriched in viable cells (about 95% excluding vital dyes), whereas most of the nonviable cells are found in the bottom pellet. With this method, about 300 mg of packed cells can be separated, and the recovery of cell protein is about

85%. For separation of more cells, several gradients may be run simultaneously.[65] The stability of the buoyant density of a population of cells by this gradient technique may be controlled by recentrifugation in a new gradient (Fig. 2B).

The density-resolved hepatocytes are divided into four bands designated P1–P4 (Fig. 2A). The distribution of intraacinar marker enzymes among these four density populations indicates that the low density cell population P1 is enriched in perivenous cells and P4 in periportal cells.[67]

In more recent experiments, enhanced separation was obtained, as shown by a P4/P1 ratio of 1.58 for alanine aminotransferase (ALAT) and of 0.85 for pyruvate kinase (PK) (Table 1). The individual variation in the marker enzyme ratios is large, but this is also true for results from microdissection studies.[68–71] By selecting the seven preparations with the highest value for the expression $(ALAT_{P4} \times PK_{P1})/(ALAT_{P1} \times PK_{P4})$, a P4/P1 ratio of 1.98 for ALAT and of 0.80 for PK is obtained (Table 1). These values approach the periportal/perivenous ratios derived from microdissection studies in fasted rats.[71–75] Also, the directions of acinar differences of lactate dehydrogenase, glutamate dehydrogenase, and isocitrate dehydrogenase in density-separated hepatocyte populations[76] agree with those in microdissected samples.[72,73] A direct comparison between the density-gradient and microdissection techniques would be necessary to better evaluate the degree of separation. Yet, the magnitude of the ratio P4/P1 for marker enzymes suggests that a considerable separation of periportal and perivenous hepatocytes occurred.

This method has been used to investigate the intraacinar heterogeneity of enzyme activities[67,77] and, in incubation experiments, to investigate protein metabolism.[76]

Studies using discontinuous "step" gradients have also been published.[50,51,78] These gradients produce pellicles of cells in the steps, which could hinder other cells from reaching their final positions. The technique is best used

Table 1. Marker Enzyme Activities in Hepatocyte Density Populations[a]

		Hepatocyte density populations				P4/ P1	Significance levels for P1 to P4 differences (2-way ANOVA)
N		P1	P2	P3	P4		
14	ALAT	300 ± 95	370 ± 60	443 ± 76	475 ± 89	1.58	$p < 0.001$
	PK	235 ± 80	220 ± 74	207 ± 57	200 ± 50	0.85	$p < 0.01$
7	ALAT	244 ± 54	366 ± 57	457 ± 48	484 ± 88	1.98	$p < 0.001$
	PK	267 ± 98	255 ± 86	228 ± 64	214 ± 57	0.80	$p < 0.005$

[a] Isolated rat hepatocytes were separated into four density populations (P1–P4) in linear metrizamide gradients (see Fig. 2). The values are means ± S.D. of the specific activities of alanine aminotransferase (ALAT) and pyruvate kinase (PK) derived from 14 different consecutive cell preparations. The values from 7 preparations with the highest ALAT/PK ratio of P4/P1 are also shown.

when it is evident that the cells form a nonbiased and reproducible density distribution in continuous gradients. For rat hepatocytes (at least from starved animals), our experience indicated that the variation in average density between individual rats is so high that the use of a standard discontinuous gradient is impractical.

Pretreatment of animals to alter the density of hepatocytes in a specific zone has been done with the aim of facilitating the separation. Thus, treatment with phenobarbital, which is known to cause proliferation of the smooth endoplasmic reticulum in perivenous cells,[48,49] has been tried.[62,79,80] The results from the study by Wanson et al.[49] indicate that better separation of periportal and perivenous hepatocytes may be achieved using this approach. The same laboratory also used pretreatment with glucose and insulin to permit separation according to glycogen content.[81] On the other hand, experimentally induced steatosis by chronic ethanol treatment caused lipid accumulation in hepatocytes scattered throughout the entire acinus.[66] Therefore, acinar separation was not achieved, although the lipid-laden cells formed a separate band in continuous metrizamide gradients. In one study, however we found an accumulation of lipid in periportal areas of both enthanol-treated and pair-fed control rats (seen on histological sections), and within a bell-shaped, single-band distribution, the low-density hepatocytes contained more than 3 times more lipid than the high-density hepatocytes.[65] To our knowledge, there is no standard way to facilitate separation of periportal and perivenous hepatocytes with density-gradient centrifugation by pretreatment of the donor animals. Furthermore, the pretreatment itself would limit the usefulness of the separated cells.

5.2.2. Velocity Sedimentation and Elutriation

While isopycnic centrifugation is based on density differences, velocity sedimentation and elutriation are based more on differences in size. The reader interested in details about theory and practice of these and related techniques is referred to a recent treatise.[82]

Several authors have fractionated hepatocytes using velocity sedimentation at unity gravity. Since cells are separated mainly on the basis of differences in size by this technique,[83] tetraploid cells, which are larger, can be separated from diploid cells.[84,85] Since there does not seem to be any clear distribution difference of ploidy within the acinus,[86] any separation of periportal and perivenous cells by this technique is doubtful.

Hepatocytes have also been separated by centrifugal elutriation,[55,87,88] but whether the isolated cell populations originated from different zones could not be established. Sumner et al.[46] attempted to label the acinar zones with fluorescent dyes, but the relationship between the elutriated cell populations and their acinar origin remains obscure.

5.2.3. Phase Partitioning and Free-Flow Electrophoresis

It is conceivable that cells from the afferent and efferent parts of the sinusoid differ with respect to their surface properties. Techniques based on such differences include free-flow electrophoresis, used by Miller et al.[52] for liver cell subfractionation, and partitioning between two aqueous polymers (for reviews, see Fisher[89] and Walter[90]). The latter technique, which is usually based on the use of a mixture of dextran and polyethyleneglycol, has been used extensively for separation of erythrocytes and other blood cells[90] and has also been used for fractionation of hepatocytes.[57] Application of this potentially useful separation method for periportal and perivenous cells must await evidence for differences in surface properties among cells from different acinar zones.

5.2.4. Receptor Affinity

Rojkind et al.[54] separated a population of hepatocytes having lectin receptors by adsorption to nylon concanavalin discs. Since these cells were reported to synthesize glycogen more effectively than unbound cells, and glycogen metabolism is known to be distributed unequally in the acinus,[91,92] the cells may have represented a specific acinar zone. Since there should be hormone concentration gradients along the sinusoid, differences in hormone-receptor density or affinity are also quite possible. Further attempts at acinar separation utilizing this principle may prove fruitful.

As discussed earlier, enchancement of separation of hepatocyte subpopulations has been attempted by pretreatment procedures that specifically alter either perivenous or periportal hepatocyte densities. Similarly, pretreatments that specifically alter cell surface properties including receptor density or affinity may become available.

5.3. Separation of Cells from Either Subacinar Zone

The methods described above for separation of subtypes of hepatocytes from a heterogeneous liver cell mixture are based on their physicochemical differences: An alternative approach to separate periportal and perivenous cells is to attempt liberation of intact cells from only one acinar zone. This can be done either by confining the digestive effect of collagenase to one acinar zone or by first selectively destroying the cells in one area and then digesting the remaining part of the liver.

5.3.1. Zone-Selective Collagenase Action

We have developed a method in our laboratory, which we call collagenase-gradient perfusion, for zone-specific collagenase digestion.[93] The essential steps of this method are summarized in Table II. The principle is to concentrate the

Table II. Outline of the Collagenase-Gradient Perfusion Technique

Step	Comment
1. Conventional portal preperfusion of the liver *in situ* with Ca^{2+}-free medium	Desmosomes are loosened. This improves the subsequent action of collagenase.
2. Collagenase-gradient perfusion: 2×6–7 ml/min for 6–7 min.	Medium is slowly pumped via both the portal and the hepatic veins. Collagenase is added to either medium.
3. Conventional portal postperfusion	To wash out the collagenase and reoxygenate the parenchyma.
4. Collection of liberated cells	The liver is rapidly sliced, the slices are agitated in buffer, and the slurry is filtered through nylon cloth.
5. Separation of intact cells	The separation of damaged and viable cells by three gentle ($30g$) centrifugations is facilitated by a brief trypsinization. Alternatively, single-step separation by centrifugation with 30% metrizamide may be used.

digestive effect of collagenase on either the afferent or the efferent part of the sinusoids. This is achieved by slow simultaneous ante-and retrograde pumping into the liver of the medium, which has to ooze out through the liver capsule. For separation of cells originating mainly from the periportal area, collagenase is added to the portally pumped medium. If cells from the perivenous area are desired, collagenase is added to the medium perfused via the hepatic veins. After partial collagenase digestion, which usually takes 5–6 min, the liver is washed with conventionally perfused oxygenated medium and then rapidly sliced. The cells from the areas affected by collagenase are liberated by shaking the slices and viable cells collected after trypsinization and purification by centrifugations.

With this method, a cell population with high viability clearly enriched from either the periportal or the perivenous area is obtained, as indicated from the activity distribution of marker enzymes (Table III). The success of separation is dependent, however, on several essential factors. Rapid, complete blanching of the liver during preperfusion with the Ca^{2+}-free medium is obligatory. Also, both the preperfusion time (usually 6–8 min) and the collagenase digestion time are critical factors, which in turn are influenced by the flow rate, the temperature, and the efficiency of the collagenase preparation. The hypoxia and the moderate swelling necessarily created during the period of slow bidirectional perfusion does not seem to cause any irreversible cell damage.

The penetration of the collagenase-containing medium into the desired area can be conveniently monitored by addition of a dye, such as blue dextran, to the medium.[94] A successful portal collagenase perfusion is characterized by a distinct polygonal dye network, visualizing the periportal areas surrounding the subcapsular terminal hepatic venules (Fig. 3A). The converse coloration is ob-

Table III. Distribution of Alanine Aminotransferase (ALAT), Glutamate Dehydrogenase (GLDH), and Pyruvate Kinase (PK) in Periportal (pp) and Perivenous (pv) Hepatocytes Isolated by the Collagenase-Gradient Perfusion Technique[a]

Enzyme	pp		pv		pp/pv ratio
	N	Content (U/mg prot.)	N	Content (U/mg prot.)	
ALAT	5	0.63 ± 0.14	5	0.33 ± 0.12[b]	1.89
GLDH	5	0.75 ± 0.07	5	1.05 ± 0.10[c]	0.71
PK	3	0.76 ± 0.14	5	1.43 ± 0.33[d]	0.53

[a] From Väänänen and Lindros.[97] Values are means ± S.D. of the numbers of experiments (N) indicated.
[b–d] Significant pp/pv differences: [b] $p < 0.1$; [c] $p < 0.0001$; [d] $p < 0.05$.

served during perfusion with collagenase and the dye from the hepatic venous direction (Fig. 3B).

Although the differences in activities of the marker enzymes analyzed from periportal and perivenous preparations, respectively, clearly demonstrate the enrichment of cells from either area, we do not know the exact magnitude of the original *in vivo* marker enzyme gradients in a particular series of experiments. The enzyme gradients vary diurnally, with the feeding state,[95] with age, and most probably among strains. Therefore, as with the density-gradient method, the degree of separation achieved can be only roughly estimated.

Although the proportion of damaged cells in the initial suspension is substantial (70–90%), the yield of intact cells obtained after purification (normally 0.1–0.5 g packed cells) is large enough to permit conventional analysis of a large number of enzyme activities.[96] Furthermore, the yield is usually large enough to permit metabolic studies by incubation experiments.[97] The yield of purified cells from the perivenous area is usually smaller than when cells from the periportal area are prepared. This may be associated with the unphysiological retrograde perfusion direction. Using a double dye infusion technique during the bidirectional perfusion, we found evidence for a distension of the portal tree relative to the hepatic venous tree, even though the portal and venous pressures were similar.[94] Thus, limited collagenase penetration could explain the lower perivenous cell yields.

5.3.2. Separation after Zone-Specific Cell Destruction

Häusing et al.[98] studied acinar heterogeniety by zone-specific destruction of the perfused liver with CCl_4. Quistorff et al.[99] used the cholesterol complexing agent digitonin for the same purpose, but in neither study were cells isolated. However, during the preparation of this review, both our laboratory[100] and Quistorff[101] demonstrated that intact cells from one acinar region are obtained by first destroying the plasma membranes of cells in one region by a brief pulse of digitonin and then collecting the remaining intact cells after conventional

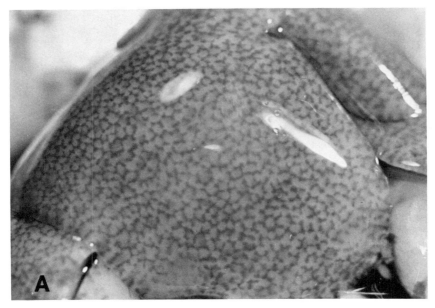

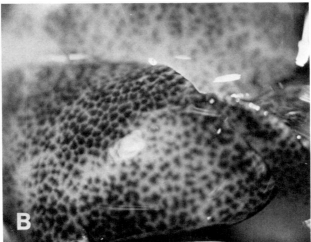

Figure 3.   Pattern of the liver surface after addition of trypan blue and collagenase to either the portal (A) or the hepatic venous (B) medium during bidirectional closed collagenase-gradient perfusion. (A) During portal collagenase addition, a distinct polygonal dye network appeared. (B) On the other hand, when the dye was added to medium perfused via the hepatic veins, a complementary pattern with dark spots appeared.

collagenase perfusion. Compared to the collagenase gradient technique, the selectivity is slightly less, but the yield is higher and it is much more reproducible. This method opens new possibilities to characterize the periportal and perivenous hepatocytes.

6. CONCLUSIONS

The different types of cells in the liver were histologically identified and characterized several decades ago, but only during the last 15 years have methods to isolate intact cells and separate the various cell types become available. With various proteolytic enzymes and/or centrifugation and sedimentation techniques, hepatocytes can be separated from the much smaller sinusoidal cells. Recently, methods for further separation of Kupffer cells, endothelial cells, and fat-storing cells have been developed. Most probably, methods for isolation of other nonhepatocyte cells such as pit cells and bile ductule cells will be developed in the near future. These methods enable us to characterize the cell types enzymatically and to study their participation and role in various vital hepatic functions by incubation and culture experiments.

Although the acinus is a histologically well-characterized entity, only recently has convincing evidence for its metabolic heterogeneity been obtained. Acinar activity gradients for a number of enzymes have been established by analysis of microdissected subacinar samples, but intact cells cannot be isolated with this technique. Most of the attempts to separate cells from a mixture of hepatocytes according to their acinar origin have been unsuccessful. Nevertheless, by careful low-speed isopycnic high-resolution density-gradient centrifugation of a hepatocyte suspension from starved male rats, populations clearly enriched in cells from either the periportal or the perivenous area have been separated. With this method, the recovery of cells is high and cells from all acinar zones are obtained from the same liver. The possible unequal acinar distribution of fat, glycogen, and other constituents that influence density may, on the other hand, restrict the use of this method.

The collagenase-gradient technique, based on regiospecific tissue digestion, produces cells highly enriched from one zone, but the yield is variable and modest. With the digitonin-collagenase technique the yield is much larger and the zone-specificity is still good. However, with either technique, only cells from one region are obtained.

These methods allow a comparision of functions of intact hepatocytes derived from either acinar zone. The two methods to isolate cells from one acinar region should also be useful for separation of sinusoidal cells from one region, thus allowing studies on the role of these cell types in acinar heterogeneity.

The possibility of obtaining reasonably pure cell preparations of a specific type opens new dimensions. For instance, by culturing specific cell populations in the presence of various xenobiotics, we will learn more about the mechanisms of cell specificity in drug toxicity. Incubation or culture of separated periportal and perivenous hepatocytes under identical conditions will establish the extent to which their initial enzyme activity differences result from their different sinusoidal microenvironments. The functional cooperation between two types of cells can be studied by their coculture. Such studies are already in progress.

It is clear that these recent methodological advances have vastly increased our possibilities for studying the interactions among cell types and within the acinus. These tools will help us to learn more about how the liver functions under normal and pathological conditions.

7. SUMMARY

This chapter has described recent development in methods to isolate or enrich the various cell types with specialized functions from the liver after its disintegration. Most commonly, a heterogeneous suspension containing various cell types is obtained after perfusing the liver with collagenase to digest the intercellular connective tissue. Hepatocytes are conveniently separated from the much smaller nonhepatocytes (sinusoidal cells) by centrifugation. Recently developed techniques base on sedimentation, on adsorption differences, or on selective enzymatic destruction enable further separation of the various nonhepatocyte types. The increased attention given to acinar metabolic heterogeneity has stimulated attempts to separate intact cells from different zones of the acinus. Partial separation of periportal and perivenous hepatocytes is achieved by careful density-gradient centrifugation. Populations highly enriched in cells from one acinar region are obtained by the collagenase gradient technique or by the high-yield digitonin-collagenase perfusion technique.

These newly developed separation techniques enable the biochemical characterization of morphologically and functionally specific cell types of the liver. Furthermore, growth, differentiation, and regulatory properties of these cell types can be studied during their culture, thereby increasing our understanding of their specific functions and their complex interactions.

REFERENCES

1. Gumucio, J. J., and Miller, D. L., 1981, Functional implications of liver cell heterogeneity, *Gastroenterology* **80:**393–403.
2. Jungermann, K., and Katz, N., 1982, Functional hepatocellular heterogeneity, *Hepatology* **2:**385–395.
3. Blowin, A., Bolender, R. P., and Weibel, E. R., 1977, Distribution of organelles and membranes between hepatocytes and nonhepatocytes in the rat liver parenchyma: A stereological study, *J. Cell Biol.* **72:**441–445.

4. Van Berkel, T. J. C., 1982, Functions of hepatic non-parenchymal cells, in : *Metabolic Compartmentation* (H. Sies ed.), pp. 437–482, Academic Press, London.
5. Zahlten, R. N., Rogoff, T. M., and Steer, C. J., 1981, Isolated Kupffer cells, endothelial cells and hepatocytes as investigative tools for liver research, Fed. Proc. *Fed. Am. Soc. Exp. Biol* **40**:2460–2468.
6. Daoust, R., 1958, The cell population of liver tissue and the cytological reference bases, in: *Liver Function: A Symposium on Approaches to the Quantitative Description of Liver Function* (R. W. Brauer, ed.), Vol. 4, pp. 3–10, American Institute of Biological Science, Washington D. C.
7. Jungermann, K., and Sasse, D., 1978, Heterogeneity of liver parenchymal cells. *Trends Biochem. Sci.* **3**:198–202.
8. Böyrum, A., Berg, T., and Blomhoff, R., 1983, Fractionation of mammalian cells, in: *Iodinated Density Gradient Media: A Practical Approach* (D. Rickwood, ed.), pp. 147–171, IRL Press, Oxford.
9. Seglen, P. O., 1979, Disaggregation and separation of rat liver cells, in: *Cell Populations,* Vol. 9 (E. Reid ed.), pp. 25–46, Ellis Horwood, Chichester, England.
10. Kleinman, H. K., Klebe, R. J., and Martin, G. R., 1981, Role of collagenous matrices in the adhesion and growth of cells, *J. Cell Biol.* **88**:473–485.
11. Waymouth, C., 1982, Methods for obtaining cells in suspension from animal tissues, in: *Cell Separation* (T. G. Pretlow and T. P. Pretlow, eds), pp. 1–31, Academic Press, New York.
12. Takeda, Y., Ichihara, A., Tanioka, H., and Inoue, H., 1964, The biochemistry of animal cells, *J. Biol. Chem.* **239**:3590–3596.
13. Ramadori, G., Lenzi, M., Dienes, H. P., and Meyer zum Büschenfelde, K. H., 1983, Binding properties of mechanically and enzymatically isolated hepatocytes for IgG and C3, *Liver* **3**:358–368.
14. Herbst, C., 1900, Über das Auseinandergehen von Furchungs und Gewebezellen in kalkfreiem Medium, *Arch. Entwicklungsmech. Org.* **9**:424–463.
15. Andersson, N., 1953, The mass isolation of whole cells from rat liver, *Science* **117**:627–628.
16. Berry, M. N., Farrington, C., Grivel, A. R., and Wallace, P. G., 1983, Preparation of isolated hepatocytes in good yield without enzyme digestion, in: *Isolation, Characterisation, and Use of Hepatocytes* (R. A. Harris and N. W. Cornell, eds.), pp. 7–10, Elsevier, Amsterdam.
17. Howard, R. B., Christensen, A., Gibbs, F. A., and Pesch, L. A., 1967, The enzymatic preparation of isolated intact parenchymal cells from rat liver, *J. Cell Biol.* **35**:675–684.
18. Howard, R. B., and Pesch, L. A., 1968, Respiratory activity of intact isolated parenchymal cells from rat liver, *J. Biol. Chem.* **243**:3105–3109.
19. Berry, M. N., and Friend, D. S., 1969, High-yield preparation of isolated rat liver parenchymal cells, *J. Cell Biol.* **43**:506–520.
20. Seglen, P. O., 1976, Preparation of isolated rat liver cells, *Methods Cell Biol.* **13**:29–83.
21. Nilsson, M., and Berg, T., 1977, Uptake and degration of formaldehyde-treated ^{125}I-labelled human serum albumin in rat liver cells *in vivo* and *in vitro, Biochim. Biophys. Acta.* **497**:171–182.
22. Munthe-Kaas, A. C., and Seglen, P. O., 1974, The use of metrizamide as a gradient medium for isopycnic separation of rat liver cells, *FEBS Lett.* **43**:252–256.
23. Seglen, P. O., 1976, The use of metrizamide for preparation of rat-liver cells, in: *Biological Separations in Iodinated Density Gradient Media* (D. Rickwood, ed.), pp. 107–221, Information Retrieval, London.
24. Pertoft, H., Rubin, K., Kjellen, L., Laurent, T. C., and Klingeborn, B., 1977, The viability of cells grown or centrifuged in a new density gradient medium, Percoll, *Exp. Cell Res.* **110**:449–458.
25. Singh, B., Borrebaek, B., and Osmundsen, H., 1983, Separation of different cell populations of rat liver by density gradient centrifugation in a vertical rotor with self-generated Percoll gradients, *Acta Physiol. Scand.* **117**:497–505.
26. Mills, D. M., and Zucker-Franklin, D., 1969, Electron microscopic study of isolated Kupffer cells, *Am. J. Pathol.* **54**:147–166.

27. Roser, B., 1968, The distribution of intravenously injected Kupffer cells in the mouse, *J. Reticuloendothel. Soc.* **5**:455–471.

28. Knook, D. L., Sleyster, E. C., and van Noord, M. J., 1975, Changes in lysosomes during ageing of parenchymal and non parenchymal liver cells, *Adv. Exp. Med. Biol.* **53**:155–169.

29. Berg, T., and Boman, D., 1973, Distribution of lysosomal enzymes between parenchymal and Kupffer cells of rat liver, *Biochim. Biophys. Acta* **321**:585–596.

30. Blomhoff, R., Smedsrod, B., Eskild, W., Granum, P. E., and Berg, T., 1984, Preparation of isolated liver endothelial cells and Kupffer cells in high yield by means of an enterotoxin, *Exp. Cell Res.* **150**:194–204.

31. Wisse, E., and Knook, D. L. (eds.), 1977, Kupffer cells and other liver sinusoidal cells, in: *Proceedings of the International Kupffer Cell Symposium,* Noordwijkerhout, The Netherlands, Elsevier/North-Holland, Amsterdam, New York, and Oxford.

32. Knook, D. L., and Wisse, E. (eds.), 1982, *Sinusoidal Liver Cells,* Elsevier/North-Holland, Amsterdam, New York, and Oxford.

33. Jones, E. A., 1983, Hepatic sinusoidal cells: New insights and controversies, *Hepatology* **3**:259–266.

34. Van Berkel, T. J. C., Kruijt, J. K., and Koster, J. F., 1975, Identity and activities of lysosomal enzymes in parenchymal and non-parenchymal cells from rat liver, *Eur. J. Biochem.* **58**: 142–152.

35. Grant, A. G, and Billing, B. H., 1977, The isolation and characterization of a bile ductule cell population from normal and bile-duct ligated rat livers, *Br. J. Exp. Pathol.* **58**:301–310.

36. Munthe-Kaas, A. C., Berg, T., Seglen, P.O., and Seljelid, R., 1975, Mass isolation and culture of rat Kupffer cells, *J. Exp. Med.* **141**:1–10.

37. Knook, D. L., and Sleyster, E. C., 1976, Separation of Kupffer and endothelial cells of the rat liver by centrifugal elutriation, *Exp. Cell Res.* **99**:444–449.

38. Knook, D. L., Blansjaar, N., and Sleyster, E. C., 1977, Isolation and characterization of Kupffer and endothelial cells from the rat liver, *Exp. Cell Res.* **109**:317–329.

39. Praaning-van Dalen, D. P., and Knook, D. L., 1982, Quantitative determination of *in vivo* endocytosis by rat liver Kupffer and endothelial cells facilitated by an improved cell isolation method, *FEBS Lett.* **141**:229–232.

40. Nagelkerke, J. F., Barto, K. P., and van Berkel, T. J. C., 1983, *In vivo* and *in vitro* uptake and degradation of acetylated low density lipoprotein by rat liver endothelial, Kupffer, and parenchymal cells, *J. Biol. Chem.* **258**:12,221–12,227.

41. De Leeuw, A. M., Barelds, R. J., de Zanger, R., and Knook, D. L., 1982, Primary cultures of endothelial cells of the rat liver, *Cell Tissue Res.* **223**:201–215.

42. Sleyster, E. C., and Knook, D. L., 1983, Relation between localization and function of rat liver Kupffer cells, *Lab Invest.* **47**:484–494.

43. Sleyster, E. C., Westerhuis, F. G., and Knook, D. L., 1977, The purification of nonparenchymal liver cell classes by centrifugal elutriation, in: *Kupffer Cells and Other Sinusoidal Cells* (E. Wisse and D. L. Knook, eds.), pp. 289–298, Elsevier, Amsterdam.

44. Knook, D. L., and de Leeuw, A. M., 1982, Isolation and characterisation of fat-storing cells from the rat liver, in: *Sinusoidal Liver Cells* (D. L. Knook and E. Wisse, eds.), pp. 45–52, Elsevier, Amsterdam.

45. Yaswen, P., Hayner, N. T., and Fansto, N., 1984, Isolation of oval cells by centrifugal elutriation and comparison with other cell types purified from normal and preneoplastic livers, *Cancer Res.* **44**:324–331.

46. Sumner, J. G., Freedman, R. B., and Lodola, A., 1983, Characterisation of hepatocyte subpopulations generated by centrifugal elutriation, *Eur. J. Biochem.* **134**:539–545.

47. Gumucio, J. J., Miller, D. L., Krauss, M. D., and Zanolli, C. C., 1981, Transport of fluorescent compounds into hepatocytes and the resultant zonal labeling of the hepatic acinus in the rat, *Gastroenterology* **80**:639–646.

48. Gumucio, J. J., De Mason, L. J., Miller, D. L., Krezoski, S. O., and Keener, M., 1978, Induction of cytochrome P-450 in a selective subpopulation of hepatocytes, *Am. J. Physiol.* **234**:C102–C109.

49. Wanson, J.-C., Drochmans, P., May, C., Penasse, W., and Popowski, A., 1975, Isolation of centrolobular and perilobular hepatocytes after phenobarbital treatment, *J. Cell Biol.* **66**:23–41.

50. Tonda, K., Hasegawa, T., and Hirata, M., 1983, Effects of phenobarbital and 3-methylcholanthrene pretreatments on monooxygenase activities and proportions of isolated rat hepatocyte subpopulations, *Mol. Pharmacol.* **23**:235–243.

51. Tonda, K., and Hirata, M., 1983, Glucuronidation and sulfation of *p*-nitrophenol in isolated rat hepatocyte subpopulations: Effect of phenobarbital and 3-methylcholanthrene pretreatment, *Chem. Biol. Interact.* **47**:277–287.

52. Miller, S. B., Saccomani, G., Pretlow, T. P., Kimball, P. M., Scott, J. A., Sachs, G., and Pretlow, T. G., 1983, Purification of cells from livers of carcinogen-treated rats by free-flow electrophoresis, *Cancer Res.* **43**:4176–4179.

53. Walter, H., Krob, E. J., Ascher, G. S., and Seaman, G. V. F., 1973, Partition of rat liver cells in aqueous dextran–polyethylene glycol phase systems, *Exp. Cell Res.* **28**:15–26.

54. Rojkind, M., Portales, M. L., and Cid, M. E., 1974, Isolation of rat liver cells containing concanavalin A receptor sites, *FEBS Lett.* **47**:11–14.

55. Bernaert, D., Wanson, J.-C., Mosselmans, R., de Paermentier, F, and Drochmans, P., 1979, Separation of adult rat hepatocytes into distinct subpopulations by centrifugal elutriation: Morphological, morphometrical and biochemical characterisation of cell fractions, *Biol. Cell.* **34**:159–174.

56. Loud, A., 1968, A quantitative stereological description of the ultrastructure of normal rat liver parenchymal cells *J. Cell Biol.* **37**:27–46.

57. Schmucker, D. L., Mooney, J. S., and Jones, A. L., 1978, Stereological analysis of hepatic fine structure in the Fisher 344 rat: Influence of sublobular location and animal age, *J. Cell. Biol.* **78**:319–337.

58. Reith, A., and Schüler, B., 1971, The ultrastructure of mitochondria in relation to the lobular distribution of hepatocytes of the normal rat, *J. Ultrastruct. Res.* **36**:550–551.

59. Jones, A. L., Schmucker, D. L., Mooney, J. S., Adler, R. D, and Ockner, R. K., 1978, A quantitative analysis of hepatic ultrastructure in rats during enhanced bile secretion, *Anat. Rec.* **192**:277–288.

60. Leif, R. C., 1970, Buoyant density separation of cells, in: *Automated Cell Identification and Cell Sorting* (G. L. Wied and G. F. Bahr, eds.), pp. 21–95, Academic Press, New York and London.

61. Drochmans, P., Wanson, J.-C., and Mosselmans, R., 1975, Isolation and subfractionation on Ficoll gradients of adult rat hepatocytes, *J. Cell Biol.* **66**:1–22.

62. Castagna, M., and Chauveau, J., 1969, Séparation des hépatocytes isolés de rat en fractions cellulaires métaboliquement distinctes, *Exp. Cell Res.* **57**:211–222.

63. Bengtsson, G., Kiessling, K.-H., and Axelsson, K., 1978, Density subpopulations of isolated rat hepatocytes differ in alanine aminotransferase activity, *IRCS Med Sci.* **6**:119.

64. Wakefield, J. St J., Gale, J. S., Berridge, M. V., Jordan, T. W., and Ford, H. C., 1982, Is Percoll innocuous to cells?, *Biochem. J.* **202**:795–797.

65. Bengtsson, G., Smith-Kielland, A., and Morland, J., 1984, Ethanol effects on protein synthesis in nonparenchymal liver cells, hepatocytes, and density populations of hepatocytes, *Exp. Mol. Pathol.* **41**:44–57.

66. Kondrup, J., Bro, B., Dich, J., Grunnet, N., and Thieden, H. I. D., 1980, Fractionation and characterisation of rat hepatocytes isolated from ethanol-induced fatty liver, *Lab. Invest.* **43**:182–190.

67. Bengtsson, G, Kiessling, K.-H., Smith-Kielland, A., and Morland, J., 1981, Partial separation and biochemical characteristics of periportal and perivenous hepatocytes from rat liver, *Eur. J. Biochem.* **118**:591–597.

68. Katz, N., Teutsch, H. F., Jungermann, K., and Sasse, D, 1977, Heterogeneous reciprocal localization of fructose-1,6-bishosphatase and of glucokinase in microdissected periportal and perivenous rat liver tissue, *FEBS Lett.* **83**:272–276.

69. Katz, N., Teutsch, H. F., Sasse, D., and Jungermann, K., 1977, Heterogeneous distribution of glucose-6-phosphatase in microdissected periportal and perivenous rat liver tissue, *FEBS Lett.* **76**:226–230.

70. Teutsch, H. F., and Rieder, H., 1979, NADP-dependent dehydrogenases in rat liver parenchyma. II. Comparison of qualitative and quantitative G6PDH distribution patterns with particular reference to sex differences, *Histochemistry* **60**:43–52.

71. Zierz, S., Katz, N. and Jungermann, K., 1983, Distribution of pyruvate kinase type L and M2 in microdissected periportal and perivenous rat liver tissue with different dietary states, *Hoppe-Seyler's Z. Physiol. Chem.* **364**:1447–1453.

72. Shank, R. E., Morrison, G., Cheng, C.H., Karl, I., and Schwartz, R., 1959, Cell heterogeneity within the hepatic lobule (quantitative histochemistry), *J. Histochem. Cytochem.* **7**:237–239.

73. Morrison, G. R., Brock, F. E., Karl, I. E., and Shank, R. E., 1965, Quantitative analysis of regenerating and degenerating areas within the lobule of the carbon tetrachloride-injured liver, *Arch Biochem. Biophys.* **111**:448–460.

74. Welsh, F. A, 1972, Changes in distribution of enzymes within the liver lobule during adaptive increases, *J. Histochem. Cytochem.* **20**:107–111.

75. Guder, W. G., and Schmidt, U., 1976, Liver cell heterogeneity: The distribution of pyruvate kinase and phosphoenolpyruvate carboxykinase (GTP) in the liver lobule of fed and starved rats, *Hoppe-Seyler's Z. Physiol. Chem.* **357**:1793–1800.

76. Smith-Kielland, A., Bengtsson, G., Svendsen, L., and Morland, J., 1982, Protein synthesis in different populations of rat hepatocytes separated according to density, *J. Cell Physiol.* **110**:262–266.

77. Bengtsson, G., and Gadeholt, G, 1981, The intra-acinar distribution of superoxide dismutase, NADPH-cytochrome *c* reductase and cytochrome *c* oxidase (using rat hepatocytes), *Acta Pharmacol. Toxicol.* **49**(Suppl. 4), Abstract 37.

78. Weigand K., Otto, I., and Schopf, R., 1974, Ficoll density separation of enzymatically isolated rat liver cells, *Acta Hepato-Gastroenterol.* **21**:245–253.

79. Burger, P. C., and Herdson, P. B., 1966, Phenobarbital-induced fine structural changes in rat liver, *Am. J. Pathol.* **48**:793–809.

80. Weigand, K., Richter, E., and Esperer, H.-D., 1977, Biochemical studies of isolated rat hepatocytes from normal and phenobarbital-treated liver as obtained by rate zonal centrifugation, *Acta Hepato-Gastroenterol.* **24**:170–174.

81. Russo, E., Drochmans, P., Penasse, W., and Wanson, J. C., 1975, Heterogeneous distribution of glycogen within the (rat) liver lobule, induced experimentally, *J. Submicrosc. Cytol.* **7**:31–45.

82. Pretlow, T. G, and Pretlow, T. P., 1982, Sedimentation of cells: An overview and discussion of artifacts, in: *Cell Separation* (T. G. Pretlow, and T. P. Pretlow, eds.), pp. 41–61, Academic Press, New York.

83. Wells, J. R., 1982, A new approach to the separation of cells at unit gravity, in: *Cell Separation* (T. G. Pretlow and T. P. Pretlow, eds.), pp. 169–191, Academic Press, New York.

84. Tulp, A., Welagen, J. J. M. N., and Emmelot, P., 1976, Separation of intact rat hepatocytes and rat liver nuclei into ploidy classes by velocity sedimentation at unit gravity, *Biochim. Biophys. Acta* **451**:567–582.

85. Deschenes, J., Valet, J.-P., and Marceau, N., 1981, The relationship between cell volume, ploidy, and functional activity in differentiating hepatocytes, *Cell Biophys.* **3**:321–334.

86. Epstein, C. J., 1967, Cell size, nuclear content, and the development of polyploidy in the mammalian liver, *Proc. Natl. Acad. Sci. U.S.A.* **57**:327–334.

87. Le Rumeur, E., Guguen-Guillouzo, C., Beaumont, C., Saunier, A., and Guillouzo, A., 1983, Albumin secretion and protein synthesis by cultured diploid and tetraploid rat hepatocytes separated by elutriation, *Exp. Cell Res.* **147**:247–256.

88. Wanson, J.-C., Bernaert, D., Penasses, W., Mosselmans, R., and Bannasch, P., 1980, Separation in distinct subpopulations by elutriation of liver cells following exposure of rats to *n*-nitrosomorpholine, *Cancer Res.* **40**:459–471.

89. Fisher, D., 1981, The separation of cells and organelles by partitioning in two-polymer aqueous phases, *Biochem. J.* **196**:1–10.

90. Walter, H., 1982, Separation and subfractionation of blood cell populations based on their surface properties by partitioning in two polymer aqueous phase systems, in: *Cell Separation* (T. G. Pretlow and T. P. Pretlow, eds.), pp. 261–301, Academic Press, New York.

91. Sasse, D., 1975, Dynamics of liver glycogen: The topochemistry of glycogen synthesis, glycogen content and glycogenolysis under the experimental conditions of glycogen accumulation and depletion, *Histochemistry* **45**:237–254.

92. Richards, W. L., and van Potter, R., 1980, Scanning microdensitometry of glycogen zonation in the livers of rats adapted to a controlled feeding schedule and to 30, 60, or 90% casein diets, *Am. J. Anat.* **157**:71–85.

93. Väänänen, H., Lindros, K. O., and Salaspuro, M., 1983, Selective isolation of intact periportal or perivenous hepatocytes by antero- or retrograde collagenase gradient perfusion, *Liver* **3**:131–139.

94. Bengtsson, G., and Lindros, K., 1984, Dye infusion to evaluate the efficiency of the collagenase gradient perfusion for isolation of periportal and perivenous hepatocytes, *Acta Pharmacol. Toxicol.* **55**:(Suppl. I):4.

95. Sasse, D. Katz, N. and Jungermann, K., 1975, Functional heterogeneity of rat liver parenchyma and of isolated hepatocytes, *FEBS Lett.* **57**:83–88.

96. Väänänen, H., Salaspuro, M., and Lindros, K., 1984, The effect of chronic ethanol ingestion on ethanol metabolizing enzymes in isolated periportal and perivenous rat hepatocytes, *Hepatology* **4**:862–866.

97. Väänänen, H. and Lindros, K., 1985, Comparison of ethanol metabolism in isolated periportal or perivenous hepatocytes: Effects of chronic ethanol treatment, *Alcoholism, Clin. Exptl. Res.* **9**:315–322.

98. Häussinger, D., and Gerok, W., 1983, Hepatocytes heterogeneity in glutamate uptake by isolated rat liver, *Eur. J. Biochem.* **136**:421–425.

99. Quistorff, B., Grunnet, N. and Cornell, N., 1985, Digitonin perfusion of rat liver. A new approach in the study of intra-acinar and intracellular compartmentation in the liver, *Biochem. J.* **226**:289–297.

100. Lindros, K., and Penttilä, K., 1985, Digitonin-collagenase perfusion for efficient separation of periportal or perivenous hepatocytes, *Biochem. J.* **228**:757–760.

101. Quistorff, B., 1985, Gluconeogenesis in periportal and perivenous hepatocytes, isolated by a new high-yield digitonin/collagenase perfusion technique, *Biochem. J.* **229**:221–226.

Chapter 7

New Micromethods for Studying Sublobular Structure and Function in the Isolated, Perfused Rat Liver

John J. Lemasters, Sungchul Ji, and Ronald G. Thurman

1. INTRODUCTION

Periportal and pericentral (centrilobular) regions of the liver lobule differ with respect to ultrastructure, metabolism, and pathology.[1–3] These differences are most striking in the response of the liver to various hepatotoxins.[4] Some toxins (e.g., ethanol and carbon tetrachloride) cause selective damage to centrilobular areas, while others (e.g., allyl alcohol) injure periportal regions predominantly. In part, these differences among various regions of the liver lobule may reflect gradients of oxygen, metabolites, and hormones that are established as blood flows through the living lobule. They may also result from intrinsic differences in enzymes, cofactors, and metabolic intermediates in different regions of the liver lobule. A better understanding of hepatic function in health and disease requires that more knowledge about microheterogeneity within the liver lobule be obtained.

JOHN J. LEMASTERS • Laboratories for Cell Biology, Department of Anatomy, School of Medicine, University of North Carolina, Chapel Hill, North Carolina 27514.   SUNGCHUL JI • Department of Pharmacology and Toxicology, College of Pharmacy, Rutgers University, Piscataway, New Jersey 08854.   RONALD G. THURMAN • Department of Pharmacology, School of Medicine, University of North Carolina, Chapel Hill, North Carolina 27514.

1.1. Criteria for Direct, Dynamic Measurements of Sublobular Events with Miniature Probes

With increasing miniaturization of biophysical and physiological probes, it is now possible to monitor directly intralobular gradients and the metabolism of cells in different parts of the liver lobule. The minimal criteria for such measurements are:

1. The probe (measuring device) must be small enough to be placed within discrete portions of the liver lobule. Since the liver lobule is 700–1000 μm in diameter, the diameter of the probe should be less than 200 μm.
2. The miniature probe must be sensitive enough to respond to changes in only a few hundred hepatocytes.
3. Last, there must be a means by which the miniaturized probe can be positioned accurately within identified regions of the liver lobule.

If these criteria can be met, then gradients within the lobule and intralobular differences in metabolism can be determined.

2. MINIATURE PROBES

We have employed two miniaturized probes in our studies of intralobular oxygen gradients and sublobular metabolism: a two-fiber micro-light guide and a miniature Clark-type oxygen electrode.

2.1. Micro-Light Guide

In 1977, Ji, working in Chance's laboratory at the Johnson Foundation, developed a two-fiber micro-light guide that enabled the measurement of NADH fluorescence from small regions of the liver surface.[5] In Chapel Hill, the design was refined by gluing the tips of two optical fibers side by side with epoxy such that the tip was fully visible and amenable to precise positioning (Fig. 1A).[6] A scanning electron micrograph of this micro-light guide is shown in Fig. 1B. The modified micro-light guide possesses an excitation–collection tip approximately 170 μm in diameter, much smaller than the average diameter of the liver lobule. For measurement of NADH fluorescence (Fig. 2), one of the two fibers is connected to a near-UV light source (100-watt mercury arc lamp, Illumination Industries, Inc., Sunnyvale, California) and the other fiber to a photomultiplier (EMI Type 9824B). The first fiber illuminates the tissue with the 366 nm mercury arc line isolated with a Corning glass filter No. 5840. The second fiber collects fluorescence ($\geq$ 450 nm), which is passed through Kodak gelatin filters 2E and 47 to a photomultiplier. The signal from the photomultiplier is amplified by conventional electronics and recorded. With the selection of appropriate wave-

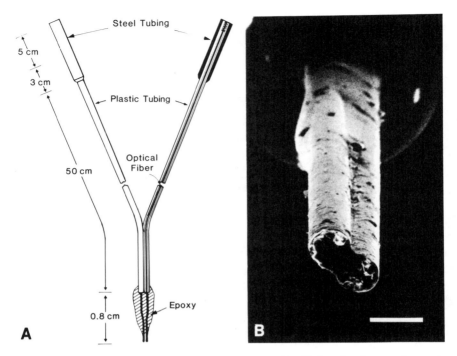

Figure 1. (A) Schematic representation of the micro-light guide. (B) Scanning electron micrograph of a retired micro-light guide. Scale bar: 100 μm.

lengths, other fluorescence signals can also be monitored from native and introduced fluorophores.

2.1.1. Tissue Volume Monitored by the Micro-Light Guide

If a single optical fiber is positioned against a tissue surface, a portion of that tissue will be illuminated by light conducted within the fiber. In liver and many other tissues, illumination with near-UV light (366 nm mercury line) causes a visible blue fluorescence with a broad peak around 450 nm originating mainly from NADH. To determine the distribution of fluorescence within hemoglobin-free, perfused livers, the tissues were cut into thick slices (3–6 mm), and an optical fiber was positioned against the liver surface just below the cut edge (Fig. 3). Near-UV light transmitted through an optical fiber produced a spot of blue light that was readily visible on the cut edge of the tissue slice. From photomicrographs of tissue slices positioned in this manner, the distribution of fluorescence excited by the micro-light guide within the tissue was quantified by densitometry (Fig. 4). Tissue fluorescence was gaussian in the plane parallel to the surface. In the axial direction, the distribution of fluorescence was skewed

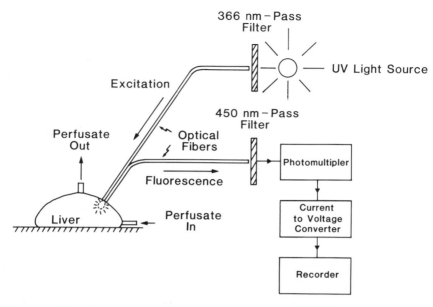

Figure 2. Schematic representation of apparatus used to measure NADH fluorescence from periportal and pericentral regions of the perfused liver. Filtered UV light is directed to the surface of the liver via a single glass optical wave guide, 80 μm in diameter. A second wave guide conducts fluorescent light to a photomultiplier, and the signal is continuously recorded.

toward the liver surface. Assuming symmetry around the axis, the tissue that absorbed 95% of the incident light formed an eccentric spheroid with dimensions of 330 μm × 225 μm × 225 μm having a total volume of about 9 nl (Fig. 5). Fluorescence was not distributed evenly within this volume. Half the emitted light originated from a region with dimensions of 170 μm × 110 μm × 110 μm and a volume of 1 nl.

To measure an optical signal from a tissue surface, two optical fibers are required, one to deliver exciting light and the other to collect reflected or fluorescent light. Assuming that the volume observed by the collection fiber is approximately the same size and shape as the volume illuminated by the excitation fiber, the dimensions of an overlap volume can be determined (Fig. 5). This overlap volume represents tissue that is both illuminated by the excitation fiber and observed by the collection fiber, i.e., the tissue that gives rise to the optical signal. The overlap of the volumes representing 95% of excitation light and 95% of collected light is a disk of tissue with dimensions of 290 μm × 120 μm × 195 μm and a total volume of about 3 nl. At about 100 hepatocytes/nl of liver parenchyma,[7] the micro-light guide collects information from an overlap volume that contains about 300 hepatocytes.

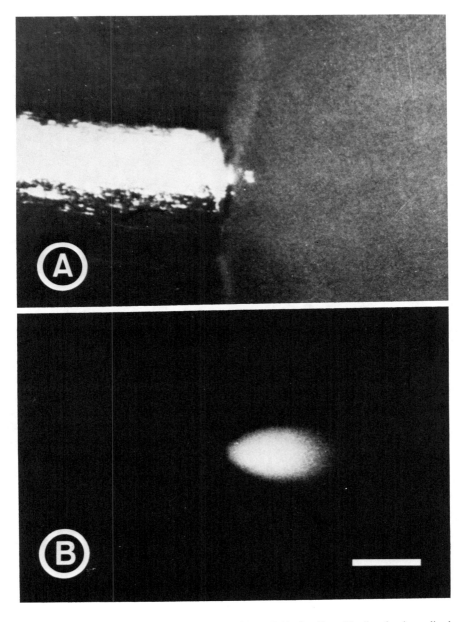

Figure 3. Micro-light guide applied to surface of hemoglobin-free liver. The liver has been sliced and is viewed from above the face of the cut. (A) Bright-field micrograph. (B) Visible fluorescence after excitation with 366 nm light through one of the optical fibers in the micro-light guide. Here, the micro-light guide is contained within steel tubing, 0.5 mm outside diameter. Scale bar: 250 μm.

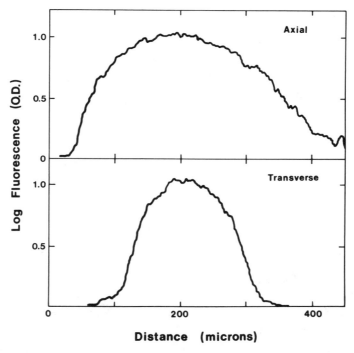

Figure 4. Densitometry of Fig. 3B illustrating the distribution of illumination from an 80-μm-diameter optical fiber.

2.2. Miniature Oxygen Electrode

For measurement of oxygen tensions within small volumes of tissue, a miniature oxygen electrode has been constructed (Fig. 6).[8] This electrode is made by inserting a 50-μm-diameter platinum wire into a glass capillary and pulling the capillary under heat with a vertical pipette puller (David Kopf Instruments, Tujunga, California, Model 700C). The middle section of the capillary stretches and breaks into needle-shaped pieces. Platinum wire fused in glass is exposed by gently tapping the tip against a smooth metal surface or by cutting the tip with a pair of scissors. An oxygen-permeable membrane is formed by covering the tip with a droplet of acrylic ester polymer (Rhoplex™, Rohm and Haas, Philadelphia, Pennsylvania) and drying it in air overnight. A connector is soldered to the platinum wire, and all but the tip of the electrode is covered with heat-shrinkable tubing to provide mechanical stability. The finished electrode has a tip diameter of 50–60 μm and is used in combination with an Ag–AgCl reference electrode. The electrodes are connected to a standard oxygen-electrode polarization and amplification circuit. Electrodes so prepared give linear calibration curves with aqueous standard solutions of varying oxygen tension. Only

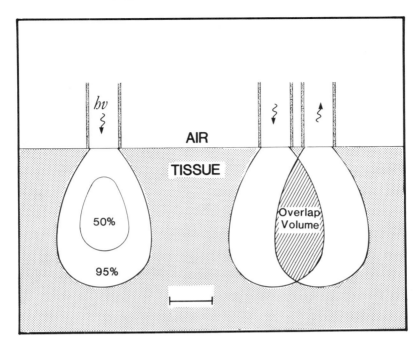

Figure 5.   Schematic representation of the volume illuminated by an 80-μm-diameter optical fiber and of the overlap volume of adjacent excitation and observation fibers. Tissue volumes receiving 95 and 50% of excitation light are 9 nl and 1 nl, respectively. The overlap of 95% of excitation light and 95% of observation light is 3 nl corresponding to the volume occupied by about 300 hepatocytes. Scale bar: 100 μm.

those electrodes with zero current less than 10% of the current generated by air-saturated saline are employed. Using these criteria, one half to three quarters of the electrodes constructed as described are discarded. Oxygen sensitivities range from 20 to 300 pA/torr at 37°C with a 90% response time of less than 10 sec.

2.2.1.   Calibration of the Miniature Oxygen Electrode

The current that flows through an oxygen-electrode polarization circuit as a result of reduction of oxygen at the platinum surface is a complex function of the geometry of the electrode and the diffusion and solubility coefficients of oxygen both in the tissue medium and in the oxygen-permeable membrane.[35,36] Since the diffusion and solubility coefficients of oxygen in tissue are different from the corresponding coefficients in dilute aqueous medium, the sensitivity of the electrode to oxygen may change when oxygen is measured at a tissue surface. To estimate electrode sensitivity at the tissue surface accurately, isolated, perfused livers were fixed with 1% paraformaldehyde to preserve microstructure

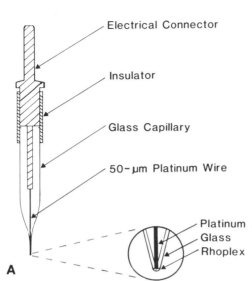

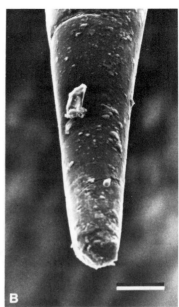

Figure 6. (A) Schematic representation of the miniature oxygen electrode. (B) Scanning electron micrograph of a retired miniature oxygen electrode. Scale bar: 100 μm.

but abolish oxygen uptake. A calibration curve for the electrode on the fixed liver surface was then obtained and compared to the calibration curve obtained in saline (Fig. 7). At equal oxygen tensions, current in the electrode circuit was about 3 times greater in saline than on the fixed tissue surface. Because of this marked difference in electrode sensitivity, each electrode must be calibrated on paraformaldehyde-fixed tissue at the conclusion of perfusion.

2.2.2. Tissue Volume Monitored by the Miniature Oxygen Electrode

Oxygen is reduced at the surface of polarized platinum with consequent movement of electrons through the polarization circuit. In the steady state, oxygen concentration at the electrode surface is virtually zero, and current through the electrode is proportional to the rate at which oxygen diffuses to its surface. Surrounding the active surface of the electrode is a small zone of low oxygen tension. The rate of oxygen diffusion to the electrode depends on the oxygen tension just outside the oxygen-depleted zone, and the size of the depleted zone corresponds to the volume monitored by the oxygen electrode.

In making sequential oxygen determinations, the miniature oxygen electrode is moved about the surface of the perfused liver (see Fig. 13). Each time the electrode makes contact with the liver, there is a transient surge of current that

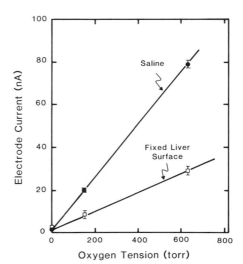

Figure 7. Calibration curves of the miniature oxygen electrode in saline and on the surface of paraformaldehyde-fixed liver. Vertical brackets indicate S.E.M.

decays rapidly to a steady-state value proportional to oxygen tension. The current surge most likely corresponds to the formation of an oxygen-depleted zone around the electrode; i.e., as oxygen is depleted in the vicinity of the electrode, extra current flows through the polarization circuit. Since two electrons flow for every atom of oxygen reduced, the oxygen extracted from the depleted zone can be calculated from the amount of extra charge flowing through the polarization circuit during this initial transient current surge. At a tissue O_2 concentration of 250 μM, this extra charge is of the order of 5×10^{-8} coulombs, corresponding to 2.5×10^{-13} g-atom of oxygen. This amount of oxygen is contained in 0.5 nl—the volume of measurement. The actual volume of measurement may be smaller than 0.5 nl, since other capacitance effects may add to the size of the initial current transient. As with the micro-light guide, the estimated volume of measurement for the miniature oxygen electrode is much smaller than the dimensions of the liver lobule and corresponds to the volume occupied by about 50 hepatocytes.

3. LOCALIZATION OF SUBLOBULAR REGIONS ON THE SURFACE OF PERFUSED LIVER

3.1. Models of Liver Lobular Structure

It has long been accepted that the liver is subdivided into histological units called lobules. This lobular structure has been interpreted in several ways, and three principal schemes have emerged: the classic lobule,[9] the portal lobule,[10] and the liver acinus[11] (see Chapter 1, Fig. 5). The classic lobule is a polyhedral prism of tissue about 0.7 mm × 2.0 mm in dimension. In humans, rodents, and many other species, the boundaries of the classic lobule are indistinct except for the more or less regular distribution of portal tracts containing branches of the portal vein, hepatic artery, and bile duct. A branch of the hepatic vein called the central vein lies at the center of the classic lobule. Radiating toward the central vein is an interconnecting system of parenchymal cell plates and specialized blood capillaries called sinusoids. Blood enters the periphery of the classic lobule from the portal tracts and flows through the lobule in sinusoids, leaving the lobule by the central vein. Bile flows in a countercurrent direction within tiny intercellular canaliculi. In cross section, the classic lobule is a hexagon. At each corner is a portal tract, and at the center is a central vein.

The portal lobule is a triangular prism of hepatic tissue derived from portions of three adjacent classic lobules. A portal tract lies at the center of the portal lobule. Central veins, now more appropriately called terminal hepatic venules, are at each of the three corners. Advocates of the portal lobule have argued that it better represents the functional unit of the liver, since all exocrine secretion of the portal lobule is drained by one duct, the bile duct of the portal duct.

The liver acinus of Rappaport[11] is the third scheme of hepatic lobular architecture. Proposed as the smallest functional unit of liver, the hepatic acinus is similar in some ways to the portal lobule. At the core of the liver acinus are tiny portal branches arising perpendicularly from portal tracts. The periphery of the liver acinus extends from the edge of one central vein (terminal hepatic venule) to another. Within the liver acinus, Rappaport identifies three concentric zones: Zone 1 (periportal), Zone 2 (midzonal), and Zone 3 (centrilobular, pericentral, or perivenular). Zone 1 is the first to receive blood-borne hormones and nutrients and Zone 3 the last. The concept of sublobular zonation has been useful for studying zone-specific pathology and for interpreting metabolic heterogeneity within the liver lobule.

The three concepts of liver lobular structure are not incompatible. Each describes the same design but from a different perspective. All provide a morphological basis for sublobular compartmentation, which is the subject of this book.

3.2. India Ink Injections and Vascular Casts

Since the average diameter of the liver lobule is on the order of a millimeter, it is evident that the two-fiber micro-light guide and miniature oxygen electrode can measure signals originating from a fraction of a single lobule. Such sublobular measurements cannot be used, however, unless the miniaturized probes can be positioned accurately over specific, identified sublobular regions. With this in mind, the relationship between liver pigmentation and lobular architecture was investigated.

The surface of perfused rat liver displays a faint pattern of dark spots and light areas that are more prominent in livers from mature animals and from animals treated with phenobarbital (Fig. 8).[6,8] The relationship of this pigmentation pattern to lobular structure was examined by infusing livers with india ink and by making acrylate casts of the vasculature (Fig. 8). When india ink or colored acrylate was injected into the vena cava (retrograde infusion), staining at the liver surface appeared first in dark areas, identifying them as pericentral (centrilobular or perivenular) regions. When dye was injected into the portal vein (anterograde infusion), staining appeared first in light areas surrounding the more darkly pigmented spots. These lighted areas were therefore identified as periportal zones. Thus, the distribution of native pigments identifies periportal and pericentral regions of the liver lobule. The identity of these pigments has not been determined, but since the intensity of pericentral pigmentation increases following treatment with phenobarbital, a phenobarbital-induced protein such as cytochrome P-450 may be responsible. This hypothesis is supported by the observation that cytochrome P-450 is induced to a greater extent in centrilobular than in periportal regions of the liver lobule.[12,13]

Tissue slices from injected livers revealed that periportal and centrilobular zones approached the liver surface in columns. Terminal branches of the portal vein were at the core of every light column, and central veins were at the center of every dark column. Portal and central venules approached the liver surface in different manners (Fig. 9). Portal veins tapered as they approached the surface until they became essentially indistinguishable from sinusoids about 200 μm from the surface. Central veins tapered less as they approached the surface and could be distinguished from sinusoids to within 50 μm of the liver surface. Light-microscopic serial sections confirmed these observations (Fig. 10). At about 200 μm from the liver surface, portal venules narrowed to the extent that they could not be distinguished from sinusoids. In contrast, central veins continued to within several microns of the surface as relatively large (≈50-μm-diameter) vessels. As little as one hepatocyte separated the terminal central venule from the liver surface.

3.3. Microcirculation at the Liver Surface

The results of these experiments indicate a distinctive pattern of microcirculation near the liver surface (Fig. 11). Blood first approaches the liver surface in portal vessels, but as these vessels narrow and terminate, the circulation is taken over by sinusoids that continue to the liver surface and radiate to adjacent central venules. In contrast to portal vessels, central veins extend to just beneath

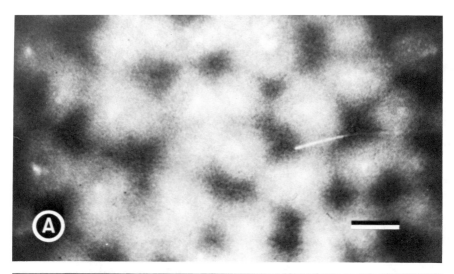

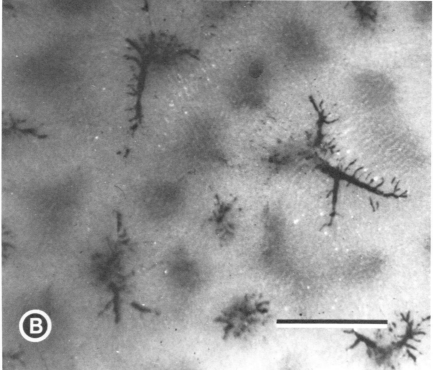

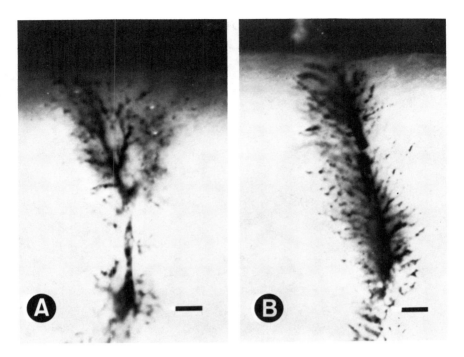

Figure 9. (A) Photomicrograph of a liver slice after acrylate injection via the portal vein. At about 200 μm from the liver surface, portal vessels cannot be distinguished from sinusoids. (B) Photomicrograph of a liver slice after acrylate injection via the vena cava. Branches of central veins project more closely to the liver surface than portal vessels. Scale bars: 100 μm.

Glisson's capsule. Thus, surface hepatocytes of pericentral regions are close to their central vein, whereas surface hepatocytes in periportal regions are at least 200 μm from their portal vein. These differences in surface anatomy need to be taken into account in interpreting data from micro-light guides and miniature oxygen electrodes.

Figure 8. (A) Photomicrograph of the surface of a hemoglobin-free, perfused liver from a phenobarbital-treated rat. Note the pigmentation pattern of dark spots and light areas. (B) Photomicrograph of the surface of perfused rat liver after acrylate injections via the portal and hepatic veins. Central veins are seen as discrete vessels often branching as they approach closely to the surface. Portal veins do not approach as closely to the surface. Portal regions are identified by the "blush" of injected sinusoids. Although the natural pigmentation is not apparent, regions around central veins correspond to dark spots, and regions over portal veins correspond to light areas. Scale bars: 500 μm.

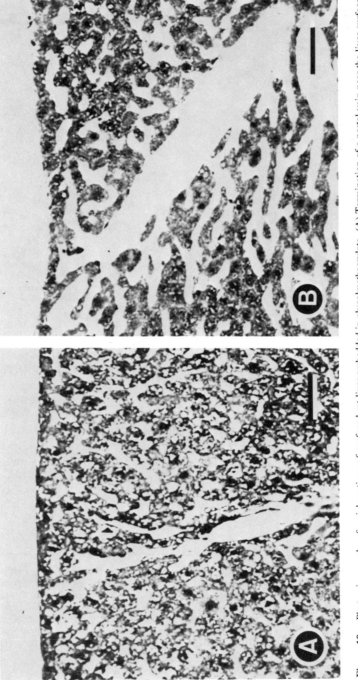

Figure 10. Photomicrographs of serial sections of perfused rat liver embedded in glycolmethacrylate. (A) Termination of a portal vein near the liver surface. The portal venule narrows to the size of a sinusoid at about 200 μm from the surface. (B) Termination of a central vein near the liver surface. The central vein continues as a relatively broad vessel to within several microns of the surface. As little as one hepatocyte separates the terminal central venule from the liver capsule. Scale bars: 50 μm.

Periportal
(light)

Pericentral
(dark)

350 torr

271 torr

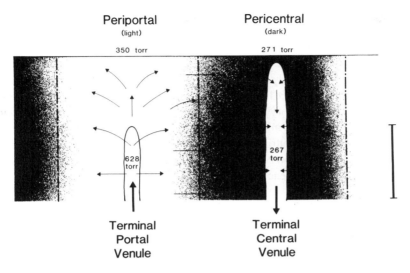

628 torr

267 torr

Terminal
Portal
Venule

Terminal
Central
Venule

Figure 11. Schematic representation of microcirculation near the liver surface. Arrows indicate the direction of flow of blood or perfusate. Oxygen tensions within the terminal portal venule and terminal central venule are assumed to equal the inflow and outflow oxygen tensions. Oxygen tensions over periportal and pericentral regions were determined with a miniature oxygen electrode. Scale bar: 200 μm.

3.4. Hepatic Lobular Continuum

The pattern of pigmentation in the liver does not describe discrete lobular units. Rather, there is a continuum of coextensive cords of periportal and pericentral tissue. At the core of each periportal cord is a portal vein, and at the core of each pericentral cord is a central vein. These periportal and pericentral cords branch with the branching of the portal and central veins to form extensive continua. In this sense, there is but a single lobule within each lobe. To describe this histological organization and to emphasize the continuous, cordlike organization of periportal and pericentral parenchyma, we introduce the term *hepatic lobular continuum*. This term emphasizes the uniformity of periportal and pericentral regions throughout the liver and reminds us that gradients and compartmentation exist within the liver despite the absence of discrete lobules.

4. LOBULAR OXYGEN GRADIENTS

4.1. Surface Measurements of NADH Fluorescence

NAD^+ and $NADP^+$ are essential cofactors in a broad variety of metabolic pathways. Their reduced forms, NADH and NADPH, are highly fluorescent when excited by wavelengths near 340 nm, whereas their oxidized forms are essentially nonfluorescent. Since NAD(H) and NADP(H) are present in high concentrations within the cell (≈ 0.5 mM), most fluorescence excited by near-UV light arises from these two nucleotides. In liver and many other tissues, $NADP^+$ is mainly reduced and NAD^+ is predominantly oxidized under normal aerobic conditions.[14] NADH is oxidized ultimately by oxygen via the action of the mitochondrial respiratory sequence. In the absence of oxygen, cellular NADH increases until essentially all cellular NAD^+ is in the reduced form. Since the apparent K_m of mitochondrial cytochrome c oxidase for oxygen is very low ($< 10^{-7}$ M), the increase in NADH during hypoxia will not occur until the tissue is virtually anoxic.[15] For each cell, this increase in NADH will occur as nearly an all-or-none phenomenon.

Two-fiber micro-light guides with tip diameters of 170 μm provide a convenient means of monitoring NADH fluorescence from different parts of the liver lobule. Typical responses of pericentral and periportal regions of the liver lobule to a cycle of anoxia are shown in Fig. 12. As the perfusate was saturated with nitrogen instead of oxygen, a rapid decrease in oxygen tension entering the

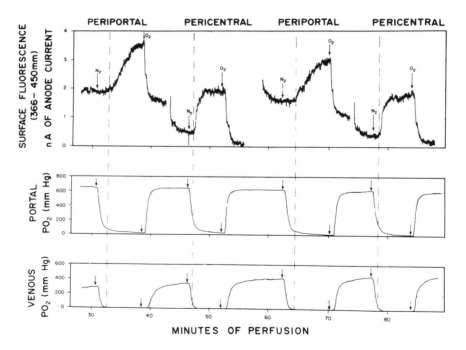

Figure 12. Dynamic fluorescence responses of periportal and pericentral areas to anoxic perfusion. A micro-light guide was positioned on light (periportal) and dark (pericentral) areas of the surface of the perfused liver using a flexible mechanical arm. Arrows indicate that the equilibrating gas mixture was changed to either 95% nitrogen–5% carbon dioxide (N_2) or 95% oxygen–5% carbon dioxide (O_2). From Ji et al.[5]

portal vein occurred, followed by a decrease in effluent oxygen tension after a short lag. As the influent oxygen tension dropped, tissue fluorescence began to increase. The rate of increase was nearly twice as fast in pericentral regions as in periportal areas. Since $NADP^+$ is already predominantly reduced in aerobic liver cells, the increase in fluorescence of anoxic liver is due predominantly to an increase in NADH. When oxygen was restored, NADH was reoxidized and fluorescence returned to basal values in both regions of the liver.

NADH fluorescence will begin to increase as soon as any tissue becomes anoxic. As oxygen delivery to the liver declines, areas of anoxia should develop first around the central vein, the region furthest removed from the oxygen supply. As the tissue becomes more hypoxic, an expanding zone of anoxia will develop until the entire lobule is depleted of oxygen. Under conditions of low flow, a steady state can be established in which pericentral zones are anoxic as evidenced by a maximal NADH fluorescence signal, whereas periportal zones remain normoxic without any increase in NADH fluorescence.[16] This finding shows that the micro-light guide measures periportal and pericentral fluorescence independently, i.e., there is no "cross talk" of signals arising from the two regions.

When a micro-light guide is positioned over a periportal zone of the liver surface, the cells that become anoxic first as influent oxygen tension decreases will be those most distant from a portal vein, i.e., those cells closest to the surface. When a micro-light guide is positioned on a pericentral region, the first cells to respond will be those immediately adjacent to the central venule (see Fig. 11). The inflow oxygen tension at which fluorescence first begins to increase in periportal regions corresponds to the oxygen gradient between the portal venule and the edge of the periportal region. This is the periportal oxygen gradient. The inflow oxygen tension at which pericentral fluorescence first begins to increase is the oxygen gradient for the portal vein to the central vein. This is the lobular oxygen gradient. The difference between the lobular gradient and the periportal gradient is the pericentral oxygen gradient. Table I provides some typical values for the lobular, periportal, and pericentral oxygen gradients of isolated, perfused rat livers determined in this manner. The periportal oxygen gradient is greater than the pericentral gradient, consistent with the higher concentration of mitochondria in periportal hepatocytes.[1] As expected, the lobular oxygen gradient at constant oxygen delivery increased as oxygen consumption by the livers increased, e.g., in livers from ethanol-treated animals.[8]

4.2. Surface Oxygen Tension

A representative experiment for measuring surface oxygen tensions with the miniature oxygen electrode is shown in Fig. 13. By moving the electrode around the liver, pairs of measurements were made from adjacent periportal and pericentral areas. Oxygen tensions were always lower in pericentral than in adjacent periportal regions, a direct demonstration of the lobular oxygen gradient.

Table I. Periportal, Pericentral, and Lobular Oxygen Gradients in Isolated, Perfused Rat Livers[a]

| | | Oxygen gradient (torr) | | |
Method	Treatment	Periportal	Pericentral	Lobular
Micro-light guide	Control	208 ± 13	67 ± 14	275 ± 20
	Ethanol	264 ± 19	136 ± 12^{b}	400 ± 23^{b}
Miniature oxygen electrode	Control	278 ± 50	79 ± 12	357 ± 50
	Ethanol	281 ± 46	143 ± 14^{b}	424 ± 47

[a] From Ji *et al.*[8] Livers from control and chronically ethanol-treated rats were perfused with hemoglobin-free medium. Oxygen gradients were determined with micro-light guides or miniature oxygen electrodes. Rates of oxygen uptake were 110 ± 7 and 144 ± 6 ($p < 0.001$) μmoles/g per hr, respectively, in livers from control and ethanol-treated rats. Values are means $\pm$ S.E.
[b] Significantly different from control: $p < 0.01$.

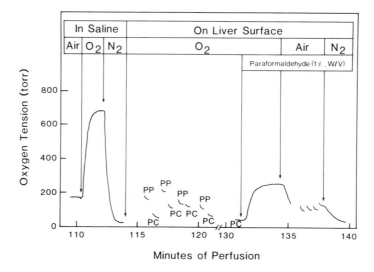

Figure 13. Tissue oxygen-tension measurements employing the miniature oxygen electrode. After calibration in saline, the electrode is positioned on periportal (PP) and pericentral (PC) areas. Each time the electrode makes contact with the liver after repositioning, there is a transient surge of current that decays to a steady-state value proportional to oxygen tension. At the conclusion of perfusion, the liver is fixed with 1% paraformaldehyde and recalibrated on the liver surface with reference to oxygen, air, and nitrogen.

Following these measurements, the liver was perfused with 1% paraformalde-hyde, and the miniature electrode was calibrated as described above (see Fig. 7). As expected, the average surface oxygen tension was intermediate between the inflow (portal) and outflow (vena caval) oxygen tensions. Earlier reports with a multiwire Clark electrode indicated that the average surface oxygen tension was lower than that of the venous outflow.[17,18] The reason for this discrepancy is not known. However, in the earlier reports, the oxygen electrode was calibrated with saline rather than tissue, which might have led to underestimation of actual tissue oxygen tensions.

In normal rat livers at an inflow oxygen tension of 628 torr, periportal oxygen tension measured with the miniature oxygen electrode was 350 torr and pericentral oxygen tension was 271 torr, close to the effluent oxygen tension of 267 torr (see Fig. 11). These are oxygen tensions at or near the liver surface. Thus, since portal venules terminate at least 200 μm from the liver surface, the periportal oxygen gradient is the influent oxygen tension minus the oxygen tension of the periportal liver surface. Since central venules terminate very close to the liver surface, the pericentral gradient is the oxygen tension at the periportal surface minus the oxygen tension at the pericentral surface. Calculated in this way, the periportal oxygen gradient was 278 torr, the pericentral oxygen gradient was 79 torr, and the total lobular gradient (periportal plus pericentral) was 357 torr (Table I). These values for the periportal, pericentral, and lobular oxygen gradients determined with the miniature oxygen electrode agree closely with those from micro-light guide measurements. This demonstrates the reliability and consistency of the two types of measurements and validates the use of paraformaldehyde-fixed tissue to calibrate the miniature oxygen electrode.

4.2.1. Stopped-Flow Measurement of Local Rates of Oxygen Uptake

Periportal oxygen gradients were greater than pericentral gradients deter-mined both by NADH fluorescence and by surface oxygen tension. This indicated that the local rate of tissue oxygen utilization was greater in periportal than in pericentral areas. Matsumura and Thurman[19] evaluated this directly using a stopped-flow oxygen-uptake technique. Miniature oxygen electrodes were placed on specific zones of the liver surface, and the flow of perfusate was stopped briefly (4–6 sec). Following cessation of flow, oxygen tension decreased rapidly as oxygen was consumed locally. The rate of decrease was more than twice as great in periportal areas as in pericentral ones. In livers from fed rats, oxygen consumption in periportal and pericentral regions was 131 and 56 μmoles/g per hr, respectively. In livers from fasted rats, rates were 141 and 89 μmoles/g per hr, increasing significantly in pericentral regions. These findings confirm that hepatocytes in periportal areas respire at a faster rate than cells in pericentral regions and demonstrate the importance of the effect of nutritional state on local rates of hepatic oxygen consumption.

4.3. Precautions and Other Considerations

Basal NADH fluorescence was greater in periportal than in pericentral regions of the liver lobule. This difference could arise from differences in the amount of NADH and other fluorophores in the two regions or from differential distribution of endogenous absorbing species. These possibilities were evaluated by infusing an exogenous fluorophore, 7-hydroxycoumarin, under conditions where it was not metabolized.[20] The increase of fluorescence in periportal and pericentral areas was proportional to the background, basal fluorescence. Since both regions were exposed to identical amounts of hydroxycoumarin but displayed different absolute changes in fluorescence, it was concluded that the quenching of fluorescence was greater in pericentral areas. The lower fluorescence in pericentral areas was probably due to absorbance of fluorescent light by a phenobarbital-induced pigment (colorimetric quenching). Such an interpretation is consistent with the observation that NADH levels are nearly equal in periportal and pericentral regions of the liver lobule.[21] Thus, periportal and pericentral regions must be compared in terms of percentage changes relative to basal fluorescence.

It is not a trivial matter to place a micro-light guide or miniature oxygen electrode accurately and reliably on a given periportal or pericentral region. Even if micromanipulators are used, there is still some uncertainty as to whether the probe has been placed in the middle or periphery of a given zone. Careful movement around a zone allows one to position an oxygen electrode at a point of highest oxygen tension in periportal zones and lowest oxygen tension in pericentral zones. These points are not necessarily the geometric centers of the various zones, but represent their physiological or metabolic centers. Lack of precision in probe placement can increase the variability of the experimental data substantially. Thus, careful placement together with multiple determinations are required to ensure collection of accurate, meaningful information.

An implicit assumption in these measurements is that perfusion is uniform throughout the liver. This seems borne out in india ink and acrylate injections, which distribute uniformly in the liver. However, vasoactive substances or toxins, especially vasoconstrictors, can lead to heterogeneous distribution of flow, with the result that some lobular cords are not perfused at all while others, even adjacent ones, are well perfused.[22] Thus, odd or contradictory data should raise the suspicion that microcirculation at the liver surface is not uniform.

5. OTHER APPLICATIONS OF MINIATURE PROBES

5.1. NAD⁺-Linked Cellular Metabolism

Many cellular processes are linked directly or indirectly to the oxidation–reduction state of cellular NAD^+. With suitable controls, NADH fluorescence can be used as an indicator of the relative activities of such pathways in periportal and pericentral regions after challenge with a metabolic substrate. In this way, the rate of ethanol metabolism has been determined in periportal and pericentral regions of the liver lobule.[23] Infusion of ethanol caused an increase of NADH fluorescence in periportal and pericentral regions that was blocked fully by inhibitors of alcohol dehydrogenase. The increases in fluorescence were proportional to the rate of alcohol or acetaldehyde metabolism by the whole liver. Since the changes in NADH fluorescence produced by ethanol in both regions were equal, it was concluded that local rates of alcohol-dehydrogenase-dependent ethanol metabolism are similar in periportal and pericentral regions of the liver lobule. In a similar fashion, other NADH-linked metabolic pathways can be monitored in periportal and pericentral tissue.[24–26]

5.2. Mixed-Function Oxidations

The micro-light guide can be employed to measure the fluorescence of not only intrinsic tissue fluorophores such as NADH but also introduced fluorophores. 7-Ethoxycoumarin, a substrate for hepatic mixed-function oxidation, is deethylated to the highly fluorescent compound 7-hydroxycoumarin. Using a large-tipped light guide, steady-state tissue fluorescence is directly proportional to the rate of 7-ethoxycoumarin O-deethylation. Thus, the sublobular fluorescence of 7-ethoxycoumarin measured by micro-light guides permits the estimation of local rates of mixed-function oxidation of 7-ethoxycoumarin.[20,27] Deethylation of 7-ethoxycoumarin was twice as great in pericentral regions as in periportal areas. The effect was not a "wash-in" effect, since identical results were obtained in livers perfused normally in the anterograde direction or in reverse perfusion via the vena cava. This approach has also been employed to determine rates of sulfation and glucuronidation of 7-hydroxycoumarin in periportal and pericentral regions.[28,29]

A novel approach using the micro-light guide is the measurement of local microcirculation using the Fick principle following a bolus injection of a fluorescent substance, e.g., fluorescein-dextran, into the perfused liver. This approach has been employed to determine the relative arterial and portal contributions to blood flow through preneoplastic hepatic nodules.[30]

6. ASSESSMENT OF LIVER INJURY AFTER TOXIC OR METABOLIC INSULT

The perfused liver lends itself well to the evaluation of metabolic and toxic insults that often affect specific regions. Dosages and exposures can be controlled precisely, and unlike isolated hepatocytes, the perfused liver retains its natural architecture. In this section, we describe briefly methods used in our laboratories to assess cellular injury in the isolated, perfused liver.

6.1. Light and Electron Microscopy

The perfused liver is readily prepared for examination by light and electron microscopy. For light-microscopic sections, perfused livers are fixed by infusion with 1 or 2% paraformaldehyde in Krebs–Henseleit–bicarbonate buffer. For transmission and scanning electron microscopy, both glutaraldehyde (2%) and paraformaldehyde (2%) are employed for adequate preservation of ultrastructural detail. Subsequent steps of preparation for either light or electron microscopy employ conventional techniques.

Light microscopy, scanning electron microscopy, and transmission electron microscopy each have advantages in the evaluation of tissue injury. Preparation for light microscopy is relatively rapid and can often be performed by service laboratories. Light-microscopic histochemistry and immunocytochemistry can provide important information about cell composition in different regions of the liver lobule. Light microscopy can also provide information concerning cell viability in specific zones of the liver lobule during short-term experiments based on trypan blue exclusion.[31] During the final 10 or 15 min of a liver perfusion, 0.2 mM trypan blue is added to the perfusate, followed by fixation. Nonviable cells will accumulate trypan blue in their nuclei, as revealed in tissue sections stained with acid dyes such as eosin (Fig. 14). The trypan blue technique has been used recently to identify cell death in periportal and pericentral regions of the perfused liver exposed to chemicals.[31]

Electron microscopy provides a greater wealth of cytological detail than light microscopy, and morphological evidence of hepatocellular injury can be detected much earlier with electron microscopy than with light microscopy. Scanning electron microscopy is particularly useful for detecting changes in cell surface topography and cell volume following hypoxic or toxic cell injury.[32,33] In anoxic liver, reversible structural changes can be observed in as little as 5 min[16,32,33] (see Chapter 12). Transmission electron microscopy completes the morphological picture and permits visualization of mitochondria, endoplasmic reticulum, and other organelles that are prone to swelling and other alterations in the early stages of toxic or metabolic cell injury.[34]

6.2. Enzyme Release

In vivo, a prominent feature of hepatocellular injury and death is the release of enzymes into the bloodstream. These enzymes include lactic dehydrogenase, transaminases, 5'-nucleotidase, and many others. When using a nonrecirculating system, enzyme release from isolated, perfused liver can be followed easily in samples of effluent. There are at least two patterns of release.[32,33] One pattern is associated with reoxygenation of reversibly injured hypoxic liver. Here, enzyme release is abrupt, short-lived, and associated with the appearance of fragments of cytoplasm in the effluent (see Chapter 12). These fragments result from

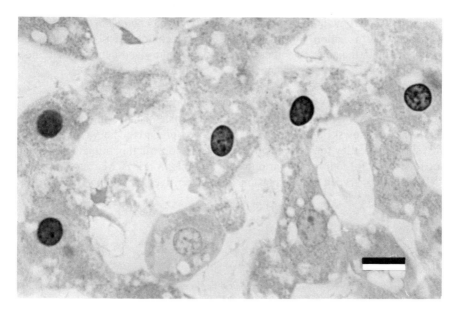

Figure 14. Light microscopy of perfused rat liver following ischemia and trypan blue infusion. The nuclei of necrotic cells are darkly labeled with trypan blue. Viable cells are unlabeled. The liver was fixed after 1 hr of ischemia at 37°C and 15 min of reflow with 0.2 mM trypan blue in Krebs–Henseleit–bicarbonate buffer, embedded in glycomethacrylate, and counterstained with eosin. Scale bar: 10 μm.

the shedding of surface projections (blebs) formed during hypoxia. A second pattern is associated with irreversible cell injury in which enzyme release is sustained and often massive.

7. CONCLUSION

The new methods described here for studying sublobular events in isolated, perfused liver represent the convergence of advances in two areas. The first is in the fabrication of miniature probes, namely, micro-light guides and miniature oxygen electrodes. The second important advance is in the understanding of liver lobular structure. No probe, however small, can be very valuable for monitoring sublobular events unless it can be positioned on identified sublobular zones. Further, the interpretation of signals from these surface probes must be made in the context of lobular structure at and near the liver surface. Especially important in these respects are lobular pigmentation, surface microcirculation, and the fashion in which cords of periportal and pericentral tissue approach the liver surface.

In showing that metabolism is indeed different in various zones of the liver lobule, these micromethods demonstrate directly the biochemical zonation of the liver lobule. Information gained with these new techniques will help us to ultimately explain the zonal specificities of hypoxic injury and hepatotoxicity due to alcohol, drugs, and other chemicals.

ACKNOWLEDGMENTS. We thank Yukio Tanaka for assistance in electron microscopy and photography, Dr. Allen E. Blaurock for assistance in densitometry, Carole J. Stemkowski and Patricia L. Hicks for preparing the vascular casts, Dr. Charles Woodley for advice and assistance in constructing miniature oxygen electrodes, Erich Lieth for preparing serial sections, Mark E. Marotto and Blair U. Bradford for trypan blue exclusion in hypoxic liver, and Gina Harrison for artwork.

REFERENCES

1. Loud, A. V., 1968, A quantitative stereological description of the ultrastructure of normal rat liver parenchymal cells, *J. Cell Biol.* **37**:27–46.
2. Jungermann, K., and Sasse, D., 1978, Heterogeneity of liver parenchymal cells, *Trends Biochem. Sci.* **3**:198–202.
3. MacSween, R. N. M., Anthony, P. P., and Scheuer, P. J., (eds.), 1979, *Pathology of the Liver*, Churchill Livingstone, Edinburgh.
4. Zimmerman, H. J., 1978, *Hepatotoxicity*, Appleton-Century-Crofts, New York.
5. Ji, S., Chance, B., Nishiki, K., Smith, T., and Rich, T., 1979, Micro-light guides, a new method for measuring tissue fluorescence and reflectance, *Am. J. Physiol.* **236**:C144–C156.
6. Ji, S., Lemasters, J. J., and Thurman, R. G., 1980, A non-invasive method to study metabolic events within sublobular regions of hemoglobin-free perfused liver, *FEBS Lett.* **113**:37–41; **114**:349.
7. Zahlten, R. N., Stratman, F. W., Lardy, H. A., 1973, Regulation of glucose synthesis in hormone-sensitive isolated rat hepatocytes, *Proc. Natl. Acad. Sci. U.S.A.* **70**:3213–3218.
8. Ji, S., Lemasters, J. J., Christenson, V., and Thurman, R. G., 1982, Periportal and pericentral pyridine nucleotide fluorescence from the surface of the perfused liver: Evaluation of the hypothesis that chronic treatment with ethanol produces pericentral hypoxia, *Proc. Natl. Acad. Sci. U.S.A.* **79**:5415–5419.
9. Kiernan, F., 1833, The anatomy and physiology of the liver, *Philos. Trans. R. Soc. London* **123**:711–770.
10. Mall, F. P., 1906, A study of the structural unit of the liver, *Am. J. Anat.* **5**:227–308.
11. Rappaport, A. M., 1976, The microcirculatory acinar concept of normal and pathological hepatic structure, *Beitr. Pathol.* **157**:215–243.
12. Baron, J., Redick, J. A., and Guengerich, F. P., 1978, Immunohistochemical localizations of cytochromes P-450 in rat liver, *Life Sci.* **23**:2627–2632.
13. Gooding, P. E., Chayen, J., Sawyer, B., and Slater, T. F., 1978, Cytochrome P-450 distribution in rat liver and the effect of sodium phenobarbitone administration, *Chem.-Biol. Interact.* **20**:299–310.
14. Sies, H., 1982, Nicotinamide nucleotide compartmentation, in: *Metabolic Compartmentation* (H. Sies, ed.), pp. 205–231, Academic Press, London.

15. Chance, B., Cohen, P., Jobsis, F., and Schoener, B., 1962, Intracellular oxidation–reduction states *in vivo, Science* **137**:499–508.
16. Lemasters, J. J., Ji, S., and Thurman, R. G., 1981, Centrilobular injury following hypoxia in isolated, perfused rat liver, *Science* **213**:661–663.
17. Kessler, M., Goernandt, L., and Lang, H., 1973, Correlation between oxygen tension in tissue and hemoglobin dissociation curve, in: *Oxygen Supply* (M. Kessler, D. F. Bruley, L. C. Clark, D. W. Lübbers, L. A. Silver, and J. Strauss, eds.), pp. 156–159, University Park Press, Baltimore.
18. Kessler, M., Höper, J., and Krumme, B. A., 1976, Monitoring of tissue perfusion and cellular function, *Anaesthesiology* **45**:184–197.
19. Matsumura, T., and Thurman, R. G., 1983, Measuring rates of O_2 uptake in periportal and pericentral regions of the liver lobule: Stop-flow experiments with perfused liver, *Am. J. Physiol.* **244**:G656–659.
20. Belinsky, S. A., Kauffman, F. C., Ji, S., Lemasters, J. J., and Thurman, R. G., 1983, Stimulation of mixed-function oxidation of 7-ethoxycoumarin in periportal and pericentral regions of the perfused rat liver by xylitol, *Eur. J. Biochem.* **137**:1–6.
21. Ghosh, A. K., Finegold, D., White, W., Zawalich, K., and Matschinsky, F. W., 1982, Quantitative histochemical resolution of the oxidation–reduction and phosphate potentials within the simple hepatic acinus, *J. Biol. Chem.* **257**:5476–5481.
22. Ji, S., Beckh, K., and Jungermann, K., 1984, Regulation of oxygen consumption and microcirculation by α-sympathetic nerves in isolated perfused rat liver, *FEBS Lett.* **167**:117–122.
23. Kashiwagi, T., Ji, S., Lemasters, J. J., and Thurman, R. G., 1982, Rates of alcohol dehydrogenase-dependent ethanol metabolism in periportal and pericentral regions of the perfused rat liver, *Mol. Pharmacol.* **21**:438–443.
24. Kashiwagi, T., Lindros, K. O., and Thurman, R. G., 1983, Aldehyde dehydrogenase-dependent acetaldehyde metabolism in periportal and pericentral regions of the perfused rat liver, *J. Pharmacol. Exp. Ther.* **224**:538–542.
25. Belinsky, S. A., Matsumura, T., Kauffman, F. C., and Thurman, R. G., 1984, Rates of allyl alcohol metabolism in periportal and pericentral regions of the liver lobule, *Mol. Pharmacol.* **25**:158–164.
26. Matsumura, T., and Thurman, R. G., 1984, Predominance of glycolysis in pericentral regions of the liver lobule, *Eur. J. Biochem.* **140**:229–234.
27. Ji, S., Lemasters, J. J., and Thurman, R. G., 1981, A fluorometric method to measure sublobular rates of mixed-function oxidation in the hemoglobin-free perfused rat liver, *Mol. Pharmacol.* **19**:513–516.
28. Conway, J. O., Kauffman, F. C., Ji, S., and Thurman, R. G., 1982, Rates of sulfation and glucuronidation of 7-hydroxycoumarin in periportal and pericentral regions of the liver lobule, *Mol. Pharmacol.* **22**:509–516.
29. Conway, J. G., Kauffman, F. C., Tsukada, T., and Thurman, R. G., 1984, Glucuronidation of 7-hydroxycoumarin in periportal and pericentral regions of the liver lobule, *Mol. Pharmacol.* **25**:487–493.
30. Conway, J. G., Popp, J. A., Ji, S., and Thurman, R. G., 1983, Effect of size on portal circulation of hepatic nodules from carcinogen-treated rats, *Cancer Res.* **43**:3374–3378.
31. Belinsky, S. A., Popp, J. A., Kauffman, F. C., and Thurman, R. G., 1984, Trypan blue uptake as a new method to investigate hepatotoxicity in periportal and pericentral regions of the liver lobule: Studies with allyl alcohol in the perfused liver, *J. Pharmacol. Exp. Ther.* **230**:755–760.
32. Lemasters, J. J., Stemkowski, C. J., Ji, S., and Thurman, R. G., 1982, Liver structure and function in hypoxia, in: *Protection of Tissues against Hypoxia* (A. Wauquier, M. Borgers, and W. K. Amery, eds.), pp. 15–30, Elsevier, Amsterdam.

33. Lemasters, J. J., Stemkowski, C. J., Ji, S., and Thurman, R. G., 1983, Cell surface changes and enzyme release during hypoxia and reoxygenation in the isolated, perfused rat liver, *J. Cell Biol.* **97**:778–786.

34. Trump, B. F., and Arstila, A. U., 1975, Cell membranes and disease processes, in: *Pathobiology of Cell Membranes,* Vol. I (B. F. Trump and A. U. Arstila, eds.), pp. 1–103, Academic Press, New York.

35. Inch, W. R., 1958, Problems associated with the use of the exposed platinum electrode for measuring oxygen tension *in vivo, Can. J. Biochem. Physiol.* **36**:1009–1021.

36. Baumgärtl, H., and Lübbers, D. W., 1983, Microaxial needle sensor for polarographic measurement of local O_2 pressure in the cellular range of living tissue: Its construction and properties, in: *Polarographic Oxygen Sensors* (E. Gtnaiger and H. Forstner, eds.), pp. 37–65, Springer-Verlag, Berlin.

Chapter 8

Redox Scanning in the Study of Metabolic Zonation of Liver

Bjørn Quistorff and Britton Chance

1. INTRODUCTION

The metabolic activity of an organ, e.g., the liver, will create gradients of oxygen, substrates, hormones, and products of metabolism along the capillaries. These concentration gradients will tend to subdivide the organ into zones of different metabolic activity at the capillary level. In many organs, e.g., muscles and brain, capillaries seem to be organized so as to minimize the zonation effect of the longitudinal capillary gradients, since adjacent parallel capillaries are perfused in opposite directions.

In the liver, however, microcirculation is organized, it seems, to obtain a maximum of zonation. Capillaries (sinusoids) in this organ form functional units in which adjacent sinusoids have adjacent exit points and flow in the same direction.[1] The response of the liver to various pathological conditions and toxic substances demonstrates clearly such a functional zonation of the parenchyma (for reviews, see Rappaport[1] and Jungermann and Katz[2]). At present, there is no clear understanding of the physiological significance of zonation.

The study of intercellular metabolic heterogeneity requires special tech-

BJØRN QUISTORFF • Department of Biochemistry, University of Copenhagen, 2200 Copenhagen, Denmark.   BRITTON CHANCE • The Johnson Research Foundation, University of Pennsylvania, Philadelphia, Pennsylvania 19104.

niques, some of which are described in Chapters 3–7. Among other new and potentially useful techniques is a recently developed column technique, in which isolated hepatocytes are packed on a polyacrylamide column, effectively transforming the liver into one "macrosinusoid."[3] Further, a digitonin perfusion technique has been developed that allows specific release of intracellular material from periportal or perivenous cells.[4,4a] Finally, nuclear magnetic resonance (NMR) spectroscopy offers the possibility of noninvasive study of both inter- and intracellular compartmentation *in vivo*. Phosphorus NMR imaging has recently been achieved *in vivo*.[5] At present, however, the technique provides a resolution in the linear dimension of only 5–10 times the length of the sinusoid.

In this chapter, we describe the use of redox-ratio scanning in the study of metabolic zonation, employing a surface fluorescence technique, designed for three-dimensional (3-D) measurement on frozen tissue with a spatial resolution of approximately 2×10^{-7} ml.[6,7]

2. INDICATORS OF THE INTRACELLULAR REDOX STATE OF PYRIDINE NUCLEOTIDES

2.1. Indicator Metabolite Method

The term "intracellular redox state" is often used to indicate the redox state of one of the pyridine nucleotide redox couples, $NAD^+/NADH$ and $NADP^+/NADPH$. According to Williamson *et al.*,[8] the redox state is defined as the ratio of the free concentrations of the reduced and oxidized pyridine nucleotide at thermodynamic equilibrium. The redox potential, E_h, is obtained by inserting this ratio into the Nernst equation employing the proper midpoint potential. Since the pyridine nucleotides are compartmentalized within the cells due to impermeability of most intracellular membranes to these molecules, the redox state must be specified for a specific intracellular compartment. In the context of this work, the relevant compartments are the mitochondrial and the cytosolic compartment. The most widely used method in assessing the redox state of the $NAD^+/NADH$ or the $NADP^+/NADPH$ redox couple is either the metabolite indicator method or direct spectrometric measurement of the fluorescence or absorption of the reduced species of the redox couple.

With the metabolite indicator method, a dehydrogenase reaction is chosen that is specific for either the mitochondrial or the cytosolic compartment and specific for the redox couple in question. Provided that thermodynamic equilibrium can be assumed in the dehydrogenase reaction, the redox ratio may be calculated from the equilibrium constant and the actual equilibrium concentrations of the substrates of the reaction. Table I shows examples of dehydrogenases that are commonly used in assessing the redox state of $NAD^+/NADH$ and

Table I. Redox Indicator Metabolite Reactions and Redox Potentials in Liver[a]

Cytosolic space	Ref.	Mitochondrial space	Ref.
NAD/NADH -214 mV Lactate dehydrogenase	10	NAD/NADH -318 mV β-Hydroxybutyrate dehydrogenase	8, 12
NADP/NADPH -393 mV Isocitrate dehydrogenase 6-P-Gluconate dehydrogenase Malic enzyme	11, 12	NADP/NADPH -415 mV Isocitrate dehydrogenase Glutamate dehydrogenase	11, 13

[a] Modified from Sies.[11] The indicator metabolite systems are discussed in the references given in the table.

NADP$^+$/NADPH redox couples for the cytoplasmic and mitochondrial compartments in liver and other tisseus (for a recent review, see Sies[9]).

2.2. Tissue Fluorescence

Fluorescence measurement on intact tissue as a way of assessing the tissue redox state was first applied by Chance and Jöbsis[14] and Chance et al.[15] for reduced pyridine nucleotide (PN) and by Ramirez and Vega[16] for flavoprotein (FP). PN fluorescence from intact tissue is obtained as a broad peak at 450 nm after excitation with UV light, usually the mercury arc line at 366 nm. The signal originates predominantly from the pyridine nucleotides NADPH and NADH, which are present in the cell in both a free and a protein-bound form within the cytosolic and the mitochondrial compartment. In addition, however, there is a chemically undefined background fluorescence excited under the same conditions, some of which is related to lipids, but which does not seem to take part in metabolic redox transitions. This latter contribution to the PN fluorescence signal varies considerably among different tissues. The white matter of brain [17] and part of the epicardium[18] are examples of tissues with high PN fluorescence background. In the liver, this background fluorescence is comparatively small.[19]

The liver cell contains several FPs. Among these, however, the flavin moeity of the dehydrolipoamide dehydrogenase has by far the highest fluorescence yield.[20,21] This flavin is coupled to the mitochondrial NAD$^+$/NADH system by the pyruvate dehydrogenase and α-ketoglutarate dehydrogenase reactions.[22] More than 90% of the flavin signal originates from the mitochondrial compartment.[23]

Since fluorescence measurements on intact tissue require excitation light of high spectral purity and intensity, most work is done with fixed-wavelength instruments. Excitation–emission spectra obtained from isolated mitochondrial preparations are useful in assigning fixed wavelengths for PN and FP measurements. Figure 1 shows the excitation–emission spectra of oxidized and reduced

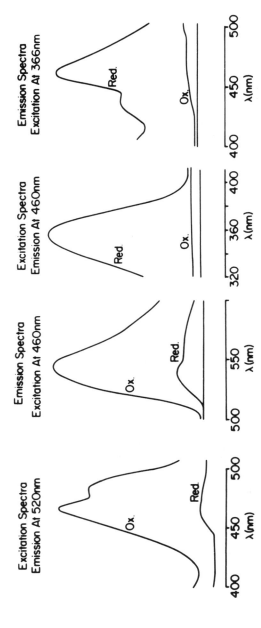

Figure 1. Low-temperature excitation–emission spectra for PN (366–460 nm) and FP (460–520 nm) for pigeon heart mitochondria. Reprinted from Chance *et al.*[24] with permission.

pigeon heart mitochondria at $-196°C$, the temperature at which the redox scanner operates. Compared with room temperature, there is a 7 to 14-fold (tissue-dependent) fluorescence enhancement of FP and PN signals with a much smaller enhancement of the background signal, thus improving the signal-to-noise ratio.[24] The PN fluorescence is attributed to NADH rather than NADPH, since cardiac mitochondria have little NADPH fluorescence.[25] The spectra of reduced mitochondria show high PN signal and very little FP signal and vice versa for oxidized mitochondria. FP may be excited between 405 and 500 nm usually with negligible excitation of PNs. Conversely, excitation of PN at 366 nm results in relatively little excitation of FP that is removed easily by appropriate secondary filters.

2.3. Different Pyridine Nucleotide Pools

2.3.1. Fluorescence Enhancement

In perfused organs, quantitative information on different PN pools may be obtained by simultaneous measurement of absorption (340 nm) and fluorescence, allowing calculation of the $\Delta F/\Delta A$ ratio, which may be taken as a measure of fluorescence quantum yield.[10,26] Since the fluorescence yield as well as the wavelength of maximum fluorescence and absorption depend on the chemical state of the reduced species of the PN redox couples, the $\Delta F/\Delta A$ ratio may be used to calibrate the response to different redox transitions. In the perfused rat liver, Bücher et al.[10] showed that the fluorescence yield changed 2.5-fold more with ethanol than with ammonium chloride. Further, the fluorescence yield of intracellular PN was 4 times larger than added, extracellular NADH.[10] Avi-Dor et al.[27] demonstrated in isolated rat liver mitochondria that the PN fluorescence yield was 4 times higher with β-hydroxybutyrate-induced redox changes than with ammonium chloride. The fluorescence enhancement of intracellular PN is due to specific binding to various dehydrogenases.[28] There are, however, exceptions: Binding to glyceraldehyde phosphate dehydrogenase in muscle decreases rather than increases the quantum efficiency of NADH fluorescence.[29]

2.3.2. Fluorescence Blue Shift

Another effect of NADH binding to protein is a shift toward the blue of the wavelength of maximum emission.[28] This blue shift of PN fluorescence is seen, however, only in isolated systems, e.g., isolated mitochondria,[30] not in intact organs.[31] Thorell and Chance[32] found large changes in the light-absorbing properties of isolated liver cells between 400 and 460 nm. It was therefore suggested[15] and later confirmed[31] that the difference between fluorescence emission peaks of isolated mitochondria and the corresponding intact tissues may be due to attenuation of the short-wavelength side of the fluorescence band by filter effect of the tissue. However, even with suitable correction for this possible filtering effect, the fluorescence emission maximum varies in different types of tissues, probably as a result of quantitative or qualitative differences in binding sites.

2.3.3. Cytosolic vs. Mitochondrial Contribution to the Pyridine Nucleotide Fluorescence Signal

In skeletal and heart muscle, it is generally agreed that a majority of the PN fluorescence signal originates from the mitochondrial compartment.[33-35] In the brain, O'Connor et al.[36] found that PN fluorescence increases to a steady-state level after 30–40 sec of anoxia; however, chemically determined total NADH continues to increase along with an increase in the lactate concentration for the next 5 min to more than 2-fold the initial value obtained at the time steady-state fluorescence was obtained. O'Connor and co-workers thus concluded that the cytoplasmic NADH does not contribute significantly to PN fluorescence in brain. In the electric organ of the electric fish, however, the PN fluorescence signal is largely cytoplasmic, apparently due to the paucity of mitochondria in this organ.[37]

In the rat liver, the situation is somewhat different. From the studies of Scholz et al.,[23] it is apparent that PN fluorescence originates from both compartments. In the rotenone-inhibited perfused rat liver, pyruvate (2 mM) reversed about 50% of the PN fluorescence. Furthermore, in the anoxic perfused liver, pyruvate perfusion reversed about 40% of the PN fluorescence, but did not change the FP fluorescence. On the contrary, in the rotenone-inhibited liver, acetoacetate reversed the FP reduction almost completely, but reversed the PN reduction only partially. This experiment suggests that approximately half the PN fluorescence originates from the cytosol and half from the mitochondria, whereas the flavin fluorescence originates predominantly from the mitochondria. It was further observed that aminopyrine does not change the flavin fluorescence in the perfused liver, but causes an oxidation of PN in agreement with the aforestated conclusion.[23] This result also suggests that cytoplasmic flavin, e.g., flavin associated with the microsomal monooxygenation system, does not contribute significantly to the fluorescence signal.

2.4. Flavoprotein/Pyridine Nucleotide Ratio Method

We have used the ratio of the FP fluorescence signal to that of PN as a redox indication.[24] As shown in Fig. 1, only the oxidized species of the FP couple is fluorescent, and only the reduced species of the PN couple is fluorescent. With the reservations discussed above, the FP/PN ratio will reflect the redox state of the mitochondrial NAD/NADH redox couple. Since the two components of the redox ratio vary in opposite directions on a redox change, sensitivity will

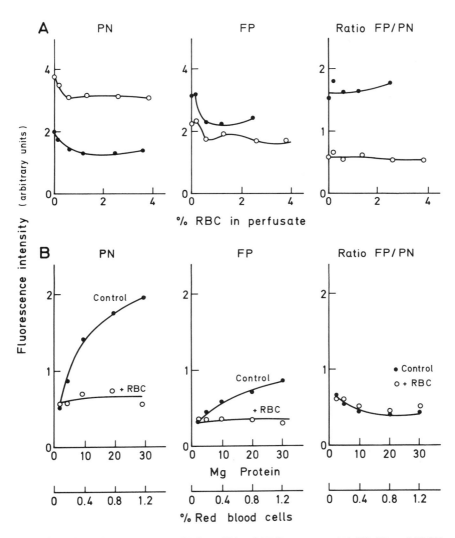

Figure 2.   Effect of red blood cells (RBC) on PN and FP fluorescence. (A) PN, FP, and FP/PN signals were recorded by surface fluorometry on the perfused liver in the normoxic, ●, and the hypoxic state, ○. RBC volume was varied as indicated on the abscissa. (B) Isolated pigeon heart mitochondria and RBC were mixed in the concentrations given on the abscissa as mg mitochondrial protein and % RBC volume, respectively. The traces labeled *Control* are those obtained in the absence of RBC. Modified from Chance *et al.*[24]

be increased compared with recording of only one of the parameters. The FP/PN ratio (called the calculated ratio) varies between 0.05 and 10 in isolated mitochondria,[24] while in intact tissue, the redox range is of the order of 2–4.[38–40]

In freeze trapping studies, the system should be stable at the trapped temperature for adequate time for precise measurement. While it might seem advantageous for redox state measurements to observe the cytochrome components of the frozen sample, particularly cytochrome oxidase, we have elected the FP/PN ratio.[24] One reason for this is that in the trapping procedure, oxygen, which is of crucial importance may not be readily trapped, and its diffusion in supercooled water may indeed greatly exceed expectations based upon freezing at 0°C.[40a] However, the FP/PN redox couple is well protected from perturbations of the cytochrome oxidase by diffusible oxygen by the 'freeze out' of electron transfer in the respiratory chain usually at the cytochrome b ubiquinone site. Thus, we have reasonable assurance that the freeze trapping of the FP/PN ratio affords fidelity of the room temperature redox state.

Another important quality of the redox ratio is its relative insensitivity to changes in mitochondrial concentration, interfering pigments, and red blood cells in the tissue. This is illustrated in Fig. 2A for a perfused rat liver in which the concentration of red blood cells (RBC) in the perfusate was varied. While FP and PN varied significantly with changes in blood concentration, the ratio was affected only slightly. Similarly, in Fig. 2B, the concentration of isolated mitochondria with or without RBC was varied. Again, the ratio was affected much less than the FP and PN signal alone. To interpret the observed changes in FP and PN fluorescence with respect to respiratory activity of the tissue being scanned, the concept of metabolic state of isolated mitochondria advanced by Chance and Williams[41] has proven very useful. Table II shows this relationship between the degree of reduction of PN and FP in five different metabolic states.

Table II. Metabolic State of Mitochondria and Associated Oxidation–Reduction Levels of Flavoprotein and Pyridine Nucleotide[a]

			Characteristics of metabolic state			Steady-state reduction (%)	
State	O	ADP level	Substrate level	Respiration rate	Rate-limiting factor	FP	PN
1	>0	Low	Low	Slow	ADP	21	90
2	>0	High	0	Slow	Substrate	0	0
3	>0	High	High	Fast	Respiratory chain	20	53
4	>0	Low	High	Slow	ADP	40	99
5	0	High	High	0	Oxygen	100	100

[a]Data from Chance and Williams[41] (modified from Jöbsis and Lamanna[52]).

3. LOW-TEMPERATURE SCANNING TECHNIQUE

3.1. General Description

The scanning instrument is shown in Fig. 3. The technique is based on automated scanning of fluorescence signals from the surface of frozen tissue with a micro-light guide. The parameters measured are the pyridine nucleotide (PN) and flavoprotein (FP) fluorescence signals as discussed above.

The frozen liver sample, which may be obtained by a number of different freeze–quenching techniques, is mechanically fixed in the Dewar flask of the instrument filled with liquid nitrogen, as shown in Fig. 4. Redox-ratio scanning is performed as follows: A flat surface on the sample is created by milling the sample at 77°K.[42] The micro-light guide is then placed over an appropriate point on the tissue sample and moved across the surface under computer control, while the optical signals from each point are read and stored by the computer. The instrument now allows for another scan of the same sample at a deeper level. This is carried out by milling away the surface of the specimen to any desired depth and repeating the scan as described. In this way, a series of consecutive scans from the same sample may be collected. The scans will be identical in size and shape and will be aligned vertically. Such a data set may thus be used for a 2- and/or 3-D reconstruction of a "metabolic representation" of the sample in terms of redox state.

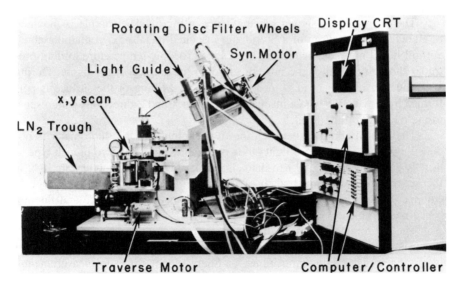

Figure 3. Redox-ratio scanning instrument. See the text for details.

TO FLUOROMETER

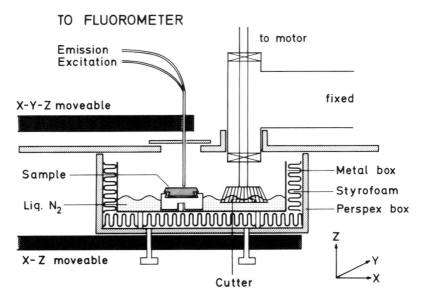

Figure 4. Simplified diagram of the redox-ratio scanning instrument. Fluorescence signals are measured from the frozen sample by moving the micro-light guide across the surface, point by point. FP and PN are recorded from each point. When a scan is completed, 50–100 μm is milled off the sample and the scan is repeated on the new surface. Reprinted from Quistorff and Chance[42] with permission.

3.2. Details of the Instrument

The instrument is shown schematically in Fig. 4. The sample is mounted in a holder in the bottom of a Styrofoam-insulated metal box, containing about 250 ml liquid nitrogen. A milling head suited for low-temperature milling protrudes through the lid of the box for grinding the surface of the tissue. During scanning, the milling head is in liquid nitrogen. Milling of the surface is performed by moving the whole insulated box in the X and Z directions with respect to the rotating milling head.[42]

The optical coupling between the liver sample and the fluorometer is obtained by a multifiber micro-light guide of the one-end-fused two-branch type,[43] usually constructed with 50-μm-diameter quartz fibers. The mercury arc light is focused on the excitation branch of the light guide. The sampling branch is equipped with a 5/95% beam splitter for simultaneous reflectance and fluorescence measurements.

The fluorometer is essentially the instrument described by Chance *et al.*[44] It consists of two synchronized disks, rotating at 60 Hz, that contain the optical filters. Each disk has four positions for filters. For redox-ratio measurements, two channels are used: for PN and FP. The reflectance signals obtained at the FP and PN excitation wavelengths may be recorded simultaneously in the two other channels. For PN, the excitation wavelength 366 nm is used; for PN emission, a filter combination is employed giving peak transmission at 450 nm. For FP, the corresponding values for excitation and emission are 436 and 520 nm, respectively.[7]

After integration and analog-to-digital conversion, the fluorescence signals are read and stored by a computer. The data may be presented in a variety of ways, e.g., as television images of single scans (see Figs. 9 and 10), in which a scan is composed of a number of pixels corresponding to the number of points scanned on the particular tissue surface. As a standard procedure, we use a gray scale for the display of the redox images in which black represents a low number (reduced) and white represents a high number (oxidized).[7]

4. SPATIAL RESOLUTION OF THE INSTRUMENT

The 2-D resolution in the scanning plane is strictly a function of light-guide size and geometry and of the distance between the tissue surface and the light guide. This relationship has been dealt with elsewhere.[43] With a fiber diameter of 50 μm and a tissue–light guide distance of 30–50 μm, which have been used in the experiments reported herein, the area covered is approximately 0.004 mm[2]. The resolution down through the tissue is somewhat more complex, being determined by a number of different factors such as the absorption of both the excitation light and the emitted fluorescence by the tissue. In addition, this internal filtering effect may be wavelength-specific, especially for the excitation light.[31] The fact that readings in vertically aligned 2-D scans separated by only 50 μm may change by more than 100% suggests that the actual reading depth may be even less than 50 μm. However, assuming 50 μm as the depth of reading, the 3-D resolution of the instrument may be calculated to 2×10^{-7} ml, corresponding to 20–30 hepatocytes.

5. FREEZE–QUENCHING OF TISSUE

The tissue scanner is designed to analyze the 2- or 3-D distribution of metabolic states in freeze–trapped tissues. Freeze trapping has several significant advantages for this type of study in the liver: It quenches (1) metabolic processes, giving a "snapshot" of the metabolic state of the tissue. (2) It fixes the sample mechanically to a holder, which allows mounting in the instrument (see Fig. 6A and B). (3) It allows an investigation of the distribution of the metabolic states in three dimensions throughout the sample. (4) The fluorescence quantum yield of the flavoprotein and especially of the pyridine nucleotide is increased sev-eralfold due to the low temperature, thus improving the signal-to-noise ratio.[24]

We have used various freezing methods, each of which was selected to suit

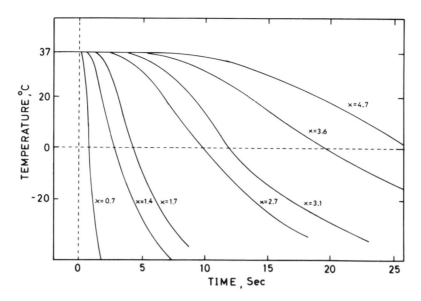

Figure 5. Time–course of freezing at different distances from the cooled surface in a freeze–clamped rat brain. Temperature was recorded with a thermocouple inserted at various positions in the brain prior to freeze–clamping. ($\times$) equals depth in mm from surface to center of thermocouple. Reprinted from Quistorff.[45]

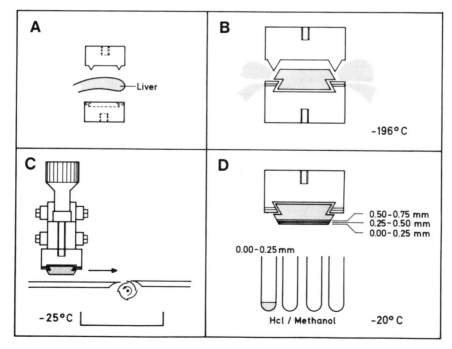

Figure 6. Steps in the procedure for freeze–clamping of rat liver and analysis of metabolites along the freezing gradient.

the particular tissue and experimental goal. If the aim of the particular experiment is to obtain measurements that reflect the *in vivo* state, the freeze–quenching procedure must be designed accordingly, i.e., to obtain the shortest possible time interval between interruption of normal circulation and quenching of metabolic processes.[45] Even under optimal conditions, this implies that only small tissue samples or thin wafers of tissue can be used, since the freezing time in the tissue increases exponentially with distance from the cooled surface, as demonstrated in Fig. 5.

For 3-D studies with the redox scanning technique, it is therefore important to know the exact manner in which each tissue is frozen and to check which part of the sample still reflects the *in vivo* state.[42,45] This may be controlled by chemical analysis of the $[ATP/(ADP \times P_i)]$ ratio along the freezing gradient of the freeze–clamped liver as by means of the technique illustrated in Fig 6. Applying this technique, Quistorff and Poulsen[46] found that freeze–clamped liver samples preserved the metabolic state to a depth of about 1 mm.

6. EXAMPLES OF SCANNING RESULTS

6.1. Histogram Distribution of Redox States

The size of the microcirculatory unit of the liver is of the order of 0.5 mm in diameter.[1] To include a reasonable number of such units, scans of liver usually cover an area of 4–16 mm^2. With 50 μm per light-guide step, this corresponds to 1600–6400 single-point readings of flavoprotein (FP) and pyridine nucleotide (PN) fluorescence. If carried out as a serial section scan to a depth of 1 mm, the total number of data points for such a 3-D scan at 50-μm resolution amounts to 32,000–128,000. Figure 7 shows the frequency distribution of the FP/PN ratio from a 13-section scan of a control liver at a resolution of 50 μm. On the x axis, the redox ratio is displayed, while the y axis shows the number of points in the scan in which a particular FP/PN value was recorded. On the z axis, the scanning depth below the sample surface is indicated.

Since the individual 2-D scans cover cross sections of 50–60 presumably functionally identical microcirculatory units at different cross-sectional levels, the redox-ratio distribution of a single 2-D scan may be regarded as a measure of the average redox-ratio distribution of the microcirculatory unit. On the basis of knowledge of the structure of the liver, one would not expect this average redox distribution to change with distance from the surface, except, perhaps, for the first 50–100 μm. Figure 8 confirms this assumption. Furthermore, the fact that no reduction of the average redox ratio is observed with increased distance from the surface suggests that the freeze–clamping of the sample was sufficiently fast to ensure quenching of all parts of the tissue block before the onset of anoxia.

A number of different redox perturbations have been tried on the perfused

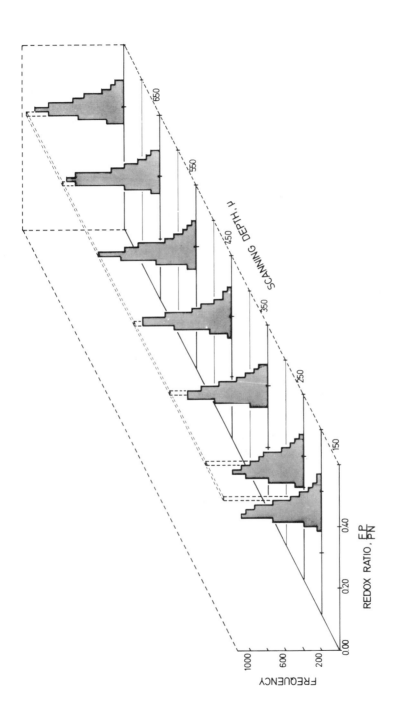

Figure 7. Frequency-distribution histogram of the FP/PN ratio for 13 consecutive scans of a freeze–clamped perfused rat liver. Prior to freezing, the liver was perfused for 20 min with Krebs–Henseleit–bicarbonate buffer, equilibriated with O_2 : Co_2 95 : 5, (vol. %). Each histogram represents one scan of 3.5 × 3.5 mm with 5041 single-point measurements of the FP/PN ratio. Only every second histogram is displayed for reasons of clarity. Reprinted from Quistorff and Chance.[39]

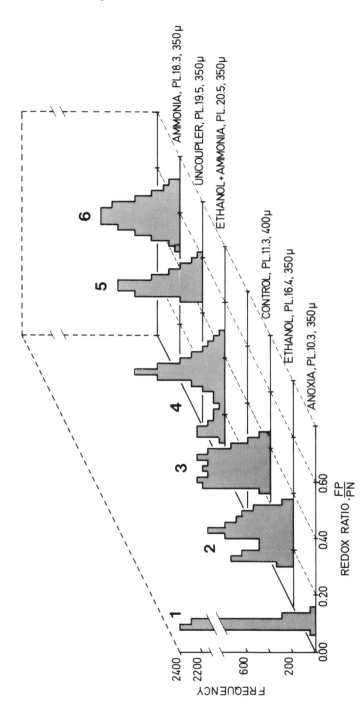

Figure 8. Frequency-distribution histograms of the FP/PN ratio. Shown are typical histograms from a number of different experiments with different redox perturbations. (1) The anoxic liver was freeze–clamped after having been left unperfused for 10 min (5 min at room temperature followed by 5 min on ice) and was covered with oxygen-impermeable foil. (2) Ethanol (6 mM) was included in the perfusate for 15 min prior to freeze–clamping. (3) Scan from control liver. (4) Ethanol (6 mM) and ammonium chloride (1 mM) were included in the perfusate 4×4 mm scan with 6561 data points at a resolution of 50 μm (5) Uncoupler [carbonylcyanide-*m*-chlorophenylhydrazone (CCCP)] (0.02 mM) was included in the perfusate for 15 min prior to freeze–clamping. (6) Ammonium chloride (1 mM) was included in the perfusate. All histograms, except histogram 4, represent 6×6 mm scans at a resolution of 100 μm, with 3721 data points per scan.

liver. Figure 8 shows examples of such experiments, presented as typical frequency-distribution histograms of the FP/PN ratio. Histogram 1, from an anoxic liver, shows a maximally reduced state and very narrow redox-ratio range. In fact, the 2-D redox ratio image of the anoxic liver (not shown) is completely without pattern. This allows the very important conclusion that liver morphology *per se* does not contribute any pattern to the redox scan.

With ethanol in the perfusate (histogram 2), the average redox ratio decreases to approximately 60% of control, in agreement with the well-known effect of ethanol on both the lactate/pyruvate and the hydroxybutyrate/acetoacetate ratio.[47] However, the histogram appears to have aquired a bimodal shape. One population of hepatocytes (25%) is highly reduced, while the majority of the readings reflect a somewhat reduced state but still within the control range.[48]

As would be expected, both uncoupler and ammonium chloride cause an increase of the average redox ratio, the increase being approximately 2-fold for ammonia (histogram 6) and 1.6-fold for uncoupler (histogram 5). Interestingly, the oxidation caused by ammonia seems to be almost completely eliminated by simultaneous addition of ammonia and ethanol (histogram 4). With this perturbation, about 25% of the readings become highly reduced, comparable to the reduced fraction of the ethanol histogram, while the remaining part is within the control range. An explanation of this result must await further experiments, but it is possible that zonation of either the metabolism of ammonia or that of ethanol plays a role. Recent work by Häussinger[49] supports the concept of zonation of the metabolism of ammonia. On the other hand, Kashiwagi *et al.*[50] do not find a zonation of the metabolism of ethanol.

6.2. Two- and Three-Dimensional Redox-Ratio Images

Figure 9 shows the 2-D redox pattern of a control liver *in vivo*. The FP/PN ratio is displayed on a gray scale covering the interval 0.48–0.22, with white as oxidized and black as reduced. The observed pattern represents a "redox image" of the particular liver section, rather than a structural image. The scan may be described as regularly scattered "reduced dots" (black) on a more or less uniformly oxidized background (white), very much resembling the well-known and characteristic lobular morphology of the liver. The reduced dots are 0.3–0.5 mm in diameter with a center-to-center distance of about 0.8 mm. We interpret the pattern as the white areas being the oxidized periportal space and the reduced black spots being the perivenous area. We have encircled what could be a classic lobule in Fig. 9, including a reduced perivenous area in the middle, surrounded by a number of "metabolic acini."[1]

On the basis of perfusion with india ink, Ji *et al.*[51] suggested that the darker spots on the surface of the hemoglobin-free perfused liver corresponded to the perivenous area in the rat liver. When FP/PN scans were compared with reflec-

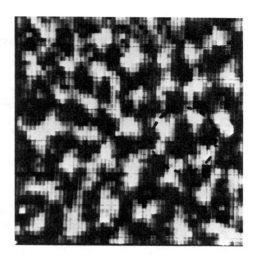

Figure 9. Television display of FP/PN scan from a control rat liver *in vivo*. The liver was freeze–clamped *in situ* as described in Quistorff and Chance.[42] The image represents a 6 × 6 mm area at a resolution of 100 μm and a depth of 400 μm, and was reconstructed from 3721 single-point measurements of the FP and PN fluorescence.

tance scans of the same surface, the lighter areas (more reflectance) of the latter corresponded to the oxidized parts of the FP/PN scans, thus supporting the aforedescribed interpretation of the redox pattern. However, the final proof will of course be an experiment in which a histological examination of the scanned surface confirms oxidized area as periportal space.

Figure 10 shows scans from freeze–clamped perfused livers. Two controls, one scanned at a resolution of 100 μm (left column) and another scanned at a resolution of 50 μm (middle column) are shown. The right-hand column shows a scan of a liver in which ethanol (6 mM) was included in the perfusate. For all three scans, the PN, the FP, and the calculated FP/PN ratio image are given. Note that different gray scales are used for the different images. In all images, however, a high number is represented in white and a low number in black. Compared with the *in vivo* scan in Fig. 9, the perfused control liver (Fig. 10, left column) shows an almost identical pattern. It is noteworthy that the FP and images actually show inverse patterns, except in a few localized spots where the signal is very low in both channels. The effect of ethanol on the 2-D redox pattern (Fig. 10, right column) is a significant increase in the reduced perivenous area and a much steeper transition between the periportal and perivenous areas. In most locations, the transition occurs within the linear resolution of the scan, i.e., 50 μm. On examination of the 2-D FP/PN scans of Fig. 10, one may recognize, in the outline of the reduced perivenous area in both the ethanol and the control liver, the so-called "starfish" shape found histologically in the liver in various pathological conditions,[1] supporting the concept of metabolic zonation.[2]

One of the virtues of the redox-ratio scanning technique is the ability to obtain information on 3-D metabolic structure. Figure 11 shows examples of

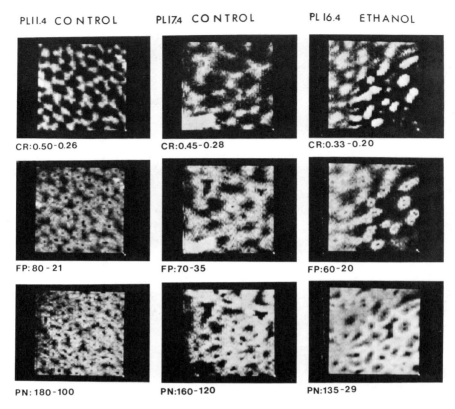

Figure 10. Television display of FP, PN, and FP/PN scans from perfused rat liver. The liver was perfused as described in the Fig 7 caption. The control liver (PL11.4) represents a 6 × 6 mm scan with 3721 data points at 100-μm resolution. The other control (PL17.4) represents a 3.5 × 3.5 mm scan with 5041 data points recorded at a resolution of 50 μm. The scan in the right-hand column is from a liver for which ethanol (6 mM) was included in the perfusate for 15 min prior to freeze–clamping. Scan size and resolution were as for control PL17.4. In all scans, the gray scale used represents a high number as white and a low number as black.

this for perfused rat liver. Figure 11A is from a control and Fig. 11B from an ethanol-perfused liver. It is obvious from the 2-D scans in Figs. 9 and 10 that there is a relatively well defined border zone in the FP/PN image. It was therefore convenient to reconstruct the 3-D data from the liver with only two gray levels, white as oxidized and black as reduced. The tissue block represented in the control (Fig. 11 A) was 2.9 × 2.9 × 0.9 mm, reconstructed from 5400 singlepoint measurements of the FP/PN ratio. For the ethanol-perfused liver (Fig. 11B), the tissue block was 1.9 × 1.9 × 0.55 mm, reconstructed from 16,000 points. Both models clearly show that the 2-D pattern of the consecutive scans forms a consistent 3-D structure, which may be interpreted as above in terms of the oxidized zones (white) and the reduced zones (black) being periportal and

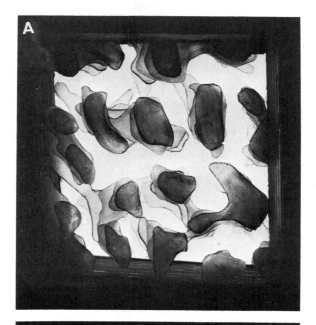

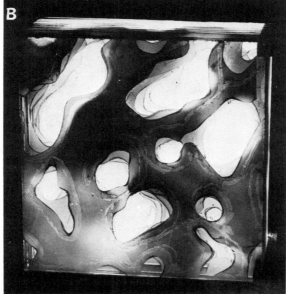

Figure 11. Three-dimensional redox-ratio model of perfused liver. (A) Control liver; (B) ethanol (6 mM)-perfused liver. Both models are seen from the surface of the liver. Modified from Quistorff and Chance.[39]

perivenous spaces, respectively. These figures demonstrated for the first time the existence of a 3-D metabolic organization of the liver.[48]

7. CONCLUSIONS

The redox-ratio scanning technique, although not nondestructive when used as a 3-D scanning technique, allows the evaluation of intercellular redox gradients. Thus, a much-needed link between biochemical examination of average organ function and physiological evaluation of the integrated metabolic function of the organ is now provided.

The data presented herein demonstrate clearly the existence of a redox gradient along the sinusoid of the normoxic perfused liver as well as for liver *in vivo*. The 3-D scans have identified the existence of a "metabolic acinus" in the liver, the shape of which is highly sensitive to redox perturbations such as those caused by alcohol metabolism.

8. SUMMARY

The intercellular compartmentation of the mammalian liver seems to play an important role in the integrated metabolic function of the organ. This chapter has discussed redox-state measurements in intact liver by means of automated surface fluorescence scanning. The spatial resolution of the current redox-ratio scanning method is about 2×10^{-7} ml, corresponding to 20–30 hepatocytes. This allows 3-D mapping of the microcirculatory unit of the liver in terms of redox state. Available 2- and 3-D redox scans of liver with various redox perturbations were summarized, demonstrating a periportal–perivenous redox gradient in the normoxic liver *in vivo* as well as in the perfused liver. Finally, the existence of a three-dimensional "metabolic acinus" was demonstrated.

ACKNOWLEDGMENTS. This research was supported in part by Grants USPHS-AA-05662 and NINCDS-10939, The Novo Foundation, and The Danish Medical Research Council, J. 12-4549 and 12-5473.

REFERENCES

1. Rappaport, A. M., 1980, Hepatic blood flow: Morphologic aspects and physiologic regulation, in: *Liver and Biliary Tract Physiology I*, Vol. 21 (N. B. Javitt, ed.), pp. 1–63, *Int. Rev. Physiol.*, University Park Press, Baltimore.
2. Jungermann, K., and Katz, N., 1982, Functional hepatocellular heterogeneity, *Hepatology* 2(3):385–395.

3. Quistorff, B., 1983, The use of a hepatocyte column in the study of metabolic zonation in the liver, in: *Isolation, Characterization, and Use of Hepatocytes* (R. A. Harris and N. W. Cornell, eds.), pp. 131–137, Elsevier, New York.

4. Quistorff, B., Grunnet, N., and Cornell, N. W., 1985, Digitonin perfusion of rat liver: A new approach in the study of intraacinar and intracellular compartmentation in the liver, *Biochem. J.* **226**: 289–297.

4a. Quistorff, B., 1985, Gluconeogenesis in periportal and perivenous hepatocytes of rat liver, isolated by a new high-yield, digitonin–collagenase perfusion technique, *Biochem. J.* **229**:221–226.

5. Haselgrove, J. C., Subramanian, V. H., Leigh, J. S., Jr., Gyulai, L., and Chance, B., 1983, *In vivo* one-dimensional imaging of phosphorus metabolites by phosphorus-31 nuclear magnetic resonance, *Science* **220**:1170–1173.

6. Quistorff, B., and Chance, B., 1977, Two- and three dimensional analysis on brain oxygen delivery, in: *Oxygen and Physiological Function* (F. F. Jöbsis, ed.), pp. 100–110, Professional Information Library, Dallas.

7. Quistorff, B., Haselgrove, J. C., and Chance, B., 1985, High spatial resolution read-out of 3-D metabolic organ structure: An automated, low-temperature redox ratio scanning instrument, *Anal. Biochem.* **148**:389–400.

8. Williamson, D. H., Lund, P., and Krebs, H. A. 1967, The redox state of free nicotinamide-adenine dinucleotide in the cytoplasm and mitochondria of rat liver, *Biochem. J.* **103**:514–527.

9. Sies, H., 1982, Nicotinamide nucleotide compartmentation, in: *Metabolic Compartmentation* (H. Sies, ed.), pp. 205–231, Academic Press, London.

10. Bücher, T., Brauser, B., Conze, A., Klein, F., Langguth, O., and Sies, H., 1972, State of oxidation–reduction and state of binding in cytosolic NADH-systems as disclosed by equili-bration with extracellular lactate/pyruvate in hemoglobin-free perfused rat liver, *Eur. J. Biochem.* **27**:301–317.

11. Sies, H., 1977, Redox compartmentation: A survey with emphasis on current problems, in: *Alcohol and Aldehyde Metabolizing Systems,* Vol. 3 (R. G. Thurman, J. R. Williamson, H. Drott, and B. Chance, eds.), pp. 47–64, Academic Press, New York.

12. Krebs, H. A., 1966, The redox state of NAD in the cytoplasm and mitochondria of rat liver, *Adv. Enzyme. Regul.* **5**:409–437.

13. Hoek, J. B., and Ernster, L., 1974, Mitochondrial transhydrogenase and the regulation of cytosolic reducing power, in: *Alcohol and Aldehyde Metabolizing Systems,* Vol. 1 (R. G. Thurman, Y. Yonetani, J. R. Williamson, and B. Chance, eds.), pp. 351–364. Academic Press, London.

14. Chance, B., and Jöbsis, F. F., 1959, Changes in fluorescence in a frog sartorius muscle following a twitch, *Nature (London)* **4681**:195–197.

15. Chance, B., Cohen, P., Jöbsis, F. F., and Schoener, B., 1962, Intracellular oxidation–reduction states *in vivo, Science* **137**:449–508.

16. Ramirez, J., and Vega, J., 1965, Cambios de la fluorescencia del musculo cardiaco durante la actividad mecanica, *Acta Physiol. Lat. Am.* **15**:239–240.

17. Welsh, F. A., O'Connor, M. J., and Langfitt, T. W., 1977, Regions of cerebral ischemia located by pyridine nucleotide fluorescence, *Science* **198**:951–953.

18. Barlow, C. H., and Chance, B., 1967, Ischemic areas in perfused rat hearts: Measurement by NADH fluorescence photography, *Science* **193**:909–910.

19. Chance, B., Schoener, B., Krejci, K., Rüssmann, W., Wessmann, W., Schnitger, H., and Bücher, T., 1965, Kinetics of fluorescence and metabolite changes in rat liver during a cycle of ischaemia, *Biochem. Z.* **341**:325–333.

20. Chance, B., and Schoener, B., 1966, Fluorometric studies of flavin component of the respi-ratory chain, in: *Flavins and Flavoproteins* (E. C. Slater, ed.), pp. 510–519, Elsevier, Am-sterdam.

21. Hassinen, I., and Chance, B., 1968, Oxidation–reduction properties of the mitochondrial flavoprotein chain, *Biochem. Biophys. Res. Commun.* **31**(6):895–900.

22. Chance, B., Mela, L., and Wong, D., 1968, Flavoproteins of the respiratory chain, in: *Flavins and Flavoproteins*, (K. Yagi, ed.), pp. 107–121, University Park Press, Baltimore.

23. Scholz, R., Thurman, R. G., Williamson, J. R., Chance, B., and Bücher, T., 1969, Flavin and pyridine nucleotide oxydation–reduction changes in perfused rat liver: Anoxia and subcellular localization of fluorescent flavoproteins, *J. Biol. Chem.* **244**(9):2317–2324.

24. Chance, B., Schoener, B., Oshino, R., Itshak, F., and Nakase, Y., 1979, Oxidation–reduction ratio studies of mitochondria in freeze-trapped samples, *J. Biol. Chem.* **254**:4764–4771.

25. Chance, B., Williamson, J. R., Jamieson, D., and Schoener, B., 1965, Properties and kinetics of reduced pyridine nucleotide fluorescence of the isolated *in vivo* rat heart, *Biochem. Z.* **341**:357–377.

26. Sies, H., Häussinger, D., and Grosskopf, M., 1974, Mitochondrial nicotinamide nucleotide systems: Ammonium chloride responses in hemoglobin-free perfused liver, *Hoppe-Seyler's Z. Physiol. Chem.* **355**:305–320.

27. Avi-Dor, Y., Olson, J. M., Doherty, M. D., and Kaplan, N. O., 1962, Fluorescence of pyridine nucleotides in mitochondria, *J. Biol. Chem.* **237**(7):2377–2383.

28. Boyer, P. D., and Theorell, H., 1956, The changes in reduced NAD (NADH) fluorescence upon combination with liver ADH, *Acta Chem. Scand.* **10**:447–450.

29. Velick, S. F., 1958, Fluorescence spectra and polarization of glyceraldehyde-3-P- and lactic dehydrogenase coenzyme complexes, *J. Biol. Chem.* **233**(6):1455–1467.

30. Chance, B., and Baltschefsky, H., 1958, Respiratory enzymes in oxidative phosphorylation. VII. Binding of intramitochondrial reduced NAD(P), *J. Biol. Chem.* **233**(3):736–739.

31. Galeotti, T., Rossum, D. V. van, Mayer, D. H., and Chance, B., 1970, On the fluorescence of NAD(P)H in whole cell preparation of tumours and normal tissues, *Eur. J. Biochem.* **17**:485–496.

32. Thorell, B., and Chance, B., 1960, Microspectrography of respiratory enzymes within the single cell under different metabolic conditions, *Exp. Cell Res.* **20**:43–55.

33. Jöbsis, F. F., and Duffield, J. C., 1967, Oxidative and glycolytic recovery metabolism in muscle, *J. Gen. Physiol.* **50**:10109–1047.

34. Chapman, J. B., 1972, Fluorometric studies of oxidative metabolism in isolated papillary muscle of the rabbit, *J. Gen. Physiol.* **59**:135–154.

35. Williamson, J. R., 1965, Glycolytic control mechanisms, *J. Biol. Chem.* **240**:2308–2318.

36. O'Connor, M. J., Welsh, F., Komarnicky, L., Davis, T., Stevens, J., Lewis, D., and Herman, C., 1977, Origin of labile NADH tissue fluorescence, in: *Oxygen and Physiological Function* (F. F. Jöbsis, ed.), pp. 90–99, Professional Information Library, Dallas.

37. Aubert, X., Chance, B., and Keynes, R. D., 1964, Optical studies of biochemical events in the electric organ of *Electrophorus*, *Proc. R. Soc. London Ser. B.* **160**:211–233.

38. Haselgrove, J. C., Barlow, C. H., and Chance, B., 1980, The 3-D distribution of metabolic states in the gerbil brain during the course of spreading depression, in: *Cerebral Metabolism and Neuronal Function* (J. V. Passonneau, R. A. Hawkins, W. D. Lust, and F. A. Welsh, eds.), pp. 72–76, Williams & Wilkins, Baltimore.

39. Quistorff, B., and Chance, B., 1982, 3-Dimensional recording of metabolic structure of rat liver: Evidence for a dynamic spatial ordering of liver metabolism, in: *Alcohol and Alcohol Metabolism: First Symposium on Alcohol* (J. Wadstein, ed.), pp. 21–39, Ferrosan, Malmö, Sweden.

40. Chance, B., and Quistorff, B., 1978, Study of tissue oxygen gradients by single and multiple indicators, in: *Oxygen Transport to Tissue—III* (I. A. Silver, M. Erecińska, and H. I. Bicher, eds.), pp. 331–338, Plenum Press, New York.

40a. Erecińska, M., and Chance, B., 1972, Studies on the electron transport chain at subzero temperatures: Electron transport at site III. *Arch. Biochem. Biophys.* **151**:304–315.

41. Chance, B., and Williams, G. R., 1957, The respiratory chain and oxidative phosphorylation, *Methods Enzymol.* **17**:65–134.

42. Quistorff, B., and Chance, B., 1980, Simple techniques for freeze–clamping and for cutting and milling frozen tissue at low temperature for the purpose of two- or three-dimensional metabolic studies *in vivo*, *Anal. Biochem.* **108**:237–248.

43. Ji, S., Chance, B., Nishiki, K., Smith, T., and Rich, T., 1979, Micro-light guide: A new method for measuring tissue fluorescence and reflectance, *Am. J. Physiol.* **236**:C144–C156.

44. Chance, B., Legallais, V., Sorge, J., and Graham, N., 1975, A versatile time-sharing multichannel spectrophotometer, reflectometer, and fluorometer, *Anal. Biochem.* **66**:498–514.

45. Quistorff, B., 1980, Guillotine freeze–clamping of rat brain: Analysis of energy metabolites along the freezing gradient, in: *Cerebral Metabolism and Neuronal Function* (J. V. Passonneau, R. A. Hawkins, W. D. Lust, and F. A. Welsh, eds.), pp.42–52, Williams & Wilkins, Baltimore.

46. Quistorff, B., and Poulsen, H., 1980, Evaluation of a freeze–clamping technique designed for two- and three-dimensional metabolic studies of rat liver *in vivo:* Quenching efficiency and effect of clamping on tissue morphology, *Anal. Biochem.* **108**:249–256.

47. Williamson, J. R., Scholtz, R., Browning, E. T., Thurman, R. G., and Fukami, M. H., 1969, Metabolic effects of ethanol in the perfused liver, *J. Biol. Chem.* **244**(18):5044–5054.

48. Quistorff, B., and Chance, B., 1977, Three-dimensional mapping of metabolic state of rat liver: Effects of high and low alcohol concentrations, *Hoppe-Seyler's Z. Physiol. Chem.* **358**:1261.

49. Häussinger, D., 1983, Hepatocyte heterogeneity in glutamine and ammonia metabolism and the role of an intracellular glutamine cycle during ureogenesis in perfused rat liver, *Eur. J. Biochem.* **133**:269–275.

50. Kashiwagi, T., Ji, S., Lemasters, J. J., and Thurman, R. G., 1981, Rates of alcohol dehydrogenase-dependent ethanol metabolism in periportal and pericentral regions of the perfused rat liver, *Mol. Pharmacol.* **21**:438–443.

51. Ji, Š., Lemasters, J. J., and Thurman, R. G., 1980, A non-invasive method to study metabolic events within sublobular regions of hemoglobin-free perfused liver, *FEBS Lett.* **113**(1):37–41.

52. Jöbsis, F. F., and Lamanna, J. C., 1978, Kinetic aspects of intracellular redox reactions, in: *Extrapulmonary Manifestations of Respiratory Disease* (E. Robin, ed.), pp. 63–106, Marcel Dekker, New York.

Distribution of Metabolic Functions

Chapter 9

Metabolism of Carbohydrates

Kurt Jungermann and Norbert Katz

1. INTRODUCTION

The liver can be regarded as the center of intermediary metabolism of the organism. It removes glucose if in excess, as after a normal carbohydrate-rich meal, via glycogen synthesis and glycolysis plus liponeogenesis, and it liberates glucose if needed, as between meals, via glycogen degradation and gluconeogenesis. It alone produces ketone bodies and has a major role in lipoprotein metabolism (see Chapter 10). The liver detoxifies ammonia and amino acid nitrogen by the synthesis of urea and glutamine (see Chapter 11). The major pathways of energy production are the β-oxidation of fatty acids and the degradation of amino acids. This chapter first reviews how the liver functions as a glucostat in different dietary situations. It then briefly summarizes the regulation of carbohydrate metabolism by the extracellular levels of substrates and hormones, and by the hepatic nerves, and finally shows how hepatocyte heterogeneity might be involved in regulation.

KURT JUNGERMANN and NORBERT KATZ • Institut für Biochemie, Universität Göttingen, D-3400 Göttingen, Federal Republic of Germany.

2. ROLE OF THE LIVER IN THE METABOLISM OF CARBOHYDRATES: INTERORGAN RELATIONSHIPS

2.1. Glucose Uptake

2.1.1. Absorption at Rest

A normal carbohydrate-rich meal contains on average of about 100 g of glucose equivalents. During the first 2 hr after the meal, the intestine absorbs glucose at a rate of approximately 45–50 g $\times$ hr^{-1}. Only 7.5 g $\times$ hr^{-1} is utilized by the brain and the erythrocytes,[1,2] leaving an excess of about 40 g $\times$ hr^{-1}. If the excess were distributed in the extracellular space, the blood glucose concentration would rise to about 20 mM. Since the threshold of the kidney for glucose is about 10 mM, freshly absorbed glucose would be lost if this value were exceeded. This, of course, does not occur. Excess glucose is "buffered" by uptake in skeletal muscle, in adipose tissue, and predominantly in the liver. More than 50% of the absorbed glucose, about 25 g $\times$ hr^{-1}, is taken up by the liver and converted to glycogen or fat or degraded to CO_2[3,4] (Fig. 1). Glycogen synthesis, glycolysis, and liponeogenesis are thus the major processes in the liver during absorption at rest.

2.2. Glucose Release

2.2.1. Short-Term Postabsorption at Rest

After several hours without food, as after a normal fast, there is a glucose requirement of 7.5 g $\times$ hr^{-1}, [6 g $\times$ hr^{-1} being utilized by the brain, and 1.5 g $\times$ hr^{-1} by the erythrocytes[1,2]]. The glucose needs of other organs can be neglected. The major energy substrates are fatty acids, e.g., for the liver and skeletal muscle. Glucose is supplied by the liver; 4.5 g $\times$ hr^{-1} is liberated from the hepatic glycogen stores and 3 g $\times$ hr^{-1} is synthesized *de novo* from lactate, amino acids, and glycerol. Lactate is produced by the erythrocytes, so there is a constant glucose–lactate–glucose cycle. Amino acids are released from the protein stores of the muscles, whereas glycerol is formed from the triglyceride stores in the adipose tissue (Fig. 2). Glycogen degradation and gluconeogenesis are thus the prevalent processes in the liver during short-term postabsorption.

2.2.2. Long-Term Postabsorption at Rest

After several days or weeks without food, the situation is similar to short-term postabsorption,[1,2] with one decisive difference. The hepatic stores of glycogen are very limited; they last for 1 day only. The protein stores of the muscle that provide amino acids as gluconeogenic precursors are also limited. Glucose becomes the limiting substrate; therefore, the organism has developed a glucose-

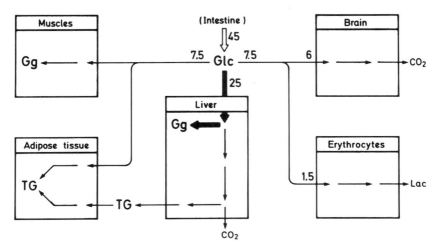

Figure 1. Substrate flow during absorption at rest. Energy turnover, 90 W. All data are given in $g \times hr^{-1}$. Abbreviations here and in Figs. 2–4. (Glc) Glucose; (Lac) lactate; (Gg) glycogen; (TG) triglycerides; (PR) protein; (AA) amino acids; (FA) fatty acids; (Gll) glycerol. For details, see Felig et al.[3] and Felig and Sherwin.[4]

saving adaptation of metabolism. The glucose requirement of the brain is drastically reduced from $6 g \times hr^{-1}$ to about $2 g \times hr^{-1}$. Glucose is replaced largely by ketone bodies, which are also supplied by the liver. The glucose need of the whole organism is reduced from $7.5 g \times hr^{-1}$ to about $3.5 g \times hr^{-1}$; $2.5 g \times hr^{-1}$ is produced by the liver via gluconeogenesis, and $1 g \times hr^{-1}$ comes from the kidney, in which gluconeogenesis is clearly increased due to metabolic acidosis

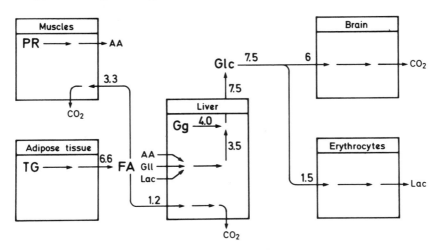

Figure 2. Substrate flow during short-term postabsorption at rest, as after an overnight fast. Energy turnover, 90 W. All data are given in $g \times hr^{-1}$. Abbreviations as in Fig. 1. For details, see Cahill et al.[1]

prevalent during fasting (Fig. 3). Thus, gluconeogenesis and ketogenesis are the major processes in the liver during long-term postabsorption.

2.2.3. Exercise during Short-Term Postabsorption

During exercise, the most important change in metabolism is the drastic increase of the carbohydrate requirement.[2,5–8] At rest in the postabsorptive situation, fatty acid oxidation contributes 80% and carbohydrate oxidation only 20% of the energy demand. At a work load of 150 W corresponding to a total energy turnover of about 800 W, carbohydrate oxidation contributes about 70% and fatty acid utilization only 30% of the energy demand, which in absolute terms is increased about 9-fold. The glucose requirement of the brain and the erythrocytes is unchanged and amounts to 7.5 g $\times$ hr^{-1}. Yet, carbohydrate utilization in muscle is enhanced from very low values of less than 2 g $\times$ hr^{-1} at rest to about 85 g $\times$ hr^{-1} during work; 63 g $\times$ hr^{-1} is derived from the breakdown of muscle glycogen and 22 g $\times$ hr^{-1} is supplied by circulating glucose. There is also an increase in the utilization of fatty acids from about 3 g $\times$ hr^{-1} to 17 g $\times$ hr^{-1}. The greatly increased requirement of free glucose during exercise is again supplied by the liver. The liver now releases glucose at a rate of 30 g $\times$ hr^{-1} instead of 7.5 g $\times$ hr^{-1} at rest, a 4-fold increase. Liver glycogen is degraded at a rate of 25 g $\times$ hr^{-1} as compared to 4.5 g $\times$ hr^{-1}, a 5- to 6-fold increase. Gluconeogenesis appears to be enhanced only slightly, from 3.5 g $\times$ hr^{-1} to 5 g $\times$ hr^{-1} (Fig. 4). Thus, enhanced glycogenolysis is the predominant process in the liver during exercise.

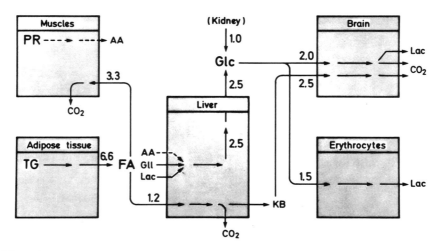

Figure 3. Substrate flow during long-term postabsorption at rest, as after 5 weeks of starvation. Energy turnover, 70 W. All data are given in g $\times$ hr^{-1}. (KB) Ketone bodies; other abbreviations as in Fig. 1. For details, see Cahill et al.[1]

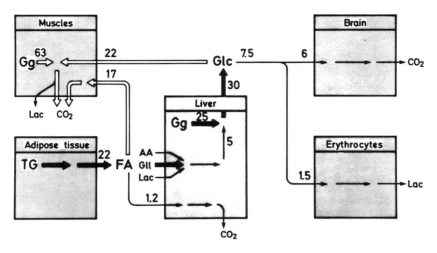

Figure 4. Substrate flow during short-term postabsorption with exercise. Work load, 150 W. Total energy turnover, 800 W. All data are given in g × hr⁻¹. Abbreviations as in Fig. 1. The data have been calculated[2] from various studies.[5-8]

In summary, in the absorptive as well as in all postabsorptive situations, the liver plays the key role in the maintenance of glucose homeostasis.

3. ROLE OF SUBSTRATES, HORMONES, AND NERVES IN THE REGULATION OF CARBOHYDRATE METABOLISM

The "everyday" problem of short-term regulation is the control of the reversible shift from glycogenolysis and gluconeogenesis during postabsorption to glycogen synthesis and glycolysis during absorption. This chapter will be able to cover only some aspects of the regulatory problems involved. There are four major factors involved in the regulation of the glucostat: substrate concentrations, hormone levels, activity of hepatic nerves, and hepatocyte heterogeneity (see Section 4).

The normal postabsorptive glucose concentration is 5 mM. After a normal meal, the concentration rises in the portal vein to 10 or 15 mM.[9,10] The major hormones involved in the regulation of hepatic carbohydrate metabolism are insulin and glucagon. After a carbohydrate-rich meal, insulin is increased and glucagon is decreased.[11] Only some effects of these two antagonists can be described here. The roles of other hormones[12] such as catecholamines, angiotensin, oxytocin, and vasopressin or gastrointestinal factors such as secretin and gastrin are beyond the scope of this overview.

The liver is innervated by both the sympathetic and the parasympathetic nervous system[13–16] (see Chapter 1). Both systems have their origin in the hypothalamus. On separate routes, the nerves reach the celiac ganglion. Then branches extend to the endocrine pancreas and the adrenal medulla, where they are involved in the regulation of the secretion of insulin, glucagon, adrenaline, and noradrenaline. Other branches extend into the liver; they reach the organ as a ramification around the hepatic artery and the portal vein. The hepatic sympathetic nerves operate at frequencies up to 20 Hz, the parasympathetic nerves at frequencies up to 50 Hz. The sympathetic tone is decreased with an increased glucose level, as after a meal, and conversely increased with a decreased glucose level, as during a work load.[17]

3.1. Glycogen Metabolism

3.1.1. Substrates and Hormones

Glucose stimulates glycogen synthesis. When high glucose concentrations were added to hepatocyte suspensions,[18] glycogen phosphorylase was inactivated and glycogen synthase was activated (Fig. 5). It is generally accepted that insulin activates the utilization of excess glucose after a meal, while glucagon stimulates the release of glucose during the postabsorptive period. Yet with respect to insulin, the picture is not so clear. As pointed out by Hue and Van de Werve[21]:

> "The study of insulin action on the liver is rather frustrating. The anti-catabolic effects are the only readily demonstrable effects. . . . Direct effects are scarce. The reason for this is not clear."

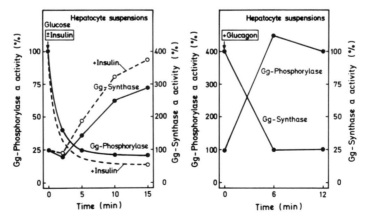

Figure 5. Effect of glucose, insulin, and glucagon on glycogen metabolism in hepatocyte suspensions. Data are redrawn from results given in Hue et al.[18,20] and Witters and Avruch.[19]

The effects of insulin and glucagon on glycogen metabolism were studied in hepatocyte suspensions. At normal glucose concentrations of 5 mM, insulin appears to be ineffective. It may be effective only in the presence of high glucose concentrations by enhancing the changes brought about by glucose itself,[19,22,23] i.e., the inhibition of glycogen phosphorylase and the activation of glycogen synthase. As expected, glucagon activates glycogen phosphorylase and inhibits glycogen synthase[20] (Fig. 5).

3.1.2. Hepatic Nerves

The role of the autonomic hepatic nerves in the regulation of liver metabolism is not as clear as that of substrates and hormones. Most studies of the nervous control of hepatic metabolism have performed preganglionic stimulation in intact animals[13,16] (references in Hartmann et al.[24]), with the conclusion that sympathetic stimulation increases glycogen breakdown and glucose output, while parasympathetic stimulation increases glycogen synthesis and glucose uptake. Studies of preganglionic stimulation, however, do not allow a clear differentiation between direct and indirect nerve effects, e.g., via the endocrine pancreas or the adrenals. This differentiation is possible in the rat liver perfused in situ with direct electrical stimulation of the hepatic nerves by placing the electrodes around the portal vein and hepatic artery. This mode of stimulation activates both sympathetic and parasympathetic nerve fibers; normally, however, sympathetic effects clearly predominate.

In livers perfused with 5 mM glucose and 2 mM lactate, electrical stimulation increased glucose output, reversed lactate uptake to output[24] (Fig. 6), reduced oxygen uptake and portal flow, and caused a redistribution of the intrahepatic circulation.[25,26] Stimulation of the nerves was accompanied by the release of norepinephrine into the hepatic vein.[27] Both the metabolic and the hemodynamic effects were mediated by α-sympathetic receptors. Apparently, parasympathetic nerves were not effective in the liver under the experimental conditions, since atropine had no influence.[24–27] The metabolic changes were due primarily to an activation of glycogen breakdown.[24]

The nerve-dependent activation of glycogenolysis was modulated by insulin and glucagon[28] (Fig. 6). If insulin was infused before nerve stimulation, the nerve-dependent glucose output was clearly reduced and the change in lactate metabolism diminished slightly. If glucagon was infused before nerve stimulation, glucose output and lactate uptake were increased first, indicating the expected activation of both glycogenolysis and gluconeogenesis. The following nerve stimulation increased glucose output further and reduced lactate uptake considerably. These data clearly show that the nerve effects are modulated by circulating hormones. Knowledge of the interaction between the hormonal and the nervous system is still very sparse; further experiments are certainly necessary.

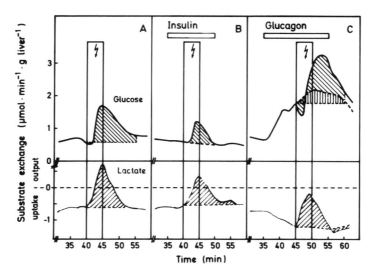

Figure 6. Effect of electrical stimulation of hepatic nerves on glucose and lactate balance in the isolated, perfused rat liver *in situ*. Modulation by insulin and glucagon. Data are redrawn from results given in Hartmann *et al.*[24] and Beckh *et al.*[28]

3.2. Glycolysis and Gluconeogenesis

3.2.1. Substrates and Hormones

Glucose stimulates its own breakdown. In hepatocyte cultures, glycolysis was clearly enhanced by an increased glucose concentration, while gluconeogenesis was unaffected[29] (Fig. 7). The autoregulatory response of glucokinase to glucose[30] and an increase of the newly discovered effector fructose-2,6-bisphosphate[31] should be involved in the activation of glycolysis by glucose.

The effect of insulin and glucagon on glycolysis and gluconeogenesis was studied in hepatocyte cultures in which direct insulin effects could be observed.[29,32] Insulin at normal glucose levels of 5 mM activated glycolysis, but had no influence on gluconeogenesis. Glucagon had inverse effects; it inhibited glycolysis and activated gluconeogenesis. The hormones were active essentially in the physiological concentration range (Fig. 7).

3.2.2. Hepatic Nerves

Glycolysis and gluconeogenesis are probably also under nervous control. In glycogen-rich livers from fed rats, α-sympathetic nerve stimulation enhanced lactate output[24,28] (see Fig. 6); in glycogen-poor livers from fasted rats, nerve stimulation increased lactate uptake and glucose output[33] (not shown).

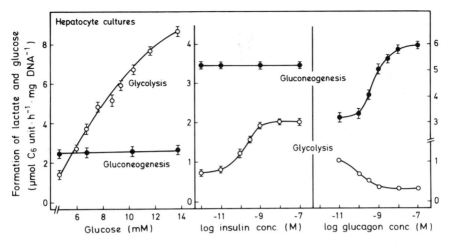

Figure 7. Effect of glucose, insulin, and glucagon on glycolysis and gluconeogenesis in hepatocyte cultures. Data are given in Probst et al.[29]

4. ROLE OF ZONAL HEPATOCYTE HETEROGENEITY IN THE REGULATION OF CARBOHYDRATE METABOLISM

Hepatocytes from the periportal (afferent) and perivenous (efferent) zones of the liver parenchyma differ in their enzyme contents and subcellular structures. This heterogeneity has been known for many years, first on a more descriptive level,[34,35] then increasingly on a more functional level.[36–38]

On the assumption that enzyme activities indicate metabolic capacities, it was proposed that the periportal cells should predominantly catalyze oxidative metabolism, β-oxidation, and glucose formation via glycogen breakdown and gluconeogenesis and that, inversely, the perivenous cells should preferentially mediate glucose utilization via glycogen sythesis, glycolysis, and liponeogenesis. This proposal became known as the model of metabolic zonation.[39]

4.1. Zonal Distribution of Enzymes

4.1.1. Oxidative Energy Metabolism

The catabolism of energy-yielding substrates such as glucose, alanine, and palmitate may be subdivided into two phases: the initial breakdown to acetyl-CoA and the final oxidation of acetyl-CoA to CO_2. All hepatocytes certainly catalyze this *final oxidation*. Yet periportal cells which receive oxygen-rich blood and thus are the more "aerobic", appear to possess the better enzymatic equipment for the final oxidative metabolism. They contain greater mitochondrial volume and cristae area per cell[40] as well as higher activities of the citrate cycle enzymes succinate dehydrogenase and malate dehydrogenase[41] and of the respiratory-chain enzyme cytochrome oxidase[34] (Table I). The *initial breakdown* of fatty acids and amino acids, on one hand, and that of glucose, on the other, appears to be distributed reciprocally. This inverse localization is in accord with the unequal distribution of the final oxidative metabolism and should be expected on the basis of theoretical considerations: Catabolism of fatty acids and of amino acids is possible only in the "more aerobic" periportal cells. The initial catabolism of glucose—at least in its glycolytic part—is possible in the absence of oxygen and should therefore be situated in the "less aerobic" perivenous cells (see below).

4.1.2. Carbohydrate Metabolism

Glycogen metabolism appears to be organized heterogeneously within the liver parenchyma. The localization of glycogen has been studied for more than a century,[42–44] yet a generally accepted view on the topochemistry of glycogen metabolism is still missing. All hepatocytes can obviously synthesize and degrade glycogen, yet the the time and rate of these processes are different in periportal and perivenous cells; major factors that determine these differences are the eating behavior during the 24-hr day–night rhythm and the type of diet, e.g., carbo-hydrate- or protein-rich food.[44] With some reservations, it may be generalized that in the rat fed a normal carbohydrate-rich diet, glycogen degradation during the light period (fasting) is more intensive in the periportal zone, so that at the end of the fasting period, more glycogen is left in the perivenous zone. Glycogen repletion during the dark period (eating) also occurs faster in the periportal zone, so that at the end of the eating period, glycogen is distributed almost equally over the parenchyma.[42–44]

Glycolysis seems to be predominant in the perivenous zone. This is indicated by the localization of the key enzymes of glycolysis, glucokinase[45–47] and py-ruvate kinase isoenzyme L[48,49] (Table I and Fig. 8). Glycolysis is functionally linked to liponeogenesis.

Liponeogenesis appears to be prevalent in the perivenous zone, as indicated by the localization of the key enzymes ATP-dependent citrate lyase,[50] acetyl-CoA carboxylase,[51] and fatty acid synthase (Katz, Ruschenburg, and Giffhorn, unpublished) and of the auxiliary NADPH-generating enzymes glucose-6-phos-phate dehydrogenase,[52–55] 6-phosphogluconate dehydrogenase,[54] and malic enzyme[43,54] (cf. Chapter 10).

Gluconeogenesis appears to be predominant in the periportal cells, as in-dicated by the localization of phosphoenolpyruvate carboxykinase,[48,55,73] fruc-tose-1,6-bisphosphatase,[45,56] and glucose-6-phosphatase[57,58] (Table I and Fig. 8). Lactate dehydrogenase[41,59] and alanine aminotransferase,[52,59,60] which me-diate the connection of lactate and alanine to the gluconeogenic pathway proper, also show higher activities in the periportal zone (Table I).

Table I. Heterogeneous Distribution of Key Enzymes and of Subcellular Structures Linked to Carbohydrate Metabolism over the Liver Parenchyma

Enzymes and structures	Periportal/ perivenous		Sex[b]	Method[c]	Ref. Nos.
	Fed[a]	Fasted[a]			
Oxidiative energy metabolism (citrate cycle, respiratory chain)					
Single mitochondrion					
Diameter	1.8	—	F	M	40
Length	0.7	—			
Volume	2.3	—			
Cristae area	2.1	—			
Total mitochondria					
Number per cell	0.7	—			
Volume per cell	1.5	—			
Cristae area	1.5	—			
Succinate dehydrogenase	1.9	—	M	KMP	41
Malate dehydrogenase	1.7	—	M	KMP	41
Cytochrome oxidase	<1	—	N.R.	HC	34
Glucose output (glycogen degradation, gluconeogenesis)					
Glucose-6-phosphatase	1.7–2.8	1.4–1.7	M, F	MMB	43, 57, 58
Fructose-1,6-bis-phosphatase	1.9–3.5	1.5–2.5	F, M	MMB	45, 56
Phosphoenolpyruvate carboxykinase	2.9	1.7	M	MMB, IHC	48, 55, 73
Lactate dehydrogenase[d]	1.3–1.8		M, N.R.	KMP, MMB	41, 59
Alanine aminotransferase[d]	1.6–5.0	3.0	F, N.R., M	MMB	52, 59, 60
Glucose uptake (glycogen synthesis, glycolysis)					
Glucokinase	0.3–0.6	0.3–0.6	M, F	MMB	45–47
Hexokinase	1.5–1.9		M, F	MMB	46, 47
Pyruvate kinase L	0.4–0.5	0.6–0.8	M, F	MMB	48, 49
Pyruvate kinase M_2	0.9	1.0	M, F	MMB	49

[a] Fed: fed *ad libitum;* Fasted: fasted 24 or 48 hr.
[b] (N.R.) Not reported.
[c] (M) Morphometry; (KMP) kinetic microsocpic photometry; (HC) histochemistry; (MMB) microdissection with microbiochemistry; (IHC) immunohistochemistry.
[d] The reason for linking this enzyme to the respective metabolic function is explained in the text (cf. Table I in Chapter 10 and in Chapter 11).

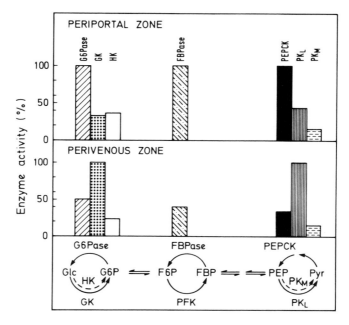

Figure 8. Distributions of the key enzymes of gluconeogenesis and glycolysis over the liver parenchyma of fed rats. Enzyme activities were determined in microdissected liver tissue with microbiochemical techniques. To facilitate comparisons, all activities were extrapolated to 37°C assuming a doubling of activity per 10°C temperature increase and converted from dry to wet weight using a factor of 0.3. The following values (μmoles $\times$ min^{-1} $\times$ g^{-1} wet weight, 37°C) were obtained: glucokinase (GK) + hexokinase (HK), 1.7 periportal (pp), 3.4 perivenous (pv)[45]; GK, 1.0 pp, 3.0 pv[47]; HK, 1.1 pp, 0.7 pv[47]; glucose-6-phosphatase (G6Pase), 10.7 pp, 4.7 pv[57]; fructose bisphosphatase (FBPase), 10.5 pp, 3.0 pv[56]; total pyruvate kinase (PK), 88 pp, 193 pv[48]; pyruvate kinase L (PK$_L$), 22 pp, 52 pv[49]; pyruvate kinase M$_2$ (PK$_M$), 6.2 pp, 7.9 pv[49]; phosphoenolypyruvate carboxykkinase (PEPCK), 7.7 pp, 2.7 pv.[48] In each case, the higher value is set equal to 100%. (Glc) Glucose; (G6P) glucose-6-phosphate; (F6P) fructose-6-phosphate; (FBP) fructose-1,6-biphosphate; (PEP) phosphoenolypyruvate; (Pyr) pyruvate; (PFK) phosphofructokinase.

The predominance of gluconeogenesis and oxidative energy metabolism in the periportal "more aerobic" zone and of glycolysis and liponeogenesis in the perivenous "less aerobic" area is in line with thermodynamic considerations.[36] Gluconeogenesis is an endergonic process (2 lactate$^-$ + 2H$^+$ $\rightarrow$ glucose, ΔG_0^l = +47.2 kcal/mole glucose) that must be driven by oxidative catabolism; it should therefore be located in cells receiving oxygen-rich blood. Glycolysis and liponeogenesis, however, are exergonic processes (4 glucose $\rightarrow$ palmitate$^-$ + H$^+$ + 8CO$_2$ + 6 H$_2$O + 2H$_2$, ΔG_0^l = -71.1 kcal/mole glucose), which are in principle independent of oxygen; they could thus be situated in hepatocytes supplied with oxygen-poor blood. An analogous functional heterogeneity also exists in the kidney cortex, where the proximal tubules are gluconeogenic and the distal ones glycolytic.[61] However, in contrast to periportal and perivenous hepatocytes, the proximal and distal tubules are supplied with oxygen equally well.

The study of liver-cell heterogeneity can be very complex. Isoenzymes, e.g., glucokinase and hexokinase[47] or pyruvate kinase L and M_2,[49] may be localized in both parenchymal and nonparenchymal cells or in only one of the two cell types. The same enzyme, e.g., glucose-6-phosphate dehydrogenase,[53] may occur with low activity in parenchymal and with very high activity in nonparenchymal cells, which are located predominantly in the periportal zone. Moreover, sex differences in the zonal distribution of enzymes have been observed: With some enzymes involved in the synthesis of fat from carbohydrates, only female rats appear to possess the periportal-to-perivenous gradient. This suggests that the female liver is especially suited to convert carbohydrate to fat (see Chapter 10).

4.2. Zonal Heterogeneity of Signals and Signal Transmission

The different equipment of hepatocytes with key enzymes and subcellular structures certainly provides the basis for different metabolic capacities, and it appears very likely that these different *capacities* are indeed realized as different metabolic rates or *activities*. However, even if the hepatocellular enzyme content were the same all over the parenchyma, different metabolic rates could occur in the different zones under two conditions. Zonal differences might exist (1) if the signals controlling metabolism such as substrate and hormone concentrations and cellular innervation differed and (2) if the signal transmission via ecto- or intracellular receptors varied. Thus, due to a possible zonal heterogeneity of signals (cf. Chapter 16) and signal transmission, the different zonal enzymatic capacities could be modulated.

4.2.1. Substrates, Hormones, and Nerves

During passage through the liver, carbon substrates such as glucose, lactate, and amino acids are either taken up or released so that concentration gradients, either decreasing or increasing from the periportal to the perivenous zone, are formed. The substrate gradients are normally relatively small (around 10–20%), and it is not clear whether they are of major regulatory importance.

In contrast to most carbon substrates, a pronounced periportal-to-perivenous oxygen gradient exists. The O_2 tension falls from about 65 mm Hg in periportal, i.e., mixed arterial (30%) and portal (70%) blood, to about 35 mm Hg in perivenous, i.e., hepatovenous blood. The O_2 gradient appears to be important for both short-term (see Section 4.3.3) and long-term regulation of the zonation of liver metabolism (cf. Chapter 16).

Hormones such as insulin, glucagon, catecholamines, and corticosteroids are degraded during passage through the liver, so that hormone concentration gradients are formed. If the rate of degradation is different for the single hormones, the hormone ratio changes from the periportal to the perivenous zone. In feeding rats, the rate of hepatic insulin degradation appears to be smaller (about 15%) than that of its antagonist glucagon (about 35%).[62] Moreover, the rate of degradation of another insulin antagonist, adrenaline, appears to be even greater [about 80% (Beckh, Balks, and Jungermann, unpublished)]. Thus, the perivenous zone is under control of a higher insulin/glucagon + adrenaline ratio than the periportal zone; this should favor glucose formation in the periportal area and glucose utilization in the perivenous area in accord with the model of metabolic zonation. Such changes in hormone ratios appear to be important not only for the short-term but also for the long-term regulation of liver metabolism (cf. Chapter 16).

Finally, the autonomic innervation of the periportal and perivenous zones may be different. In rat and mouse, sympathetic nerves appear to reach only the outer periportal cells, from which a signal might be propagated through gap junctions via electrotonic coupling; in guinea pig, rabbit, cat, dog, and man, almost all hepatocytes exhibit nerve contacts.[13–15,24]

4.2.2. Hormone Receptors

The zonal distribution of the ectocellular receptors for insulin, glucagon, and catecholamines or of the intracellular receptors for glucocorticoids is not known. It is feasible that the periportal cells have a lower and the perivenous cells a higher density of insulin receptors due to a down-regulation. The distribution of the adenylate cyclase system has recently been studied[74]; it was found that in the fed state, the basal and the glucagon − , NaF − , and forskolin-stimulated activities were equally distributed in the two zones. In the fasted state, the glucagon-stimulated activity was higher in the perivenous zone.

4.3. Functional Significance of Zonal Hepatocyte Heterogeneity: Metabolic Zonation

4.3.1. Dynamics of Zonal Heterogeneity

The zonal heterogeneity is dynamic or functional rather than static or structural. The zonation may change on longer-lasting changes in the metabolic situation or on pathological alterations of the liver (cf. Chapter 16). This dynamic behavior is the strongest *in vivo* evidence for a functional significance of zonal cell heterogeneity. Moreover, the heterogeneity is not an inherent property of liver parenchyma *per se;* in the rat, it develops only gradually during the second week of life before the intake of carbohydrate-rich food when the liver gets prepared for the glycolytic–gluconeogenic and glycogen-forming and -degrading function of a glucostat.[63,64]

During *starvation,* the glucogenic zone seems to be enlarged and the glycolytic zone seems to be diminished due to an increase of the gluconeogenic and a decrease of the glycolytic enzymes (Table I). During *regeneration* after partial hepatectomy, the glucogenic zone seems to be moved transiently to the intermediate or even the perivenous zone, while the periportal area, the site of proliferation, apparently becomes glycolytic.[65,66] In experimentally induced *cirrhosis*, the normal heterogeneity of carbohydrate metabolism was found to be preserved in nearly all cirrhotic nodules, in which the centers correspond to the periportal zone. It was concluded that the heterogeneity is required for the regulatory "altruistic" functions of the organ as a "metabolitostat." The loss of heterogeneity in some nodules was interpreted as the first step in the direction of "autistic" malignancy.[67] In alloxan *diabetes*, the heterogeneity is essentially preserved; it appears to be similar though not identical to the zonation observed during starvation.[73]

4.3.2. Zonal Flux Differences Calculated from Enzyme and Metabolite Distributions

According to the model of metabolic zonation, the *periportal* hepatocytes under normal feeding conditions may be *glucose-forming;* they may operate as a net one-way street from pyruvate to glucose and glycogen, which if required is degraded in these cells to glucose. The *perivenous* hepatocytes may normally be *glucose-utilizing;* they may function as a net one-way street from glucose and glycogen, which is formed from glucose in these cells, to pyruvate and triglycerides. This proposal would explain a number of results that are as yet unexplained, as outlined previously,[36] mainly that two thirds of newly formed glycogen is derived from C_3 compounds (in periportal cells?) and only one third from glucose (in perivenous cells?) and that glycogen and lactate are major precursors for fatty acid synthesis (in perivenous cells?). When the model of metabolic zonation was first proposed,[78] a major consequence was already pointed out, namely that C_3 substrates should be important precursors of liver glycogen. This view was repeatedly expressed.[36,38] Recently, the problem whether glucose is directly (glucose $\rightarrow$ glucose-6-phosphate $\rightarrow$ glucose-1-phosphate $\rightarrow$ glycogen) or indirectly (glucose $\rightarrow$ lactate $\rightarrow$ glucose-6-phosphate $\rightarrow$ $\rightarrow$ glucogen) the precursor of liver glycogen received considerable attention.[76] A major question is whether the C_3 substrates for glycogen synthesis, mainly lactate and pyruvate, are formed from glucose in extrahepatic organs such as skeletal muscle or in the liver itself, e.g. in the perivenous zone as suggested by the zonation moded.[77]

To gain insight into the metabolism of the periportal and perivenous area, the flux rate (v) of the glucose/glucose-6-phosphate cycle was calculated on the basis of the Michaelis–Menten equation using the measured zonal concentrations of glucose and glucose-6-phosphate, the zonal activities of glucokinase and glucose-6-phosphatase (Fig. 8), and the half-saturating substrate concentrations (K_M) of the two enzymes found in the literature. The concentrations of glucose were obtained as a first approximation by measuring the concentrations in portal (= periportal) and hepatovenous (= perivenous) blood; those of glucose-6-phosphate were calculated from the levels determined in microdissected periportal and perivenous liver tissue.[68] This procedure was regarded as permissible for three reasons: (1) Neither glucokinase nor glucose-6-phosphatase appears to be regulated under physiological conditions by allosteric effectors or chemical modification; (2) it appears likely that the kinetics of the two enzymes are the same under intracellular and *in vivo* conditions; and (3) it can be assumed that each of the two enzymes was saturated with its second substrate, ATP and H_2O, respectively.[68]

The calculations showed that the periportal zone during the absorptive as well as the postabsorptive phase of the 24-hr feeding rhythm should always release glucose (via glycogenolysis and gluconeogenesis) and that inversely the perivenous zone in the two situations should always take up glucose (for glycogen synthesis and glycolysis) (Fig. 9). In the perivenous zone, net flux would be more sensitive to changes in glucose-6-phosphate (steeper curves in the left panel of Fig. 9 as compared to the right panel); in the perivenous zone, net flux would be more sensitive to changes in glucose concentrations (greater spread of curves in the right panel of Fig. 9 as compared to the left panel). During the shift from the absorptive to the postabsorptive phase, the periportal glucose output would be increased and the perivenous glucose uptake would be decreased. Averaged

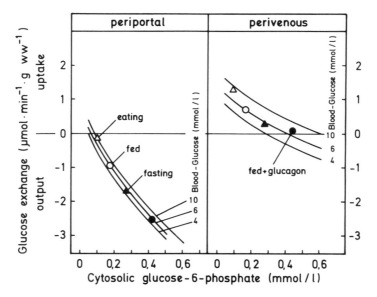

Figure 9. Dependence of the net flux of glucose in the periportal and perivenous zones of rat liver parenchyma on the concentrations of blood glucose and cytosolic glucose-6-phospate.[68] Net flux is given by the difference between the flux of the glucokinase and that of the glucose-6-phospate reaction, as calculated by the Michaelis–Menten equation (see the text). The range of substrate concentrations considered for glucose was 4–10 mM and for glucose-6-phosphate (0.1–0.5 mM. Specific physiological conditions during a 24-hr day–night rhythm (19 hr–7 hr night and access to food): fed, 9 hr, no net change in liver glycogen; fed + glucagon-treated, 9 hr, active glycogenolysis; eating, 2 hr, glycogen synthesis; fasting, 16 hr, glycogenolysis.

over the total parenchyma, the expected shift from net glucose uptake to net glucose release would result. The validity of the calculations is indicated by the finding that the overall cycling rates agreed remarkably well with those reported for intact animals.[68] The results (Fig. 9) do not prove the model of metabolic zonation; they simply serve to illustrate it. Under normal conditions, the function of a zone would not be changed. The futile cycles might serve primarily for control of amplification[69]; they might vary the rate rather than the direction of flow on changes in effector concentrations and activities of interconvertible enzymes.

4.3.3. Flux Differences in "Periportal" and "Perivenous" Hepatocytes Induced in Cell Culture

Since isolated hepatocytes could be separated only insufficiently into periportal and perivenous cells (see Jungermann and Katz[38] and Chapter 6), an attempt was made to induce an enzyme pattern typical of periportal cells in cultured hepatocytes.[29] With glucagon as the major hormone, it was possible to obtain hepatocytes that possessed approximately the ratio of glucokinase to phosphoenolpyruvate carboxykinase activity of periportal cells as determined by microbiochemical techniques. Inversely, with insulin as the major hormone, liver cells were induced that contained the enzyme activities in a ratio characteristic of perivenous hepatocytes (Fig. 10).

Glycolysis and gluconeogenesis were measured in these induced "periportal" and "perivenous" liver cells under various hormonal conditions with 5 mM glucose and 2 mM lactate as substrates. In the absence of insulin and glucagon, the glycolytic rate was 2-fold higher in the "perivenous" cells, while the gluconeogenic rate was 1.6-fold higher in the "periportal" cells. This finding demonstrates clearly that the incubation of the different enzymes of the two cell types under identical substrate and product concentrations leads to quite different metabolic rates. These rates were subject to hormonal control. In both "periportal" and "perivenous" cells, insulin decreased the glycolytic rate 3-fold, while it had no effect on gluconeogenesis. Glucagon decreased glycolysis to about 25% in both cell types, yet it enhanced the gluconeogenic rate by approximately 70% only in the "periportal" cells (Fig. 10).

In a first approximation, these results may be extrapolated to the situation *in vivo*. Since "periportal" cells were obtained with glucagon and "perivenous" cells with insulin as the major hormone, it can be assumed that the short-term regulation of glycolysis and gluconeogenesis should be governed predominantly by glucagon in "periportal" and by insulin in "perivenous" hepatocytes. It should furthermore be considered that the glycolytic rate is enhanced 2 to 3-fold by an increase of the glucose concentration from postabsorptive (5 mM) to absorptive (10 mM) levels, while the gluconeogenic rate is not affected.[29] Thus, in "periportal" cells (Fig. 10) under the major influence of glucagon, rates of gluconeogenesis of about 4.2 μmoles $\times$ hr^{-1} $\times$ mg DNA^{-1} would clearly exceed

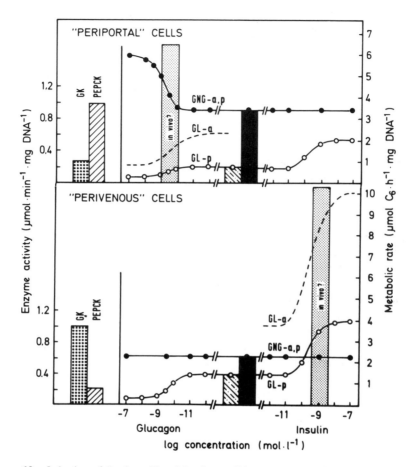

Figure 10. Induction of "periportal" and "perivenous" hepatocytes in primary cultures of rat hepatocytes.[29] Cells were cultured under standard conditions in the presence of insulin (0.5 nM) and dexamethasone (10 nM) under 13% (vol./vol.) oxygen. At 4 hr after plating, the medium was changed: "Perivenous" cells were induced for the following 44 hr with another medium change after 20 hr in the presence of insulin (10 nM) and dexamethasone (100 nM); "periportal" cells were induced in the presence of glucagon (10 nM), dexamethasone (100 nM), and insulin (0.5 nM). Metabolic rates were determined radiochemically by incubating the washed cells for another 2 hr in media containing both glucose (5 mM) and lactate (2 mM), which were labeled reciprocally, and hormones as indicated. Glycolysis (GL) was quantitated by measuring [^{14}C]lactate formation from [U^{14}C]glucose and gluconeogenesis (GNG) by determining [^{14}C]glucose production from [U^{14}C]lactate. Enzyme activities [(GK) glucokinase; (PEPCK) phosphoenolpyruvate carboxykinase] were assayed both before and after the incubation for the study of metabolic rates; no difference was observed. (a) Absorptive conditions: glucose 10 mM, lactate 2 mM; (p) postabsorptive conditions: glucose 5 mM, lactate 2 mM. Data are redrawn from results presented in Probst *et al.*[29] Values are means of 3 cultures from a representative experiment.

rates of glycolysis of about 0.6 μmole $\times$ hr^{-1} mg DNA^{-1} in the postabsorptive and 1.6 μmoles $\times$ hr^{-1} $\times$ mg DNA^{-1} in the absorptive state. Inversely, in "perivenous" cells under the major influence of insulin, rates of glycolysis of about 3.6 μmoles $\times$ hr^{-1} $\times$ mg DNA^{-1} in the postabsorptive and 8.4 μmoles $\times$ hr^{-1} $\times$ mg DNA^{-1} in the absorptive state would exceed rates of gluconeogenesis of 2.2 μmoles $\times$ hr^{-1} $\times$ mg DNA^{-1}.

In the *postabsorptive situation*, a net glucose release of 4.2 $-$ 0.6 = 3.6 μmoles $\times$ hr^{-1} $\times$ mg DNA^{-1} in "periportal" cells would be counterbalanced by a net glucose uptake of 3.6 $-$ 2.2 = 1.4 μmoles $\times$ hr^{-1} $\times$ mg DNA^{-1} in "perivenous" cells. In the *absorptive situation*, a net glucose uptake of 8.4 $-$ 2.2 = 6.2 μmoles $\times$ hr^{-1} $\times$ mg DNA^{-1} in "perivenous" cells would be counterbalanced by a net glucose release of 4.2 $-$ 1.6 = 2.6 μmoles $\times$ hr^{-1} $\times$ mg DNA^{-1} in "periportal" cells. The extrapolated values are in good agreement with the net rates of the glucose/glucose-6-phosphate cycle in the periportal and perivenous zones (see Fig. 9).

The metabolic differences between periportal and perivenous cells should be further accentuated by the different average oxygen tensions prevailing in the two zones. It was found in studies with cultured hepatocytes[70,75] that in the range of physiological oxygen levels (30mm Hg hepatovenous, 95 mm Hg arterial), gluconeogenesis remained almost constant, while glycolysis was increased by about 70% at the lower O_2 concentration.

4.3.4. Zonal Flux Differences Studied by Noninvasive Techniques in the Perfused Liver

Hepatic oxygen uptake can be linked functionally to gluconeogenesis and glycolysis. The rate of oxygen consumption was measured with miniature oxygen electrodes placed on periportal and perivenous areas on the surface of isolated, perfused livers catalyzing gluconeogenesis or glycolysis.[71,72] The lactate-dependent increase of O_2 uptake, which is related to gluconeogenesis, was found to be higher in the periportal zone; the ethanol-sensitive, glucose-dependent increase of O_2 consumption, which can be related to glycolysis, was greater in the perivenous zone. These findings indicate that gluconeogenesis and glycolysis are distributed reciprocally within the parenchyma and thus corroborate the model of metabolic zonation.

4.4. Comparison of the Non-zonation and Zonation Models for the Regulation of Carbohydrate Metabolism

In the non-zonation model (Fig. 11) based on one type of hepatocyte possessing the same enzyme activities, the shift from net glucose uptake via glycogen synthesis and glycolysis during the absorptive phase to net glucose release via glycogen degradation and gluconeogenesis would require a change of the direction of carbon flux in the single cells. The liver would function like a narrow country road with a single lane that allows traffic at a given time to proceed in one direction only, *either* glucose to lactate with a parking site glycogen *or* lactate to glucose with the same parking site glycogen.

In the zonation model (Fig. 11) based on the glucogenic periportal and the glycolytic perivenous hepatocytes, the reversible shift between glucose uptake and release would not require a change of direction of flux in single cells. On the contrary, the liver would function like a divided two- or even four-lane highway, which allows traffic to proceed at any given time at different rates in both directions: glucose to lactate *and* lactate to glucose, with both directions allowing a "stop" at the parking site glycogen. The shift between glucose uptake and release would be brought about by acceleration of traffic in one direction, including filling or emptying the parking site, and by simultaneous yet independent slowing down of traffic in the opposite direction, again including filling or emptying the parking site. The rates of traffic or metabolism will be regulated by substrate or hormone concentrations and by nerve signals. Since hormone and substrate concentrations vary during passage through the liver and since zonal innervation might be heterogeneous, a different regulation can be envisaged for the two zones or opposite directions of traffic. Perhaps the zonal organization

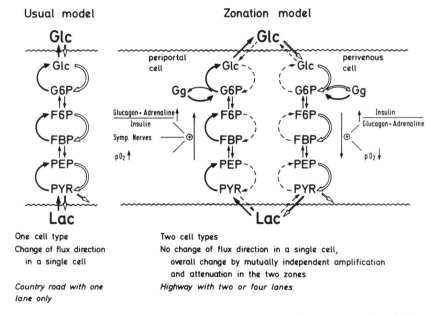

Figure 11. Comparison of the non-zonation and zonation models for the reversible shift from glucose uptake to release. (Gg) Glycogen; (Glc) glucose; (G6P) glucose-6-phosphate; (F6P) fructose-6-phosphate; (FBP) fructose-1,6,-bisphosphate; (PEP) phosphoenolypyruvate; (PYR) pyruvate; (Lac) lactate.

of metabolism, i.e., the divided highway, is more efficient than the country road.

5. SUMMARY

The liver is the glucostat of the organism. After a normal carbohydrate-rich meal, it removes about 50% of the excess nutritional glucose via glycogen synthesis and glycolysis plus liponeogenesis. During short- and long-term post-absorptive periods, as after a short fast between meals and after a longer fast for several days, as well as during exercise, it supplies, via glycogenolysis and gluconeogenesis, over 90%, about 70%, and almost 100%, respectively, of the glucose needed by the brain, the erythrocytes, and the working muscles.

The "everyday" problem of short-term regulation of carbohydrate metabolism is the control of the reversible shift from glycogen synthesis and glycolysis to glycogenolysis and gluconeogenesis. Four major factors are involved in the regulation of the glucostat: substrate concentrations, hormone levels, activity of hepatic nerves, and hepatocyte heterogeneity. Glycogen synthesis is stimulated predominantly by increases in the portal glucose concentration, with insulin and probably parasympathetic hepatic nerve activity being auxiliary signals. Glycogen breakdown is activated primarily by both glucagon and α-sympathetic hepatic nerve activity. Glycolysis is stimulated predominantly by the increase of the portal levels of glucose and insulin, and gluconeogenesis is activated primarily by glucagon. The effects of the hormonal and the nervous system are subject to mutual modulations.

Hepatocytes from the periportal (afferent) and perivenous (efferent) zones of the liver parenchyma differ in their enzyme content and subcellular structures. The key enzymes of glucose uptake, glucokinase and pyruvate kinase type L, are localized predominantly in the perivenous zone; the key enzymes of glucose release, glucose-6-phosphatase, fructose-1,6-bisphosphatase, and phosphoenol-pyruvate carboxykinase, are situated preferentially in the periportal zone. Zonal differences also exist in the signals that control metabolism, such as hormone concentrations and innervation, and probably also in signal transmission via ecto- and intracellular receptors.

The model of "metabolic zonation" proposes that the zonal heterogeneity of enzyme content, subcellular structures, signals, and signal transmission is functionally significant: Glucose release is catalyzed predominantly by periportal and glucose uptake by perivenous hepatocytes. The evidence for the model rests on the dynamics of heterogeneity upon longer-lasting changes of the metabolic situation and on zonal flux differences calculated from enzyme and metabolite distributions *in vivo*, measured in "periportal" and "perivenous" hepatocytes induced in cell culture and determined by noninvasive techniques in the perfused liver.

In the non-zonation model, the reversible shift from glucose uptake to release would depend on the change in direction of flux in each single cell. In the zonation model based on periportal and perivenous cell types, the shift would *not* depend on a change of flux direction in single cells, but on an overall change by mutually independent amplification and attenuation of the antagonistic pathways in the two zones.

ACKNOWLEDGMENTS.The investigations reported herein were supported by grants from the Deutsche Forschungsgemeinschaft, D-5300 Bonn. We thank Dr. B. Anderson, Dr. K. Beckh, Dr. W. Fischer, Dr. H. Hartmann, Dr. I. Probst, and Dr. D. Wölfle for their collaboration during various stages of this work.

REFERENCES

1. Cahill, G. F., Morliss, E. B., and Aoki, T. T., 1970, Fat and nitrogen metabolism in fasting man, B. Jeanrenaud and D. Hepp, eds., in: *Adipose Tissue: Regulation and Functions* pp. 181–185, Thieme, Stuttgart.
2. Jungermann, K., and Möhler, H., 1980, *Biochemie,* Springer-Verlag, Heidelberg. pp. 168–172 and 242–251.
3. Felig, P., Wahren, J., and Hendler, R., 1975, Influence of oral glucose ingestion on splanchnic glucose and gluconeogenic substrate metabolism in man, *Diabetes* **24:**468–475.
4. Felig, P., and Sherwin, R., 1976, Carbohydrate homeostasis, liver and diabetes, in: *Progress in Liver Diseases,* Vol. 5, H. Popper, and F. Schaffner, eds., pp. 149–171, Grune & Stratton, New York.
5. Hultman, E., and Nilsson, L. H., 1971, Liver glycogen in man: Effect of different diets and muscular exercise, *Adv. Exp. Med. Biol.* **11:**143–151.
6. Hultman, E., Bergstrom, J., and Roch-Norlund, A. E., 1971, Glycogen storage in human skeletal muscle, *Adv. Exp. Med. Biol.* **11:**273–288.
7. Saltin, B., and Karlsson, J., 1971, Muscle glycogen utilization during work of different intensities, *Adv. Exp. Med. Biol.* **11:**189–199.
8. Froberg, S., Carlson, L., and Ekelund, L., 1971, Local lipid stores and exercise, *Adv. Exp. Med. Biol.* **11:**307–313.
9. Hed, R., Nygren, A., Röjdmark, R., Sundblad, L., and Wiechel, K. L. 1979, Insulin in the portal, hepatic and peripheral venous blood after glucose, tolbutamide and glipizide stimulation, *Acta Med. Scand.***205:**221–225.
10. Strubbe, J. H., and Steffens, A. B., 1977, Blood glucose levels in portal and peripheral circulation and their relation to food intake in the rat, *Physiol. Behav.* **19:**303–107.
11. Unger, R. H., 1971, Pancreatic glucagon in health and disease, *Adv. Intern. Med.* **17:**265–273.
12. Whitton, P. D., 1981, Hormonal regulation of glycogenolysis, in: *Short-Term Regulation of Liver Metabolism,* (L. Hue and G. Van de Werve, eds.), pp. 45–62, Elsevier North-Holland, Amsterdam.
13. Lautt, W. W., 1980, Hepatic nerves, *Can J. Physiol. Pharmacol.* **58:**105–123.
14. Forssmann, W. G., 1980, Introduction and historical remarks on the innervation of the liver, in: *Communications of Liver Cells* (H. Popper, L. Bianchi, F. Gudat, and W. Reutter, eds.), pp. 109–114, MTP Press, Lancaster.
15. McCuskey, R. S., 1980, Intrahepatic distribution of nerves: A review, in: *Communications of Liver Cells* (H. Popper, L. Bianchi, F. Gudat, and W. Reutter, eds.), pp. 115–120, MTP Press, Lancaster.

16. Shimazu, T., 1981, Central nervous system regulation of liver and adipose tissue metabolism, *Diabetologia* **20:**343–356.

17. Niijima, A., 1979, Control of liver function and neuroendocrine regulation of blood glucose levels, in: *Integrative Functions of the Autonomic Nervous System* (C. McC. Brooks, K. Koizumi, and A. Sato, eds.), pp. 68–83, Elsevier, Amsterdam.

18. Hue, L., Bontemps, F., and Hers, H. G., 1975, The effect of glucose and of potassium ions on the two forms of glycogen phosphorylase and of glycogen synthetase, *Biochem. J.* **152:**105–114.

19. Witters, L. A., and Avruch, J., 1978, Insulin regulation of hepatic glycogen synthase and phosphorylase, *Biochemistry* **17:**406–410.

20. Hue, L., Feliu, J. E., and Hers, H. G., 1978, Control of gluconeogenesis and of enzymes of glycogen metabolism in isolated rat hepatocytes, *Biochem. J.* **176:**791–797.

21. Hue, L., and Van de Werve, G., 1981, *Short-term Regulation of Liver Metabolism*, pp. 453–456, Elsevier North-Holland, Amsterdam.

22. Nyfeler, F., Fasel, P., and Walter, P., 1981, Short-term stimulation of net glycogen production by insulin in rat hepatocytes, *Biochim. Biophys. Acta* **675:**17–23.

23. Beynen, A. C., and Geelen, M. J. H., 1981, Control of glycogen metabolism by insulin in isolated hepatocytes, *Horm. Metab. Res.* **13:**376–378.

24. Hartmann, H., Beckh, K., and Jungermann, K., 1982, Direct control of glycogen metabolism in the perfused rat liver by the sympathetic innervation, *Eur. J. Biochem.* **123:**521–526.

25. Beckh, K., Hartmann, H., Jungermann, K., and Scholz, R., 1984, Regulation of oxygen consumption in perfused rat liver: Decrease by α-sympathetic nerve stimulation and increase by the α-agonist phenylephrine, *Pfluegers Arch. Eur. J. Physiol.* **401:**104–106.

26. Ji, S., Beckh, K., and Jungermann, K., 1984, Regulation of oxygen consumption and microcirculation by α-sympathetic nerves in isolated perfused rat liver, *FEBS Lett.* **167:**117–122.

27. Beckh, K., Balks, H. J., and Jungermann, K., 1982, Activation of glycogenolysis and norepinephrine overflow in the perfused rat liver during repetitive nerve stimulation, *FEBS Lett.* **149:**261–265.

28. Beckh, K., Hartmann, H., and Jungermann, K., 1982, Modulation by insulin and glucagon of the activation of glycogenolysis by perivascular nerve stimulation in the perfused rat liver, *FEBS Lett.* **146:**69–72.

29. Probst, I., Schwartz, P., and Jungermann, K., 1982, Induction in primary culture of "gluconeogenic" and "glycolytic" hepatocytes resembling periportal and perivenous cells, *Eur. J. Biochem.* **126:**271–278.

30. Bontemps, F., Hue, L., and Hers, H. G., 1976, Phosphorylation of glucose in isolated rat hepatocytes, *Biochem. J.* **174:**603–611.

31. Hers, H. G., and van Schaftingen, E., 1982, Fructose-2,6-bisphosphate 2 years after its discovery, *Biochem. J.* **206:**1–12.

32. Probst, I., and Jungermann, K., 1983, Short-term regulation of glycolysis by insulin and dexamethasone in cultured rat hepatocytes, *Eur. J. Biochem.* **135:**151–156.

33. Powis, G., 1970, Perfusion of rat's liver with blood: Transmitter overflows and gluconeogenesis, *Proc. R. Soc. London Ser. B* **174:**503–515.

34. Novikoff, A. B., 1959, Cell heterogeneity within the hepatic lobule of the rat (staining reactions), *J. Histochem. Cytochem.* **7:**240–244.

35. Rappaport, A. M., 1960, Betrachtungen zur Pathophysiologie der Leberstruktur, *Klin. Wochenschr.* **38:**561–577.

36. Jungermann, K., and Sasse, D., 1978, Heterogeneity of liver parenchymal cells, *Trends Biochem. Sci.* **3:**198–202.

37. Gumucio, J. J., and Miller, D. L., 1981, Functional implications of liver cell heterogeneity, *Gastroenterology* **80:**393–403.

38. Jungermann, K., and Katz, N., 1982, Functional hepatocellular heterogeneity, *Hepatology* **2:**385–395.

39. Katz, N., and Jungermann, K., 1976, Autoregulatory shift from fructolysis to lactate gluco-neogenesis in rat hepatocyte suspensions: The problem of metabolic zonation of liver paren-chyma, *Hoppe-Seyler's Z. Physiol. Chem.* **357**:359–375.
40. Loud, A. V., 1968, Quantitative stereological description of the ultrastructure of normal rat liver parenchymal cells, *J. Cell. Biol.* **37**:27–46.
41. Wimmer, M., and Pette, D., 1979, Microphotometric studies on intraacinar enzyme distribution in rat liver, *Histochemistry* **64**:23–33.
42. Sasse, D., 1975, Dynamics of liver glycogen, *Histochemistry* **4**:237–254.
43. Teutsch, H. F., 1981, Chemomorphology of liver parenchyma, *Prog. Histochem. Cytochem.* **14**(3):1–92.
44. Richards, W. L., and Potter, V. R., 1980, Scanning microdensitometry of glycogen zonation in livers of rats adapted to a controlled feeding schedule and to 30, 60 or 90% casein diets, *Am. J. Anat.* **157**:71–85.
45. Katz, N., Teutsch, H. F., Jungermann, K., and Sasse, D., 1977, Heterogeneous reciprocal localization of fructose-1,6-bisphosphatase and glucokinase in microdissected periportal and perivenous rat liver tissue, *FEBS Lett.* **83**:272–276.
46. Trus, M., Zawalich, H., Gaynor, D., and Matschinsky, F., 1980, Hexokinase and glucokinase distribution in the liver lobule, *J. Histochem. Cytochem.* **28**:579–581.
47. Fischer, W., Ick, M., and Katz, N., 1982, Reciprocal distribution of hexokinase and glucokinase in periportal and perivenous rat liver tissue, *Hoppe-Seyler's Z. Physiol. Chem.* **363**:375–380.
48. Guder, W. G., and Schmidt, U., 1976, Liver cell heterogeneity: The distribution of pyruvate kinase and phosphoenolpyruvate carboxykinase (GTP) in the lobule of fed and starved rats, *Hoppe-Seyler's Z. Physiol. Chem.* **357**:1793–1800.
49. Zierz, S., Katz, N., and Jungermann, K., 1983, Distribution of pyruvate kinase type L and M_2 in microdissected periportal and perivenous rat liver tissue with different dietary states, *Hoppe-Seyler's Z. Physiol. Chem.* **364**:1447–1453.
50. Katz, N. R., Fischer, W., and Ick, M., 1983, Heterogeneous distribution of ATP citrate lyase in rat-liver parenchyma, *Eur. J. Biochem.* **130**:297–301.
51. Katz, N. R., Fischer, W., and Giffhorn, S., 1983, Distribution of enzymes of fatty acid and ketone body metabolism in periportal and perivenous rat liver tissue, *Eur. J. Biochem.* **135**:103–107.
52. Morrison, G. R., Brock, F. E., Karl, I. E., and Shank, R. E., 1965, Quantitative analysis of regenerating and degenerating areas within the lobule of the carbon tetrachloride-injured liver, *Arch. Biochem. Biophys.* **111**:448–464.
53. Teutsch, H. F., and Rieder, R., 1979, NADP-dependent dehydrogenases in rat liver parenchyma II, *Histochemistry* **60**:43–52.
54. Rieder, R., 1981, NADP-dependent dehydrogenases in rat liver parenchyma III, *Histochemistry* **72**:579–615.
55. Andersen, B., Nath, A., and Jungermann, K., 1982, Heterogeneous distribution of phospho-enolpyruvate carboxykinase in rat liver parenchyma, isolated and cultured hepatocytes, *Eur. J. Cell. Biol.* **28**:47–53.
56. Schmidt, U., Schmid, H., and Guder, W., 1978, Liver cell heterogeneity: The distribution of fructose-bisphosphatase in fed and fasted rats and in man, *Hoppe-Seyler's Z. Physiol. Chem.* **359**:193–198.
57. Katz, N., Teutsch, H. F., Sasse, D., and Jungermann, K., 1977, Heterogeneous distribution of glucose-6-phosphatase in microdissected periportal and perivenous rat liver tissue, *FEBS Lett.* **76**:226–230.
58. Teutsch, H. F., 1978, Quantitative determination of G6Pase activity in histochemical defined zones of the liver acinus, *Histochemistry* **58**:281–288.
59. Shank, R. E., Morrison, G., Cheng, C. H., Karl, I., and Schwartz, R., 1959, Cell heterogeneity within the hepatic lobule (quantitative histochemistry), *J. Histochem. Cytochem.* **7**:237–239.
60. Welsh, F. A., 1972, Changes in distribution of enzymes within the liver lobule during adaptive increase, *J. Histochem. Cytochem.* **20**:107–111.

61. Guder, W. G., and Ross, B. D., 1982, Heterogeneity and compartmentation in the kidney, in: *Metabolic Compartmentation* (H. Sies, ed.), pp. 363–409, Academic Press, London.
62. Balks, H. J., and Jungermann, K., 1984, Regulation of the peripheral insulin/glucagon ratio by the liver, *Eur. J. Biochem.* **141:**645–650.
63. Katz, N., Teutsch, H., Jungermann, K., and Sasse, D., 1976, Perinatal development of the metabolic zonation of hamster liver parenchyma, *FEBS Lett.* **69:**23–28.
64. Andersen, B., Zierz, S., and Jungermann, K., 1983, Perinatal development of the distribution of phosphoenolpyruvate carboxykinase and succinate dehydrogenase in rat liver parenchyma, *Eur. J. Cell Biol.* **30:**126–131.
65. Brinkmann, A., Katz, N., Sasse, D., and Jungermann, K., 1978, Increase of the gluconeogenic and decrease of the glycolytic capacity of rat liver with a change of the metabolic zonation after partial hepatectomy, *Hoppe-Seyler's Z. Physiol. Chem.* **359:**1561–1571.
66. Andersen, B., Zierz, S., and Jungermann, K., 1984, Alteration in zonation of succinate dehydrogenase, phosphoenolpyruvate carboxykinase and glucose-6-phosphatase in regenerating rat liver, *Histochemistry* **80:**97–101.
67. Nuber, R., Teutsch, H. F., and Sasse, D., 1980, Metabolic zonation in thioacetamide-induced liver cirrhosis, *Histochemistry* **69:**277–288.
68. Jungermann, K., Heilbronn, R., Katz, N., and Sasse, D., 1982, The glucose/glucose-6-phosphate cycle in the periportal and perivenous zone of rat liver, *Eur. J. Biochem.* **123:**429–436.
69. Newsholme, E. A., and Start, C., 1973, *Regulation in Metabolism,* pp. 71–76, 121–126, and 248, Wiley, London.
70. Wölfle, D., Schmidt, H., and Jungermann, K., 1983, Short-term modulation of glycogen metabolism, glycolysis and gluconeogenesis by physiological oxygen concentrations in hepatocyte cultures, *Eur. J. Biochem.* **135:**405–412.
71. Matsumura, T., and Thurman, R. G., 1984, Predominance of glycolysis in pericentral regions of the liver lobule, *Eur. J. Biochem.* **140:**229–234.
72. Matsumura, T., Kashiwagi, T., Meren, H., and Thurman, R. G., 1984, Gluconeogenesis predominates in periportal regions of the liver lobule, *Eur. J. Biochem.* **144:**409–415.
73. Miethke, H., Wittig, B., Nath, A., Zierz, S., and Jungermann, K., 1985, Metabolic zonation in liver of diabetic rats, *Biol. Chem. Hoppe-Seyler* **366:**493–501.
74. Zierz, S., and Jungermann, L., 1984, Alteration with dietary state of the activity and zonal distribution of adenylate cyclase stimulated by glucagon, fluoride and forskolin in microdissected rat liver tissue, *Eur. J. Biochem.* **145:**499–504.
75. Wölfle, D., and Jungermann, K., 1985, Long-term effects of physiological oxygen concentrations on glycolysis and gluconeogenesis in hepatocyte cultures. *Eur. J. Biochem.* **151:**299–303.
76. Kate, J., and McGarry, J. D., 1984, The glucose paradox. Is glucose a substrate for liver metabolism? *J. Clin. Invest.* **74:**1901–1909.
77. Pilkis, S. J., Regen, D. M., Claus, T. H., and Cherrington, A. D., 1985, Role of hepatic glycolysis and gluconeogenesis in glycogen synthesis. *Bioassays* **2:**273–276.
78. Jungermann, K., Katz, N., Teutsch, H., and Sasse, D., 1977, Possible metabolic zonation of liver parendyma into glucogenic and glycolytic hepatocytes, in: *Alcohol and Aldehyde Metabolizing Systems* (R. G. Thurman, J. R. Williamson, H. Drott, and B. Chance, eds.), pp. 65–76, Academic Press, New York.

Chapter 10

Metabolism of Lipids

Norbert Katz

1. INTRODUCTION

The integration of lipid metabolism is maintained predominantly by the liver. Excessive dietary glucose can be converted to fatty acids that are esterified and exported in triglyceride-rich very-low-density lipoproteins. Excessive fatty acids provided by lipolysis in adipose tissue are either reesterified or converted to ketones via β-oxidation in the liver. Cholesterol is transferred by lipoproteins from peripheral organs to the liver for excretion into the bile. This is the main mechanism by which cholesterol is eliminated. The chapter reviews the pathways of lipid metabolism in the liver, including interorgan relationships and lipoprotein turnover. The short- and long-term regulation by substrates and hormones is described along with aspects of the zonal heterogeneity of lipid metabolism.

2. ROLE OF THE LIVER IN THE METABOLISM OF LIPIDS: INTERORGAN RELATIONSHIPS

2.1. Fatty Acid Synthesis

During absorption, excess carbohydrate can be converted to fat by liver and adipose tissue. Thus, carbohydrate-dependent fatty acid synthesis is involved in

NORBERT KATZ • Institut für Biochemie, Universität Göttingen, D-3400 Göttingen, Federal Republic of Germany.

glucose homeostasis. Newly synthesized fatty acids are esterified with glycerol to triglycerides that are exported from the liver in very-low-density lipoproteins (VLDL). The glucose-dependent formation of fatty acids is low in the presence of 5 mM glucose, but it is increased markedly in the presence of high glucose concentrations.[1,2] However, lactate, fructose, and glycogen seem to be better substrates for liponeogenesis, which for the latter two compounds may be due to their more rapid glycolytic degradation.[3] For experimental animals such as the rat and chick, the metabolic significance of hepatic fatty acid synthesis is indicated by the very effective long- and short-term regulation of this pathway (see Section 3). The role of hepatic liponeogenesis in man is uncertain. Under normal feeding conditions, the human liver exhibits a low lipogenic capacity that appears to be unchanged even after administration of a carbohydrate-rich diet for a few days.[4]

2.2. Lipolysis and β-Oxidation

During postabsorption, fatty acids are the predominant energy substrate of the liver. There are two sources: exogenous triglycerides from adipose tissue and endogenous hepatic triglycerides. In man at rest, 6.6 g $\times$ hr^{-1} fatty acids and 0.7 g $\times$ hr^{-1} glycerol are released from adipose tissue.[5] In liver, 1.7 g $\times$ hr^{-1} fatty acids are reesterified or degraded via mitochondrial (90%) and peroxisomal (10%) β-oxidation to acetyl-CoA.[6] In muscle, 3.3 g $\times$ hr^{-1} fatty acids are oxidized. During exercise, lipolysis in adipose tissue is drastically increased; 22 g $\times$ hr^{-1} fatty acids are released during a total energy turnover of 800 W. Fatty acids (17 g $\times$ hr^{-1}) are taken up by the working muscles, but no significant alteration of the hepatic catabolism of fatty acids occurs.[7] The level of fatty acids bound to albumin in plasma is increased significantly during exercise. Endogenous triglyceride stores, which represent 1–3% of the liver mass,[8] appear to be hydrolyzed by a lysosomal acid lipase to fatty acids and monoglycerides, which are processed further by microsomal monoacyl glycerol hydrolase.[9] However, no conclusive information is available about the quantitative contribution of endogenous triglycerides to hepatic fatty acid turnover.

2.3. Ketogenesis

In contrast to other organs, the liver utilizes acetyl-CoA not only as a substrate for energy supply, but also as a substrate for ketogenesis.[10–12] The rate of ketogenesis is low during feeding; however, it is increased slightly to 0.5 g $\times$ hr^{-1} after an overnight fast and to 2.0 g $\times$ hr^{-1} or more during prolonged starvation,[13] which results in an increase of ketone bodies in serum from 0.2 to 3 mM.

Acetoacetate and 3-hydroxybutyrate are excellent energy-yielding substrates for muscle during short-term postabsorption. Yet during prolonged starvation or diabetes, the uptake of ketone bodies is decreased in muscle, possibly due to the low insulin concentration.[13] This results in a further increase of ketone bodies in serum. On the other hand, the uptake of ketone bodies in brain depends exclusively on the level of ketone bodies in the serum. Thus, the utilization of ketone bodies in the central nervous system is increased markedly during starvation. Essentially all ketone bodies formed in this metabolic state are utilized by the brain, where they are responsible for up to 60% of the energy supply.[5]

2.4. Esterification

Under all metabolic conditions, the uptake of fatty acids in the liver exceeds the rate of degradation. During absorption, about 80% of fatty acids taken up by the liver are esterified, 8% are catabolized to CO_2, and 12% are transformed into ketone bodies. During starvation, about 30% are esterified, 10% are catabolized, and 60% are metabolized to ketone bodies.[10,12] Triglycerides formed by esterification of fatty acids are exported from the liver as VLDL.

The coordination of esterification, β-oxidation, and ketogenesis in liver is essential for the integration of fat and carbohydrate metabolism in the intact organism.[14] During starvation, glucose has to be replaced by fatty acids as the main energy substrate of the organism; however, the glucagon-dependent release of fatty acids in adipose tissue by hormone-sensitive lipases is not under precise control in relation to the energy requirements by other tissues. Thus, the release of fatty acids may exceed the demand for energy production in muscle and kidney. Under these conditions, the liver can remove a large proportion of surplus fatty acids by esterification or ketogenesis, which avoids an increase of fatty acids to toxic concentrations in the serum.

2.5. Lipoprotein Formation and Processing

Lipids such as triglycerides, phospholipids, cholesterol, and cholesterol esters are transported in blood in the form of lipoproteins. There are five major classes of lipoproteins: chylomicrons (CM), very-low-density lipoproteins (VLDL), intermediate-density lipoproteins (IDL), low-density lipoproteins (LDL), and high-density lipoproteins (HDL). They differ in their content of lipids and apoproteins as well as in their function.

2.5.1. Chylomicron Processing

A normal meal contains 35 g of fat on average, predominantly as triglycerides. After digestion and absorption, nutritional fat is transported in the form of CM from the intestine to the adipose tissue for final storage of triglycerides. During transit in the blood, CM undergo a rapid exchange with HDL: Some phospholipids and apoprotein (Apo) A are lost from the CM surface to HDL, while cholesterol and Apo C and E are transferred from HDL to CM[15] (Fig. 1). Some of these alterations, e.g., the transfer of Apo C II, enable the interaction

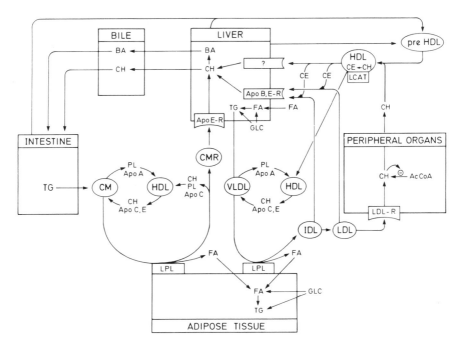

Figure 1. Lipoprotein metabolism. (CM) Chylomicrons; (CMR) chylomicron remnants; (VLDL) very-low-density lipoproteins; (IDL) intermediate-density lipoproteins; (LDL) low-density lipoproteins; (HDL) high-density lipoproteins; (TG) triglycerides; (FA) fatty acids; (PL) phospholipids; (CH) cholesterol; (CE) cholesterol ester; (BA) bile acids; (AcCoA) acetyl-CoA; (GLC) glucose; (Apo) apoprotein; (LPL) lipoprotein lipase; (LCAT) lecithin cholesterol acyl transferase; (R) receptor.

of the lipoprotein with lipoprotein lipase on endothelial cell membranes followed by hydrolysis of triglyceride from the core and shrinking of the particle. The resulting fatty acids are taken up mainly by the adipose tissue for reesterification to triglycerides. During this shrinking, redundant cholesterol, phospholipids, and Apo C are lost to HDL, and CM remnants result.[15] The remnants are recognized by the Apo E binding CM remnant receptor on the hepatocyte membrane.[16] After endocytosis, the remnants are degraded by interaction with lysosomes. Thus, a small part of the nutritional triglycerides and a large amount of the exogenous cholesterol are delivered to liver.[17] The triglycerides are reexported in VLDL; cholesterol is excreted directly or, after transformation to cholic acids, into the bile.

2.5.2. Synthesis and Processing of Other Lipoproteins (VLDL, IDL, LDL, and HDL)

Triglycerides formed from exogenous and newly synthesized, endogenous fatty acids are secreted by the liver in VLDL. These particles contain the liver-specific Apo B-100 among other apoproteins, but no intestine-specific Apo B-

48.[17] Analogous to CM, VLDL transport triglycerides predominantly to the adipose tissue (Fig. 1). Therefore, both lipoproteins exhibit a similar exchange with HDL and hydrolysis by lipoprotein lipase. In the rat and the rabbit, VLDL remnants are apparently cleared by the liver via a receptor-mediated process.[18] In man, where these remnants are usually called IDL, they are taken up by the liver or transformed into LDL in the plasma. LDL transport cholesterol to peripheral organs for membrane formation. Furthermore, a significant part of LDL is catabolized in the liver. The specific endocytosis of LDL is mediated by an Apo B and E binding receptor at the plasma membrane. Within the cell, the particles are fused with lysosomes for degradation. Since cholesterol cannot by degraded in mammalian cells, a steady-state level of circulating cholesterol is maintained only if cholesterol uptake and synthesis are balanced by hepatic cholesterol excretion into the bile. HDL are involved in cholesterol transport from peripheral organs to the liver. These particles are synthesized by liver in a nascent, Apo-E-rich form and by intestine in a nascent, Apo-A- and C-rich form.[19,20] Cholesterol is transferred from the plasma membrane as well as from CM and VLDL to nascent HDL, where it is esterified by associated lecithin cholesterol acyl transferase (LCAT). The apolar cholesterol ester moves from the surface into the core of the particle, forming a gradient for the further transfer of cholesterol from cells to HDL. Different subclasses of HDL are involved in this process, but only Apo-E-rich particles appear to be taken up by the liver.[18,20] Similar to other lipoproteins, HDL are fused with lysosomes after internalization, and the liberated cholesterol can be excreted into the bile. Another, indirect way of cholesterol transport to the liver involves the transfer of cholesterol ester from HDL to VLDL, IDL, or LDL by the combined actions of LCAT and cholesterol ester transfer protein. When these particles are processed, cholesterol is cleared by the hepatic uptake of IDL and LDL.

3. ROLE OF METABOLITES AND HORMONES IN THE REGULATION OF LIPID METABOLISM

The "everyday" problem of short-term regulation of fatty acid metabolism is the reversible shift from high rates of β-oxidation and ketogenesis during postabsorption to high rates of fatty acid synthesis and esterification during absorption. Besides the short-term regulation, lipid metabolism must adapt to longer-lasting alterations of the dietary condition. Moreover, formation and processing of VLDL, IDL, LDL, and HDL must be regulated.

3.1. Liponeogenesis

Acetyl-CoA carboxylase can be regarded as the rate-limiting enzyme due to its low activity *in vivo*. It exists in two forms: a protomeric or oligomeric form with low activity and a polymeric form with high activity. The enzyme is regulated by allosteric effectors and phosphorylation–dephosphorylation. Citrate is known to be a very effective allosteric activator, which increases the catalytic activity without causing any change in the affinity for substrates. This alteration is accompanied by polymerization of the enzyme and can be antagonized by long-chain fatty acyl-CoA.[21] However, maximal allosteric activation by citrate is obtained at 5–10 mM, which is an order of magnitude higher than the cellular citrate concentration. Furthermore, only small fluctuations in the citrate level are observed during the change between absorption and postabsorption.[22,23] Thus, the physiological significance of citrate-dependent regulation is highly questionable. Due to large fluctuations in the cellular fatty acyl-CoA level, the allosteric inhibition by these metabolites may be more important. Coenzyme A activates the enzyme by allosteric enhancement of the affinity for acetyl-CoA. This results in a reduction of the apparent K_m from 200 to 4 μM, which is in the range of the cytosolic acetyl-CoA concentration.[24] Activation by CoA is also accompanied by polymerization of acetyl-CoA carboxylase.

Glucagon and cyclic AMP (cAMP) decrease the acetyl-CoA carboxylase activity by phosphorylation, which reduces the V_{max} without changing the apparent K_m values for substrates.[25] This inactivation is accompanied by enzyme depolymerization. A corresponding regulation is obtained by catecholamines.[26] Dephosphorylation by various phosphatases in turn activates the enzyme.[27] Yet the regulatory concept is complicated by the observation of an insulin-dependent phosphorylation.[28] Similar to acetyl-CoA carboxylase, ATP citrate lyase is phosphorylated by glucagon as well as by insulin. In this case, however, neither of the two modifications appears to change the enzyme activity.[29,30]

Hepatic fatty acid synthesis is adapted to longer-lasting changes of the metabolic situation by enzyme synthesis and degradation. During prolonged starvation as well as in diabetes, the levels of the lipogenic enzymes ATP citrate lyase, acetyl-CoA carboxylase, and fatty acid synthase are reduced significantly by more than 70%.[31,32] Refeeding a carbohydrate-rich diet[31] and insulin therapy[32] are both followed by an increase of the enzyme levels above the normal range. These observations indicate that insulin or glucose or both are major signals for the induction of the enzymes.

In the intact animal, however, it is not possible to decide definitively whether carbohydrates increase enzyme synthesis directly or via a secondary increase in the insulin concentration. Studies using primary cultures of rat hepatocytes demonstrate clearly a glucose-dependent induction of ATP citrate lyase, acetyl-CoA carboxylase, and fatty acid synthase even in the absence of hormones (Fig. 2).[33–35] Since the glucose-dependent induction is reduced drastically by inhibitors of glycolysis and since it is enhanced significantly by insulin, this induction seems to be due to a metabolite of glucose rather than to glucose itself.

The rate of fatty acid synthesis correlates under all conditions with the activity of acetyl-CoA carboxylase. Its decrease during starvation is due to reduced enzyme synthesis as well as to enhanced enzyme degradation[36]; the latter

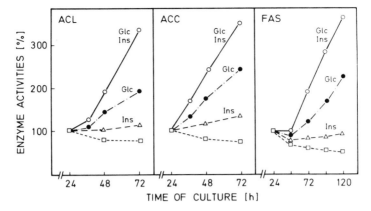

Figure 2. Effect of glucose and insulin on the levels of liponeogenic enzymes in primary cultures of rat hepatocytes. Glucose (Glc) (20 mM), insulin (Ins), (10^{-7} M), or Glc (20 mM) plus Ins (10^{-7} M) was added to cultures as indicated beginning 24 hr after preparation of hepatocytes. (ACL) ATP citrate lyase; (ACC) acetyl-CoA carboxylase; (FAS) fatty acid synthase.

is observed mainly in the presence of high levels of fatty acids in serum. The increase of the enzyme level during refeeding is due to induction as well as to decreases in enzyme degradation.[36]

3.2. Lipolysis and β-Oxidation

Hepatic lipolysis appears to be stimulated by glucagon, which enhances autophagocytosis, a process believed to be involved in the breakdown of liver triglycerides.[37]

Short-term regulation of fatty acid utilization occurs first of all at the branch point between esterification and mitochondrial uptake of fatty acids. The transport across the inner mitochondrial membrane involves the exhange of CoA and carnitine at the fatty acid moiety catalyzed by carnitine acyl transferases I and II. The carnitine acyl transferase I at the outer surface of the inner mitochondrial membrane is largely inhibited by micromolar concentrations of malonyl-CoA.[38] The intracellular concentration of malonyl-CoA varies between 0.5 and 7 nmoles/g liver depending on the hormonal or nutritional state of the animal. The level is high during fatty acid synthesis, resulting in inhibition of fatty acid degradation.[39] The inhibitory effect of malonyl-CoA is antagonized by elevation of the substrate long-chain acyl-CoA, as observed during enhanced lipolysis. The carnitine acyl transferase activity is furthermore regulated by the level of the cosubstrate, carnitine. The overall hepatic concentration of carnitine varies with the metabolic state of the animal and is enhanced during ketogenesis.[40] Addition of carnitine to perfused liver or isolated hepatocytes of fed rats results in a moderate increase of ketogenesis due to the enhanced mitochondrial uptake of fatty acids.[41]

Results of the long-term regulation of β-oxidation are contradictory. Whether the level of carnitine acyl transferase I is enhanced during starvation or not is not clear (for a review, see Zammit[42]).

3.3. Ketogenesis

Glucagon dependent lipolysis in adipose tissue can be regarded as the main trigger for the enhancement of ketogenesis due to an enhanced supply of fatty acids to the liver. An interorgan feedback regulation of ketogenesis is achieved by ketone bodies themselves, since they antagonize the lipolysis in adipose tissue directly as well as by stimulating insulin secretion from the pancreas.[42]

The intrahepatic regulation of ketogenesis occurs primarily via the regulation of carnitine acyl transferase (see Section 3.2) and glycerolphosphate acyl transferase at the branch point of fatty acyl-CoA between esterification and mitochondrial uptake. Furthermore, regulation exists at the branch point of acetyl-CoA between the formation of citrate for the tricarboxylate cycle and the formation of acetoacetyl-CoA for ketogenesis. Citrate synthase, which competes for acetyl-CoA, is apparently not saturated with the cosubstrate, oxaloacetate. This might explain the antiketogenic effect of gluconeogenic substrates, which increase the level of oxaloacetate.[42,43] On the other hand, enhanced oxidation of fatty acids raises the mitochondrial $NADH/NAD^+$ ratio, which shifts the malate–oxaloacetate reaction to a more reduced state followed by a decrease in oxaloacetate and hence increased ketogenesis.[43] Furthermore, hepatic citrate synthase is inhibited *in vitro* by ATP. Since the ATP–ADP translocation at the inner mitochondrial membrane is apparently inhibited by high levels of cytosolic acyl-CoA, the mitochondrial ATP concentration should be increased during lipolysis. Therefore, inhibition of citrate synthesis may also enhance ketogenesis.[44]

A third point of intrahepatic regulation exists at the level of the ketogenic enzymes themselves. The activity of acetyl-CoA acetyl transferase (thiolase), the first enzyme of ketogenesis, is subject to short-term regulation by physiological concentrations of CoA and acetoacetyl-CoA. The covalent modification of the enzyme by CoA at a specific regulatory binding site significantly decreases the affinity for the substrate acetyl-CoA.[45] Acetoacetyl-CoA may be of regulatory significance, since it inhibits mitochondrial acetyl-CoA acetyl transferase as well as hydroxymethylglutaryl-CoA synthase activity.[46,47] Acetyl-CoA acetyl transferase apparently does not exhibit any long-term adaptation to different metabolic states.

3.4. Esterification

The first step in the esterification of fatty acids is catalyzed by glycerolphosphate acyl transferase, which exists in a microsomal and an ectomitochondrial form. Insulin exhibits a short-term control by increasing the enzyme activity within 30 min,[48] which might be due to interconversion similar to that observed in adipose tissue.[30] Besides short-term regulation, the overall activity of acyl transferase is decreased during starvation and restored after refeeding, probably by a change in the enzyme level.[49]

3.5. Lipoprotein Metabolism

Synthesis and secretion of VLDL depends mainly on the rate of triglyceride synthesis. This is correlated with the cellular level of acyl-CoA as well as with the activity of glycerolphosphate acyl transferase and probably with the activities of phosphatidate phosphohydrolase and diglyceride acyl transferase.[50] Insulin increases and glucagon or cAMP decreases the secretion of VLDL.[51]

Not only exocytosis but also the specific uptake of lipoproteins by the liver seem to be regulated. The Apo B and E binding LDL receptor is suppressed when the hepatic cholesterol level is increased or the demand for cholesterol in liver is reduced. This is the case during cholesterol feeding[52] or infusion of lymph or bile acids.[53] On the other hand, the receptor level increases when cholesterol synthesis is blocked by compactin or mevinolin or if cholesterol absorption is reduced by cholestyramine. Furthermore, the receptor number is increased by thyroxine as well as by estrogen (for a review, see Brown and Goldstein[16]). The Apo E binding CM remnant receptor does not appear to respond to different metabolic states.

4. ZONAL HEPATOCYTE HETEROGENEITY OF LIPID METABOLISM

Hepatocytes from the periportal region (Zone 1) and from the perivenous area (Zone 3) of the liver acinus differ in their enzyme activities and subcellular structures. This heterogeneity can be regarded as the expression of a metabolic zonation of the liver parenchyma, which is true for some but not for all metabolic pathways.

4.1. Liponeogenesis

Fatty acid synthesis appears to be catalyzed predominantly in the perivenous zone, as indicated by the localization of the key enzymes ATP citrate lyase,[54] acetyl-CoA carboxylase,[55] and fatty acid synthase[56] and of the auxiliary NADPH-generating enzymes glucose-6-phosphate dehydrogenase,[57–61] 6-phosphogluconate dehydrogenase,[61,62] and malic enzyme[60,61] (Table I).

Liver-cell heterogeneity is very complex, as evidenced by the localization of glucose-6-phosphate dehydrogenase.[59,60] The results obtained with the microdissection technique must be corrected for the very high enzyme activity in nonparenchymal cells, which are preferentially located in the periportal zone.

Table I. Heterogeneous Distribution of Key Enzymes and of Subcellular Structures Linked to Lipid Metabolism over the Liver Parenchyma.

Enzymes and structures	Periportal/perivenous		Sex	Method[b]	Ref.
	Fed[a]	Fasted[a]			
Fatty acid synthesis (liponeogenesis) ATP-dependent					
citrate lyase	0.4–0.5	0.6–0.7	M, F	MMB	54
Acetyl-CoA-carboxylase	0.6	0.8	M, F	MMB	55
Fatty acid synthase	0.5	0.9	F	MMB	56
	0.9	1.2	M		
Glucose-6-phosphate	0.7	—	F	MMB	59
dehydrogenase[c]	0.4 cor	—	F		59
	2.1	—	M		59
	1.0 cor	—	M		59
	0.7	0.7	F, M		57, 58
6-Phosphogluconate dehydrogenase[c]	0.7	—	M	MMB	62
Malic enzyme[c]	1.2	—	M	MMB	60
	0.5	—	F		
Alcohol dehydrogenase[c]	0.6	—	F	MMB	63
Fatty acid utilization (β-oxidation, ketogenesis) β-Hydroxybutyryl-CoA					
dehydrogenase	1.1–1.2	1.3	F, M	MMB	57, 55
β-Hydroxybutyrate dehydrogenase	0.6	0.5–0.6	F, M	MMB	55
Bile acid excretion Volume of Golgi-rich					
area per cell	2.3	—	M	M	65
Volume of bile canaliculi per cell	2.2	—	M	M	65
Canalicular ATPase	1	—	M	HC	66

[a] Fed: fed *ad libitum* or re-fed for 48 hr after starvation; Fasted: fasted for 24–48 hr.
[b] (MMB) Microdissection and microbiochemical analysis; (M) morphology; (HC) histochemistry.
[c] The reason for linking this enzyme to the respective pathway is explained in the text.

After this correction is made, sex differences become evident. Female rats contain higher activities than male animals. Only female rats appear to possess a periportal-to-perivenous gradient (Table I). This as well as the more pronounced gradient of fatty acid synthase in female compared to male rats might indicate that the female liver is especially suited to convert carbohydrate to fat.

Similar to the zonation of gluconeogenic and glycolytic enzymes, the heterogeneous distribution of liponeogenic enzymes is dynamic rather than static, indicating the metabolic significance of zonation. Since the adaptation of the liponeogenic capacity occurs mainly in the perivenous zone, the perivenous-to-periportal gradient is decreased during starvation, when the liponeogenic capacity is low. On the other hand, it is increased during refeeding with a carbohydrate-rich diet, when the liponeogenic capacity is enhanced strongly. Moreover, the simultaneous predominance of liponeogenesis and of acetyl-CoA formation from glucose (see Chapter 9), or from ethanol[63] in the perivenous zone appears to be metabolically significant.

The heterogeneous distribution is apparently due to the predominance of the induction of liponeogenic enzymes in the perivenous zone. As mentioned above, liponeogenic enzymes seem to be induced by a metabolite of glucose that is formed in the presence of insulin. Due to the higher glycolytic capacity in the perivenous compared to the periportal zone, the formation of this metabolite might prevail in perivenous hepatocytes, resulting in a heterogeneous expression of the genome.

4.2. β-Oxidation

It was speculated that energy is supplied in the periportal zone mainly by β-oxidation and in the perivenous zone mainly by glycolysis. This proposal was supported by the 1.5-times higher mitochondrial volume in the periportal compared to the perivenous zone.[64] However, the essentially homogeneous distribution of 3-hydroxyacyl-CoA dehydrogenase[56,57] does not support this hypothesis (Table I). With regard to the glucostat function of the liver, it seems to be reasonable that β-oxidation is not restricted to the periportal zone, since glucose formed by periportal hepatocytes during starvation should not be utilized by perivenous liver cells.

Thus, periportal hepatocytes might utilize fatty acids as energy substrate, while perivenous hepatocytes might utilize excess glucose during absorption but fatty acids during postabsorption. In contrast to gluconeogenesis and glycolysis, futile cycling between acetyl-CoA and fatty acids is unlikely due to intracellular compartmentation of liponeogenesis and β-oxidation. Therefore, no zonal separation of the two antagonistic processes seems to be necessary.

4.3. Ketogenesis

Histochemical studies[61] and microbiochemical analysis of microdissected tissue[56] indicate that 3-hydroxybutyrate dehydrogenase predominates in the perivenous zone. This distribution pattern suggests but does not prove the predominance of ketogenesis in the perivenous zone, since formation of 3-hydroxybutyrate from acetoacetate is an additional, non-compulsory step in ketogenesis. Nevertheless, one can hypothesize that β-oxidation supplies acetyl-CoA mainly for energy production in periportal hepatocytes and provides acetyl-CoA mainly

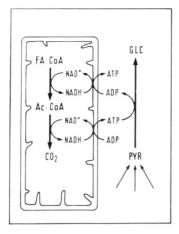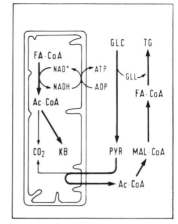

PERIPORTAL HEPATOCYTE   PERIVENOUS HEPATOCYTE

Figure 3. Model of mainly gluconeogenic periportal hepatocytes and of mainly glycolytic, lipo-
neogenic, and ketogenic perivenous hepatocytes. (Ac-CoA) Acetyl-CoA; (FA-CoA) fatty acyl-CoA;
(GLC) glucose; (GLL) glycerol; (MAL-CoA) malonyl-CoA; (PYR) pyruvate; (TG) triglycerides;
(KB) ketone bodies.

for ketogenesis in perivenous hepatocytes (Fig. 3). This hypothesis is supported
by recent studies using the micro-light-guide technique; these studies demonstrate
that ketogenesis is about 50% higher in the perivenous compared to the periportal
zone of livers perfused with octanoate (R. Thurman, personal communication).

4.4. Lipoprotein Metabolism

Since liponeogenesis appears to be catalyzed predominantly in the perivenous zone, it is possible that VLDL containing triglycerides formed from excess
glucose are secreted mainly by perivenous hepatocytes. No information appears
to be available on whether this is also true for VLDL that contain triglycerides
formed from fatty acids derived from intestine or adipose tissue. On the other
hand, the predominance of Golgi-rich areas, bile canaliculi, and canalicular
ATPase in the periportal zone indicates that cholic acids might be secreted mainly
by periportal hepatocytes.[65,66] Since cholesterol is excreted into the bile directly
or after transformation to cholic acids, the cholesterol-rich lipoproteins HDL,
LDL, and IDL should be taken up predominantly by periportal hepatocytes.
However, further studies will be necessary to test this hypothesis by determination
of the distribution of specific lipoprotein receptors in the liver acinus.

5. SUMMARY

During absorption, the liver catalyzes carbohydrate-dependent liponeogenesis, which is involved in glucose homeostasis. This is true mainly during administration of a diet low in triglycerides. During postabsorption, excess fatty acids supplied by enhanced lipolysis in the adipose tissue are taken up by the liver and converted to ketones or reesterified. Newly synthesized triglycerides are exported as very-low-density lipoproteins (VLDL). Chylomicron remnants and VLDL remnants, as well as the cholesterol-rich low-density lipoproteins (LDL) and high-density lipoproteins (HDL), are cleared by the liver via receptor-mediated endocytosis. Cholesterol is excreted into the bile either directly or after its conversion to cholic acids.

Short-term regulation of liponeogenesis, VLDL secretion, β-oxidation, and ketogenesis is mediated by metabolites and hormones. Under physiological conditions, the key liponeogenic enzyme, acetyl-CoA carboxylase, is activated by CoA and inactivated by long-chain acyl-CoA. Furthermore, the enzyme is inactivated by glucagon-dependent phosphorylation. Short-term regulation of β-oxidation is due to activation of carnitine acyl transferase by the substrate acyl-CoA and to inhibition by malonyl-CoA. An increased rate of β-oxidation, as observed during lipolysis, is followed by enhancement of ketogenesis. This is due to an increased supply of acetyl-CoA as well as to a decreased rate of citrate synthesis, the alternative pathway of acetyl-CoA metabolism in mitochondria.

Long-term regulation of liponeogenesis is achieved by alteration of the levels of ATP citrate lyase, acetyl-CoA carboxylase, and fatty acid synthase. During starvation, the levels are decreased by enhancement of enzyme degradation; during refeeding with a carbohydrate-rich diet, the levels are greatly increased by insulin- and glucose-dependent induction.

The predominance of glycolytic as well as of liponeogenic enzymes in perivenous hepatocytes supports the view that carbohydrate-dependent fatty acid synthesis is catalyzed mainly in the perivenous zone of the liver acinus. On the other hand, bile acids and cholesterol appear to be secreted by periportal hepatocytes. The distribution patterns of 3-hydroxyacyl-CoA dehydrogenase and of 3-hydroxybutyrate dehydrogenase support the hypothesis that β-oxidation supplies acetyl-CoA mainly as an energy source in periportal regions and predominantly for ketogenesis in perivenous hepatocytes. The first indirect measurements of β-oxidation and ketogenesis in the periportal and perivenous zones support this hypothesis, but further studies will be necessary.

REFERENCES

1. Clark, D. G., Rognstad, R., and Katz, J., 1974, Lipogenesis in rat hepatocytes, *J. Biol. Chem.* **249:**2028–2036.

2. Brunnengraber, H., Boutry, M., and Lowenstein, J. M., 1973, Fatty acid and 3-β-hydroxysterol synthesis in the perfused rat liver, *J. Biol. Chem.* **248:**2656–2669.

3. Walli, R., 1978, Interrelation of aerobic glycolysis and lipogenesis in isolated perfused liver of well fed rats, *Biochim. Biophys. Acta* **539:**62–80.

4. Hoffmann, G. E., Andres, H., Weiss, L., Kreissel, C., and Sander, R., 1980, Lipogenesis in man, *Biochim. Biophys. Acta* **620:**151–158.

5. Cahill, G. F., Marliss, E. B., and Aoki, T. T., 1970, Fat and nitrogen metabolism in fasting man, in: *Adipose Tissue: Regulation and Functions* (B. Jeanrenaud and D. Hepp, eds., pp. 181–185, Thieme, Stuttgart.

6. Mannaerts, G. P., Debeer, L. J., Thomas, J., and De Schepper, P. J., 1979, Mitochondrial and peroxisomal fatty acid oxidation in liver homogenates and isolated hepatocytes from control and clofibrate-treated rats, *J. Biol. Chem.* **254:**4585–4595.

7. Jungermann, K., 1983, Role of the liver in metabolism of carbohydrates, in: *Liver in Metabolic Diseases* (L. Bianchi, W. Gerok, L. Landmann, K. Sickinger, and G. A. Stalder, eds.), pp. 207–220, MTP Press, Boston.

8. Hems, D. A., 1977, Short-term hormonal control of hepatic carbohydrate and lipid metabolism, *FEBS Lett.* **80:**237–245.

9. Debeer, L. J., Beynen, A. C., Mannaerts, G. P., and Geelen, M. J. H., 1982, Lipolysis of hepatic triacylglycerol stores, *FEBS Lett.* **140:**159–164.

10. Mayes, P. A., 1970, Studies of the major pathways of hepatic lipid metabolism using the perfused liver, in: *Adipose Tissue: Regulation and Functions,* B. Jeanrenaud and D. Hepp, eds.), pp. 186–195, Thieme, Stuttgart.

11. Ontko, J. A., 1972, Metabolism of free fatty acids in isolated liver cells, *J. Biol. Chem.* **247:**1788–1800.

12. Shafrir, E., 1978, Absence of ketosis during glucocorticoid induced fat mobilization, in: *Biochemical and Clinical Aspects of Ketone Body Metabolism* (H. D. Soeling and C. D. Seufer, eds.), pp. 127–136, Thieme, Stuttgart.

13. Owen, O. E., Patel, M. S., and Boden, G., 1978, Ketone body metabolism in humans during health and disease, in: *Biochemical and Clinical Aspects of Ketone Body Metabolism* (H. D. Soeling and C. D. Seufer, eds.), pp. 155–165, Thieme, Stuttgart.

14. Newsholm, E. A., 1976, Role of the liver in integration of fat and carbohydrate metabolism and clinical implications in patients with liver disease, in: *Progress in Liver Diseases,* Vol. 5 (H. Popper and F. Schaffner, eds.), pp. 125–135, Grune and Stratton, New York.

15. Owen, J. S., and McIntyre, N., 1982, Plasma lipoprotein metabolism and lipid transport, *Trends Biochem. Sci.* **7:**95–98.

16. Brown, M. S., and Goldstein, J. L., 1983, Lipoprotein receptors in the liver, *J. Clin. Invest.* **72:**743–747.

17. Sherill, B. C., and Ditschy, J. M., 1978, Characterization of the sinusoidal transport process responsible for uptake of chylomicrons by the liver, *J. Biol. Chem.* **253:**1859–1867.

18. Brown, M. S., Kovanen, P. T., and Goldstein, J. L., 1981, Regulation of plasma cholesterol by lipoprotein receptors, *Science* **212:**628–635.

19. Tall, A. R., and Small, D. M., 1979, Body cholesterol removal: Role of plasma high density lipoproteins, *Adv. Lipid Res.* **17:**1–51.

20. Nicoll, A., Miller, N. E., and Lewis, B., 1979, High density lipoprotein metabolism, *Adv. Lipid Res.* **17:**53–106.

21. Ogiwara, H., Tanabe, T., Nikawa, J., and Numa, S., 1978, Inhibition of rat liver acetyl-CoA carboxylase by palmitoyl-coenzyme A, *Eur. J. Biochem.* **89:**33–41.

22. Halestrap, A. P., and Denton, R. M., 1974, Hormonal regulation of adipose tissue acetyl-CoA carboxylase by changes in the polymeric state of the enzyme, *Biochem. J.* **142:**365–377.

23. Siess, E. A., Brocks, D. G., Lattke, H. K., and Wieland, O., 1977, Effect of glucagon on metabolite compartmentation in isolated rat liver cells during gluconeogenesis from lactate, *Biochem. J.* **166:**225–235.

24. Yeh, L.-A., Song, C.-S., and Kim K.-H., 1981, Coenzyme A activation of acetyl-CoA carboxylase, *J. Biol. Chem.* **256:**2289–2296.

25. Witters, L. A., Moriarity, D., and Martin, D. B., 1979, Regulation of hepatic acetyl coenzyme A carboxylase by insulin and glucagon, *J. Biol. Chem.* **254:**6644–6649.

26. Ly, S., and Kim K.-H., 1981, Inactivation of hepatic acetyl-CoA carboxylase by catecholamine and its agonists through the α-adrenergic receptors, *J. Biol. Chem.* **256:**11,585–11,590.

27. Krakower, G. R., and Kim, K.-H., 1980, Dephosphorylation and activation of acetyl-CoA carboxylase by phosphorylase phosphatase, *Biochem. Biophys. Res. Commun.* **92:**389–395.

28. Witters, L. A., 1981, Insulin stimulates phosphorylation of acetyl-CoA carboxylase, *Biochem. Biophys. Res. Commun.* **100:**872–878.

29. Janski, A. M., Srere, P. A., Cornell, P. A., and Veech, R. L., 1979, Phosphorylation of ATP citrate lyase in response to glucagon, *J. Biol. Chem.* **254:**9365–9368.

30. Hardie, G., 1981, Fat and phosphorylation—the role of the covalent enzyme modification in lipid synthesis, *Trends Biochem. Sci.* **6:**75–77.

31. Gibson, D. M., Lyons, R. T., Scott, D. F., and Muto, Y., 1972, Synthesis and degradation of lipogenic enzymes of rat liver, *Adv. Enzyme Regul.* **10:**187–204.

32. Nepokroeff, C. M., Lakshmanan, M. R., Ness, G. D., Muesing, R. A., Kleinsek, D. A., and Porter, J. W., 1974, Coordinate control of rat liver lipogenic enzymes by insulin, *Arch. Biochem. Biophys.* **162:**340–344.

33. Spence, J. T., and Pitot, H. C., 1982, Induction of lipogenic enzymes in primary cultures of rat hepatocytes, *Eur. J. Biochem.* **128:**15–20.

34. Katz, N. R., and Giffhorn, S., 1983, Glucose- and insulin-dependent induction of ATP citrate lyase in primary cultures of rat hepatocytes, *Biochem. J.* **212:**65–71.

35. Giffhorn, S., and Katz, N. R., 1984, Glucose-dependent induction of acetyl-CoA carboxylase in rat hepatocyte cultures, *Biochem. J.* **221:**343–350.

36. Nakanishi, S., and Numa, S., 1970, Purification of rat liver acetyl-CoA carboxylase and immunochemical studies on its synthesis and degradation, *Eur. J. Biochem.* **16:**161–173.

37. Deter, R. I., and De Duve, C., 1967, Influence of glucagon, an inducer of cellular autophagy, on some physical properties of rat liver lysosomes, *J. Cell Biol.* **33:**437–449.

38. McGarry, J. D., Mannaerts, G. P., and Foster, D. W., 1977, A possible role for malonyl-CoA in the regulation of hepatic fatty acid oxidation and ketogenesis, *J. Clin. Invest.* **60:**265–270.

39. McGarry, J. D., and Foster, D. W., 1979, In support of the roles of malonyl-CoA and carnitine acyltransferase I in the regulation of hepatic fatty acid oxidation and ketogenesis, *J. Biol. Chem.* **254:**8163–8168.

40. Snoswell, A. M., and Henderson, G. D., 1970, Aspects of carnitine ester metabolism in sheep liver, *Biochem. J.* **119:**59–65.

41. McGarry, J. D., Robles-Valdes, C., and Foster, D. W., 1975, Role of carnitine in hepatic ketogenesis, *Proc. Natl. Acad. Sci. U.S.A.* **72:**4385–4388.

42. Zammit, V. A., 1981, Intrahepatic regulation of ketogenesis, *Trends Biochem. Sci.* **6:**46–49.

43. Weiss. L., and Löffler, G., 1970, Interrelationship between adipose tissue and liver: Gluconeogenesis and ketogenesis, in: *Adipose Tissue: Regulation and Functions* (B. Jeanrenaud and D. Hepp, eds.), pp. 196–203, Thieme, Stuttgart.

44. Newsholm, E. A., and Start, C., 1973, *Regulation in Metabolism*, pp. 315–323, Wiley, London.

45. Quandt, L., and Huth, W., 1984, Modulation of rat liver mitochondrial acetyl-CoA acetyl transferase activity by a reversible chemical modification with coenzyme A, *Biochim. Biophys. Acta* **784:**168–176.

46. Reed, W. D., Clinkenbeard, K. D., and Lane, M. D., 1975, Molecular and catalytic properties of mitochondrial 3-hydroxy-3-methylglutaryl-CoA synthase of liver, *J. Biol. Chem.* **250:**3117–3125.

47. Menahan, L. A., Hron, W. T., Hinkelman, D. G., and Miziorko, H. M., 1981, Interrelationships between 3-hydroxy-3-methylglutaryl-CoA synthase, acetoacetyl-CoA and ketogenesis, *Eur. J. Biochem.* **119:**287–294.

48. Saggerson, E. D., and Bates, E. J., 1981, Regulation of glycerolipid synthesis, in: *Short Term Regulation of Liver Metabolism* (L. Hue and G. Van de Werve, eds.), pp. 247–262, Elsevier, Amsterdam.

49. Bates, E. J., and Saggerson, E. D., 1979, A study of the glycerol phosphate acyltransferase and dihydroxyacetone phosphate acyltransferase activities in rat liver mitochondrial and microsomal fractions, *Biochem. J.* **182:**751–762.

50. Balint, J. A., 1982, Lipid metabolism in relation to liver physiology and disease, in: *(The Liver Annual 2* (I. M. Arias, M. Frenkel, and J. H. P. Wilson, eds.), pp. 16–27, Excerpta Medica, Amsterdam.

51. Beynen, A. C., Haagsman, H. P., Van Golde, L. M. G., and Geelen, M. J. H., 1981, The effects of insulin and glucagon on the release of triacylglycerols by isolated rat hepatocytes, *Biochim. Biophys. Acta* **665:**1–7.

52. Hui, D. Y., Innerarity, T. L., and Mahley, R. W., 1981, Lipoprotein binding to canine hepatic membranes, *J. Biol. Chem.* **256:**5646–5655.

53. Angelin, B., Raviola, C. A., Innerarity, T. L., and Mahley R. W., 1983, Regulation of hepatic lipoprotein receptors in the dog, *J. Clin. Invest.* **71:**816–831.

54. Katz, N. R., Fischer, W., and Ick, M., 1983, Heterogeneous distribution of ATP citrate lyase in rat liver parenchyma, *Eur. J. Biochem.* **130:**297–301.

55. Katz, N. R., Fischer, W., and Giffhorn, S., 1983, Distribution of enzymes of fatty acid and ketone body metabolism in periportal and perivenous rat liver tissue, *Eur. J. Biochem.* **135:**103–107.

56. Katz, N., and Giffhorn, S., 1985, Predominance of liponeogenesis in the perivenous zone of the rat liver acinus, *J. Hepatol. Suppl.* **1:**S74.

57. Morrison, G. R., Brock, F. E., Karl, I. E., and Shank, R. E., 1965, Quantitative analysis of regenerating and degenerating areas within the lobule of carbon tetrachloride-injured liver, *Arch. Biochem. Biophys.* **111:**448–460.

58. Welsh, F. A., 1972, Changes in distribution of enzymes within the liver lobule during adaptive increases, *J. Histochem. Cytochem.* **20:**107–111.

59. Teutsch, H. F., and Rieder, H., 1979, NADP$^+$-dependent dehydrogenases in rat liver parenchyma. II. Comparison of qualitative and quantitative G6PDH distribution patterns with particular reference to sex differences, *Histochemistry* **60:**43–52.

60. Teutsch, H. F., 1981, Chemomorphology of liver parenchyma: Qualitative histochemical distribution patterns and quantitative sinusoidal profiles of G6Pase, G6PDH and malic enzyme activity and of glycogen content, *Prog. Histochem. Cytochem.* **14**(3)**:**1–92.

61. Rieder, H., 1981, NADP$^+$-dependent dehydrogenases in rat liver parenchyma. III. The description of a lipogenic area on the basis of histochemically demonstrated enzyme activities, *Histochemistry* **72:**579–615.

62. Hildebrand, R., 1980, Nuclear volume and cellular metabolism, *Adv. Anat. Embryol. Cell Biol.* **60:**1–54.

63. Morrison, G., and Brock, F. E., 1967, Quantitative measurement of alcohol dehydrogenase in the lobule of normal livers, *J. Lab. Clin. Med.* **70:**116–120.

64. Loud, A. V., 1968, Quantitative stereological description of the ultrastructure of normal rat liver parenchymal cells, *J. Cell Biol.* **37:**27–46.

65. Jones, A. L., Schmucker, D. L., Mooney, J. S., Adler, R. D., and Ockner, R. K., 1978, A quantitative analysis of hepatic ultrastructure in rats during enhanced bile secretion, *Anat. Rec.* **192:**227–228.

66. Daoust, R., 1979, Histochemical comparison of local losses of RNase and ATPase activities in preneoplastic rat livers, *J. Histochem. Cytochem.* **27:**653–656.

Chapter 11

Metabolism of Amino Acids and Ammonia

Dieter Häussinger and Wolfgang Gerok

1. INTRODUCTION

Amino acids are not only essential building blocks for the synthesis of peptides, proteins, amino sugars, purines, and pyrimidines, but also a major source of energy in different organs. Apart from this, several amino acids or their derivatives are important for organ-specific functions, such as neurotransmission in the brain or stimulation of hormone secretion by endocrine glands.

About 14,000 g of amino acids is present in normal man in the form of peptide bonds ("amino acid reservoir"), whereas free amino acids account for only about 5% of the total body amino acid pool. The size of this pool is kept fairly constant, indicating a remarkable equilibrium of amino acid output and input during both catabolic and anabolic states or under different nutritional conditions. The importance of the liver in maintaining this amino acid balance rapidly becomes evident after hepatectomy or in fulminant hepatic failure, in which the plasma levels of nearly all amino acids are considerably elevated and the plasma amino acid pattern becomes disarranged. The isolated, perfused rat liver releases amino acids, and after 90 min, almost constant levels are established for all individual amino acids, which resembles the pattern found in the plasma *in vivo*.[1]

DIETER HÄUSSINGER and WOLFGANG GEROK • Medizinische Universitätsklinik, D-7800 Freiburg, Federal Republic of Germany.

A thorough examination of the role and regulation of hepatic amino acid and ammonia metabolism must deal with more than 20 different chemical compounds, an approach that is beyond the scope of this chapter. Therefore, in the following discussion, some principal aspects of hepatic amino acid and ammonia metabolism, its interorgan relationships, and its regulation in liver with special reference to the role of zonal hepatocyte heterogeneity will be presented. Examples of alanine, glutamine, glutamate, branched-chain amino acid, and ammonia metabolism will be considered.

2. ROLE OF THE LIVER IN THE METABOLISM OF AMINO ACIDS AND AMMONIA

2.1. Interorgan Relationships in Amino Acid Metabolism

The liver has important catabolic and anabolic functions in the metabolism of amino acids. In the anabolic direction, the liver synthesizes most plasma proteins and peptides, such as glutathione, nonessential and essential amino acids, if the ketoanalogues are available, and amino acid conjugates for biliary excretion. The catabolic role includes the deamination of amino acids to provide carbon for gluconeogenesis, ketogenesis, or fatty acid synthesis. The highest rates of hepatic amino acid extraction are observed for the gluconeogenic amino acids alanine, serine, and threonine, and their nitrogen is released mainly as urea. Most of the essential amino acids appear to be degraded predominantly in the liver, except for the branched-chain amino acids, which are rapidly metabolized in other tissues, especially muscle. However, the liver will extract large amounts of their ketoanalogues, which are produced by muscle. Amino acid concentrations in portal venous blood of rats may increase up to 20-fold after ingestion of a protein meal,[2] and the liver is the first organ to process absorbed amino acids. Under these conditions, the liver extracts a large fraction of nearly all amino acids, except for branched-chain amino acids.[2,3] This explains the only slight fluctuations of most arterial plasma amino acids during absorption from the intestine. On the other hand, after feeding a protein-free diet, only small fractions of amino acids are extracted from portal venous blood,[2] and during amino-acid-free liver perfusion, there is even a release of amino acids.[1] Thus, the liver acts as a metabolic buffer in the control of the levels of plasma amino acids; however, other organs will also contribute significantly to amino acid homeostasis.

Several studies on arteriovenous concentration differences across various organs have provided insight into interorgan amino acid fluxes in man (for reviews, see Felig,[4] Cahill et al.,[5] and Christensen[6]). These studies have been performed mainly by measurement of arterial–hepatic venous concentration differences, giving information on hepatic plus extrahepatic splanchnic amino acid exchange, whereas there are only limited data available on arterial–portal venous concentration differences in man.

2.1.1. Alanine Metabolism

Muscle is a major site of alanine release in man, amounting to about 30–40% of total α-amino-nitrogen release.[7] Muscle alanine production is increased during short-term starvation and exercise.[7] Alanine nitrogen in muscle derives mainly from branched-chain amino acids, and about 70% of total alanine released is newly synthesized *in situ*.[4,8] Also, the gut releases alanine in the postabsorptive state at rates comparable to those of muscle (Fig. 1A). In the gut, alanine nitrogen is derived from glutamine, whereas 80% of alanine carbon is derived from glucose.[9,10] Alanine release by muscle and gut accounts fully for hepatic alanine uptake and its conversion to glucose in liver. Because glucose is taken up by the muscle and its carbon skeleton is converted to alanine and transported to the liver, a glucose–alanine cycle[4,11] has been suggested. The importance of alanine as a precursor of hepatic gluconeogenesis is emphasized by the finding that the rate of glucose synthesis from alanine (and serine) is far higher than that from any other amino acid.[12] Further, gluconeogenesis from alanine increases linearly with increasing alanine concentrations up to levels 10-fold higher than the physiological concentration.[11] In addition, there is also a slight release of alanine by the kidney (Fig. 1A).

Alanine is an important product in carbon and nitrogen metabolism of extrahepatic tissues and provides a nontoxic transport form for α-amino-nitrogen release from skeletal muscle and intestine. Repletion of the nitrogen stores in muscle and gut may occur by the predominant utilization of branched-chain amino acids and glutamine in these organs, respectively.

2.1.2. Glutamine Metabolism

Skeletal muscle is the major site of glutamine production, and the amounts released are similar to those of alanine in the postabsorptive state.[4,17] Glutamine is taken up by the intestine, where it is a major respiratory fuel. Splanchnic glutamine uptake, as indicated by the positive arterial–hepatic venous concentration difference in man, is due largely to an uptake by the nonhepatic splanchnic bed.[13] Glutamine nitrogen is released mainly from the intestine in the form of ammonia, alanine, and citrulline; the latter is taken up predominantly by the kidney (for a review, see Windmueller[10]). Alanine nitrogen and ammonia are converted to urea in the liver. Another site of glutamine uptake in normal man in the postabsorptive state is the kidney (Fig. 1B), whereas in the rat, the kidneys have no significant effect on circulating glutamine.[15] During acidosis, however, in man and in the rat, glutamine uptake by the kidney is increased and its nitrogen is excreted into urine as ammonium ions.[15,16] Under these conditions, glutamine

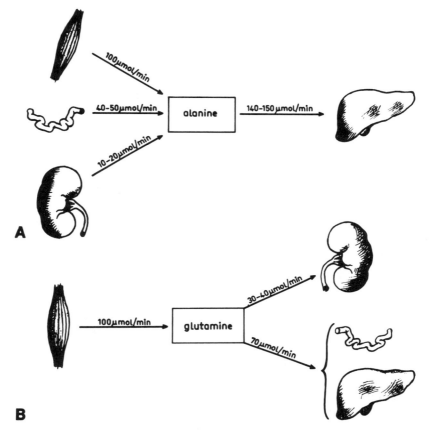

Figure 1. Interorgan fluxes in alanine (A), glutamine (B), and ammonia, and urea (C) metabolism in man. Calculation of data for the postabsorptive state (A, B) was based on arteriovenous concentration differences given in Felig[4] and Tizianello *et al.*[14] and measured rates of blood flow. Mesenteric vein blood flow was assumed to be about 70% of hepatic blood flow. Dashed lines denote increased metabolite fluxes in acidosis.

release by muscle may increase up to 2-fold, and the liver becomes a site of glutamine production[15] (Fig. 1C).

Apart from this, the role of the liver in glutamine metabolism is controversial. Depending on nutritional and experimental conditions, data indicate that there is either a slight net glutamine uptake or release by the liver.[15,18–21] This apparent discrepancy is explained by the complex and sensitive regulation of hepatic glutamine-metabolizing enzymes by portal glutamine and ammonia concentrations, hormones, and pH, with the consequence of either net glutamine uptake or release.[22–25] The role of the liver in glutamine metabolism is presented in more detail in Section 4.3.

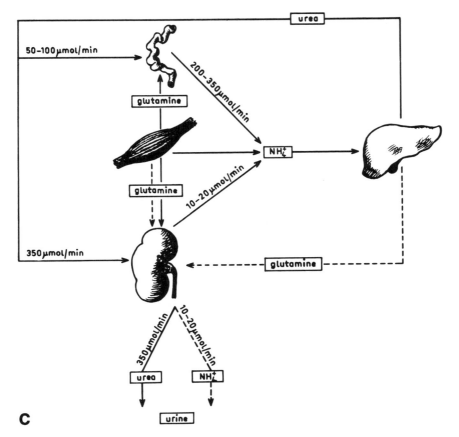

50–100 µmol/min

200–350 µmol/min

glutamine

glutamine

10–20 µmol/min

350 µmol/min

urea

NH₄⁺

glutamine

NH₄⁺

350 µmol/min

10–20 µmol/min

urea   NH₄⁺

urine

C

Figure 1. (*continued*)

2.1.3. Branched-Chain Amino Acids

In the postabsorptive state in man, there is only slight extraction of branched-chain amino acids by the total splanchnic bed; however, there is a slight release of these amino acids from the gut.[4,13] Muscle releases significant amounts of branched-chain amino acids at rates about 20–30% as fast as alanine in the postabsorptive state. A significant exchange for these amino acids is not observed in the kidney, and it was suggested that the brain could be a site of uptake; however, the brain seems to play a minor role in the metabolism of other amino acids.[5,26]

After ingestion of a protein meal, branched-chain amino acids are increasingly taken up by muscle,[4,21] whereas alanine release by muscle is almost unaffected. However, increased alanine release by muscle during exercise is accompanied by an increased uptake of branched-chain amino acids.[27] Branched-chain amino acid release by muscle is reduced by insulin.[28]

These data point to a predominant role of skeletal muscle in the metabolism of branched-chain amino acids, providing an important nitrogen source for alanine and glutamine production by muscle. In addition, the ketoanalogues of branched-chain amino acids are released by extrahepatic tissues[29] and are oxidized rapidly in the liver.

2.2. Interorgan Relationships in Ammonia Metabolism

The physiological ammonia concentration in arterial blood is in the range of 30 μM. At high concentrations, ammonia is toxic and hyperammonemia is recognized as one of the factors in the pathogenesis of hepatic encephalopathy, a syndrome of neuropsychiatric disturbance of various grades of severity developing in advanced liver disease (for a review, see Gerok and Häussinger[30]). The important role of the liver in maintaining low, nontoxic concentrations of ammonia was demonstrated in animals with Eck's fistula or after hepatectomy. These and similar studies showed that blood ammonia concentration is determined by the balance resulting from the rate of ammonia production in different tissues and the rate of hepatic and extrahepatic substrate-driven ammonia removal.

2.2.1. Sources of Ammonia

An important site of ammonia production is the gut. In the dog, ammonia release into mesenteric venous blood from the gut is about 0.16 mmole/hr per kg body weight. About one half of intestinal ammonia production is derived from the colon, whereas about 30 and 20% are released from the jejunum and the ileum, respectively.[31] Ammonia formation by the small intestine can be largely accounted for by the metabolism of glutamine, the major respiratory fuel (for a review, see Windmueller[10]), and there is a linear relationship between glutamine uptake and ammonia release. On the other hand, glutamine uptake by the colon accounts for only 9% of ammonia release by the colon.[31] Large-bowel ammonia production is due predominantly to the hydrolysis of other nitrogenous compounds under the influence of colonic bacteria. About 40% of ammonia production from the colon arises from hydrolysis of urea by bacterial urease. In man, about 20–30% of urea synthesized by the liver is hydrolyzed in the gut under normal condition[32] (Fig. 1C).

The kidney also releases ammonia into the renal vein at a rate of about 1 mmole/hr in normal man.[14] This is due to ammonia generation in the tubular epithelia and its redistribution by nonionic diffusion into the blood according to the pH difference between these compartments. Renal ammonia release into the blood is enhanced during hypokalemia[33] and under conditions of increased renal ammoniagenesis and ammonia excretion into the urine during acidosis.[34]

In normal man, the arterial–venous concentration difference for ammonia across resting skeletal muscle is about zero.[35] Studies with ^{15}N-labeled ammonia in man demonstrated a metabolic trapping of ^{15}N in resting muscle,[36] indicating simultaneous ammonia production and uptake. However, during exercise, skeletal muscle releases ammonia in proportion to the amount of work done.[37,38] In muscle, most of the ammonia is generated by the action of the purine nucleotide cycle (for a review, see Lowenstein[37]). On the other hand, in studies of arterial–venous concentration differences across the resting human forearm in the presence of elevated arterial ammonia concentrations, considerable ammonia uptake by muscle has been demonstrated.[38] These data point to an important role of skeletal muscle in ammonia production and uptake.

Under normal conditions, human brain releases or extracts negligible amounts of ammonia. There is a linear relationship between the arterial–venous concentration difference for ammonia across the brain and the arterial ammonia concentration,[39] resulting in a cerebral ammonia uptake during hyperammonemia. Similar results were obtained in studies on human brain [^{15}N]ammonia metabolism.[36]

Although measurements of portal–hepatic vein concentration differences indicate a substantial net hepatic ammonia uptake, considerable ammonia must also be produced as an intermediate by the liver during gluconeogenesis from amino acids. In the liver, during amino acid degradation, ammonia is generated predominantly by oxidative deamination of glutamate and glutamine hydrolysis, whereas ammoniagenesis by the purine nucleotide cycle is of minor importance.[40] However, hepatic ammonia formation represents an intermediate step in hepatic nitrogen catabolism, the major end product being urea.

2.2.2. Ammonia Detoxification

In normal man ingesting a 100-g protein diet, more than 95% of excess nitrogen is removed by urea formation, whereas renal ammonia excretion into the urine is only about 0.03 mole/24 hr,[14] i.e., about 2% of total nitrogen excretion. During acidosis, however, the proportion of nitrogen elimination in the form of urea decreases at the expense of urinary ammonia excretion.[41] Ammonia detoxification by urea synthesis is a liver-specific, irreversible process. Although all urea-cycle enzymes are also present in the brain, cerebral urea production has never been observed. In man, the maximal rate of urea synthesis *in vivo* is about 4 moles urea/24 hr[42] and exceeds by far the average rate of urea excretion of about 0.5 mole/24 hr, even if urea hydrolysis by the intestinal flora is taken into account.

The second important pathway of ammonia detoxification is glutamine synthesis. Glutamine synthetase activity is found not only in the liver but also in other tissues, such as muscle, brain, and kidney. In the rat, the total body capacities for glutamine and urea synthesis are of the same order of magnitude.[43] The overall rate of metabolic ammonia clearance from the vascular compartment in man is a linear function of its arterial concentration. The importance of ammonia removal by glutamine synthesis was demonstrated by Duda and Handler.[43] After injection of ^{15}N-labeled ammonia into rats, most of the isotope was recovered in the amide group of glutamine within about 20 min, and it was shown that the rate of ^{15}N loss from glutamine is of the same order as the fixation of ammonia into urea under normal conditions. Ammonia fixation by glutamine synthesis is reversible, because ammonia can be liberated from glutamine by the action of glutaminases, enzymes present in the liver, kidney, and gut. Hydrolysis of glutamine in the intestine and liver yields ammonia, which serves as a substrate for hepatic urea synthesis. Therefore, glutamine may act as a buffer for ammonia and may be considered as a nontoxic transport form of ammonia between different tissues (Fig. 1C).

Under conditions of impaired urea synthesis, such as severe liver injury, hepatectomy, or decreased hepatic blood flow, extrahepatic ammonia fixation by glutamine synthesis increases, leading to elevated plasma glutamine levels. Under these conditions, however, especially if the pH is normal, urinary ammonia excretion as a consequence of renal glutamine hydrolysis does not provide a sufficient compensatory mechanism for elimination of excess nitrogen from the organism, and hyperammonemia develops.

3. REGULATION OF HEPATIC AMINO ACID AND AMMONIA METABOLISM: ROLE OF TRANSPORT, SUBSTRATES, AND HORMONES

3.1. Amino Acid Metabolism

In general, regulation of metabolism can occur at the level of substrate availability and by control of the activity of the metabolizing enzymes. Both sites are influenced by hormones. Therefore, the role of amino acid transport across biological membranes, some regulatory features of amino-acid-metabolizing enzymes, and the influence of hormones on the control of hepatic amino acid metabolism need to be considered regarding alanine, glutamine, and glutamate metabolism.

3.1.1. Regulation by Transport

Hepatic gluconeogenesis and ureagenesis from amino acids are largely dependent on intracellular amino acid pools. To be metabolized, amino acids must be transported across the plasma membrane of hepatocytes. Studies on perfused rat liver, isolated hepatocytes, hepatocyte cultures, and isolated plasma membrane vesicles have shown the existence of different transport systems in the plasma membrane for neutral amino acids. These transport systems have been characterized by their ion dependence, by the transport of system-specific model substrates (nonmetabolizable amino acid analogues), and by their competition with the transport of naturally occurring amino acids. They were termed systems L, A, ASC, and N, and apart from the latter, they are found in a great variety of different mammalian cells (for reviews, see Guidotto et al.[44] and Shotwell et al.[45]). System L is sodium-independent, whereas systems A, ASC, and N are sodium-dependent. Amino acid transport by these carriers in liver shows an overlapping specificity for physiological amino acids and competition of different amino acids for transport by one system. The preferred natural substrates for these systems are Leucine and other branched-chain and aromatic amino acids (system L); Alanine, serine, glycine (system A); Alanine, Serine, Cysteine (system ASC); and glutamine, histidine, asparagine (system N).

Several studies have shown that alanine transport across the plasma membrane of rat liver is rate-controlling for its metabolism.[46–48] Thus, alanine transport is expected to be a major regulatory site for hepatic alanine metabolism. The K_m(alanine) of its transport is about 2–4 mM,[46] i.e., above the physiological portal alanine concentration during the absorptive phase of 1–2 mM.[47] This indicates that hepatic alanine uptake depends on variations in portal alanine supply. The alanine–sodium symport is an electrogenic process, and electroneutrality is brought about by countertransport of other cations or cotransport of anions. The latter strongly influence alanine transport in isolated plasma membrane vesicles of rat liver as a consequence of the relative permeability of plasma membrane to them.[48] However, there is no evidence for a regulatory role of anions in alanine transport under physiological conditions. Alanine transport is inhibited strongly by other amino acids transported in a sodium-dependent way, such as proline, serine, cysteine, and glutamine. The rate of alanine transport is increased in hepatocytes from rats ingesting a high-protein diet and to a lesser extent during starvation.[47] This is in line with an increased hepatic alanine utilization observed under these conditions. Sodium-dependent transport of alanine and other amino acids is increased in the postnatal period and declines gradually with progressive development to rates similar to those found in normal adult animals.[49] Similar results have been obtained during compensatory growth in the regenerating liver *in vivo*.

Transport of alanine and other amino acids via system A across the hepatocyte plasma membrane is increased by thyroid hormones, glucagon, cyclic AMP (cAMP), insulin, and glucocorticoids (for reviews, see Guidotto et al.[44] and Shotwell et al.[45]). Some regulatory properties of alanine transport across liver plasma membrane are given in Fig. 2. The effects of glucagon and cAMP on amino acid transport system A in hepatocytes are due partly to the induction

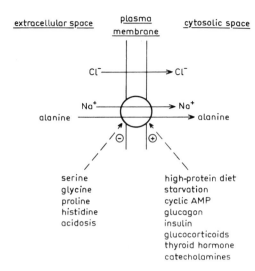

Figure 2. Scheme of some regulatory aspects of alanine transport across rat liver plasma membrane. Sodium-dependent alanine transport is electrogenic; electroneutrality is brought about by cotransport of anions, e.g., Cl⁻, or countertransport of cations.

of a high-affinity component of this transport system,[50] probably by *de novo* synthesis of carrier proteins. The high turnover of these high-affinity carriers should provide a mechanism for adjustment of amino acid transport to the increased needs for amino acids during gluconeogenesis or hepatic protein synthesis. On the other hand, there are no effects of glucagon and insulin on transport systems ASC and N.[51]

Glutamine transport across the plasma membrane of hepatocytes is mediated by system N.[51] The transport rate of glutamine was stimulated 2-fold after cultivation of hepatocytes for 8 hr in an amino-acid-free medium, also suggesting an adaptive regulation of this system.[51] For comparison, under these conditions, the transport capacity of system A was increased about 16-fold. However, starvation did not increase glutamine transport in rat hepatocytes compared to normal fed controls,[52] as was the case for alanine transport. This indicates independent regulation of the transport of glutamine and alanine. Evidence has been presented that glutamine transport across the plasma membrane of hepatocytes is rate-controlling for its metabolism but as yet not for glutamine transport across the mitochondrial membrane.[113] Glutamine transport system N is unique to liver and some hepatoma cell lines.[45] Its possible physiological role will be discussed in Section 5 in relation to hepatocyte heterogeneity in glutamine and glutamate metabolism.

Acidic amino acids, such as glutamate and aspartate, are transported by a sodium-dependent transport system in liver plasma membrane with a high substrate affinity but a low transport capacity.[53] Glutamate uptake by the liver is rate-controlling for its metabolism,[53,54] and in isolated perfused rat liver, the

K_m(glutamate) is in the range of the physiological portal glutamate concentration. In recent studies, glutamate uptake by cultured hepatocytes was found to occur not only by a sodium-dependent, but also by a sodium-independent, transport system.[55] The sodium-dependent transport system was induced by glucocorticoids, in agreement with enhanced hepatic glutamate uptake after ingestion of a high-protein diet.[20] Na^+-dependent glutamate uptake in isolated hepatocytes and perfused rat liver is slow compared to the Na^+-independent portion.[55,121] Interestingly, glutamate release from the liver is considerably increased by the keto analogues of leucine and methionine.[120] This effect is not related to the metabolism of these ketoacids and represents probably a direct effect on the sodium-independent glutamate transport system.

3.1.2. Regulation by Substrates and Hormones

In vivo and *in vitro* studies have shown that hepatic amino acid uptake depends on the rate of their release from peripheral tissues. In livers of fasted rats, perfused with a mixture of amino acids at various multiples of their normal plasma concentration, glucose production was half-maximal at normal amino acid concentrations and approached saturation at 3 times the normal concentrations.[11] Under these conditions, gluconeogenesis and ureagenesis increased almost linearly with amino acid supply up to levels twice the normal concentrations. If alanine was added alone, gluconeogenesis increased linearly up to alanine concentrations of about 10 mM, underlining again the importance of this amino acid in hepatic metabolism and in gluconeogenesis. Because the reactions of alanine aminotransferase, aspartate aminotransferase, and glutamate dehydrogenase in liver are near equilibrium in the presence of physiological amino acid concentrations, transamination or deamination is a minor rate-controlling or regulatory site in the catabolism of intracellular alanine, aspartate, or glutamate. The rate-controlling steps in the breakdown of these amino acids are localized in the gluconeogenic or oxidative pathway starting from pyruvate, oxalacetate, or α-oxoglutarate and are under the control of various hormones such as glucagon, cAMP, glucocorticoids, catecholamines, thyroid hormone, and insulin (see also Chapter 9). However, these hormones influence hepatic amino acid metabolism not only indirectly by regulation of the rate of gluconeogenesis, but also directly by affecting amino acid transport across the plasma membrane of the hepatocyte, induction of amino-acid-metabolizing enzymes in liver, release of amino acids by extrahepatic tissues, and regulation of hepatic protein synthesis and degradation. For example, glucagon enhances gluconeogenesis and ureagenesis from alanine and other amino acids by stimulation of amino acid transport across the hepatocyte plasma membrane and by increasing the hepatic levels of tyrosine aminotransferase, serine dehydratase, aspartate and phenylalanine aminotransferase, and other enzymes of amino acid metabolism. Further, glucagon decreases protein synthesis in extrahepatic tissues, increases amino acid output, and stimulates hepatic proteolysis.

For the catabolism of some other amino acids, the rate-controlling and regulatory step is proximal to the reactions that lead to the production of a central metabolite of the citric acid cycle or the gluconeogenic or ketogenic pathway. This is suggested for the conversion of proline to glutamate, where the flux through proline oxidase and 1-pyrroline-5-carboxylate dehydrogenase may be controlled by the subcellular NADH/NAD$^+$ ratios[56] and is stimulated by glucagon.[57] Similarly, hepatic glutamine degradation is controlled by the activity of hepatic glutaminase. Flux through this enzyme is stimulated by increasing substrate supply within the physiological concentration range[24] and is under the control of portal ammonia. Half-maximal stimulation of glutaminase flux by ammonia is observed at the physiological portal ammonia concentration of 0.2–0.3 mM, and flux is maximal at a concentration of about 0.6 mM.[22–24] Because the intestine releases ammonia derived from the metabolism of glutamine into the portal vein, hepatic glutaminase flux will be affected by the rate of glutamine utilization by the gut. This triggering of hepatic glutamine degradation by intestinal ammonia release is an example of an interorgan feed-forward regulation system[23] that provides an effective means for removal of surplus glutamine by splanchnic tissues. Effectors that control glutaminase flux in the liver are given schematically in Section 4 (Fig. 8).

Amino acid supply for the liver not only determines the rate of amino acid catabolism, but also is of regulatory importance for hepatic protein balance. Ammonia and several amino acids (for review see ref. 58), especially glutamine, glutamate, and alanine, have been shown to be potent inhibitors of hepatic proteolysis. Since glucagon and α-adrenergic activators stimulate glutaminase flux and are capable of decreasing the intracellular concentration of glutamine, glutamate, and alanine, the deprivation of glutamine or other gluconeogenic amino acids might provide an important link between gluconeogenesis and intrahepatic proteolysis (for a review, see Mortimer and Pösö[58]) induced by these hormones. On the other hand, hepatic synthesis of secretory and nonsecretory proteins is regulated by the amino acid concentration.[59–61] In perfused rat liver, decreased rates of protein synthesis in the absence of added amino acids were shown to be due to reduced rates of peptide-chain initiation, as evidenced by elevated concentrations of ribosomal subunits and a loss of polysomal material. This response to amino acid deprivation could be reversed by readdition of amino acids.[61] Hepatic amino acid utilization for protein synthesis is also under hormonal control, as shown by decreased rates of protein synthesis after experimental thyroidectomy or hypophysectomy and in diabetes.

In summary, these few data indicate that hepatic amino acid metabolism is under the complex control of amino acid supply and metabolizing enzymes and that both sites are influenced by the action of various hormones.

3.2. Ammonia Metabolism

3.2.1. Regulation of Urea Synthesis

Urea is the major end product of amino acid nitrogen, and the regulatory properties of the urea cycle guarantee the maintenance of low, nontoxic ammonia concentrations, even after ingestion of large amounts of protein. The maintenance of nontoxic ammonia concentrations instead of a complete removal of ammonia is important, because ammonia also serves as a precursor of glutamate and therefore of all nonessential amino acids and is also a key metabolite in the mitochondrial redox systems. Urea synthesis consumes stoichiometric amounts of aspartate and ammonia, the latter being provided by hepatic glutamate dehydrogenase reaction or glutamine hydrolysis or via the portal vein. If urea is formed predominantly from portal ammonia, urea synthesis is accompanied by an oxidation in the mitochondrial NADPH system and a reduction of the mitochondrial NADH system, and to maintain urea-cycle flux, the activity of energy-linked transhydrogenase is required.[25,62] If urea is synthesized from alanine, ammonia must be formed by oxidative deamination of glutamate by glutamate dehydrogenase. This implies the production of reducing equivalents in the mitochondrial NADPH and NADH system, and reoxidation of these compounds is required. This may explain the inhibition of urea synthesis from alanine by ethanol.[63] Thus, the rate of urea synthesis may be influenced by the redox state of mitochondrial nicotineamide nucleotide systems.[25,63]

The activities of all five urea-cycle enzymes are increased in an adaptive manner under conditions of increased amino acid catabolism, such as ingestion of high-protein diets, fasting, or corticosteroid or glucagon administration.[64–66] Besides this long-term regulation of urea synthesis, several mechanisms of short-term regulation have been demonstrated (for a review, see Meijer and Hensgens[67]). With saturating substrate concentrations, the rate of ureagenesis is limited by the capacity of argininosuccinate synthase, as was shown by the accumulation of the substrates of this reaction *in vitro* and *in vivo*.[68] However, under physiological conditions, when the available ammonia concentrations are far below the $K_m(NH_4^+) = 1$–2 mM[69] for carbamoyl phosphate synthetase I, flux through this enzyme becomes rate-controlling.[67,121,122] This is evidenced by the finding of an almost linear increase of urea production after injection of $^{15}NH_3$ up to toxic concentrations.[43]

The activity of carbamoyl phosphate synthetase I depends strongly on the presence of its activator, N-acetylglutamate.[70,71] The rate of citrulline synthesis is also correlated closely with the intramitochondrial N-acetylglutamate concentration.[72] This cofactor is synthesized within the mitochondria by N-acetylglutamate synthase, which is activated by arginine. The $K_a(arginine)$ is 5–10 μM,[73] about one order of magnitude below the arginine levels in tissue. However, this must not reflect the mitochondrial concentration of arginine, and an increase of N-acetylglutamate content was shown in mice after injection of arginine.[74] The activity of N-acetylglutamate synthase is enhanced after long-term protein feeding, and the mitochondrial levels of N-acetylglutamate rise with increasing protein content of the diet.[72] Increased mitochondrial N-acetylglutamate levels were also observed after glucagon administration.[75] Propionyl-CoA, arising during the oxidation of ketoisovalerate, decreased the N-acetylglutamate concentration in the mitochondria, leading to an inhibition of urea synthesis.[76] Degradation of N-acetylglutamate occurs rapidly in the cytosol, and the $T_{1/2}$ of N-acetylglutamate in the mouse is about 20 min.[74] Therefore, rapid changes of the mitochondrial concentration of N-acetylglutamate provide effective short-term regulation of ammonia metabolism by positive feedback control of carbamoyl phosphate synthetase flux by arginine. Such regulatory properties of carbamoyl phosphate synthetase are also important to guarantee the supply of stoichiometric amounts of aspartate and carbamoylphosphate for urea synthesis, because the aspartate aminotransferase and glutamate dehydrogenase reactions are near equilibrium in liver, and the concentrations of aspartate and ammonia therefore are linked closely by these equilibria.[63] In addition, carbamoyl phosphate synthetase is activated by Mg^{2+} and inhibited by Ca^{2+}[77]; at present, however, it is not clear whether this is of physiological importance. Rate control of carbamoyl phosphate synthesis by bicarbonate and the activity of carbonic anhydrase has been demonstrated in isolated guinea pig liver mitochondria and in the isolated perfused rat liver.[22,123,124] This may be of interest in severe metabolic acidosis, when the bicarbonate concentration is below the reported $K_m(HCO_3^-) = 5.3$ mM[78] for carbamoyl phosphate synthetase.

Besides ammonia, bicarbonate and aspartate availability and the control of carbamoyl phosphate synthetase activity, the rate of urea synthesis is also affected by the concentration of ornithine.[79] Hepatic ornithine content increases with increasing dietary protein uptake, possibly as a consequence of an increased arginine ingestion or due to an inhibition of ornithine aminotransferase by ingested branched-chain amino acids.[80] Ornithine aminotransferase activity is increased after feeding a high-protein diet, but is decreased during starvation.[81] This might help to save this urea-cycle intermediate during starvation, i.e., under conditions without nutritional arginine supply. Ornithine is transported into the mitochondria either by ornithine–citrulline exchange or by ornithine–H$^+$ exchange.[82] At present, however, it is unclear whether this is an additional step of urea cycle control *in vivo*. Ornithine stimulates net flux through carbamoyl phosphate synthetase, possibly by increasing carbamoyl phosphate removal by citrulline synthesis and therefore deinhibition of carbamoyl phosphate synthetase by its product.[83] However, the K_i(carbamoyl phosphate) for carbamoyl phosphate synthetase is about 10–20 mM, and it is unlikely that such high intramitochondrial concentrations occur *in vivo*.[121,125] Other studies have shown that ornithine, like cysteine and histidine, activates carbamoyl phosphate synthetase by chelating divalent cations, which inhibit this enzyme.[77] On the other hand, the stimulatory effect of ornithine on net carbamoyl phosphate synthesis may be explained partly by degradation of carbamoyl phosphate in the absence of its physiological acceptor, ornithine. Such a cycle of carbamoyl phosphate synthesis and degradation, catalyzed by carbamoyl phosphate synthetase, has been demonstrated in isolated rat liver mitochondria.[84]

Several amino acids affect urea-cycle flux. Alanine, isoleucine, and valine are competitive inhibitors of argininosuccinate synthetase with respect to citrulline, whereas inhibition by histidine is noncompetitive.[85,86]

The rate of urea synthesis is stimulated by hormones such as glucagon, catecholamines, angiotensin II, vasopressin, and thyroid hormone, partly due to increased substrate supply. In the case of glucagon, this is explained by a stimulation of proteolysis, amino acid uptake and catabolism, increased intramitochondrial levels of N-acetylglutamate, and a long-term induction of urea-cycle enzymes. Some aspects of the short-term regulation of urea synthesis are given in Fig. 3.

3.2.2. Regulation of Glutamine Synthesis

In the presence of various substrates for glutamine synthesis, the rate of glutamine production by the isolated perfused rat liver was found to be very low, amounting to only about 1/40th of the assayable glutamine synthetase

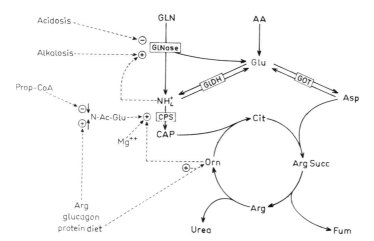

Figure 3. Regulation of urea synthesis. Dashed lines denote activating (+) or inhibitory effects (−) of effectors on urea synthesis. (CPS) Carbamoylphosphate synthetase I; (GIDH), glutamate dehydrogenase; (GINase) glutaminase; (GOT) glutamate oxalacetate transaminase; (AA) amino acids; (Arg) arginine; (ArgSucc) argininosuccinate; (Asp) aspartate; (CAP) carbamoylphosphate; (Cit) citrulline; (Glu) glutamate; (GIN) glutamine; (Fum) fumarate; (N-Ac-Glu) N-acetylglutamate; (Prop-CoA) propionyl-coenzym A; (orn) ornithine.

activity in tissue extracts.[87] This was explained partly by the occurrence of glutamine cycling, i.e., the simultaneous synthesis and degradation of glutamine in rat liver.[23,24] Isolated rat liver glutamine synthetase is activated by α-oxoglutarate, but is inhibited by glycine, alanine, carbamoylphosphate, and Mn^{2+}.[88–90] Glutamine synthetase flux in perfused liver depends on the portal glutamine and ammonia concentration and is influenced by glucagon. Further, glutamine synthetase flux is inhibited during alkalosis or by phenylephrine and is increased during acidosis.[24,91] Glutamine synthetase is subject to product inhibition [89] and it was suggested that low rates of glutamine synthesis in the intact liver might be explained by limitation of glutamine export from hepatocytes with the consequence of intracellular glutamine accumulation and therefore product inhibition of glutamine synthetase.[25,113] Further details concerning the importance of zonal hepatocyte heterogeneity in glutamine metabolism are given in Section 4.

4. ROLE OF ZONAL HEPATOCYTE HETEROGENEITY IN THE REGULATION OF AMINO ACID AND AMMONIA METABOLISM IN THE LIVER

The functional units of the liver are the so-called acini[92] extending from the terminal portal venules to the terminal hepatic venules. Hepatocyte heterogeneity in oxygen, substrate and hormone supply, and different enzyme activities from the periportal and perivenous area led to the concept of metabolic zonation, i.e., the different localization of metabolic pathways in the liver acinus (for a review, see Jungermann and Katz[93]). As shown previously for glutamine and ammonia metabolism, such compartmentation offers important additional regulation in amino acid and ammonia metabolism.[24,95]

4.1. Zonal Distribution of Enzymes

The inhomogeneous distribution of enzymes and metabolic pathways between the periportal and perivenous zones in the liver lobule has been studied with histochemical, immunohistochemical, and microdissection techniques and by direct measurement of metabolic flux differences in the intact perfused rat liver (see various other chapters). Data on the predominant localization of enzymes and metabolic steps of amino acid and ammonia metabolism are given in Table I. In general, these enzyme activities exhibit a more or less steep gradient along the acinus from the periportal to the perivenous area. Only for rat liver glutamine synthetase has an exclusive perivenous localization without immunohistochemical staining in the periportal area been demonstrated.[95] Such a circumscribed enzyme localization may not be identical with a very general perivenous distribution, but may represent a subzone of the perivenous area in the liver lobule. The borderline between periportal and perivenous regions in

Table I. Zonal Distribution of Enzymes and Metabolic Pathways of Amino Acid and Ammonia Metabolism in Liver Parenchyma[a]

Enzymes	Method[b]	Ref. Nos.
Predominant periportal localization		
Alanine aminotransferase	M, H	96, 98, 99
Aspartate aminotranserase	H	96
Tyrosine aminotransferase	H	98
Glutaminase	F	94
γ-Glutamyl transpeptidase	H	101
Carbamoylphosphate synthetase	H	102
Ornithine carbamoyl transferase	H	103
Arginosuccinate synthetase	H	104
Arginase	H	104
Ammonia production from endogenous proteins and amino acids	F	94
Urea synthesis from ammonia and amino acids	F	94
Proline degradation	F	54
Predominant perivenous localization		
Glutamate dehydrogenase	M, H	96, 97, 99, 100
Glutamine synthetase	H	95
Glutamine synthesis from ammonia	F	94
Ornithine aminotransferase	H	110
Glutamate uptake system in plasma membrane	F	54

[a] The data are from studies on rat liver.
[b] (H) Histochemical or immunohistochemical; (M) microdissection and microbiochemistry; (F) metabolic flux measurements in isolated, perfused rat liver.

the acinus is not defined clearly and must be considered to be rather dynamic from the functional point of view. Quantitative histochemical and microdissection measurements have shown the ratios of periportal/perivenous enzyme activities to be about 0.5–0.8 for glutamate dehydrogenase, 1.6–5.0 for alanine aminotransferase, 1.6 for tyrosine aminotransferase, and 1.4 for aspartate aminotransferase.[96–100]

The data in Table I suggest a preferential periportal localization of amino acid utilization. Because the enzymes of gluconeogenesis are found predominantly in the periportal zone (see Chapter 9), the carbon skeleton of various amino acids, especially alanine, should be readily available for gluconeogenesis. This shows that functionally linked processes are localized in the same area of the acinus.[93] In addition, the periportal zone exhibits high enzyme activities for ammonia and amino acid nitrogen detoxification, as shown by the predominant periportal localization of urea-cycle enzymes and predominant periportal urea production in the structurally and metabolically intact perfused rat liver in the presence of different substrate gradients along the liver lobule.[94] Ureagenesis requires stoichiometric amounts of aspartate and ammonia, and during ureagenesis from amino acids, ammonia must be generated by periportal glutamate dehydrogenase activity. Although this enzyme is found at 1.3- to 2-fold higher amounts in the perivenous zone,[97] glutamate dehydrogenase is present in sufficient amounts in the periportal area for ammonia production in view of the high activity of this enzyme in total liver tissue.

Studies on the metabolically and structurally intact perfused rat liver have shown a complimentary distribution of the two hepatic ammonia-fixating systems, urea and glutamine synthesis.[94] This is also illustrated by the strictly complementary immunohistochemical localization of argininosuccinate synthase and arginase in the periportal area and of glutamine synthetase in the perivenous area (Fig. 4).

Evidence for a zonal distribution of amino acid transport systems in the plasma membrane of hepatocytes has been reported.[54] Vascular glutamate is utilized predominantly for perivenous glutamine synthesis, and a glutamate transport capacity about 15- to 20-fold higher in the plasma membrane of glutamine-synthesizing hepatocytes compared to controls has been calculated.[54] The common localization of glutamine synthetase and the glutamate transport system in the plasma membrane is another example of the concept of a similar localization of functionally linked processes in the liver acinus.

4.2. Dynamics of Zonal Hepatocyte Heterogeneity in Amino Acid and Ammonia Metabolism

As mentioned above, zonal hepatocyte heterogeneity in amino acid and ammonia metabolism is a dynamic process that is influenced by developmental, nutritional, and hormonal conditions. Further, several hepatotoxins exert their effects predominantly in the periportal or perivenous area of the acinus with the consequence of a more or less selective impairment of metabolic pathways in amino acid and ammonia metabolism.

4.2.1. Development

In fetal rat liver, γ-glutamyl transpeptidase is distributed throughout the lobule without apparent zonal distribution. After birth, γ-glutamyl transpeptidase in hepatocytes declines rapidly and is found only in clusters of hepatocytes predominantly in the periportal area. From the 7th day after birth, there is essentially no γ-glutamyl transpeptidase detectable in hepatocytes, and remaining enzyme activity is found only in the bile duct epithelia.[101] Similarly, at birth,

Figure 4. Immunohistochemical localization of argininosuccinate synthase (A), arginase (B), and glutamine synthetase (C) in the liver lobule. (D) Light microscopy of (C). The figures were kindly provided by Prof. T. Saheki[104] (A, B) and Dr. Gebhardt[55] (C, D).

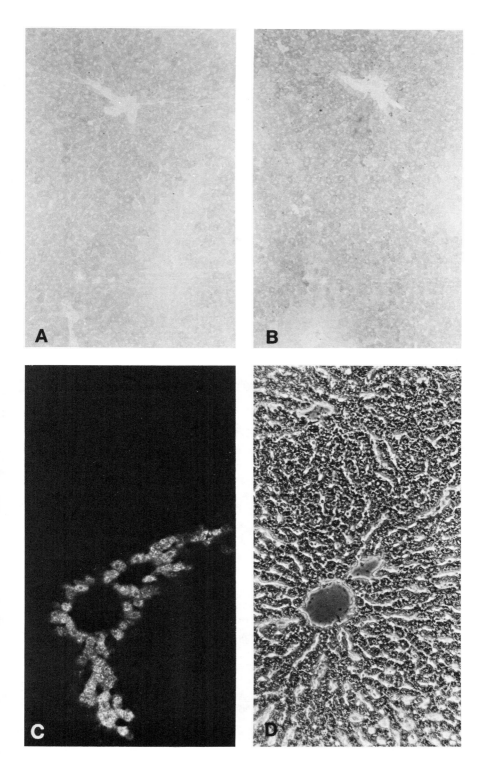

ornithine carbamoyltransferase in mouse liver is evenly distributed in the acinus. However, 4 days later, there is a slightly uneven distribution of this enzyme reaching the predominant periportal localization within 10–12 days, as is observed in the adult animal.[105] Such developmental changes in zonal hepatocyte heterogeneity have been attributed to changes of the nutritional state and to different alterations of the microenvironment of the hepatocytes, depending on their localization in the liver acinus, as a consequence of the marked changes of hepatic blood circulation at birth. In addition, there are also species differences. Whereas in spiny mouse liver at birth carbamoyl phosphate synthetase and glutamine synthetase exhibit the adult type of enzyme distribution, in the newborn rat liver only glutamine synthetase shows the adult localization, while carbamoyl phosphate synthetase is found throughout the acinus.[128]

4.2.2. Nutrition and Hormones

Starvation increases alanine aminotransferase activity in the liver about 3- to 4-fold, not only in the periportal area, but also, and even more markedly, in the perivenous hepatocytes.[98] With respect to liver function, such changes are in agreement with an enlargement of the gluconeogenic zone under these conditions.[106]

Hydrocortisone causes an approximate 6-fold increase of tyrosine aminotransferase activity within a few hours in perivenous hepatocytes, but only a 4-fold increase in periportal hepatocytes.[98] Induction of this enzyme by glucagon depends greatly on oxygen supply, indicating also a modulating effect of different physiological oxygen tensions on the dynamics of hepatocyte heterogeneity in amino acid metabolism.[107] There are also diurnal rhythms that influence enzyme gradients along the acinus. In the rat, tyrosine aminotransferase activity in the periportal zone was twice as high at 5:00 P.M. as at 9:00 A.M., whereas the activity of this enzyme in perivenous hepatocytes was almost unchanged.[98]

The exclusive immunohistochemical localization of glutamine synthetase in a small number of hepatocytes surrounding the terminal hepatic venule *in situ* is also maintained during isolation of parenchymal cells and persists in cultured cells for at least 3 days.[95] Even induction of glutamine synthetase in cultured hepatocytes by addition of dexamethasone and growth hormone[108] did not change the number of glutamine-synthetase-containing cells. Therefore, in contrast to other enzymes in amino acid metabolism, the stability of glutamine synthetase distribution in the acinus may reflect a phenotypic difference between two distinct subpopulations of liver parenchymal cells, rather than an adaptational response to different environmental conditions.[95]

4.2.3. Carbon Tetrachloride Intoxication

Hepatocyte heterogeneity in oxygen supply, glutathione content, and activities of microsomal monooxygenases and glutathione peroxidase is taken as an explanation of the development of perivenous liver cell necrosis in the presence of various drugs, such as CCl_4 (for a review, see Jungermann and Katz[93]). Perivenous liver cell necrosis after CCl_4 pretreatment of the rat is followed by a decreased rate of hepatic ammonia removal (Fig. 5). This decrease is due to an almost complete loss of hepatic glutamine synthesis, whereas urea synthesis is not affected (Fig. 5). The different response to CCl_4-induced perivenous hepatocyte damage of the two hepatic mechanisms for ammonia detoxification reflects the periportal and perivenous localization of urea synthesis and glutamine synthesis, respectively, in the liver lobule.[109] Similarly, the predominant peri-

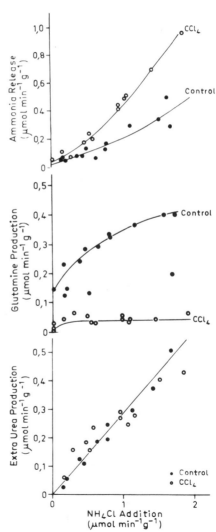

Figure 5. Effect of CCl_4-induced perivenous liver cell necrosis on ammonia detoxification and glutamine and urea production from added NH_4Cl. A portal ammonia addition of 1 μmole/g per min corresponds to a physiological portal ammonia concentration of about 0.25 mM. From Häussinger and Gerok.[109]

venous localization of the glutamate transport system in the plasma membrane explains the marked inhibition of $^{14}CO_2$ production from portal $[1-^{14}C]$glutamate after CCl_4 treatment.[54] On the other hand, $^{14}CO_2$ production from $[1-^{14}C]$proline is affected only slightly under these conditions as a consequence of a predominant periportal uptake and metabolism of proline.[54] Conversely, in the presence of periportal necrosis induced by allylformate, the activity of urea-cycle enzymes was decreased by about 50%, whereas glutamine synthetase activity was almost unaffected.[108]

Microdissection studies showed that glutamate dehydrogenase activity in the periportal area was not influenced by CCl_4 treatment of the rat, whereas the activity of this enzyme was decreased by about 70–80% in the perivenous hepatocytes.[99] Similar findings were also obtained for alanine aminotransferase.[99]

These data show that different drugs may influence hepatic amino acid and ammonia metabolism in different ways as a consequence of zonal toxicity.

4.3. Functional Significance of Zonal Hepatocyte Heterogeneity in Amino Acid and Ammonia Metabolism

Histochemical and microdissection studies of the zonal distribution of enzymes imply severe structural and metabolic disturbances of the liver and give no information on the actual metabolic fluxes at different subacinar compartments. Therefore, methods for investigation of zonal hepatocyte heterogeneity in the metabolically and structurally intact liver have been developed. They include the use of micro-light guides and microoxygen electrodes for measuring fluorescence and oxygen tension in different zones of the liver lobule[111,112] and direct measurements of metabolic flux rates in isolated, perfused liver employing antegrade (portal to hepatic vein) and retrograde (hepatic to portal vein) perfusion techniques.[94] The latter method has been used to study amino acid and ammonia metabolism in rat liver. The underlying idea is as follows: If two metabolic pathways are competing for the same substrate and are present at different activities in different subacinar zones, under conditions of a rate-limiting substrate supply, one of these pathways will be favored against the other, depending on the direction of perfusion (Fig. 6). These studies on the metabolically and structurally intact perfused rat liver demonstrated the predominant periportal localization of urea synthesis, glutaminase activity, proline metabolism, and ammonia production from endogenous proteins and the perivenous localization of glutamine synthetase and the glutamate transport system in the plasma membrane.[54,94]

4.3.1. Zonal Flux Differences in Ammonia Metabolism and Urea and Glutamine Formation

In isolated, perfused rat liver, added ammonium ions are converted mainly to urea during physiological antegrade perfusion, but are preferentially utilized

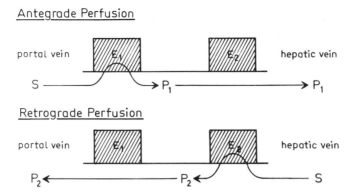

Figure 6. Effect of perfusion direction on the contribution of two differently localized metabolic pathways (E_1, E_2) in converting a common substrate (S) to the respective products (P_1, P_2) under conditions of a limiting substrate supply. Urea and glutamine synthesis from ammonium ions are such competing pathways.

for glutamine synthesis during retrograde perfusion (Fig. 7). This effect of perfusion direction on the rates of urea and glutamine synthesis is not observed after inhibition of one of these pathways or after addition of excess ammonia, i.e., conditions under which the competition between both pathways is abolished.[94] The data in Fig. 7 indicate the periportal and perivenous localization of urea and glutamine synthesis in the liver lobule. If ammonia, urea, and glutamine are formed during the catabolism of endogenous hepatic amino acids or proteins, the liver releases large amounts of glutamine and small amounts of ammonia during antegrade perfusion (Table II). Conversely, during retrograde perfusion,

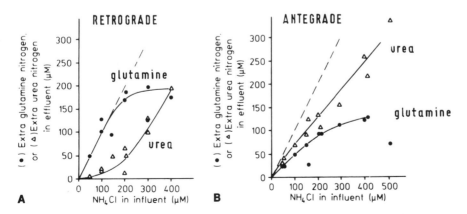

Figure 7. Effect of perfusion direction on urea and glutamine synthesis from added ammonium ions in isolated, perfused rat liver. (A) Retrograde perfusion; (B) antegrade perfusion. (— — — —) Theoretical curve for complete conversion of added ammonia to urea or glutamine. From Häussinger.[94]

Table II.   Effect of Direction of Perfusion Flow on Glutamine, Ammonia, and Urea Production from Endogenous Substrates by Perfused Rat Liver in the Absence and in the Presence of Methionine Sulfoximine, an Inhibitor of Glutamine Synthetase[a]

	Glutamine release	Ammonia release	Urea release
Condition		(nmoles/g per min)	
Control			
Antegrade	152 ± 15 (8)	18 ± 2(9)	99 ± 9 (8)
Retrograde	54 ± 8 (12)	124 ± 15 (7)	91 ± 11 (7)
Methionine sulfoximine			
Antegrade	15 ± 4 (5)	164 ± 16 (5)	171 ± 13 (5)
Retrograde	12 ± 3 (6)	190 ± 17 (6)	168 ± 10 (6)

[a] From Häussinger.[94] The perfusion direction had no effect on glutamate release by the liver. (N) Number of experiments.

ammonia release is high at the expense of glutamine production. After inhibition of glutamine synthetase by methionine sulfoximine,[126] hepatic ammonia release is high regardless of the direction of perfusion (Table II). This shows that the liver produces and releases ammonia during the catabolism of endogenous substrates from the periportal area of the liver lobule, in agreement with the histochemical localization of various amino-acid-catabolizing enzymes. However, in physiological antegrade perfusions, ammonium ions are again taken up by perivenous hepatocytes and are utilized for glutamine synthesis. They are washed out during inhibition of glutamine synthetase by methionine sulfoximine or during retrograde perfusion, when the perfusate first passes perivenous glutamine-synthesizing hepatocytes before periportal ammonia-producing hepatocytes. This shows a metabolic interaction of hepatocytes from different subacinar zones with a continuous periportal ammonia release of about 120–200 nmoles/g per min and a perivenous ammonia uptake at a similar rate. Under these conditions, periportal ammonia production requires glutamate dehydrogenase to operate in the direction of ammonia formation and NADPH production.[25] Simultaneously, perivenous glutamine synthesis from periportally released ammonia implies an increased glutamate formation and NADPH utilization at glutamate dehydrogenase. These postulated different directions of flux point to converse roles of glutamate dehydrogenase in the sublobular periportal and perivenous compartments during nitrogen metabolism from endogenous substrates.

Recent studies have shown that glutamate is simultaneously released and taken up by perfused rat liver.[54,120] Hepatic glutamate uptake occurs predominantly in the perivenous hepatocytes; and there is evidence for a simultaneous glutamate release from periportal hepatocytes.[120]

Ammonia elimination by urea synthesis is restricted to ammonia concentrations above 50 μM.[94] This is also shown by a comparatively high rate of ammonia release of about 160–200 nmoles/g per min by perfused rat liver during inhibition of glutamine synthetase, while urea synthesis is unaffected under these conditions (Table II).

On the other hand, with glutamine synthetase active, hepatic ammonia release is only 18 nmoles/g per min. Also, when ammonium ions are added to the portal perfusate at a physiological concentration of 0.2–0.3 mM, a marked ammonia extraction is observed only with glutamine synthetase active.[94] This indicates that glutamine synthesis, but not urea synthesis, removes ammonia at concentrations below 50 μM. This important difference between the two ammonia-utilizing pathways is explained by the different $K_m(NH_4^+)$ values of isolated rat liver carbamoylphosphate synthetase I and glutamine synthetase of 1–2 mM[69] and 0.3 mM,[89] respectively. In the isolated perfused rat liver, the $K_{0.5}(NH_4^+)$ for glutamine synthesis (measured during retrograde perfusion) and urea synthesis (measured during antegrade perfusion) was 0.1 mM and 0.6 mM,[22] respectively. Therefore, the zonal distribution of urea and glutamine synthesis represents the sequence of a high-K_m system and low-K_m system with respect to ammonia elimination. Urea synthesis will remove the bulk of ammonia in the periportal zone, whereas perivenous glutamine synthetase will extract the remaining low concentrations of ammonia that were not available for urea synthesis. Thus, glutamine synthetase has a scavenger role for ammonium ions before the bloodstream enters the systemic circulation. Such a mechanism should guarantee an efficient hepatic ammonium elimination. The relative rates of ammonium ion detoxication in the periportal and perivenous zones by urea and glutamine synthesis, respectively, are given in Fig. 7.

Label dilution experiments showed that endogenously synthesized glutamine was only available for glutaminase reaction, when the livers were perfused in the retrograde direction and demonstrated the periportal localization of glutaminase activity in the liver acinus.[91] A different subacinar localization of glutaminase and glutamine synthetase has also been suggested by the finding that labeled glutamate derived from added 1-^{14}C-glutamine was not utilized as substrate for glutamine synthesis.[24]

Whereas glutaminase and glutamine synthetase are heterogeneously distributed in the liver acinus, glutamine transaminase reaction was shown to occur as well in the periportal as well in the perivenous compartment.[127] Thus, endogenously synthesized glutamine may not exclusively be destined for export. However, in view of the low physiological concentrations of ketoacid acceptors, flux through glutamine transaminases is considered to be negligible compared to flux through glutaminase.

4.3.2. Intercellular Glutamine Cycle

Studies in the isolated, perfused rat liver during retro- and antegrade perfusions have demonstrated that glutaminase is located in the periportal zone.[91] Periportal glutaminase and perivenous glutamine synthetase are simultaneously active in liver,[23,24,91] resulting in an energy-consuming intercellular (as opposed to intracellular) cycling of glutamine with periportal glutamine uptake and perivenous glutamine resynthesis and release.[94] Energy requirements of this glutamine cycle have been shown in the isolated perfused rat liver by an increased extra oxygen uptake that could not be accounted for by energy requirements of urea synthesis.[23] In the presence of physiological portal glutamine concentrations, the rate of this intercellular glutamine cycle is in the range of about 0.1 μmole/g per min, and its flux is under the control of portal glutamine and ammonia concentrations, of hormones such as glucagon and phenylephrine, and of pH (for a review, see Sies and Häussinger[25]) (Table III and Fig. 8). These effectors of the glutamine cycle influence flux through periportal glutaminase as well through perivenous glutamine synthetase to different extents, resulting in either a net uptake or a net release of glutamine by the liver. The zonal glutamine flux differences in perfused rat liver in the presence of a physiological portal glutamine concentration of 0.6 mM[18,21] under the influence of the aforementioned effectors are given in Table III. The highest rates of this cycle are observed at physiological pH in the presence of ammonium ions, i.e., conditions of increased rates of urea synthesis.

The restriction of glutamine synthetase to a small population of perivenous hepatocytes implies that the glutamine transport system in these hepatocytes must bring about glutamine export, whereas it should mediate net glutamine input in the periportal zone. Periportal glutamine uptake as well as perivenous glutamine release are sodium-dependent and are inhibited by histidine at near-physiological concentrations.[113] Studies on the glutamine content of perfused rat liver[113] in the absence and in the presence of methionine sulfoximine, an inhibitor of glutamine synthetase, have shown that the glutamine content is about 17 μmoles/g dry weight in the perivenous glutamine synthetase containing hepatocytes, even when no glutamine was added to the perfusion medium. This value was about twice the average liver glutamine content in the presence of physiological portal glutamine and ammonia concentrations.[113] These observations suggest that the opposite net glutamine movements across the plasma membrane of periportal and perivenous hepatocytes are probably due to different glutamine concentration gradients across the plasma membrane at the respective subacinar locations. However, the existence of two different glutamine transport systems in the plasma membrane, being heterogeneously distributed in the acinus, cannot be excluded. In addition, evidence has been provided that not only periportal glutamine import is rate-controlling for its metabolism, but that also a control of glutamine synthetase flux by glutamine export must be considered[25,113] as a consequence of product inhibition of this enzyme.[89]

4.3.3. Role of the Intercellular Glutamine Cycle during Ureagenesis from Portal Ammonia

Because periportal urea synthesis ("low affinity system") and perivenous glutamine synthesis ("high affinity system") are two sequential pathways of

Table III. Effect of Ammonium Ions, Glucagon, and Phenylephrine on Simultaneous Periportal Glutamine Degradation (Glutaminase Flux) and Perivenous Glutamine Synthesis (Glutamine Synthetase Flux) in Perfused Rat Liver in the Presence of a Physiological Portal Glutamine Concentration (0.6 mM)[a]

Additions	Periportal glutaminase flux	Perivenous glutamine synthetase flux	Glutamine cycle	Net glutamine release (+) or uptake (−)	Number of perfusion experiments
			(nmoles/g per min)		
None	67 ± 3	148 ± 10	67 ± 3	+81 ± 11	15
NH₄Cl (0.6 mM)	168 ± 9	248 ± 12	168 ± 9	+80 ± 8	7
Glucagon (10⁻⁷ M)	231 ± 32	84 ± 20	84 ± 20	−147 ± 30	7
Phenylephrine (5 µM)	88 ± 4	113 ± 9	88 ± 4	+25 ± 8	6
NH₄Cl + phenylephrine	299 ± 7	83 ± 5	83 ± 5	−216 ± 15	4
NH₄Cl + glucagon	379 ± 36	122 ± 27	122 ± 27	−254 ± 33	5
Phenylephrine + glucagon	152 ± 15	64 ± 13	64 ± 13	−88 ± 22	4

[a] The rate of glutamine cycling corresponds to the flux through the enzyme with the lower flux. Values are means ± S.E.M. and are from Häussinger et al.[24] and Häussinger and Sies.[91]

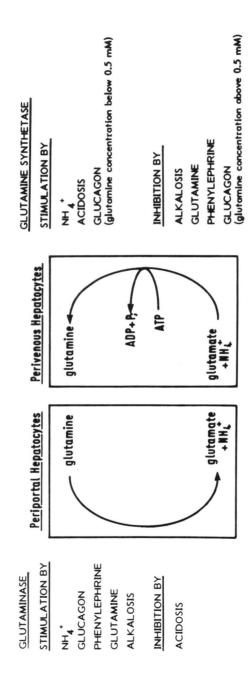

Figure 8. Regulation of glutaminase and glutamine synthetase flux in perfused rat liver. Glutaminase and glutamine synthetase are simultaneously active, but are differently localized in the liver lobule, resulting in an intercellular (as opposed to intracellular) glutamine cycle. The "intercellular cycle" is defined as a sequence of metabolic reactions in an organ that lead to the regeneration of an initial substrate, whereby the metabolic steps are heterogeneously distributed among two or more parenchymal cell populations in this organ. Compared to intracellular cycles, the pool of products formed in a given reaction of an intercellular cycle need not necessarily be identical with the substrate pool for the following reaction.

ammonia detoxification in the liver and only the latter removes ammonium ions at low concentrations, hepatic ammonia removal could cause a net glutamine production (see Fig. 7B) that is normally not observed under physiological conditions. However, in the presence of physiological portal glutamine concentrations of about 0.6 mM, periportal urea synthesis is increased by additional glutamate plus ammonia supply derived from glutamine by the action of periportal glutaminase, a mitochondrial enzyme like carbamoylphosphate synthetase I.[69] This is shown by the data in Table IV. Urea production from portal ammonia at physiological concentrations is increased by about 50% by further addition of glutamine (0.5 mM), whereas there is a slight net glutamine uptake. Since periportal glutaminase flux exceeds by far net glutamine uptake by the liver, glutamine must be resynthesized in perivenous areas. Therefore, the intercellular glutamine cycle provides an effective means for complete conversion of portal ammonia to urea by periportal urea formation from portal ammonia and glutamine and by the perivenous resynthesis of glutamine from ammonia that was not available for urea synthesis. This is schematically depicted in Fig. 9. Such a mechanism is in line with the finding that glutamine cycling increases with increasing portal ammonia concentrations.[24]

4.3.4. Role of the Intercellular Glutamine Cycle in Hepatic pH Regulation

Maintainance of pH homeostasis in higher organisms requires mechanisms for stabilization of the HCO_3^-/CO_2 ratio in blood. The complete oxidation of amino acids and proteins at physiological pH values will yield H_2O, CO_2, HCO_3^-, and NH_4^+. In man, oxidation of a daily ingested 100-g protein meal will produce about 1 mole HCO_3^-, an amount that cannot be disposed of by the kidney in view of a limited urine volume. According to Oliver et al.[114] and Atkinson and Camien,[115] the major pathway for disposal of HCO_3^- is hepatic urea synthesis, consuming stoichiometric amounts of HCO_3^- and NH_4^+:

Table IV. Effect of a Physiological Portal Glutamine Concentration (0.5 mM) on Urea and Net Glutamine Production from Added Ammonium Ions at a Physiological Concentration of 0.3 mM[a]

Condition	Urea production	Net glutamine production	Periportal glutaminase flux
	(μmoles/g per min)		
NH_4Cl	0.65 ± 0.01	0.30 ± 0.01	—
NH_4Cl + glutamine	0.97 ± 0.01	-0.07 ± 0.01	0.21 ± 0.01

[a] Influent perfusate contained NH_4Cl (0.3 mM) and glucagon (50 nM). At 40 min of perfusion, [1-^{14}C]glutamine (0.5 mM) was further added to influent perfusate. Glutaminase flux was determined according to Häussinger et al.[24] as [14]CO_2 production from [1-^{14}C]glutamine. Net glutamine production is negative when glutamine is net taken up.

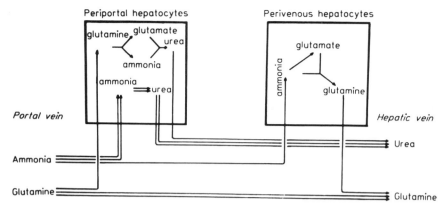

Figure 9. Role of the intercellular glutamine cycle during ureogenesis from portal ammonia. The periportal glutaminase reaction feeds additional substrate into the urea cycle, whereas glutamine is resynthesized in the perivenous area from ammonia that was not available for periportal urea synthesis. Without intercellular glutamine cycling, i.e., in the absence of portal glutamine, ammonia detoxification would imply a considerable net glutamine production by the liver. From Häussinger.[94]

$$HCO_3^- + 2\ NH_4^+ \rightarrow H_2NCONH_2 + H^+ + 2\ H_2O$$

$$HCO_3^- + H^+ \rightleftharpoons H_2O + CO_2$$

$$\overline{2\ HCO_3^- + 2\ NH_4^+ \rightarrow H_2NCONH_2 + CO_2 + 3\ H_2O}$$

In contrast to urea synthesis, elimination of ammonium ions by glutamine synthesis does not remove HCO_3^-, and ammonium ions may then be excreted as such after glutamine hydrolysis in the kidney. Therefore, to maintain pH balance, the fixation of NH_4^+ by synthesis of either urea or glutamine must be regulated, because the route of hepatic NH_4^+ removal determines the rate of HCO_3^- disposal (Fig. 10). As shown in the preceding section, the intercellular glutamine cycle provides an effective means for almost complete conversion of portal NH_4^+ to urea, although urea synthesis is restricted to NH_4^+ concentrations above 50 μM. Complete conversion of portal NH_4^+ to urea without an accompanying net glutamine production, however, represents a situation that obtains at physiological pH values. During acidosis, there is a decreased rate of periportal urea synthesis and an increased rate of perivenous glutamine formation (Fig. 11). Such a mechanism should favor pH homeostasis by decreasing HCO_3^- removal by urea synthesis, whereas efficient NH_4^+ detoxification is maintained by increased net glutamine synthesis. This is in agreement with the *in vivo* finding of an increased urinary NH_4^+ excretion accompanied by a decreased urinary urea excretion during acidosis.[41] Conversely, during alkalosis, HCO_3^- removal by urea synthesis is increased, and there is even net glutamine uptake by the liver, providing additional substrate for urea synthesis. This shift from NH_4^+ removal by urea synthesis

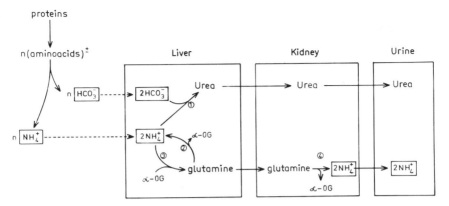

Figure 10. Relationships between ammonia and bicarbonate metabolism. Complete oxidation of proteins yields HCO_3^- and NH_4^+ in almost stoichiometric amounts. Whereas urea synthesis consumes HCO_3^-, glutamine synthesis and subsequent excretion of NH_4^+ as such does not. Thus, the route of hepatic NH_4^+ detoxication will determine the rate of HCO_3^- removal. In acidosis, flux through the pathways 1 (ureogenesis) and 2 (hepatic glutaminase) is decreased, whereas flux through the pathways 3 (hepatic glutamine synthesis) and 4 (renal glutaminase) is increased. Therefore HCO_3^- is spared in acidosis, when NH_4^+ are excreted as such into urine at the expense of urea. Other sites of increased glutamine formation from NH_4^+ in acidosis, such as muscle, are not included in the scheme. (α-OG; α-oxoglutarate)

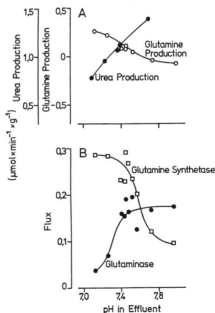

Figure 11. Effect of perfusate pH on urea and net glutamine production (A) and on periportal glutaminase and perivenous glutamine synthetase flux (B) in isolated perfused rat liver. Livers were perfused with NH_4Cl (0.6 mM) and glutamine (0.6 mM) in influent perfusate. During acidosis, bicarbonate removal by urea synthesis is decreased primarily as a consequence of a decreased glutaminase flux. Conversely, bicarbonate removal by urea synthesis is increased during alkalosis when glutaminase flux is increased, providing additional substrate for urea synthesis. From Häussinger et al.[116]

to net glutamine synthesis during acidosis and vice versa during alkalosis is performed by the regulation of the intercellular glutamine cycle.[25] During acidosis, there is a strong inhibition of periportal glutaminase flux, whereas perivenous glutamine synthetase flux is increased (Fig. 10). Conversely, during alkalosis, glutaminase flux is increased and glutamine synthetase flux is decreased. This shows that the pH-induced changes in urea formation are[116] due predominantly to activity changes of periportal glutaminase, which provides additional substrate for urea synthesis by glutamine degradation. Inhibition of glutaminase during acidosis[24,117,118] is due to an increased $K_a(NH_4^+)$ for glutaminase.[119] The role of perivenous glutamine synthetase may be seen in the removal of ammonium ions not available for urea synthesis.

In addition, acid–base control of urea cycle flux is also exerted by the rate of portal CO_2 and HCO_3^- supply and the carbonic anhydrase dependent HCO_3^- provision for mitochondrial carbamoylphosphate synthetase, whereas there seems to be no control at the level of the 5 urea cycle enzymes.[124] Because urea and glutamine synthesis represent 2 sequent pathways, acid base control of urea cycle flux will determine the ammonium supply for perivenous, glutamine-synthesizing hepatocytes and thereby regulate hepatic glutamine synthesis.

These data point to an important role of the liver in maintaining pH homeostasis by regulating the rate of HCO_3^- removal during ammonium detoxication by either urea or glutamine synthesis.

The role of the liver in pH regulation also explains the alkalosis in severe liver disease as a consequence of a decreased rate of HCO_3^- removal by impaired urea synthesis.

5. SUMMARY

Some aspects of amino acid and ammonia metabolism and its regulatory features, presumably in the liver, have been presented at the interorgan and inter- and intracellular levels. Metabolic cycles are involved at each level, as shown by the glucose–alanine cycle (interorgan cycle), the urea cycle (intracellular cycle), and the glutamine cycle between periportal and perivenous hepatocytes (intercellular cycle).

Interorgan amino acid and ammonia fluxes depend on hormonal and nutritional conditions and on the state of organ-specific functions. Alanine and glutamine are the most important nitrogen vehicles in interorgan amino acid metabolism and are the major products of amino acid metabolism in skeletal muscle. The intestine releases alanine, too, but utilizes glutamine as a respiratory fuel. Alanine serves as an important precursor of hepatic gluconeogenesis. Apart from branched-chain amino acids, which are metabolized predominantly by skeletal muscle, the liver takes up nearly all amino acids and converts their nitrogen, as well as ammonia released from the intestine, kidney, or muscle, to urea.

Hepatic amino acid metabolism is controlled by portal substrate supply, the activity of amino acid carriers in the plasma membrane of hepatocytes, and the activity of amino-acid-metabolizing enzymes. Each site is of different regulatory importance for the metabolism of the individual amino acid and is influenced by hormones and the nutritional state. These factors also affect hepatic urea synthesis, which is governed by ammonia supply, the intracellular concentrations of urea-cycle intermediates, and the activity of carbamoylphosphate synthetase.

Zonal hepatocyte heterogeneity in amino acid and ammonia metabolism is a dynamic process with respect to developmental, hormonal, and nutritional influences. The different localization of metabolic pathways in the liver lobule provides the basis for metabolic interactions of different hepatocyte populations in amino acid and ammonia metabolism. It also offers additional regulatory sites for maintenance of amino acid and ammonia homeostasis and, possibly more important, for systemic pH regulation by the liver.

REFERENCES

1. Schimassek, H., and Gerok, W., 1965, Control of the levels of free amino acids in plasma by the liver, *Biochem. Z.* **343**:407–415.
2. Ishikawa, E., 1975, The regulation of uptake and output of amino acids by rat tissues, *Adv. Enzyme Regul.* **14**:117–136.
3. Krebs, H. A., and Lund, P., 1977, Aspects of the regulation of the metabolism of branched chain amino acids, *Adv. Enzyme Regul.* **15**:375–394.
4. Felig, P., 1975, Amino acid metabolism in man, *Annu. Rev. Biochem.* **44**:933–955.
5. Cahill, G. F., Aoki, T. T., and Smith, R. J., 1981, Amino acid cycles in man, *Curr. Topics Cell. Regul.* **18**:389–399.
6. Christensen, H. N., 1982, Interorgan amino acid nutrition, *Physiol. Rev.* **62**:1193–1233.
7. Felig, P., and Wahren, J., 1971, Amino acid metabolism in exercising man, *J. Clin. Invest.* **50**:2703–2714.
8. Odessy, R., Khairalla, E., and Goldberg, A. L., 1975, Origin and possible significance of alanine production by skeletal muscle, *J. Biol. Chem.* **249**:7623–7629.
9. Windmueller, H. G., and Spaeth, A. E., 1980, Respiratory fuels and nitrogen metabolism *in vivo* in small intestine of fed rats: Quantitative importance of glutamine, glutamate and aspartate, *J. Biol. Chem.* **255**:107–112.
10. Windmueller, H. G., 1984, Metabolism of vascular and luminal glutamine by intestinal mucosa *in vivo*, in: *Glutamine Metabolism in Mammalian Tissues* (D. Häussinger and H. Sies, eds.), pp. 61–77, Springer-Verlag, Heidelberg.
11. Mallette, L. E., Exton, J. H., and Park, C. R., 1969, Control of gluconeogenesis from amino acids in the perfused rat liver, *J. Biol. Chem.* **244**:5713–5723.
12. Ross, B. D., Hems, R., and Krebs, H. A., 1967, The role of gluconeogenesis from various percursors in the perfused rat liver, *Biochem J.* **102**:942–951.
13. Felig, P., Wahren, J., and Räf, L., 1973, Evidence of inter-organ amino acid transport by blood cells in humans, *Proc. Natl. Acad. Sci. U.S.A.* **70**:1775–1779.
14. Tizianello, A., De Ferrari, G., Garibotto, G., Gurreri, G., and Robaudo, C., 1980, Renal metabolism of amino acids and ammonia in subjects with normal renal function and in patients with chronic renal insufficiency, *J. Clin. Invest.* **65**:1162–1173.

15. Schröck, H., and Goldstein, L., 1981, Interorgan relationships for glutamine metabolism in normal and acidotic rats, *Am. J. Physiol.* **240:**E519–E525.

16. Van Slyke, D. D., Phillips, R. A., Hamilton, P. B., Archibald, R. M., Futcher, P. H., and Hiller, A., 1943, Glutamine as a source material of urinary ammonia, *J. Biol. Chem.* **150:**481–482.

17. Marliss, E. B., Aoki, T. T., Pozefsky, T., Most, A. S., and Cahill, G. F., 1971, Muscle and splanchnic glutamine and glutamate metabolism in postabsorptive and starved man, *J. Clin. Invest.* **50:**814–817.

18. Lund, P., and Watford, M., 1976, Glutamine as a precursor of urea, in: *The Urea Cycle* (S. Grisolia, R. Baguena, and F. Mayor, eds.), pp. 479–488, Wiley, New York and London.

19. Aikawa, T., Matsutaka, H., Yamamoto, H., Okuda, T., Ishikawa, E., Kawano, T., and Matsumura, E., 1973, Gluconeogenesis and amino acid metabolism: Inter-organal relations and roles of glutamine and alanine in the amino acid metabolism in the fasted rat, *Biochem. J.* **74:**1003–1017.

20. Rémésy, C., Demigné, E., and Aufrère, J., 1978, Interorgan relationships between glucose, lactate and amino acids in rats fed on high-carbohydrate or high-protein diets, *Biochem. J.* **170:**321–329.

21. Yamamoto, H., Aikawa, T., Matsutaka, H., Okuda, T., and Ishikawa, E., 1974, Interorganal relationships of amino acid metabolism in fed rats, *Am. J. Physiol.* **226:**1428–1433.

22. Häussinger, D., Weiss, L., and Sies, H., 1975, Activation of pyruvate dehydrogenase during metabolism of ammonium ions in hemoglobin-free perfused rat liver, *Eur. J. Biochem.* **52:**421–431.

23. Häussinger, D., and Sies, H., 1979, Hepatic glutamine metabolism under the influence of the portal ammonia concentration in the perfused rat liver, *Eur. J. Biochem.* **101:**179–184.

24. Häussinger, D., Gerok, W., and Sies, H., 1983, Regulation of flux through glutaminase and glutamine synthetase in isolated perfused rat liver. *Biochim. Biophys. Acta* **755:**272–278.

25. Sies, H., and Häussinger, D., 1984, Hepatic glutamine and ammonia metabolism: Nitrogen and redox balance and the intercellular glutamine cycle, in *Glutamine Metabolism in Mammalian Tissues* (D. Häussinger and H. Sies, eds.), pp. 78–97, Springer-Verlag, Heidelberg.

26. Felig, P., Wahren, J., and Ahlborg, G., 1973, Uptake of individual amino acids by the human brain, *Proc. Soc. Exp. Biol. Med.* **142:**230–231.

27. Ahlborg, G., Felig, P., Hagenfeldt, L., Hendler, R., and Wahren, J., 1974, Substrate turnover during prolonged exercise in man: Splanchnic and leg metabolism of glucose, free fatty acids, and amino acids, *J. Clin. Invest.* **53:**1080–1090.

28. Pozefsky, T., Felig, P., Tobin, J., Soeldner, J. S., and Cahill, G. F., 1969, Amino acid balance across the tissues of the forearm in postabsorptive man: Effects of insulin at two dose levels, *J. Clin. Invest.* **48:**2273–2282.

29. Livesey, G., and Lund, P., 1980, Enzymic determination of branched chain amino acids and oxoacids in rat tissues: Transfer of oxoacids from skeletal muscle to liver *in vivo, Biochem. J.* **188:**705–713.

30. Gerok, W., and Häussinger, D., 1984, Ammonia detoxication and glutamine metabolism in severe liver disease and its role in the pathogenesis of hepatic encephalopathy, in: *Glutamine Metabolism in Mammalian Tissues* (D. Häussinger and H. Sies, eds.), pp. 257–277, Springer-Verlag, Heidelberg.

31. Weber, F. L., and Veach, G. L., 1979, The importance of the small intestine in gut ammonia production in the fasting dog, *Gastroenterology* **77:**235–240.

32. Walser, M., and Bodenlos, L. J., 1959, Urea metabolism in man, *J. Clin. Invest.* **38:**1617–1626.

33. Baertl, J. M., Sancetta, S. M., and Gabuzda, G. J., 1963, Relation of acute potassium depletion to renal ammonium metabolism in patients with cirrhosis, *J. Clin. Invest.* **42:**696–706.

34. Welbourne, T., 1975, Mechanism of renal ammonia production adaptation to chronic acidosis, *Med. Clin. North Am.* **59:**629–648.

35. Ganda, O. P., and Ruderman, N. B., 1976, Muscle nitrogen metabolism in chronic hepatic insufficiency, *Metabolism* **25:**427–435.

36. Lockwood, A. H., McDonald, J. M., Reiman, R. E., Gelbard, A. S., Laughlin, J. S., Duffy, T. E., and Plum, F., 1979, The dynamics of ammonia metabolism in man: Effects of liver disease and hyperammonemia, *J. Clin. Invest.* **63:**449–460.

37. Lowenstein, J. M., 1972, Ammonia production in muscle and other tissues: The purine nucleotide cycle, *Physiol. Rev.* **52:**382–414.

38. Dawson, A. M., 1978, Regulation of blood ammonia, *Gut* **19:**504–509.

39. Deferrari, G., Garibotto, G., Robaudo, C., Ghiggeri, G. M., and Tizianello, A., 1981, Brain metabolism of amino acids and ammonia in patients with chronic renal insufficiency, *Kidney Int.* **20:**505–510.

40. Krebs, H. A., Hems, R., Lund, P., Halliday, D., and Read, W. W. C., 1978, Sources of ammonia for mammalian urea synthesis, *Biochem. J.* **176:**733–737.

41. Fine, A., Carlyle, E., and Bourke, E., 1975, Adaptations in nitrogen metabolism in acidosis in man, *Kidney Int.* **8:**338–339.

42. Rudman, D., DiFulco, T. J., Galambos, J. T., Smith, R. B., Salam, A. A., and Warren, D. W., 1973, Maximal rates of excretion and synthesis of urea in normal and cirrhotic subjects, *J. Clin. Invest.* **52:**2241–2249.

43. Duda, G. D., and Handler, P., 1958, Kinetics of ammonia metabolism *in vivo, J. Biol. Chem.* **232:**303–314.

44. Guidotto, G. G., Borghetti, A. F., and Gazzola, G. C., 1978, The regulation of amino acid transport in animal cells, *Biochim. Biophys. Acta* **515:**329–366.

45. Shotwell, M. A., Kilberg, M. S., and Oxender, D. L., 1983, The regulation of neutral amino acid transport in mammalian cells, *Biochim. Biophys. Acta* **737:**267–284.

46. Sips, H. J., Groen, A. K., and Tager, J. M., 1980, Plasma membrane transport of alanine is rate-limiting for its metabolism in rat liver parenchymal cells, *FEBS Lett.* **119:**271–274.

47. Fafournoux, P., Rémésy, C., and Demigné, C., 1983, Control of alanine metabolism in rat liver by transport processes or cellular metabolism, *Biochem. J.* **210:**645–652.

48. Sips, H. J., Van Amelsvoort, M. M., and Van Dam, K., 1980, Amino acid transport in plasma-membrane vesicles from rat liver, *Eur. J. Biochem.* **105:**217–224.

49. Bellemann, P., 1981, Amino acid transport and rubidium-ion uptake in monolayer cultures of hepatocytes from neonatal rats, *Biochem. J.* **198:**475–483.

50. Fehlmann, M., and Freychet, P., 1981, Hormonal regulation of amino acid transport in isolated rat hepatocytes: Properties of a high affinity transport component induced by glucagon and cyclic AMP, in: *Advances in Cyclic Nucleotide Research* (J. E. Dumont, P. Greengard, and G. A. Robinson, eds.), Vol. 14, pp. 521–527, Raven Press, New York.

51. Kilberg, S. M., Handlogten, M. E., and Christensen, H. N., 1980, Characteristics of an amino acid transport system in rat liver for glutamine, asparagine, histidine and closely related analogs, *J. Biol. Chem.* **255:**4011–4019.

52. Hayes, M. R., and McGivan, J. D., 1982, Differential effects of starvation on alanine and glutamine transport in isolated rat hepatocytes, *Biochem. J.* **204:**365–368.

53. Sips, H. J., DeGraaf, P. A., and Van Dam, K., 1982, Transport of L-aspartate and L-glutamate in plasma-membrane vesicles from rat liver, *Eur. J. Biochem.* **122:**259–264.

54. Häussinger, D., and Gerok, W., 1983, Hepatocyte heterogeneity in glutamate uptake by isolated perfused rat liver, *Eur. J. Biochem.* **136:**421–425.

55. Gebhardt, R., and Mecke, D., 1983, Glutamate uptake by cultured rat hepatocytes is mediated by hormonally inducible, sodium-dependent transport systems, *FEBS Lett.* **161:**275–278.

56. Hensgens, H. E. S. J., Hensgens, L. A. M., Meijer, A. J., Gimpel, J. A., and Tager, J. M., 1976, Ureogenesis and gluconeogenesis from proline: The respiratory chain as site of metabolic control, in: *Use of Isolated Liver Cells and Kidney Tubules in Metabolic Studies* (J. M. Tager, H. D. Söling, and J. R. Williamson, eds.), pp. 331–338, North-Holland, Amsterdam.

57. Häussinger, D., Gerok, W., and Sies, H., 1982, Inhibition of pyruvate dehydrogenase during the metabolism of glutamine and proline in hemoglobin-free perfused rat liver, *Eur. J. Biochem.* **126:**69–76.

58. Mortimore, G. E., and Pösö, A. R., 1984, Mechanism and control of deprivation-induced protein degradation in liver: Role of glucogenic amino acids, in: *Glutamine Metabolism in Mammalian Tissues* (D. Häussinger and H. Sies, eds.), pp. 138–157, Springer-Verlag, Heidelberg.

59. Jefferson, L. S., and Korner, A., 1969, Influence of amino acid supply on ribosomes and protein synthesis of perfused rat liver, *Biochem. J.* **111**:703–712.

60. McGown, E., Richardson, A. G., Henderson, L. M., and Swan, P. B., 1973, Effect of amino acids on ribosome aggregation and protein synthesis in perfused rat liver, *J. Nutr.* **103**:109–116.

61. Flaim, K. E., Liao, W. S. L., Peavy, D. E., Taylor, J. M., and Jefferson, L. S., 1982, The role of amino acids in the regulation of protein synthesis in perfused rat liver. II. Effects of amino acid deficiency on peptide chain initiation, polysomal aggregation, and distribution of albumin mRNA, *J. Biol. Chem.* **257**:2939–2946.

62. Sies, H., Summer, K. H., Häussinger, D., and Bücher, T., 1976, NADPH utilization in mitochondria: Urea synthesis from ammonia in rat liver cells, in: *Use of Isolated Liver Cells and Kidney Tubules in Metabolic Studies* (J. M. Tager, H. D. Söling, and J. R. Williamson, eds.), pp. 311–316, North-Holland, Amsterdam.

63. Krebs, H. A., Hems, R., and Lund, P., 1972, Some regulatory mechanisms in the synthesis of urea in the mammalian liver, *Adv. Enzyme Regul.* **11**:361–377.

64. Schimke, R. T., 1962, Adaptive characteristics of urea cycle enzymes in the rat, *J. Biol. Chem.* **237**:459–468.

65. Schimke, R. T., 1962, Differential effects of fasting and protein-free diets on levels of urea cycle enzymes in rat liver, *J. Biol. Chem.* **237**:1921–1924.

66. Schimke, R. T., 1963, Studies on factors affecting the levels of urea cycle enzymes in rat liver, *J. Biol. Chem.* **238**:1012–1018.

67. Meijer, A. J., and Hensgens, H. E. S. J., 1982, Ureogenesis, in: *Metabolic Compartmentation* (H. Sies, ed.), pp. 259–286, Academic Press, New York.

68. Saheki, T., and Katunuma, N., 1975, Analysis of regulatory factors for urea synthesis by isolated perfused rat liver. I. Urea synthesis with ammonia and glutamine as nitrogen sources, *J. Biochem.* **77**:659–669.

69. Lusty, C. J., 1978, Carbamoylphosphate synthetase I of rat liver mitochondria, *Eur. J. Biochem.* **85**:373–383.

70. Grisolia, S., and Cohen, P. P., 1953, Catalytic role of glutamate derivatives in citrulline biosynthesis, *J. Biol. Chem.* **204**:753–757.

71. Shigesada, K., and Tatibana, M., 1971, Role of acteylglutamate in ureotelism. II. Occurrence and biosynthesis of acetylglutamate in mouse and rat tissues. *J. Biol. Chem.* **246**:5588–5595.

72. McGivan, J. D., Bradford, N. M., and Mendes-Mourao, J., 1976, The regulation of carbamoylphosphate synthetase activity in rat liver mitochondria, *Biochem. J.* **154**:415–421.

73. Shigesada, K., and Tatibana, M., 1978, *N*-Acetylglutamate synthetase from rat-liver mitochondria, *Eur. J. Biochem.* **84**:285–291.

74. Shigesada, K., Aoyagi, K., and Tatibana, M., 1978, Role of acetylglutamate in ureotelism: Variations in acetylglutamate level and its possible significance in control of urea synthesis in mammalian liver, *Eur. J. Biochem.* **85**:385–391.

75. Hensgens, H. E. S. J., Verhoeven, A. J., and Meijer, A. J., 1980, The relationship between intramitochondrial *N*-acetylglutamate and activity of carbamoyl-phosphate synthetase (ammonia): The effect of glucagon, *Eur. J. Biochem.* **107**: 197–205.

76. Martin-Requero, A., Corkey, B. E., Cerdan, S., Walajitis-Rode, E., Parrilla, R. L., and Williamson, J. R., 1983, Interactions between ketoisovalerate metabolism and the pathways of gluconeogenesis and urea synthesis in isolated hepatocytes, *J. Biol. Chem.* **258**:3673–3681.

77. Powers, S., 1981, Regulation of rat liver carbamoylphosphate synthetase I: Inhibition by metal ions and activation by amino acids and other chelating agents, *J. Biol. Chem.* **256**:11,160–11,165.

78. Guthörlein, G., and Knappe, J., 1969, Structure and function of carbamoylphosphate synthetase: On the mechanism of bicarbonate activation, *Eur. J. Biochem.* **8**:207–214.

79. Chamalaun, R. A. F. M., and Tager, J. M., 1970, Nitrogen metabolism in the perfused rat liver, *Biochim. Biophys. Acta* **222:**119–134.
80. Katunuma, N., Okada, M., and Nishii, Y., 1966, Regulation of the urea cycle and the TCA cycle by ammonia, *Adv. Enzyme Regul.* **4:**317–335.
81. Volpe, P., Sawamura, R., and Strecker, H. J., 1969, Control of ornithine transaminase in rat liver and kidney, *J. Biol. Chem.* **244:**719–726.
82. Bradford, N. M., and McGivan, J. D., 1980, Evidence for the existence of an ornithine/citrulline antiporter in rat liver mitochondria, *FEBS Lett.* **113:**294–298.
83. Elliot, K. R. F., and Tipton, K. F., 1974, Product inhibition studies on bovine liver carbamoylphosphate synthetase, *Biochem. J.* **141:**817–824.
84. Lof, C., Wanders, R. J. A., and Meijer, A. J., 1982, Activity of carbamoyl-phosphate synthetase (ammonia) in isolated rat-liver mitochondria: [Cycling] of carbamoyl-phosphate in the absence of ornithine, *Eur. J. Biochem.* **124:**89–94.
85. Hensgens, H. E. S. J., and Meijer, A. J., 1980, Inhibition of urea-cycle activity by high concentrations of alanine, *Biochem. J.* **186:**1–4.
86. Takada, S., Saheki, T., Igarashi, Y., and Katsunuma, T., 1979, Studies on rat liver argininosuccinate synthetase: Inhibition by various amino acids, *J. Biochem.* **85:**1309–1314.
87. Lund, P., 1971, Control of glutamine synthesis in rat liver, *Biochem. J.* **124:**653–660.
88. Tate, S. S., and Meister, A., 1971, Regulation of rat liver glutamine synthetase: Activation by ketoglutarate and inhibition by glycine, alanine and carbamoylphosphate, *Proc. Natl. Acad. Sci. U.S.A.* **68:**781–785.
89. Deuel, T. F., Louie, M., and Lerner, A., 1978, Glutamine synthetase from rat liver, *J. Biol. Chem.* **253:**6111–6118.
90. Joseph, S. K., Bradford, N. M., and McGivan, J. D., 1979, Inhibition of glutamine synthetase activity by manganous ions in a cytosol extract of rat liver, *Biochem. J.* **184:**477–480.
91. Häussinger, D., and Sies, H., 1984, Effect of phenylephrine on glutamate and glutamine metabolism in isolated perfused rat liver, *Biochem. J.* **221:**651–658.
92. Rappaport, A. M., 1976, The microcirculatory acinar concept of normal and pathological hepatic structure, *Beitr. Pathol.* **157:**215–243.
93. Jungermann, K., and Katz, N., 1982, Metabolic heterogeneity of liver parenchyma, in: *Metabolic Compartmentation* (H. Sies, ed.), pp. 411–435, Academic Press, New York.
94. Häussinger, D., 1983, Hepatocyte heterogeneity in glutamine and ammonia metabolism and the role of an intercellular glutamine cycle during ureogenesis in perfused rat liver, *Eur. J. Biochem.* **133:**269–275.
95. Gebhardt, R., and Mecke, D., 1983, Heterogeneous distribution of glutamine synthetase among rat liver parenchymal cells *in situ* and in primary culture, *EMBO J.* **2:**567–570.
96. Shank, R. E., Morrison, G., Cheng, C. H., Karl, I., and Schwartz, R., 1959, Cell heterogeneity within the hepatic lobule (quantitative histochemistry), *J. Histochem. Cytochem.* **7:**237–239.
97. Guder, W. G., Habicht, A., Kleissl, J., Schmidt, U., and Wieland, O. H., 1975, The diagnostic significance of liver cell inhomogeneity: Serum enzymes in patients with central liver necrosis and the distribution of glutamate dehydrogenase in normal human liver, *Z. Klin. Chem. Klin. Biochem.* **13:**311–318.
98. Welsh, F. A., 1972, Changes in distribution of enzymes within the liver lobule during adaptive increases, *J. Histochem. Cytochem.* **20:**107–111.
99. Morrison, G. R., Brock, F. E., Karl, I., and Shank, R. E., 1965, Quantitative analysis of regenerating and degenerating areas within the lobule of the carbon tetrachloride-injured liver, *Arch. Biochem. Biophys.* **111:**448–464.
100. Wimmer, M., and Pette, D., 1979, Microphotometric studies on intraacinar enzyme distribution in rat liver, *Histochemistry* **64:**23–33.
101. Iannaccone, P. M., and Koizumi, J., 1983, Pattern and rate of disappearance of gamma-glutamyl transpeptidase activity in fetal and neonatal rat liver, *J. Histochem. Cytochem.* **31:**1312–1316.

102. Gaasbeeek Janzen, J. W., Lamers, W. H., Moorman, A. F. M., DeGraaf, A., Los, J. A., and Charles, R., 1984, The localization of carbamoylphosphate synthase in adult rat liver, *Histochem. Cytochem.* **32:**557–564.

103. Mizutani, A., 1968, Cytochemical demonstration of ornithine carbamoyltransferase activity in liver mitochondria of rat and mouse, *J. Histochem. Cytochem.* **16:**172–180.

104. Saheki, T., and Yagi, Y., 1983, Unpublished.

105. Kanamura, S., and Asada-Kubota, M., 1980, The heterogeneity of hepatocytes during the postnatal development of the mouse, *Anat. Embryol.* **158:**151–159.

106. Sasse, S., Katz, N., and Jungermann, K., 1975, Functional heterogeneity of rat liver parenchyma and of isolated hepatocytes, *FEBS Lett.* **57:**83–88.

107. Nauck, M., Wölfle, D., Katz, N., and Jungermann, K., 1981, Modulation of the glucagon-dependent induction of phosphoenolpyruvate carboxykinase and tyrosine aminotransferase by arterial and venous oxygen concentrations in hepatocyte cultures, *Eur. J. Biochem.* **119:**657–661.

108. Gebhardt, R., and Mecke, D., 1984, Cellular distribution and regulation of glutamine synthetase in liver, in: *Glutamine Metabolism in Mammalian Tissues* (D. Häussinger and H. Sies, eds.), pp. 98–121, Springer-Verlag, Heidelberg.

109. Häussinger, D., and Gerok, W., 1984, Hepatocyte heterogeneity in ammonia metabolism: Impairment of glutamine synthesis in CCl_4 induced liver cell necrosis with no effect on urea synthesis. *Chem.-Biol. Interact.* **48:**191–194.

110. Swick, R. W., Tollaksen, S. L., Nance, S. L., and Thomson, J. F., 1970, The unique distribution of ornithine aminotransferase in rat liver mitochondria, *Arch. Biochem. Biophys.* **136:**212–218.

111. Ji, S., Lemasters, J. J., Christenson, V., and Thurman, R. G., 1982, Periportal and pericentral pyridine nucleotide fluorescence from the surface of the perfused liver: Evaluation of the hypothesis that chronic treatment with ethanol produces pericental hypoxia, *Proc. Natl. Acad. Sci. U.S.A.* **79:**5415–5419.

112. Ji, S., Lemasters, J. J., and Thurman, R. G., 1980, A non-invasive method to study metabolic events within sublobular regions of hemoglobin-free perfused liver, *FEBS Lett.* **113:**37–41.

113. Häussinger, D., Soboll, S., Meijer, A. J., Tager, J. M., and Sies, H., 1985, Role of plasma membrane transport in hepatic glutamine metabolism, *Eur. J. Biochem.,* **152:**597–603.

114. Oliver, J., Koelz, A. M., Costello, J., and Bourke, E., 1977, Acid–base induced alterations in glutamine metabolism and ureogenesis in perfused muscle and liver of the rat, *Eur. J. Clin. Invest.* **7:**445–449.

115. Atkinson, D. E., and Camien, M. N., 1982, The role of urea synthesis in the removal of metabolic bicarbonate and the regulation of blood pH, *Curr. Top. Cell. Regul.* **21:**261–302.

116. Häussinger, D., Gerok, W., and Sies, H., 1984, Hepatic role in pH regulation: Role of the intercellular glutamine cycle, *Trends Biochem. Sci.* **9:**300–302.

117. Lueck, J. D., and Miller, L. L., 1970, The effect of perfusate pH on glutamine metabolism in the isolated perfused rat liver, *J. Biol. Chem.* **245:**5491–5497.

118. Häussinger, D., Akerboom, T. P. M., and Sies, H., 1980, The role of pH and the lack of a requirement for hydrogen carbonate in the regulation of hepatic glutamine metabolism, *Hoppe-Seyler's Z. Physiol. Chem.* **361:**995–1001.

119. Verhoeven, A. J., Van Iwaarden, J. F., Joseph, S. K., and Meijer, A. J., 1983, Control of rat liver glutaminase by ammonia and pH, *Eur. J. Biochem.* **133:**241–244.

120. Häussinger, D., and Gerok, W., 1984, Regulation of hepatic glutamate metabolism. Role of 2-oxoacids in glutamate release from isolated perfused rat liver, *Eur. J. Biochem.* **143:**491–497.

121. Meijer, A. J., Lof, C., Ramos, I. C., and Verhoeven, A., 1985, Control of ureogenesis, *Eur. J. Biochem.* **148:**189–196.

122. Cohen, N. S., Kyan, F. S., Kyan, S. S., Cheung, C. W., and Raijman, L., 1985, The apparent K_m of ammonia for carbamoyl phosphate synthetase (ammonia) *in situ*, *Biochem. J.* **229:**205–211.

123. Dodgson, S. J., Forster, R. E., Schwed, D. A., and Storey, B. T., 1983, Contribution of matrix carbonic anhydrase to citrulline synthesis in isolated guinea pig liver mitochondria, *J. Biol. Chem.* **258**:7696–7701.

124. Häussinger, D., and Gerok, W., 1985, Hepatic urea synthesis and pH regulation: role of CO_2, HCO_3^-, pH and the activity of carbonic anhydrase, *Eur. J. Biochem.*, **152**:381–386.

125. Pausch, J., Rasenack, J., Häussinger, D., and Gerok, W., 1985, Hepatic carbamoylphosphate metabolism. Role of cytosolic and mitochondrial carbamoylphosphate in *de novo* pyrimidine synthesis, *Eur. J. Biochem.* **150**:189–194.

126. Meister, A., 1974, Glutamine synthesis in mammals, in: *The Enzymes* (P. D., Boyer, ed.), Vol. 10, pp. 699–754, Academic Press, New York.

127. Häussinger, D., Stehle, T., and Gerok, W., 1985, Glutamine metabolism in isolated perfused rat liver. The transamination pathway, *Biol. Chem. Hoppe-Seyler* **366**:527–536.

128. Gaasbeek Janzen, J. W., Gebhardt, R., te Kortschot, A., ten Vorde, G. H. J., Lamers, W. H., Moorman, A. F. M., and Charles, R., 1985, The distribution of carbamoylphosphate synthetase and glutamine synthetase in perinatal liver, *Abstr. Commun. 13th UIB Congress*, Mo-296.

Chapter 12

Lobular Oxygen Gradients: Possible Role in Alcohol-Induced Hepatotoxicity

Ronald G. Thurman, Sungchul Ji, and John J. Lemasters

1. INTRODUCTION

Alcoholic liver disease is a major health problem, and specific therapies are lacking because we still do not understand how alcohol causes liver damage. The purpose of this chapter is to evaluate the evidence for and against the hypothesis that hypoxia is involved in this disease. We shall review hepatic oxygen uptake, ethanol metabolism and adaptations, and hypoxic tissue damage in general briefly.

2. OXYGEN UPTAKE

The powerhouse of the cell is the mitochondrion, which converts the energy stored in chemical bonds of cellular foodstuffs into phosphate-bond energy as adenosine triphosphate. During this process, oxygen is reduced to water. Thus, organs that carry out considerable metabolic work, such as the liver, have high demands for oxygen for mitochondrial respiration. On the basis of studies with

RONALD G. THURMAN and SUNGCHUL JI • Department of Pharmacology, School of Medicine, University of North Carolina at Chapel Hill, North Carolina 27514. JOHN J. LEMASTERS • Department of Anatomy, School of Medicine, University of North Carolina at Chapel Hill, North Carolina 27514.

inhibitors of mitochondrial oxidative phosphorylation, it is estimated that about 85% of all hepatic oxygen uptake is involved in mitochondrial respiration.[1]

According to the now widely accepted "chemiosmotic hypothesis" of Peter Mitchell,[2] the common high-energy intermediate of oxidative phosphorylation is an electrochemical potential difference of protons, $\Delta\mu_{H^+}$, across the mitochondrial inner membrane. $\Delta\mu_{H^+}$ has two components—a membrane potential and a pH gradient.

The overall reaction of oxidative phosphorylation involves quite a large number of individual reactions catalyzed almost entirely by mobile protein complexes and electron carriers embedded in a fluid phospholipid bilayer[2a] (Fig. 1). Basically, NADH produced from carbohydrate metabolism via the citric acid cycle or from the β-oxidation of fatty acyl-CoA compounds passes reducing equivalents (electrons) to oxygen via a series of flavoproteins and cytochromes arranged in a sequence of increasing oxidation–reduction potential. The order of the respiratory sequence was worked out mainly by Chance and his colleagues in the 1950s using a double-beam spectrophotometer to record spectra from mitochondria.[3] It is now clear that energy transduction in the respiratory sequence is due to the activity of three proton- or charge-translocating redox-linked pumps that exist as large integral membrane protein complexes (complexes I, III, and IV). The proton gradient created by these pumps drives ATP synthesis catalyzed by the proton-translocating F_1-F_0-ATPase.[3a] The proton gradient also acts as a common high-energy intermediate to drive other reactions such as ion and me-

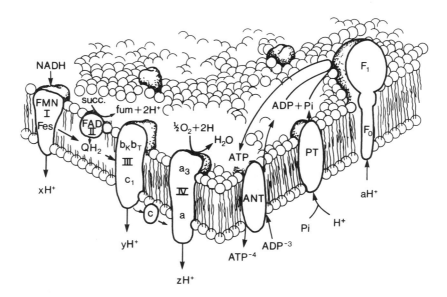

Figure 1. Scheme depicting membrane-bound oxidative phosphorylation components.

tabolite transport across the inner membrane as well as transhydrogenation reactions. For all these processes, ATP and proton stoichiometries are controversial and the focus of ongoing investigations.[3b] Although the precise regulation of mitochondrial oxidative phosphorylation is also still unclear,[3c,d] it is generally accepted that in the presence of excess substrate and oxygen, the usual physiological condition, electron flux is regulated by the supply of ADP and P_i as shown for isolated mitochondria by Chance and Williams[3] in the 1950s.

3. ETHANOL METABOLISM

Although only a few enzymes metabolize alcohol in the liver, general agreement on the quantitative contribution of these enzyme systems to alcohol uptake has not yet been reached. Three enzymes or enzyme systems have been identified or postulated to be involved in hepatic alcohol metabolism: alcohol dehydrogenase, catalase, and cytochrome P-450.

3.1. Alcohol Dehydrogenase

The most predominant enzyme involved in hepatic ethanol metabolism is clearly the zinc-containing alcohol dehydrogenase. Alcohol dehydrogenase requires NAD^+ as a cofactor and catalyzes the following reaction to near equilibrium:

$$\text{Ethanol} + NAD^+ \rightleftharpoons \text{acetaldehyde} + NADH + H^+ \qquad (1)$$

The $\Delta G'$ for the conversion of ethanol to acetaldehyde is highly unfavorable ($+4.9$ kcal/mole); however, the product, acetaldehyde, is removed rapidly by the action of aldehyde dehydrogenase in an essentially irreversible manner as follows:

$$\text{Acetaldehyde} + H_2O + NAD^+ \rightarrow NADH + H^+ + \text{acetate} \qquad (2)$$

Thus, the sum of this coupled reaction sequence is energetically favorable ($\Delta G' = -13$ kcal/mole) for the oxidation of ethanol to acetate, producing two moles of NADH by the following equation:

$$\text{Ethanol} + 2NAD^+ + H_2O \rightarrow 2NADH + 2H^+ + \text{acetate} \qquad (3)$$

The mechanism ("Theorell–Chance"[4]) of action of alcohol dehydrogenase *in vitro* is well understood. The rate-limiting step is the rate of dissociation of the binary enzyme–NADH complex [see equation (4) below] depicted for the reaction in the direction of acetaldehyde to ethanol (i.e., in the reverse direction) as in the following equations:

$$\text{NADH} + \text{enzyme} \rightleftharpoons \text{enzyme–NADH} \tag{4}$$

$$\text{Enzyme–NADH} + \text{acetaldehyde} + H^+ \rightleftharpoons \text{enzyme–NAD}^+ + \text{ethanol} \tag{5}$$

$$\text{Enzyme–NAD}^+ \rightleftharpoons \text{enzyme} + \text{NAD}^+ \tag{6}$$

Brändén et al.[5] studied the X-ray crystal structure of alcohol dehydrogenase and provided a wealth of insight into the tertiary and quaternary structure of this protein. The active site consists of a lipophilic-substrate-binding site and a nucleotide-binding site. Once substrate is bound, it is coordinated by zinc into a position favorable for hydride transfer to occur.

The action of alcohol dehydrogenase has been studied in detail in perfused organs. The half-maximal value for oxidation of alcohol is around 0.1 mM, analogous to the concentrations needed to produce half-maximal reduction in pyridine nucleotides,[6] but lower than the K_m of isolated alcohol dehydrogenase for ethanol (0.5–3 mM).[7] At low* alcohol concentrations (<2 mM), both ethanol and butanol oxidation are almost completely (over 90%) abolished by the addition of 4-methylpyrazole, an effective inhibitor of alcohol dehydrogenase.[8] Thus, in the whole organ, both ethanol and butanol are oxidized at low alcohol concentrations predominantly via alcohol dehydrogenase. Thus, hepatic alcohol metabolism, with the exception of methanol, is almost completely, if not totally, alcohol-dehydrogenase-dependent at low alcohol concentrations.

Ethanol oxidation is stimulated by artificial electron acceptors,[9] by uncoupling agents,[10] by gluconeogenic precursors,[11] and by fructose.[12] All these agents have one thing in common: They enhance the rate of reoxidation of NADH. Since these agents all stimulate ethanol uptake, it has been concluded that the rate-limiting step in ethanol oxidation, at least in livers from well-fed animals, is the rate of reoxidation of NADH. The notion that the activity of alcohol dehydrogenase is also important in the control of the rate of ethanol metabolism was postulated because the rate of ethanol metabolism, which is diminished markedly by fasting, correlates with a decrease in the activity of alcohol dehydrogenase measured in vitro.[13] However, this correlation may not be as important as cofactor reoxidation, since humans with atypical alcohol dehydrogenase have much higher enzyme activities[14] but eliminate alcohol in vivo at the same rate as normals.[15] Further, fructose stimulates ethanol metabolism in the fasted state.[12] Thus, the activity of alcohol dehydrogenase is most likely not the slowest step in alcohol metabolism, unless it is greatly diminished by chronic administration of a low-protein diet[16] or manipulated by androgens.[17] The evidence points strongly to regulation of alcohol-dehydrogenase-dependent ethanol metabolism by cofactor reoxidation.

---

*For comparison, the reader is reminded that the legal limit for blood ethanol in most of the United States is 100 mg%. This is equivalent to 22 mM.

The substrate-shuttle mechanisms responsible for transferring reducing equivalents produced by ethanol oxidation into the mitochondrial space appear to be rate-limiting for ethanol oxidation in livers from fasted animals.[18] Decreased ethanol metabolism is in all likelihood a result of depletion of essential shuttle intermediates following fasting, since uncoupling agents fail to stimulate ethanol oxidation in the fasted state and higher rates are observed when shuttle intermediates are restored.[18,19]

It seems inconsistent that the slowest step of ethanol oxidation *in vitro* should be the dissociation of the binary alcohol dehydrogenase–NADH complex, while *in vivo* it is the rate of reoxidation of NADH. However, increasing NAD$^+$ 6-fold *in vivo* by feeding nicotinamide did not stimulate ethanol oxidation, whereas stimulation of the reoxidation of NADH by addition of uncoupling agents, fructose, and gluconeogenic precursors produced marked stimulation. If one assumes that the reoxidation of NADH accelerates the dissociation of the alcohol dehydrogenase–NADH complex through equilibrium, then the rate-limiting step for alcohol oxidation *in vitro* could well be influenced *in vivo* (i.e., cofactor reoxidation may facilitate dissociation of the binary NADH–enzyme complex). If this is the case, then there is no inconsistency. Thus, the rate-limiting step for alcohol oxidation via alcohol dehydrogenase is ultimately the rate of electron flux in the mitochondrial respiratory sequence, a process that is controlled by the supply of ADP.[3] The rate of ethanol oxidation is influenced indirectly by the rate of hepatocellular biosynthetic processes.

3.2. Catalase

Catalase is a hemoprotein located in the peroxisomes in nearly all tissues.[20] It decomposes hydrogen peroxide as follows:

$$\text{Catalase} + H_2O_2 \rightarrow \text{catalase–}H_2O_2 \tag{7}$$

$$\text{Catalase–}H_2O_2 + H_2O_2 \rightarrow \text{catalase} + 2H_2O + O_2 \tag{8}$$

$$\text{Catalase–}H_2O_2 + \underset{H}{\overset{OH}{C}} \rightarrow \text{catalase} + 2H_2O + C = O \tag{9}$$

Peroxisomes contain not only high concentrations of catalase, but also a number of flavoprotein oxidases that generate hydrogen peroxide in the presence of a number of hydrogen donors (urate, glycolate, and D-amino acids) and oxygen. Hydrogen peroxide generated from the reaction of oxygen with these oxidases forms an intermediate with catalase, catalase–H_2O_2 [equation (7)]. Catalase–H_2O_2 may then undergo a subsequent reaction with another molecule of hydrogen peroxide to generate oxygen and water [equation (7) and (8)], the so-called "catalatic" reaction, or it may react with a variety of small molecules [equation (7) and (9)] to generate water and the corresponding keto compounds. This latter "peroxidatic" reaction of catalase probably represents a detoxification mechanism for a large number of small molecules, including methanol, ethanol, nitrite, and formate.[21]

Spectral techniques have been developed that allow the catalase–H_2O_2 complex to be measured directly, both in the intact hemoglobin-free perfused rat liver and *in situ*.[22] This technique has been employed to determine the rate of hydrogen peroxide production in the intact organ. A large number of agents stimulate hydrogen peroxide production in the liver[23]; however, substrates for the peroxisomal flavoproteins (e.g., fatty acids, urate, glycolate) are by far the most effective H_2O_2 generators in the liver cell.

The rate of the peroxidatic reaction of catalase is determined by complex interactions between the supply of hydrogen peroxide, the amount of catalase heme, and the concentration of the alcohol.[24] In general, however, one would not expect catalase to be an efficient ethanol oxidase at low alcohol concentrations at which alcohol dehydrogenase can operate maximally *in vivo*. At any given fixed concentration of alcohol and catalase heme, the rate-limiting step in the peroxidatic conversion of ethanol to acetaldehyde via catalase–H_2O_2 is the rate of supply of H_2O_2.

The specificity of catalase for alcohols is much different from that of alcohol dehydrogenase. Alcohol dehydrogenase oxidizes ethanol, propanol, and butanol with increasing velocities, but does not react with methanol. Conversely, catalase oxidizes ethanol and metahnol at about the same rate, but activity decreases markedly as the chain length of the alcohol is increased.[25,26]

3.3. Cytochrome P-450

When microsomes are incubated with NADPH or an NADPH-generating system and oxygen, ethanol is oxidized to acetaldehyde.[27] Alcohols also bind to cytochrome P-450, although the concentrations needed to produce spectral changes are unphysiologically high.[28] These observations led Lieber and his co-workers to postulate that a unique cytochrome-P-450-dependent alcohol oxidation occurs in liver microsomes.[29] Moreover, when rats are fed a diet containing alcohol, the endoplasmic reticulum proliferates,[29] a phenomenon observed following chronic treatment with many drug substrates for cytochrome P-450. This observation has been useful in explaining the unusual reactions of the alcoholic to drugs such as barbiturates. When ethanol is present, drug hydroxylation is inhibited, and blood levels of barbiturates remain high, resulting in the well-documented hypersensitivity of the alcoholic to barbiturates. Conversely, once the patient is sober, drug metabolism is accelerated as a result of induction of microsomal components due to alcohol intake, rendering the alcoholic subsensitive to many drugs.[30]

However, the precise mechanism(s) by which ethanol is metabolized by microsomes remains controversial. Ethanol has been shown to be a direct substrate for a pure cytochrome P-450$_{LM3a}$ isolated from rabbit liver.[31] In contrast, microsomal ethanol oxidation was inhibited largely by substrates for catalase,[32] by catalase inhibitors,[32,33] and by H_2O_2-utilizing systems,[32] supporting the involvement of catalase–H_2O_2 in that process. Moreover, microsomes incubated with NADPH and oxygen produced hydrogen peroxide at rates sufficient to account for microsomal ethanol oxidation.[32] There are several characteristics common to both microscomal ethanol oxidation and microsomal hydrogen peroxide production: Both require NADPH, both have similar K_m's for oxygen, and both processes are inhibited to the same degree by carbon monoxide.[29,32] These observations led one of us a number of years ago to propose that a major portion of microsomal ethanol oxidation was due to cytochrome-P-450-dependent hydrogen peroxide production and a subsequent peroxidatic reaction of ethanol via catalase (i.e., some process in addition to direct catalysis via cytochrome P-450 was involved.) Moreover, since inhibition of microsomal ethanol oxidation by sodium azide was incomplete,[32] the direct involvement of cytochrome P-450 is also likely in species other than the rabbit.

More work is clearly needed before the quantitative contribution of catalase and cytochrome P-450 to ethanol oxidation under physiological conditions is worked out clearly. One useful model for such work may be the alcohol-dehydrogenase-deficient deermouse.[34]

3.4. Swift Increase in Alcohol Metabolism

The prolonged consumption of alcohol leads to an accelerated rate of ethanol oxidation in both experimental animals and man.[35,36] This so-called "metabolic tolerance" has been studied in detail in liver slices[37] and perfused livers.[38] The increase in ethanol metabolism due to ethanol treatment is associated with an increase in oxygen uptake by the hepatocyte.

All three pathways of ethanol metabolism require oxygen either directly or indirectly. However, while catalase and cytochrome P-450 have direct requirements for O_2, the link between alcohol dehydrogenase and O_2 is less direct (Fig. 2). Thus, ethanol oxidation should increase oxygen uptake. However, acute addition of ethanol to perfused livers from fasted rats does not alter oxygen uptake,[39] presumably because ethanol does not alter ADP supply acutely and because ethanol is oxidized mainly via alcohol dehydrogenase.

Following chronic treatment with ethanol, however, a number of studies have demonstrated that ethanol can increase oxygen uptake. Liver slices and perfused livers from rats fed ethanol consume more oxygen than controls.[37,38] Moreover, Iturriaga et al.[40] showed that seven alcoholic patients with mild hepatic necrosis had an elevated arteriovenous oxygen concentration difference. Thus, there exists the possibility that chronic treatment with ethanol, by elevating

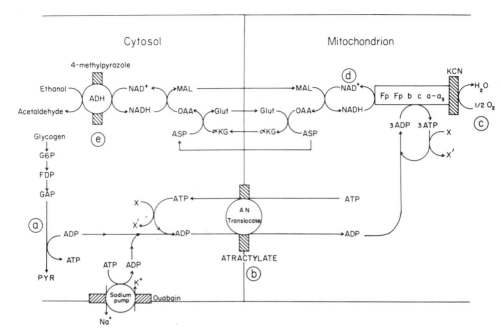

Figure 2. Scheme depicting rapid increase in hepatic oxygen uptake caused by ethanol treatment. (ADH) Alcohol dehydrogenase; (MAL) malate; (OAA) oxaloacetate; (Glut) glutamate; (αKG) α-oxoglutarate; (Asp) aspartate; (G6P) glucose-6-phospate (FDP) fructose-1,6,-bisphosphate (GAP) glyceraldehyde-3-phosphate; (PYR) pyruvate; (AN) adenine nucleotide; (X, X′) unknown ATPases; (Fp) flavoprotein; (b, c, a–a₃) cytochromes b, c, a–a₃.

oxygen uptake, produces pericentral hypoxia and subsequent liver disease (see below).

Yuki and Thurman[41] showed that the increase in oxygen uptake following treatment with ethanol was very rapid (Fig. 3). Basal rates of oxygen uptake by the ethanol-free perfused livers were between 100 and 110 μmoles/hr per g. Oxygen uptake increased swiftly in livers from rats treated previously with ethanol, and was nearly doubled 2.5 hr after the initial dose (Fig. 3).

Previously, it has been assumed that the activation of ethanol metabolism by ethanol treatment requires considerable time. For example, 3–5 weeks of treatment with diets containing ethanol have been routine.[29] The data in Fig. 3 indicate clearly, however, that the oxygen uptake by the ethanol-free perfused liver and subsequent ethanol metabolism can be nearly doubled only 2–3 hr after one large dose of ethanol to the rat. This activation of oxygen uptake persisted in the absence of ethanol, but tended to return to the basal value at 5 hr after the dose, indicating that the effect of ethanol was transient (Fig. 3).

Several studies have demonstrated a direct relationship between oxygen uptake and ethanol uptake.[38] Enhanced oxygen uptake results in an activation

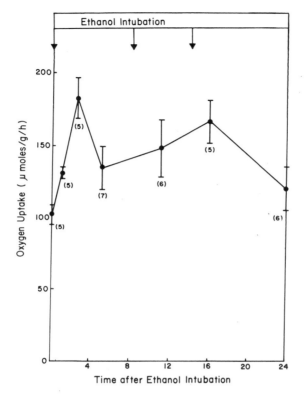

Figure 3.   Time–course of the effect of ethanol treatment in vivo on oxygen uptake by the perfused liver. Ethanol (5.0 g/kg) was administered to rats via gastric intubation at times 0, 8, and 14 hr (↓). Thus, animals at longer time points received multiple doses of ethanol. Untreated rats were intubated with 0.9% NaCl. At the times indicated (●), livers were perfused with ethanol-free Krebs–Henseleit–bicarbonate buffer, pH 7.4. After 20–30 min of preperfusion, steady-state rates of oxygen uptake were calculated from the influent–effluent oxygen concentration difference, the flow rate, and the liver weight. Results are means ± S.E.M. for the numbers of experiments in parentheses.

of NADH reoxidation. Thus, ethanol is oxidized more rapidly when the liver is respiring at a more rapid rate. The observation that ethanol uptake was greater in the perfused liver 2.5 hr after ethanol treatment than in livers from untreated rats is consistent with this hypothesis.[41] It is also likely that the rapid increase in oxygen uptake caused by ethanol treatment is responsible for the observation that rates of ethanol metobolism increase as [ethanol] is elevated *in vivo*,[42] since that process is also "remembered" (i.e., the accelerated rate of ethanol elimination is linear with time) and occurs as soon as 2 hr after the administration of ethanol. Thus, taken together, these experiments suggest strongly that a repeated acute rather than a chronic action of ethanol is responsible for the "adaptive increase" in ethanol metabolism caused by chronic prior treatment with ethanol.

3.5. Physiological Trigger for the Increase in Oxygen Uptake Caused by Ethanol Administration

Because the activation of oxygen uptake was rapid (2–3 hr) in these experiments, involvement of hormonal factors in the mechanism was expected. This hypothesis was supported by several observations. First, adrenaline injected into the rat partially mimicked the increase observed with ethanol, confirming previous observations with liver slices by Bernstein *et al.*[43] Second, the increase in hepatic respiration observed 2.5 hr after treatment with ethanol could be blocked by both α- and β-adrenergic blocking agents.[41] Third, the actions of ethanol and adrenaline were not additive, indicating that the rapid increase in hepatic oxygen uptake is triggered, at least in part, via an ethanol-mediated release of adrenaline. The observation that blood glucose concentrations increased[41] and hepatic glycogen concentrations declined with a time–course similar to the increase in oxygen uptake observed in these studies is consistent with this hypothesis, since the stimulation of glycogenolysis by adrenaline is well documented.[44]

3.6. Mechanism of Increase in Hepatic Oxygen Uptake Caused by Treatment with Ethanol

What is responsible for the increase in hepatic respiration after acute treatment with ethanol? Several possibilities seem unlikely. First, induction of ethanol-metabolizing enzymes probably does not occur within the short time frame of these experiments (2.5 hr). This hypothesis is supported by the observations that activities of alcohol dehydrogenase and ethanol oxidation by the microsomal fraction were unaltered 2.5 hr after ethanol treatment. It is also unlikely that catalase activity or H_2O_2-generating flavoproteins are induced in only 2.5 hr.

Second, an induction or activation at the Na^+,K^+-activated ATPase has been postulated to be a primary event in the mechanisms of the "adaptive increase" in ethanol metabolism caused by prior pretreatment with ethanol in liver slices[45] and perfused liver.[38] This conclusion rests primarily on the observation that oxygen and ethanol uptake by slices or perfused livers was diminished to a larger degree by ouabain in tissues from alcohol-treated than in tissues from control rats.[38,45] This postulate has, however, subsequently been challenged.[46] It was demonstrated that the inhibition by ouabain was a slow process resulting most likely from the accumulation of ions in the liver as a consequence of inhibition of the Na^+,K^+-activated ATPase.[46] Inhibition of ethanol and oxygen uptake did not correlate with the inhibition of the sodium pump as judged kinetically from the rapid change in ionic composition of the perfusion fluid. Therefore, it is unlikely that an induction of the sodium pump is involved in the mechanism of the "adaptive increase." Furthermore, it is also improbable that it could adapt in only 2.5 hr.

Enhanced ethanol oxidation due to chronic treatment with ethanol could be blocked largely by an alcohol dehydrogenase inhibitor, 4-methylpyrazole. This shows clearly that alcohol dehydrogenase is involved in the increased rate of ethanol elimination observed after 2.5 hr of treatment with ethanol despite the observation that the activity of alcohol dehydrogenase was not changed by ethanol treatment.

The mitochondrial respiratory chain is also implicated in this increase in oxygen uptake, on the basis of sensitivity to an inhibitor of cytochrome oxidase, KCN. Partial inhibition of the increased oxygen uptake by atractyloside, an inhibitor of the adenine nucleotide translocase, suggests that an ATPase of cytosolic origin is responsible for increasing ADP and thereby stimulating oxygen uptake after treatment with ethanol.

3.7. Role of Glycolysis in the Mechanism of Increased Oxygen Uptake Caused by Treatment with Ethanol

It is well known that ethanol inhibits glycolysis through redox inhibition of glyceraldehyde-3-phosphate dehydrogenase.[47] Thurman and Scholz[39] demonstrated that the diminished rate of ATP generation after inhibition of glycolysis by ethanol is responsible for the small (5–10%) increase in hepatic oxygen uptake observed when ethanol is infused into the liver; however, this phenomenon has an absolute requirement for the presence of ethanol in the liver.

4. ROLE OF HYPOXIA IN LIVER DAMAGE

It has long been recognized that mammalian tissues are damaged if oxygen supplies are inadequate. This phenomenon has received considerable attention with regard to the heart, in which hypoxic damage can result from coronary artery insufficiency. In addition, hypoxic insult plays a genuine role in a variety of diseases and is involved in pathophysiology in liver, skeletal muscle, vascular tissue, heart, and brain (stroke). Considerable interest in pharmacological intervention, particularly with calcium-channel blockers, now exists.[48,49]

In the liver, ischemia *in vivo* can produce both reversible and irreversible changes in the cell. Ischemia for longer than 30 min usually results in necrosis, while shorter periods of ischemia cause enzyme release and produce less damaging, reversible changes.[50]

The cell biology of hypoxic injury has been studied in detail by Trump and Arstila.[50] Although the precise mechanism(s) of hypoxic damage has not been elucidated, considerable insight into changes in morphology exists. As soon as 1 min after oxygen tension falls, ATP levels fall precipitately.[50] Subsequently, within 15 min, glycogen and mitochondrial matrix granules disappear. Changes in mitochondrial shape are apparent between 15 and 30 min of ischemia. By 1 hr, the polysomal arrangements on the rough endoplasmic reticulum are lost, the lysosomes lose content, and the mitochondrial membrane appears to aggregate. Mitochondrial swelling is maximal in 2–4 hr, and fragmentation of the endoplasmic reticulum is apparent.[50] By this time, ischemic changes are irreversible.

Associated changes include loss of potassium and magnesium and influx of calcium and sodium. Recently, the role of calcium in the mechanism of hepatotoxicity has received considerable attention. Farber and his colleagues, working with isolated hepatocytes, have accumulated data in general support of the notion that calcium influx precedes and precipitates cell death.[51] On the other hand, Orrenius and his colleagues suggest that cell injury, as measured by surface bleb formation in hepatocytes, occurs more frequently in the absence than in the presence of extracellular calcium.[52] More work is needed to clarify the role of calcium in hepatotoxicity.

When liver cells are damaged, enzymes are released. Following ischemic insult to the heart or liver, enzyme release is accelerated on "reflow."[53,53a] This is illustrated for the perfused liver in Fig. 4. Samples of effluent perfusate were

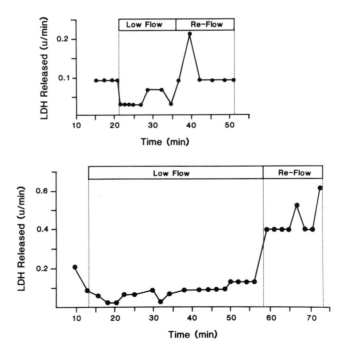

Figure 4. Lactate dehydrogenase (LDH) and protein release after reoxygenation. Hypoxia was induced for variable times by low flow (1 ml/min per g), and LDH release into the effluent measured on resumptin of normal flow. Reperfusion (4 ml/min per g) led to abrupt enzyme release, the severity of which was proportional to the duration of hypoxia.

analyzed for lactate dehydrogenase (LDH), an enzyme abundant in hepatocellular cytosol (Fig. 4). After reflow, LDH release increased sharply: The greater the period of hypoxia, the greater the release. A similar pattern was observed for the release of protein.

4.1. Hepatic Oxygen Supply

The liver is supplied with a mixture of blood via the hepatic artery and the portal vein. The ratio of blood flows from these two routes can vary depending on, for example, hormonal status and disease state, but are normally around 25% via the artery and the remainder via the vein. The dissolved oxygen is around 135 μM in arterial blood and 65–78 μM in the portal vein. Thus, if complete mixing of influent blood supplies occurred at the beginning of the sinusoid, the dissolved oxygen concentration reaching the first cells *in vivo* would be around 85 μM.

As blood flows through the liver lobule, oxygen and nutrients are extracted and metabolites are generated, establishing gradients between the portal vessels and the central vein (Fig. 5). Evidence exists, however, that the hepatic artery may supply oxygen-rich blood to the biliary system, possibly to support the concentration of bile. Thus, dissolved oxygen at the sinusoid is most likely greater than 70 and less than 85 μM oxygen *in vivo*. Since the difference between portal and venous dissolved oxygen is about 50 μM *in vivo* (Fig. 5), an oxygen gradient within the liver lobule from the portal to the central region must exist.

As early as 1918, Krough[54] postulated that oxygen gradients exist in tissue. Such gradients depend on the rate of transport in the vascular bed, the solubility of oxygen in tissue, the diffusion coefficient for oxygen, and the rate of oxygen consumption by the tissue. (For a detailed discussion of gradients, see Chapter 4).

By using a multiwire surface oxygen electrode, Kessler *et al.*[55,56] demonstrated that the distribution of oxygen tension on the liver surface is heterogeneous; oxygen tension values ranged from 0 to 60 torr in the liver *in situ* and from 100 to 500 torr in the hemoglobin-free perfused liver. Although these observations were consistent with the postulate that oxygen gradients exist in liver tissue, no attempt was made to correlate oxygen tension with the anatomical structure of the liver lobule.

Chance *et al.*[57,58] demonstrated that pyridine nucleotide fluorescence can be used to monitor tissue oxygenation. This technique is based on the fact that bound and free intracellular reduced pyridine nucleotides (NADH and NADPH), but not their oxidized counterparts, are fluorescent at 450 nm on excitation with light at 366 nm (see Chapter 8). This fluorescence is indirectly dependent on the intracellular oxygen tension, since NADH is oxidized predominantly via the mitochondrial electron-transport sequence. Cytochrome *c* oxidase, the terminal element of the electron-transfer sequence, has an extremely high affinity for

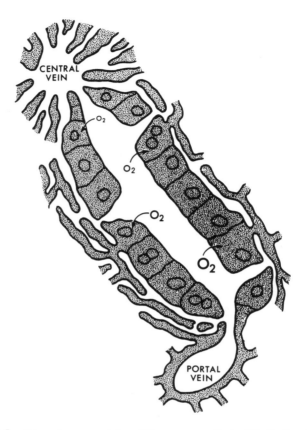

Figure 5. Schematic representation of the oxygen gradient within the liver lobule.

oxygen. In isolated mitochondria, the concentration of oxygen required for half-maximal electron transport is much less than 1 μM.[59] Thus, if mitochondria in the perfused liver tissue behave similarly to isolated mitochondria, an increase in pyridine nucleotide fluorescence can be equated with a virtual absence of oxygen within the tissue.

Chance *et al.*[60] measured the distribution of pyridine nucleotide fluorescence intensities in small cubes of tissue isolated from freeze–trapped liver. They observed an inhomogeneous distribution of fluorescence intensities, but did not correlate the optical data with the anatomical structure of the liver. In contrast, NAD^+ and NADH contents determined by quantitative histochemistry were distributed uniformly over the liver lobule.[61]

In addition to the lobular oxygen gradient, an intracellular oxygen gradient also exists. Chance and co-workers[62,63] estimated the intracellular oxygen gradient in isolated, hemoglobin-free perfused rat heart by monitoring two oxygen-sensitive intracellular pigments, cytochrome a/a_3 and myoglobin. On the basis of the observation that both these probes exhibited identical half-maximal responses when the oxygen tension was altered despite a 10-fold difference in their affinities for oxygen (0.1 vs. 1 torr), it was concluded that the intracellular oxygen gradient was very steep. Sies[64] carried out similar experiments using cytochrome a/a_3 and urate oxidase as intracellular probes for oxygen in the perfused liver and arrived at similar conclusions. Jones and Mason[65] used yet another method to estimate the intracellular oxygen gradient. They compared the apparent K_m values of cytochrome a/a_3 for oxygen in isolated hepatocytes and mitochondria. Since the values were about one order of magnitude higher in hepatocytes than in mitochondria, they also concluded that a steep intracellular oxygen gradient exists. Jones was able to shift the K_m for oxygen in hepatocytes by modifying the rate of oxygen uptake with inhibitors or uncouplers of oxidative phosphorylation (e.g., the K_m for oxygen decreased in hepatocytes treated with antimycin A but increased in the presence of uncoupling agents such as FCCP). Moreover, the K_m for oxygen in hepatocytes was decreased by digitonin treatment. However, several important questions with respect to intracellular oxygen gradients remain unanswered, not the least of which is the fact that the K_m of mixed-function oxidases for oxygen was not different in microsomes and hepatocytes, as would be expected if a steep intracellular oxygen gradient exists.

4.2. Is Hypoxia Involved in the Mechanism of Alcohol-Induced Liver Damage?

The existence of an oxygen gradient together with differential distribution of enzymes may underlie the differing sensitivities of regions of the liver lobule to various hepatotoxins and disease states. In particular, alcohol causes liver damage preferentially in centrilobular regions.[66]

Ethanol treatment enhances the rate of oxygen uptake by the liver. This occurs both acutely after a single administration of ethanol,[41] and chronically.[38,45] Ethanol and oxygen metabolism are related directly in the liver. The oxidation of ethanol produces NADH, which is then oxidized by the mitochondrial respiratory chain with the concomitant consumption of oxygen. One consequence of the alcohol-induced increase in oxygen uptake may be a steeper oxygen gradient within the liver lobule. Israel et al.[66] postulated that ethanol-induced liver injury is caused by centrilobular hypoxia resulting from such an exaggerated oxygen gradient; i.e., the oxygen gradient becomes so steep that centrilobular regions, those regions furthest removed from the oxygen supply, are not supplied sufficient oxygen. In support of this postulate, they demonstrated that brief exposure to hypoxia produced more centrilobular necrosis in ethanol-treated than in control rates. Pretreatment of rats with the antithyroid drug propylthiouracil abolished the ethanol-induced increase in oxygen uptake and diminished the tissue damage.[66]

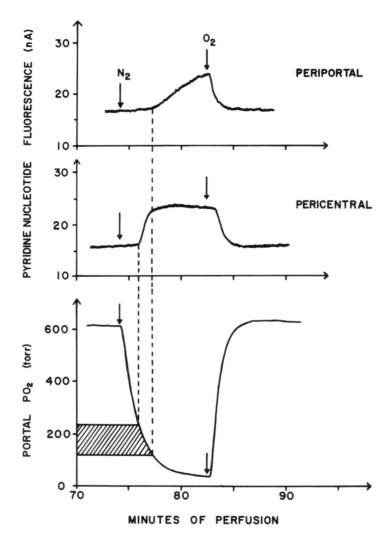

Figure 6. Measurement of the lobular oxygen gradient with micro-light guides in perfused liver from the ethanol-treated rat. The liver was perfused via the portal vein at 37°C with Krebs–Henseleit buffer. The inflow oxygen tension was monitored continuously with a Clark-type oxygen electrode located near the portal vein. A pair of micro-light guides were placed on periportal and pericentral regions, and the increase in the pyridine nucleotide fluorescence was measured when inflow oxygen was removed.

One of the goals of our laboratories has been to obtain evidence for or against this interesting hypothesis. For this purpose, we have developed several new methods to measure lobular oxygen gradients, rates of local oxygen uptake, and tissue injury (see Chapter 7).

To estimate the lobular oxygen gradient, micro-light guides were placed on periportal and pericentral regions of the liver, and the oxygen tension of the perfusing medium was reduced progressively (Fig. 6). This caused an increase in NADH fluorescence in pericentral regions that preceded any increase in periportal areas (Fig. 6). Pyridine nucleotide fluorescence began to increase when oxygen tension in the influent perfusate decreased below about 300 torr. The influent pO_2 at which pyridine nucleotide fluorescence first begins to increase in pericentral areas is the oxygen gradient across the liver lobule (Table I), since NADH fluorescence begins to increase only when local pO_2 is virtually zero due to the high affinity of cytochrome oxidase for oxygen. Similarly, the influent pO_2 at which pyridine nucleotide fluorescence begins to increase in periportal areas is the periportal oxygen gradient. The difference between the lobular gradient and the periportal gradient represents the pericentral gradient.

In sucrose-treated control livers, the lobular oxygen gradient was about 275 torr, the periportal gradient was 208 torr, and the pericentral gradient was 67 torr (Table I). This observation is consistent with the presence of larger mitochondria with more abundant cristae in hepatocytes located in periportal areas and suggests that local rates of respiration are greater in periportal tissue. In livers from rats treated chronically with ethanol, the lobular oxygen gradient increased to 400 torr. This increase was accompanied by a similar increase in hepatic oxygen uptake (Table I). The increase of the oxygen gradient was confined to the pericentral regions of the lobule, a finding of some interest, since ethanol causes injury to pericentral hepatocytes in experimental animals and man. These results present direct physical evidence that the increased oxygen

Table I. Effects of Chronic Ethanol Treatment on Oxygen Gradients in the Liver Lobule[a]

| Treatment | N | Oxygen gradient (torr) | | | Rate of O_2 uptake (μmoles/g per hr) |
		Periportal	Pericentral	Lobular	
Sucrose	12	208 ± 13	67 ± 14	275 ± 20	110 ± 7
Ethanol	15	264 ± 19	136 ± 12^b	400 ± 23^b	144 ± 6^c
Ethanol/PTU	3	177 ± 27	53 ± 16	230 ± 19	118 ± 4

[a] Control rats were given 25% (wt./vol.) sucrose in drinking water for 4–6 weeks. Ethanol-treated rats were fed the Porta diet for 4–6 weeks. Ethanol/propylthiouracil (PTU)-treated rats were given the Porta diet for 6 weeks and then given PTU plus the Porta diet for 3 or 4 more weeks. PTU was suspended in 1 ml corn oil and administered by gastric intubation (50 mg/kg body wt.). Results are means $\pm$ S.E.
[b,c] Significantly different from control; $^b p < 0.01$; $^c p < 0.001$.

uptake that results from chronic ethanol treatment indeed increases the oxygen gradient within the liver lobule.

Propylthiouracil prevents hypoxia-induced pericentral necrosis in livers from ethanol-treated rats.[66,67] We found that treatment of rats with propylthiouracil abolished both the increased tissue respiration and the enchanced pericentral oxygen gradient in perfused livers caused by chronic ethanol treatment (Table I). This demonstrates that the rate of tissue respiration plays an important role in establishing the oxygen gradient within the liver lobule. Consequently, an increase in respiration could render pericentral regions more susceptible to hypoxia. These results support the hypothesis that chronic ethanol treatment causes pericentral regions of the liver to become susceptible to hypoxia-induced cellular injury as postulated by Israel et al.[66] Tissue oxygen tensions in periportal and pericentral regions were also measured directly employing a miniature oxygen electrode (Fig. 6). At a constant inflow Po_2 of 630 torr, tissue Po_2 values in periportal regions from sucrose- and ethanol-treated rats were both approximately 350 torr (Table II). Pericentral tissue oxygen tensions were 271 and 204 torr from sucrose- and ethanol-treated rats, respectively. Oxygen gradients measured with the oxygen electrode agreed closely with the oxygen gradients calculated from NADH fluorescence measurements made with the micro-light guide (Table II).

4.2.1. Centrilobular Damage Due to Low-Flow Hypoxia

In light of Israel's proposal that ethanol produces centrilobular liver injury due to hypoxia, it was of considerable interest to learn the pattern, progression, and reversibility of hypoxia-induced liver injury. We first established that cir-

Table II. Direct Measurement of the Lobular Oxygen Gradients with Miniature Oxygen Electrode in Perfused Livers from Sucrose- and Ethanol-Treated Rats[a]

Treatment	Tissue Po_2 (torr)		Oxygen gradient[b] (torr)		
	Periportal	Pericentral	Periportal	Pericentral	Lobular
Sucrose	350 ± 49	271 ± 50	278 ± 50	79 ± 12	357 ± 50
Ethanol	347 ± 46	204 ± 47	281 ± 46	143 ± 14^c	424 ± 47

[a] Rats were treated and livers perfused as in Table I. Tissue oxygen tensions were measured on the perfused liver surface using an oxygen electrode. For each liver, 16 pairs of Po_2 measurements were made in adjacent periportal and pericentral regions and were averaged to obtain a single pair of mean periportal and pericentral tissue Po_2 values. These individual pairs of mean tissue Po_2 values from seven livers were then averaged. Results are means $\pm$ S.E.

[b] The gradients were calculated by assuming that the oxygen tension in the terminal portal venule is identical with the oxygen tension in the portal vein, which was 628 ± 11 torr. The mean venous oxygen tensions were 267 ± 23 and 228 ± 17 torr, respectively, for the sucrose- and ethanol-treated groups.

[c] Significantly different from sucrose control: $p < 0.01$.

cumscribed, anoxic zones developed in pericentral regions when the rate of oxygen delivery was reduced to approximately one quarter that employed normally. By contrast, periportal regions remained normoxic.[68] Since anoxia was confined to pericentral regions and was stable over a relatively long period, it became possible to evaluate the structural changes induced by progressively longer periods of anoxia using adjacent normoxic periportal tissue as an internal control for nonspecific changes. In this low-flow model of hypoxia, periportal tissue remained normal in appearance even after 45 min of hypoxia (Fig. 7). After as little as 15 min, however, striking alterations in cell structure were observed in centrilobular regions. Most prominent were blebs of hepatocyte plasma membrane and cytoplasma projecting into the sinusoidal lumen through fenestrations in the endothelium. These blebs remained connected to hepatocytes via slender necks. After 45 min of low-flow hypoxia, hepatocytes were distorted grossly by surface blebs that covered both the sinusoidal and the intercellular surfaces of the hepatocytes (Fig. 8). In addition, the endothelium was torn and fragmented.

It was clear from these observations that perfusion of the isolated, hemoglobin-free liver at low flow rates produced anoxic stress only in portions of the

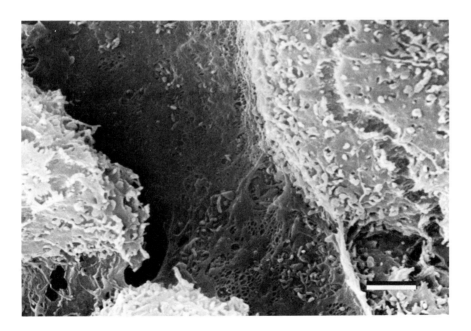

Figure 7. Scanning electron micrograph of isolated, perfused rat liver. Periportal regions after 45 min of low-flow hypoxia. The structure in periportal regions is indistinguishable from that of livers perfused under normoxic conditions. Scale bar: 2 μm.

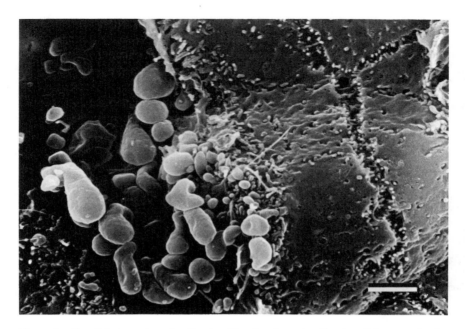

Figure 8. Centrilobular region after 15 min of low-flow hypoxia. Abundant blebs cover the sinusoidal surfaces of hepatocytes. Adjacent periportal regions were normal in appearance. Scale bar: 2 μm.

liver lobule near the central vein. In experiments in which flow was reduced further, the amount of injured tissue increased; however, those areas proximal to terminal portal venules were spared.

Reoxygenation by resumption of the original flow rate resulted in disappearance of the blebs[53a] (Fig. 9). There was also substantial shrinkage of the hepatocytes, expansion of the sinusoids, and dilation of the sinusoidal fenestrations. Thus, centrilobular regions of the liver lobule were vulnerable to hypoxic injury and were damaged rapidly. These observations are consistent with the proposal that ethanol-induced tissue hypoxia plays an important role in alcoholic liver disease.

Blebs disappeared after reoxygenation, and the question arose whether they were resorbed or released into the circulation. To distinguish between these possibilities, LDH was measured in the effluent perfusate (see Fig. 4). As noted above, after reflow, LDH release increased sharply: The greater the period of hypoxia, the greater the release. A similar pattern was observed for the release of protein. The release of LDH and protein on reoxygenation suggested that blebs were not resorbed but were released. To recover any blebs that may have entered the effluent, we filtered perfusate through polylysine-treated Nucleopore filters of 0.2-μm pore size and examined the filters by scanning electron micro-

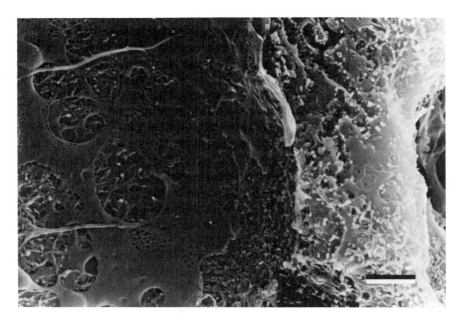

Figure 9. Centrilobular region after 15 min of low-flow hypoxia and 15 min of reflow. Blebs have disappeared and hepatocytes have decreased markedly in volume. Scale bar: 2 μm.

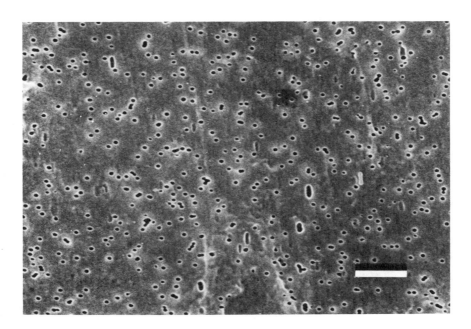

Figure 10. Nucleopore filter after passage of effluent from normoxic liver. Negligible material was released. Scale bar: 2 μm.

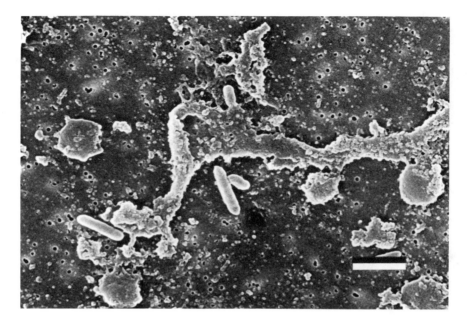

Figure 11. Nucleopore filter after passage of effluent from reoxygenated liver. On reoxygenation, substantial polymorphic cellular debris was recovered on the filter surface. Scale bar: 2 μm.

scopy. During normoxic perfusions, virtually no material was collected on the filters. Also, during the low-flow period, little material was collected on the filters (Fig. 10); however, after reflow, much more material was recovered (Fig. 11). Since this material corresponded in size and shape to blebs, it appears that blebs were released from hypoxic hepatocytes on reoxygenation.[53a]

Recently, a new method was developed to study zonal hepatotoxicity in specific regions of the liver lobule in perfused liver.[69] This method is based on exposure to a hepatotoxic chemical or procedure followed by the subsequent infusion of trypan blue, which stains nuclei in damaged cells. With this new method, comparison of the temporal relationship between metabolic changes and the onset of cellular damage induced by allyl alcohol was possible.[69] With this method, we have demonstrated that 90 min of low-flow hypoxia followed by 30 min of reflow causes dye uptake exclusively in pericentral regions of the liver lobule. It is also possible to rapidly produce hypoxic damage in fasted liver with N_2 (Fig. 12). Experiments can now be performed in the perfused liver during

Figure 12. Effect of hypoxia on perfused livers from fasted rats. (A) Rats were starved for 24 hr prior to perfusion, and livers were perfused at flow rates of 4 ml/g per min for 120 min. (B, C) Liver was perfused with perfusate saturated with 95% N_2 and 5% CO_2 for 30 min at normal flow rates. (PP) Periportal; (PC) pericentral. (A, B) × 125, scale bar: 80 μm; (C) × 250, scale bar: 40 μm.

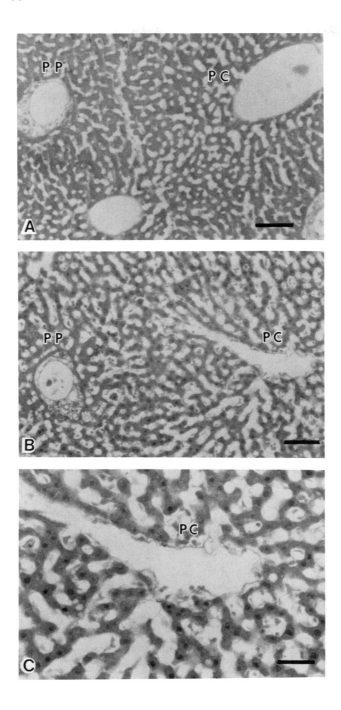

short-term exposure to hypoxia in pericentral regions of the liver lobule. Thus, nonspecific changes that may occur with models that require longer time periods can be avoided. This new dye-uptake method should have wide application in studies of the toxicity of many hepatotoxins that affect specific zones of the liver lobule.

4.2.2. Clinical Implications

Our findings suggest that alcoholic liver injury needs to be considered in the same light as ischemic heart disease. Theoretically, actions that would decrease oxygen demand by the liver and/or increase oxygen delivery to the liver should be beneficial. One such treatment is the administration of the antithyroid drug propylthiouracil (PTU), which decreases the oxygen uptake by the liver.

Two clinical trials have been carried out on alcoholic patients with PTU. In one study, patients receiving 300 mg PTU daily recovered faster than controls.[70] In another study, no effect of PTU was found.[71] Both these studies were small and have been criticized.[72] Thus, the role of thyroid hormones in alcoholic liver disease, if any, remains to be established clearly.

Since hepatic respiration and oxygen delivery are influenced by a great number of hormonal, nutritional, hemodynamic, and pharmacological factors, there are many potential therapeutic possibilities to be explored. For example, propranolol, the β-adrenergic blocker, prevents the increase in hepatic oxygen uptake caused by ethanol[41] and might ultimately prove useful in the clinic. Calcium-channel blockers have also been shown to be effective in preventing or reducing hypoxic injury.[49] Finally, these considerations may one day help to explain individual differences in susceptibility to alcoholic liver disease and may possibly allow identification of those most vulnerable. Advances in our understanding of the basic mechanisms that underlie alcohol metabolism will create new opportunities for clinical investigation. Obviously, considerable work needs to be carried out in the laboratory before a clear understanding of predisposing and protective factors in alcohol-related liver disease is reached.

One area that clearly needs work is to establish that ethanol indeed does or does not produce its detrimental effects on the liver via oxygen–hypoxia interactions. For this, it will be necessary to develop new animal models.

REFERENCES

1. Thurman, R. G., and Scholz, R., 1969, Mixed-function oxidation in perfused rat liver: The effect of aminopyrine on oxygen uptake, *Eur. J. Biochem.* **10**:459–467.
2. Mitchell, P., 1966, Chemiosmotic coupling in oxidative and photosynthetic phosphorylation, *Biol. Rev.* **41**:445–502.

2a. Schneider, H., Lemasters, J. J., Höchli, M., and Hackenbrock, C. R., 1980, Liposome–mitochondrial inner membrane fusion: Lateral diffusion of integral electron transfer components, *J. Biol. Chem.* **255**:3748–3756.

3. Chance, B., and Williams, G. R., 1955, Respiratory enzymes in oxidative phosphrylation I–V, *J. Biol. Chem.* **217**:383–438.

3a. Boyer, P. D., Chance, B., Ernst, L., Mitchell, P., Racker, E., and Slater, E. C., 1977, Oxidative phosphorylation and photophorylation, *Annu. Rev. Biochem.* **46**:955–1026.

3b. Lemasters, J. J., 1985, The ATP/oxygen and ATP/site ratios of oxidative phosphorylation: An analysis by nonequilibrium thermodynamics, *Comments Molec. Cell. Biophysics* (in press).

3c. Grunwald, R., and Lemasters, J. J., 1982, Rate-limitation of mitochondrial oxidative phosphorylation, *EBEC Short Rep.* **2**:269–270.

3d. Groen, A. K., Wanders, R. J., Westerhoff, H. V., van der Meer, R., and Tager, J. M., 1982, Quantification of the contribution of various steps to the control of mitochondrial respiration, *J. Biol. Chem.* **257**:2754–2757.

4. Theorell, H., and Chance, B., 1951, Studies on liver alcohol dehydrogenase. II. The kinetics of the compound of horse liver alcohol dehydrogenase and reduced diphosphopyridine nucleotide, *Acta Chem. Scand.* **5**:1127–1144.

5. Brändén, E.-I., Eklund, H., Zeppezauer, E., Nordström, B., Bowie, J., Söderland, G., and Ohlsson, I., 1974, Three-dimensional structure of the horse liver alcohol dehydrogenase molecule, in: *Alcohol and Aldehyde Metabolizing Systems* (R. G. Thurman, T. Yonetani, J. R. Williamson, and B. Chance, eds.), pp. 7–21, Academic Press, New York.

6. Williamson, J. R., Scholz, R., Thurman, R. G., and Chance, B., 1969, Transport of reducing equivalents across the mitochondrial membrane in rat liver, in: *The Energy Level and Metabolic Control in Mitochondria* (S. Papa, J. M. Tager, E. Quagliariello, and E. C. Slater, eds.), pp. 411–429, Adriatica Editrice, Bari.

7. Theorell, H., Nygaard, A. P., and Bonnichsen, R., 1969, On the effect of some heterocyclic compounds on the enzymatic activity of liver alcohol dehydrogenase, *Acta Chem. Scand.* **23**:255.

8. Thurman, R. G., McKenna, W. R., Brentzel, H. J. and Hesse, S., 1975, Significant pathways of hepatic ethanol metabolism, *Fed. Proc. Fed. Am. Soc. Exp. Biol.* **34**:2075–2081.

9. Madison, L., Lochner, A., and Wolff, J., 1967, Ethanol-induced hypoglycemia. II. Mechanism of suppression of hepatic gluconeogenesis, *Diabetes* **16**:252–258.

10. Videla, L., and Israel, Y., 1970, Factors that modify the metabolism of ethanol in rat liver and adaptive changes produced by its chronic administration, *Biochem. J.* **118**:275–281.

11. Williamson, J. R., Scholz, R., Browning, E. T., Thurman, R. G., and Fukami, M. H., 1969, Control mechanisms of gluconeogenesis and ketogenesis. III. Metabolic effects in perfused rat liver, *J. Biol. Chem.* **244**:5044.

12. Scholz, R., and Nohl, H., 1976, Mechanism of the stimulatory effect of fructose on ethanol oxidation in perfused rat liver, *Eur. J. Biochem.* **63**:449–458.

13. Lumeng, L., Bosron, W. F., and Li, T.-K., 1979, Quantitative correlation of ethanol elimination rates *in vivo* with liver alcohol dehydrogenase activities in fed, fasted and food-restricted rats, *Biochem. Pharmacol.* **28**:1547–1551.

14. von Wartburg, J. P., and Scharch, P. M., 1968, Atypical human liver alcohol dehydrogenase, *Ann. N. Y. Acad. Sci.* **151**:936.

15. von Wartburg, J. P., 1971, The metabolism of alcohol in normals and alcoholics: Enzymes, in: *The Biology of Alcoholism,* Vol. 1 (B. Kissin and H. Begleiter, eds.), pp. 63–102, Plenum Press, New York.

16. Goebell, H., and Bode, C., 1971, Influence of ethanol and protein deficiency on the activity of alcohol dehydrogenase in the rat liver, in: *Metabolic Changes Induced by Alcohol* (G. A. Martini and C. Bode, eds.), pp. 23–31, Springer-Verlag, Berlin.

17. Rachamin, G., MacDonald, J. A., Wahid, S., Clapp, J. L., Khanna, J. M., and Israel, Y., 1980, Modulation of alcohol dehydrogenase and ethanol metabolism by sex hormones in the spontaneously hypertensive rat, *Biochem. J.* **186:**483–490.
18. Meijer, A. J., Van Woerkom, T. C., Williamson, J. R., and Tager, J. M., 1975, Rate-limiting factors in the oxidation of ethanol by rat liver cells, *Biochem. J.* **150:**205–209.
19. Thurman, R. G., and Scholz, R., 1975, Effect of octanoate on ethanol metabolism, *Fed. Proc. Fed. Am. Soc. Exp. Biol.* **34:**634.
20. DeDuve, C., and Baudhuin, P., 1966, Peroxisomes (microbodies and related particles), *Physiol. Rev.* **46:**323–357.
21. Thurman, R. G., and Chance, B., 1969, Inhibition of catalase in perfused rat liver by sodium azide, *Ann. N. Y. Acad. Sci.* **168:**348–353.
22. Sies, H., and Chance, B., 1970, The steady state level of catalase compound I in isolated hemoglobin-free perfused rat liver, *FEBS Lett.* **11:**172–176.
23. Oshino, N., Chance, B., Sies, H., and Bücher, T., 1973, The role of H_2O_2 generation in perfused rat liver and the reaction of catalase compound I and hydrogen donors, *Arch. Biochem. Biophys.* **154:**117–131.
24. Chance, B., and Oshino, N., 1971, Kinetics and mechanisms of catalase in peroxisomes of the mitochondrial fraction, *Biochem. J.* **122:**225–233.
25. Nichols, P., and Schonbaum, G. R., 1963, Catalases, in: *The Enzymes,* 2nd ed. (P. D. Boyer, H. A. Lardy, and K. Myrback, eds.), pp. 147–225, Academic Press, New York.
26. Shore, J. D., and Theorell, H., 1966, A kinetic study of ternary complexes in the mechanism of action of liver alcohol dehydrogenases, *Arch. Biochem. Biophys.* **116:**255–260.
27. Orme-Johnson, W. H., and Ziegler, D. M., 1965, Alcohol mixed-function oxidase activity of mammalian liver microsomes, *Biochem. Biophys. Res. Commun.* **21:**78–84.
28. Imai, Y., and Sato, R., 1967, Studies on the substrate interactions with P-450 in drug hydroxylation by liver microsomes, *J. Biochem. (Tokyo)* **62:**239–249.
29. Lieber, C. S., and DeCarli, L. M., 1970, Hepatic microsomal ethanol-oxidizing system *in vitro:* Characteristics and adaptive properties *in vivo, J. Biol. Chem.* **245:**2505–2512.
30. Lieber, C. S., 1976, The metabolism of alcohol, *Sci. Am.* **234**(3):25–33.
31. Koop, D. R., Morgan, E. T., Tarr, G. E., and Coon, M. J., 1982, Purification and characterization of a unique isoenzyme of cytochrome P-450 from liver microsomes of ethanol-treated rabbits, *J. Biol. Chem.* **257:**13,951–13,957.
32. Thurman, R. G., Ley, H. G., and Scholz, R., 1972, Hepatic microsomal ethanol oxidation: Hydrogen peroxide formation and the role of catalase, *Eur. J. Biochem.* **25:**420–430.
33. Isselbacher, K. J., and Carter, E. A., 1970, Ethanol oxidation by liver microsomes: Evidence against a separate and distinct enzyme system, *Biochem. Biophys. Res. Commun.* **39:**530–537.
34. Burnett, K. G., and Felder, M. R., 1980, Ethanol metabolism in *Peromyscus* genetically deficient in alcohol dehydrogenase, *Biochem. Pharmacol.* **29:**125–130.
35. Hawkins, R., and Khanna, J. M., 1966, Effect of chronic intake of ethanol on rate of ethanol metabolism, *Can. J. Physiol. Pharmacol.* **44:**241–257.
36. Mendelson, J., and Mello, N. K., 1966, Experimental analysis of drinking behavior of chronic alcoholics, *Ann. N. Y. Acad. Sci.* **133:**828–845.
37. Videla, L., Bernstein, J., and Israel, Y., 1973, Metabolic alteration produced in the liver by chronic alcohol administration: Increased oxidative capacity, *Biochem. J.* **134:**507–514.
38. Thurman, R. G., McKenna, W. R., and McCaffrey, T. B., 1976, Pathways responsible for the adaptive increase in ethanol utilization following chronic treatment with ethanol: Inhibitor studies with the hemoglobin-free perfused rat liver, *Mol. Pharmacol.* **12:**156–166.
39. Thurman, R. G., and Scholz, R., 1977, Interactions of glycolysis and respiration in perfused rat liver: Changes in O_2 uptake following addition of ethanol, *Eur. J. Biochem.* **75:**13–21.

40. Iturriaga, H., Ugarte, G., and Israel, Y., 1980, Hepatic vein oxygenation, liver blood flow, and the rate of ethanol metabolism in recently abstinent alcoholic patients, *Eur. J. Clin. Invest.* **10:**211–218.

41. Yuki, T., and Thurman, R. G., 1980, Swift increase in alcohol metabolism: Time course and involvement of glycolysis, *Biochem. J.* **186:**119.

42. Wendell, G. D., and Thurman, R. G., 1979, Effect of ethanol concentration on rates of ethanol elimination in normal and alcohol-treated rats *in vivo, Biochem. Pharmacol.* **28:**273–279.

43. Bernstein, J., Videla, L., and Israel, Y., 1974, Hormonal influences in the development of the hypermetabolic state of the liver produced by chronic administration of ethanol, *J. Pharmacol. Exp. Ther.* **192:**583–591.

44. Sutherland, E. W., Oye, I., and Butcher, R. W., 1965, The action of epinephrine and the role of the adenyl cyclase system in hormone action, *Recent Prog. Horm. Res.* **21:**623–646.

45. Israel, Y., Videla, L., MacDonald, A., and Bernstein, J., 1973, Metabolic alterations produced in the liver by chronic alcohol administration. III. Comparison between the effects produced by ethanol and by thyroid hormones, *Biochem. J.* **134:**523–529.

46. Yuki, T., Thurman, R. G., Schwabe, U., and Scholz, R., 1980, Metabolic changes after prior treatment with ethanol: Evidence against an involvement of the $Na^+ + K^+$-activated ATPase in the increase in ethanol metabolism, *Biochem. J.* **186:**997–1000.

47. Rawat, A. K., and Lundquist, F., 1968, Influence of thyroxine on the metabolism of ethanol and glycerol in rat liver slices, *Eur. J. Biochem.* **5:**13–17.

48. Fleckenstein, A., Kammermeier, H., Döring, H., and Freund, H. J., 1967, Zum Wirkungsmechanismus neuartiger Koronardiktatoren mit gleichzeitig Sauerstoff-einsparenden Myokardeffekten, Prenylomin und Prorenatid, *Z. Kreislaufforsch* **56:**716–744 and 839–835.

49. Peck, R. C., and Lefer, A. M., 1981, Protective effect of Nifedipine in the hypoxic perfused rat liver, *Agents Actions* **11:**421–424.

50. Trump, F. G., and Arstila, A. U., 1975, Cell members and disease processes, in: *Pathobiology of Cell Membranes* (F. G. Trump and A. U. Arstila, eds.), pp. 1–103, Academic Press, New York.

51. Farber, J. L., and Young, E. E., 1981, Accelerated phospholipid degradation in anoxic rat hepatocytes, *Arch. Biochem. Biophys.* **211:**312–320.

52. Jewell, S. A., Bellomo, G., Thor, H., Orrenius, S., and Smith, M. T., 1982, Bleb formation in hepatocytes during drug metabolism is caused by disturbances in thiol and calcium ion homeostatis, *Science* **207:**1257–1259.

53. Poole-Wilson, P. A., Harding, D., Bourdillion, P., and Fleetwood, G., 1982, Mechanism of myocardial protection through Ca^{+2} blocade, in: *Protection of Tissues against Hypoxia* (A. Wauquier, ed.), pp. 351–364, Elsevier, Amsterdam.

53a. Lemasters, J. J., Stemkowski, C. J., Ji, S., and Thurman, R. G., 1983, Cell surface changes and enzyme release during hypoxia and reoxygenation in the isolated, perfused rat liver, *J. Cell Biol.* **97:**778–786.

54. Krough, A., 1918, The number and distribution of capillaries in muscles with calculations of the oxygen pressure head necessary for supplying the tissue, *J. Physiol. (London)* **52:**409–415.

55. Kessler, M., Höper, J., Lübbers, D. W., and Ji, S., 1981, Local factors affecting regulation of microflow, O_2 uptake and energy metabolism, *Adv. Physiol. Sci.* **25:**155–162.

56. Kessler, M., Höper, J., and Kramel, B. A., 1976, Tissue perfusion and cellular function, *Anaesthesiol* **45:**186–199.

57. Chance, B., Mayevsky, A., Goodwin, C., and Mela, L., 1974, Factors in oxygen delivery to tissue, *Microvasc. Res.* **8:**276–282.

58. Chance, B., Cohen, P., Jöbsis, F., and Schoener, B., 1962, Intracellular oxidation–reduction states *in vivo:* The microfluorometry of pyridine nucleotide gives a continuous measurement of the oxidation state, *Science* **137:**1–10.

59. Chance, B., 1965, Reaction of oxygen with the respiratory chain in cells and tissues, *Gen. Physiol.* **49**:163–188.

60. Chance, B., Barlow, C., Haselgrove, J., Nakase, Y., Quistorff, B., Matschinsky, F., and Mayevsky, A., 1978, Microheterogeneities of redox states of perfused and intact organs, in: *Microenvironments and Metabolic Compartmentation* (P. A. Srere and R. W. Estabrook, eds.), pp. 131–148, Academic Press, New York.

61. Matschinsky, F. M., Hintz, C. S., Reichlmeier, K., Quistorff, B., and Chance, B., 1978, The intralobular distribution of oxidized and reduced pyridine nucleotides in the liver of normal and diabetic rats, in: *Microenvironments and Metabolic Compartmentation* (P. A. Srere and R. W. Estabrook, eds.), pp. 149–166, Academic Press, New York.

62. Tamura, M., Oshino, N., Chance, B., and Silver, I., 1978, Optical measurements of intracellular oxygen concentration of rat heart *in vivo*, *Arch. Biochem. Biophys.* **191**:8–22.

63. Oshino, N., Jamieson, D., and Chance, B., 1975, Optical measurements of the catalase–hydrogen peroxide intermediate (compound I) in the liver of anaesthetized rats and its implication to hydrogen peroxide production *in situ*, *Biochem. J.* **146**:53–65.

64. Sies, H., 1978, Cytochrome oxidase and urate oxidase as intracellular O_2 indicators in studies of O_2 gradients during hypoxia in liver, *Adv. Exp. Med. Biol.* **94**:561–566.

65. Jones, D. P., and Mason, H. S., 1978, Gradients of O_2 concentration in hepatocytes, *J. Biol. Chem.* **253**:4874–4880.

66. Israel, Y., Kalant, H., Orrego, H., Khanna, J. M., Videla, L., and Phillips, J. M., 1975, Experimental alcohol-induced hepatic necrosis: Suppression by propylthiouracil, *Proc. Natl. Acad. Sci. U.S.A.* **72**:1137–1141.

67. Ji, S., Lemasters, J. J., Christenson, V., and Thurman, R. G., 1982, Periportal and pericentral pyridine nucleotide fluorescence from the surface of the perfused liver: Evaluation of the hypothesis that chronic treatment with ethanol produces pericentral hypoxia, *Proc. Natl. Acad. Sci. U.S.A.* **79**:5415–5419.

68. Lemasters, J. J., Ji, S., and Thurman, R. G., 1981, Centrilobular injury following hypoxia in isolated, perfused rat liver, *Science* **213**:661–663.

69. Belinsky, S. A., Popp, J. A., Kauffman, F. C., and Thurman, R. G., 1984, Trypan blue uptake as a new method to study zonal hepatotoxicity in the perfused liver, *J. Pharmacol. Exp. Ther.* **230**:755–760.

70. Israel, Y., Walfish, P. G., Orrego, H., Blake, J., and Kalant, H., 1979, Thyroid hormones in alcoholic liver disease, *Gastroenterology* **76**:116–122.

71. Hallé, P., Paré, P., and Kapstein, E., 1982, Double-blind, controlled trial of propylthiouracil in patients with severe acute alcoholic hepatitis, *Gastroenterology* **82**:925–931.

72. Szilagyi, A., Lerman, S., and Resnick, R. S., 1983, Ethanol, thyroid hormones and acute liver injury: Is there a relationship?, *Hepatology* **3**:593–600.

Chapter 13

Biotransformation and Zonal Toxicity

Ronald G. Thurman, Frederick C. Kauffman, and Jeffrey Baron

1. ZONAL TOXICITY

1.1. General Considerations

1.1.1. Introduction

Hepatotoxins are ubiquitous in nature. Chemical injury to the liver is dependent on the nature of the hepatotoxic agent and the circumstances of exposure (for a comprehensive review, see Zimmerman[1]). Products of plant, fungal, and bacterial metabolism, minerals,[2–4] chemicals and pharmaceuticals, industrial by-products, and waste materials can damage the liver.[5] The types of hepatic injury that result from exposure to hepatotoxins are quite diverse. Some agents cause necrosis, fat accumulation, cirrhosis, or carcinoma,[2] while others interfere with bile secretion, cause jaundice, and produce little or no injury to hepatocytes.[2,5] Exposure to hepatotoxins can be encountered under a variety of conditions.

RONALD G. THURMAN • Department of Pharmacology, School of Medicine, University of North Carolina at Chapel Hill, North Carolina 27514.   FREDERICK C. KAUFFMAN • Department of Pharmacology and Experimental Therapeutics, University of Maryland School of Medicine, Baltimore, Maryland 21201.   JEFFREY BARON • The Toxicology Center, Department of Pharmacology, The University of Iowa College of Medicine, Iowa City, Iowa 52242.

Some natural toxins, such as the pyrolidizine alkaloids, the toxin of the cycad nut, and other phytotoxins or mycotoxins, may be ingested in ignorance[3,5] or because of cultural practices. Domestic exposure to toxins may also occur either by contamination of food through careless storage or production or by accidental ingestion of solvents such as carbon tetrachloride.[5,6] Environmental contamination by industrial by-products and waste and by insecticides poses a serious threat to man and domestic animals if these contaminants are incorporated into the food chain. Hepatotoxic agents are sometimes encountered in the course of industrial operations, notably the chlorinated hydrocarbons and vinyl chloride.[7] Still another form of exposure results when toxic agents are synthesized within the body (e.g., "autogenic" hepatotoxicity). There is growing concern that contamination of livestock feed and preservation of food with nitrites[8,9] may lead to the formation of nitrosamines by intestinal bacteria with subsequent exposure *in vivo* to potent hepatotoxic and hepatocarcinogenic compounds.

Probably the most important factor that determines the susceptibility of the liver to chemical injury is its role in the metabolism of foreign compounds.[10] Although the metabolic transformation of xenobiotics by the liver has traditionally been considered a detoxification pathway, many inert chemicals are often converted into toxic products by the liver. Indeed, it appears that most hepatotoxins and hepatocarcinogens must be activated to a toxic[11,12] or carcinogenic metabolite[13] to exert their effects. For example, bromobenzene,[12] carbon tetrachloride,[11] dimethylnitrosamine,[14] and allyl compounds[15] are all toxic to the liver only after biotransformation to active metabolites.

Hepatotoxins have been classified as either intrinsic or idiosyncratic.[1] With intrinsic toxins, hepatotoxicity is predictable and is characterized by a high incidence, dose-dependence, experimental reproducibility, and a short latency period. In contrast, idiosyncratic agents produce toxicity only in susceptible individuals; their toxic effects result more from the vulnerability of the affected individual, presumably for genetic reasons, than from any inherent toxicity of the agent itself. Idiosyncratic toxicity occurs rarely and is unpredictable. One example of idiosyncratic toxicity involves the drug isoniazid; subjects who are "rapid acetylators" were found to be more susceptible to hepatic injury seen after administration of this agent.[16]

There are three major categories of hepatic injury, and they are classified on the basis of the perturbations induced. Cytotoxic injury results from damage to functional or structural components of the hepatocyte that are responsible for maintaining cellular integrity. Cholestatic injury, expressed mainly as arrested bile flow with little or no injury to the hepatocyte, results from interference with energy sources and key molecular components that are essential for bile formation and flow. Alteration of the genetic machinery (DNA, RNA) of the cell by mutagens and carcinogens represents the third type of hepatic injury. The majority of intrinsic toxins produce mainly cytotoxic and genotoxic injury.

Hepatotoxins produce either necrosis or steatosis of hepatocytes. Hepatic necrosis may be zonal, massive, or diffuse. In general, intrinsic hepatotoxins induce toxicity within specific zones of the liver lobule. Toxins may affect the central, midzonal, or periportal area of the liver lobule exclusively. Necrosis within centrilobular regions is characteristic of chemicals such as carbon tetra-chloride, chloroform, and bromobenzene, while periportal necrosis is observed with allyl alcohol, ferrous sulfate, and phosphorus.[1] A large number of agents such as acetamide, carbon disulfide, ethanol, and ethionine produce fatty liver.[1] Some toxins cause fat to accumulate only in specific zones of the liver lobule. For example, ethionine leads primarily to fat accumulation in the periportal zone,[2] while ethanol causes fat to accumulate largely within pericentral areas.[17]

1.1.2. Proposed Mechanisms of Hepatotoxins

Despite considerable work over the last decade, the precise molecular mech-anism of hepatotoxicity induced by drugs or chemicals is unknown. The path-ogenesis of steatosis is thought to result from disruption of processes involved in the synthesis and transfer of triglycerides from the liver. Normal movement of triglycerides out of the liver involves coupling acyl-CoA compounds with apoprotein and phospholipids to form very-low-density lipoproteins.[18] Trigly-cerides are formed in the liver from fatty acids that are either stored in the body, absorbed from the gut, or synthesized in the liver.[18] Steatosis most likely results from impaired egress of triglycerides from the liver either by interference with the formation of very-low-density lipoproteins[18,19] or by defective movement of the lipoprotein across damaged plasma membranes.[19] Inhibition of β-oxidation by toxins has also been attributed to the development of fatty liver.[17]

The mechanisms by which chemical agents produce necrosis remain unclear. Early studies attributed pericentral necrosis induced by carbon tetrachloride to anoxia secondary to decreased hepatic sinusoidal blood flow.[20] However, sub-sequent experiments demonstrated that pericentral perfusion remained unim-paired until necrosis had occurred.[21,22] Subcellular organelles such as mito-chondria,[22] lysosomes,[23] and endoplasmic reticulum[11] have been implicated as primary sites of injury. Recent studies directed toward determining the role of the plasma membrane in the pathogenesis of hepatic necrosis have shown that many hepatotoxins, including carbon tetrachloride,[24] phalloidin,[25] and galacto-samine,[26] damage the plasma membrane. Farber and El-Mofty[26] have hypoth-esized that damage to the plasma membrane leads to an intracellular accumulation of calcium ion that in turn enhances plasma membrane injury. This permits more calcium ion to enter and leads ultimately to necrosis. In contrast, Smith et al.[27] have presented data suggesting that toxic injury to hepatocytes is not dependent on extracellular calcium.

Several theories exist to explain the molecular basis for membrane injury. Carbon tetrachloride is thought to enhance peroxidation of lipids,[11] while phalloidin may produce injury to the plasma membrane by reacting with specific receptors.[25] In addition, alkylation of macromolecules[28] has also been proposed as a mechanism by which a number of toxins disrupt plasma membranes. Additional work is required to establish the precise sequence of events that lead to either massive or zonal necrosis by any hepatotoxin or hepatocarcinogen. To study zone-specific damage, methods are needed that allow metabolic events to be monitored in periportal and pericentral regions of the liver lobule after acute or chronic exposure to hepatotoxins. Information on the distribution of isoenzymes and metabolites has been obtained from classic histochemistry, immunohistochemistry, and autoradiography. The recent development of micro-light guides and miniature oxygen electrodes by Thurman, Ji, Lemasters, and Matsumura[29–31] allows metabolic processes to be studied in distinct regions of the liver lobule in the intact organ (see Chapter 7).

1.2. Agents That Cause Damage in Periportal Regions of the Liver Lobule

Allyl compounds, ferrous sulfate, and phosphorus damage only periportal areas. The oxidation of allyl alcohol has been shown to require NAD^+-linked alcohol dehydrogenase.[32] Using liver homogenates and isolated mitochondria, Serafini-Cessi[33] demonstrated that allyl alcohol was converted into acrolein, an aldehyde that can be subsequently oxidized to acrylic acid by aldehyde dehydrogenase.[34] Acrolein is a reactive intermediate that may account for hepatotoxicity caused by allyl alcohol[33,35]; however, only 5% of added allyl alcohol is converted to acrolein by liver homogenates.[33] Since metabolism of allyl alcohol *in vitro* occurred at very low rates and alcohol dehydrogenase was thought to be greatest in periportal regions of the lobule,[36,37] the hypothesis was advanced that metabolism of allyl alcohol to acrolein occurred exclusively in periportal regions, and this accounted for the selective damage to these regions.

Recently, Belinsky *et al.*[38] showed that a linear correlation exists between rates of allyl alcohol uptake and increases in NADH fluorescence measured with a large-tipped light guide. They used this relationship to determine rates of allyl alcohol metabolism from fluorescence changes detected in periportal and pericentral regions with micro-light guides. The increase in NADH fluorescence due to infusion of 150 μM allyl alcohol was larger in pericentral than in periportal regions of the liver lobule during both anterograde and retrograde perfusions, indicating that the capacity to metabolize allyl alcohol in the intact liver is slightly greater in pericentral regions of the liver lobule. Since allyl alcohol is metabolized in both periportal and pericentral regions of the liver lobule, the hypothesis that the zone-specific hepatotoxicity of allyl alcohol results from its exclusive metabolism to acrolein only in periportal regions of the liver lobule seems unlikely.

Thus, some other factor(s) unique to either the periportal or pericentral regions must account for the zonal toxicity.

One possibility is that uptake of allyl alcohol *in vivo* occurs mainly in periportal regions (i.e., the regions of the liver lobule first exposed to flow). This notion is also unlikely, because the concentration of allyl alcohol leaving the perfused liver (i.e., vena cava) 30 min following injection of a necrogenic dose of allyl alcohol is about one half of that entering via the portal circulation.[38]

Results of previous studies indicate that acrolein, but not allyl alcohol, inhibited succinate-linked oxygen uptake in isolated mitochondria.[32] Furthermore, when mitochondria were isolated from rats 1 hr after intraperitoneal injection of allyl alcohol, a marked inhibition of oxygen uptake was observed. Addition of glutathione and dithiothreitol to the incubation mixture completely protected mitochondrial respiration from inhibition by acrolein.[32] Since histological changes were not seen in these livers until 1 hr after allyl alcohol poisoning, biochemical alterations induced by this toxin are likely due to generation of the highly reactive aldehyde acrolein. When local rates of oxygen uptake were measured using miniature oxygen electrodes placed on periportal and pericentral regions of the liver, allyl alcohol diminished oxygen uptake selectively in periportal regions. Rates of oxygen uptake were 3 times greater in periportal than in pericentral regions,[39] possible due to more condensed mitochondria in that region. Therefore, the mitochondrial respiratory chain in the periportal cells may be more sensitive to the toxic effects of acrolein.

The carcinogen N-hydroxy-2-acetyl aminofluorene (N-OH AAF) is also hepatotoxic to cells in the periportal region of the liver lobule.[40] This effect can be prevented by pentachlorophenol and 2,6-dichloro-4-nitrophenol (DCNP), agents that inhibit sulfation.[41] Sulfation has been implicated in the carcinogenic effects of N-OH AAF[42]; however, it is not known whether or not the cytotoxic effects of N-OH AAF are involved in the carcinogenic action of N-OH AAF.

1.3. Agents That Cause Damage in Pericentral Regions of the Liver Lobule

1.3.1. Carbon Tetrachloride

Haloalkanes, with some exceptions, all appear to produce either steatosis or necrosis within pericentral regions of the liver lobule. A comprehensive review of the vast literature on haloalkane hepatotoxicity is beyond the scope of this chapter. Readers are referred to some excellent reviews.[43–45] A few of the salient details are presented below.

The hepatotoxicity of haloalkanes is inversely proportional to the chain length and directly proportional to the number of halogen atoms and their atomic number (e.g., $BrCl_3C > CCl_4 > CHCl_3$).[46]

Detailed work over the past 30 years has shown that pericentral hypoxia and the release of catecholamines are not major components of the mechanism of CCl_4 hepatotoxicity.[1] This conclusion rests in large part on the observation that $CHCl_3$ is toxic to the isolated, perfused liver, in which altered blood flow and autonomic factors are not present.[47] It is now generally accepted that CCl_4 is metabolized reductively to the CCl_3^- radical via microsomal cytochrome P-450,[48-49] In fact, many species, sex, and age differences in CCl_4 susceptibility are probably due to differences in cytochrome P-450 levels. For example, phenobarbital and DDT, agents that induce specific cytochrome P-450 isoenzymes, both potentiate hepatotoxicity due to CCl_4. Small doses of CCl_4 apparently protect the liver from larger toxic doses by destroying cytochrome P-450.[44]

CCl_3^- radicals presumably react with oxygen to form highly toxic peroxyl radicals ($CCl_3O_3^-$) that initiate lipid peroxidation. Lipid peroxidation of the endoplasmic reticulum occurs within minutes, and there is a decrease in unsaturated fatty acids within 1 hr.[44] The stimulation of malondialdehyde production by CCl_4 is proportional to the $\sqrt{CCl_4}$, a dependency often characteristic of free-radical processes. It suggests that CCl_4 is metabolized to a free-radical initiator of lipid peroxidation.[45] Early consequences of these changes are inactivation of the microsomal Ca^{++} pump and depletion of cellular NADPH. The oxidation–reduction state of thiols may be a key factor, since cystine and cysteine can block CCl_4-induced toxicity.[1] The ultimate cause of necrosis, however, remains to be elucidated. Potentiation of CCl_4-induced necrosis by acute alcohol treatment[55] and fasting[2,7,55] also remains unexplained.

It is generally accepted that CCl_4 increases fat in the liver by decreasing lipoprotein export; however, it is not clear why this occurs predominantly in pericentral regions of the liver lobule.

1.3.2. Acetaminophen

Acetaminophen is a mild analgesic that in therapeutic doses is quite safe, but at high doses is a potent hepatotoxin. At usual therapeutic doses, acetaminophen is largely converted to harmless glucuronides and sulfates, with only a small fraction being converted to a reactive imidoquinone.[56] At higher doses, greater amounts of the active metabolite are formed and bind with macromolecules or intracellular glutathione (GSH) and are then converted into a mercapturic acid. When GSH is depleted by more than 85%, covalent binding to tissue proteins increases.[56] Necrosis is ultimately observed in the area of greatest binding; however, a clear link between binding of the electrophile and necrosis is still lacking. Toxicity is potentiated by depletion of GSH. One possible explanation for the pericentral locus of acetaminophen action may be related to the lower content of GSH in that region of the liver lobule.[286]

2. MIXED-FUNCTION OXIDATION

2.1. General Considerations

2.1.1. Introduction

Considerable progress has been made in the identification of the sequence of events involved in operation of the mixed-function oxidase system. The three major components consist of NADPH-cytochrome P-450 reductase, cytochrome P-450, and phospholipid, which are components of the membranes of the endoplasmic reticulum. Many cytochromes (e.g., at least six in rabbit liver) are present for each flavoprotein, and this may account for the wide substrate specificity of the mixed-function oxidase system. Oxidation of compounds via this system involves the following sequence of events: An oxidized cytochrome binds the drug substrate, which is reduced by the flavoprotein in an NADPH-dependent reaction. This $P-450^{2+}$–drug complex then reacts with oxygen to form a $P-450^{2+}$–O_2–drug complex, which is further reduced by the second electron from NADPH. The breakdown of this second complex releases hydroxylated drug and water regenerates oxidized cytochrome P-450. Work that has led to elucidation of the foregoing sequence of events *in vitro* has been dealt with in a number of papers and reviews.[58-63]

In intact cells, the mixed-function oxidation system is intimately related to other cellular events involved in the generation of the reduced cofactor and the provision of activated biosynthetic intermediates needed for conjugation of oxidized products of this system. A scheme that illustrates some of the interactions that may occur is presented in Fig. 1. NADPH is generated by highly regulated multienzyme systems that exist in several intracellular compartments. For example, the major dehydrogenases of the pentose phosphate shunt are cytosolic, whereas fatty acid oxidation and the citric acid cycle are intramitochondrial. The former enzymes provide reducing equivalents in the cytosol directly, whereas the latter furnish substrates for malic enzyme and isocitrate dehydrogenase, which then form NADPH in the cytosol. Movement of reducing equivalents from the mitochondrial to the cytosolic space via specific substrates involves complex shuttle mechanisms. Until recently, scant attention has been given to interactions that occur between these systems and rates of mixed-function oxidation in whole cells.

There are at least four types of regulation that can be imposed on mixed-function oxidation in intact cells: induction, substrate and cofactor supply, activation and inhibition by effectors, and competing reactions. Competing reactions for substrates and cofactors (e.g., fatty acid synthesis) undoubtedly play a major role in determining the availability of NADPH for mixed-function oxidation in intact cells.

Induction of enzyme components is a generally slow form of regulation;

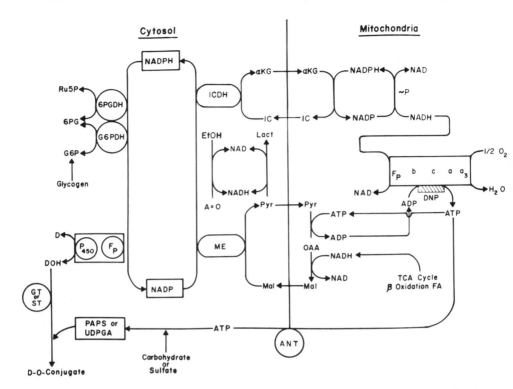

Figure 1. Interactions between drug and intermediary metabolism in intact cells. Cystolic reduced nicotinamide adenine dinucleotide phosphate (NADPH) may be generated by the pentose phosphate pathway in a series of reactions starting with glucose-6-phosphate (G6P) and involving the enzymes glucose-6-phosphate dehydrogenase (G6PDH) and 6-phosphogluconate dehydrogenase (6PGDH). In addition, cytosolic NADPH may be generated by a malate (Mal), egress of malate into the cytosol, and NADPH production via malic enzyme (ME). Alternatively, mitochondrial NADPH is generated by an energy (P)-requiring transhydrogenase that carries out the reduction of NADP$^+$ from NADH. A shuttle mechanism involving isocitrate dehydrogenase (ICDH) transfers hydrogen from NADPH to α-ketoglutarate (αkg) in the mitochondria and regenerates NADPH in the cytosol. Activated intermediates for conjugation reactions [e.g., adenosine 3'-phosphate 5'-phosphosulfate (PAPS) and uridine diphosphogalactase (UDPGA)] are formed from carbohydrate and sulfate in energy-dependent reactions. (IC) Isocitrate; (DNP) dinitrophenol; (GT) glucuronosyltransferase; (ST) sulfotransferase; (ANT) adenine nucleotide translocase; (D) drug substrate for cytochrome P-450; (DOH) hydroxylated product; (D-O-conjugate) conjugated hydroxydrug; (Ru5P) ribulose 5-phosphate; (6PG) 6-phosphogluconate; (Lact) lactate; (Pyr) pyruvate); (OAA) oxalacetate; (Fp) flavoprotein; (b, c, a, a$_3$) cytochromes b, c, a, and a_3.

however, under some conditions, it can occur in a few hours. In most cases, induction does not appear to be specific for components of the mixed-function oxidase system. For example, phenobarbital tends to induce several forms of cytochrome P-450,[64] glucuronyltransferase,[65] and several NADPH-generating enzymes as well.[66,67]

A second form of regulation involves the supply of substrate and cofactor. Diffusion of oxygen, transport of a drug to binding sites on cytochrome P-450, and delivery of NADPH to the flavoprotein may be rate-controlling. Of these three possibilities, regulation via the supply of reduced cofactor may be the most important, since maintenance of the oxidation–reduction state of the NADP : NADPH couple is a highly regulated process in intact cells. NADPH is formed in the cytosol via oxidation of substrates for intermediary metabolism such as glucose-6-phosphate, malate, and isocitrate. This cofactor may also arise in the mitochondrial space via transhydrogenation. Reactions that compete for reduced cofactor must be taken into account in explaining regulation of mixed-function oxidation in whole cells. In addition to fatty acid synthesis, reduction of oxidized glutathione is another reaction recognized to compete for NADPH. At the cytochrome P-450 level, substrates that compete for binding sites include a wide array of xenobiotics as well as endogenous substrates such as steroid hormones, vitamin D, bilirubin, fatty acids, and prostaglandins.

Modulation of rates of drug oxidation by small molecules derived from intermediary metabolism is a subject that has not been extensively studied. However, this form of regulation is suggested by strong inhibition of NADPH-generating enzymes and NADPH-cytochrome c reductase by ATP.[66] Interactions of this nature suggest that the generation of reducing equivalents and their utilization for mixed-function oxidation and conjugation may be regulated in a concerted manner in intact cells.

Alteration of the formation of specific intermediates such as NADPH and activated substrates used in conjugation reactions provides mechanisms whereby nutritional and endocrine factors may regulate mixed-function oxidation in whole cells on both an acute and a chronic basis. The review by Campbell and Hayes[68] dealt at length with effects of nutritional factors on levels of the components of mixed-function oxidases; however, acute alterations of rates of drug metabolism and conjugation by nutritional factors that involve changes in substrate and cofactor supply had not been studied extensively at that time.

2.1.2. Regulation of Mixed-Function Oxidation in Intact Cells

Work under way in several laboratories has begun to provide insight into metabolic events that regulate mixed-function oxidation in whole cells. Factors that influence rates of drug oxidation in intact hepatocytes are reviewed below.

2.1.2a. Rate Control by NADPH Supply. Information on the catalytic properties of mixed-function oxidases *in vitro* suggests that a rate-controlling step in drug oxidation in microsomes is probably the reduction of cytochrome P-450.[58,69] In reconstituted mixed-function oxidase systems from phenobarbital-treated rabbits, the activity of the flavoprotein NADPH-cytochrome P-450 reductase appears not to be rate-limiting. Experiments with stopped-flow techniques indicate that the rate-limiting step *in vitro* is after the introduction of the second electron.[69–71]

Thus, factors that influence this activity in whole cells, such as NADPH supply, must be taken into account as determinants of rates of drug oxidation. It is important to point out that experiments *in vitro* differ markedly from physiological conditions in intact cells, in which NADPH is largely bound to various dehydrogenases.

Thurman and Scholz[72] showed that the respiration of the perfused liver from a fed rat is markedly increased on infusion of aminopyrine, a classic substrate for the mixed-function oxidation system. However, an increase was not observed when the experiment was performed in the liver of a fasted rat in the presence of an inhibitor of the mitochondrial respiratory chain, antimycin A. On the other hand, microsomes prepared from livers in these two metabolic states oxidized aminopyrine at similar rates[73] when supplied with an active NADPH-generating system, suggesting that NADPH supply is rate-controlling for mixed-function oxidation in intact cells. This conclusion is further supported by the observation that rates of *p*-nitroanisole O-demethylation by the perfused liver vary over a 3-fold range in different metabolic conditions even though cytochrome P-450 levels are constant.[74]

Recently, more support for the hypothesis that NADPH supply is rate-controlling for mixed-function oxidation in the intact cell under some conditions has been forthcoming. When *p*-nitroanisole was infused into livers from normal well-fed rats or added to microsomes in the presence of NADPH, linear rates of *p*-nitrophenol production were observed. In contrast, high rates of *p*-nitrophenol production by perfused livers from phenobarbital-treated rats were linear for less than 2 min and then declined rapidly to about 25% of the control value. In this acute experiment, amounts of microsomal components did not change during perfusion when oxygen and *p*-nitroanisole were supplied in excess. While a small part of the decline in rate could be related to conjugation reactions, a decline in NADPH supply accounts for most of the decrease in rates of mixed-function oxidation in livers from fed, phenobarbital-treated rats. Further support for this hypothesis comes from the observation that the rate of mixed-function oxidation was directly correlated with $NADPH/NADP^+$ ratios calculated from substrates assumed to be in near equilibrium with malic enzyme and isocitrate dehydrogenase in three different metabolic states.[75]

2.1.2b. Relationship among Nutritional State, NADPH Supply, and Mixed-Function Oxidation. Campbell and Hayes[76] have stated:

> There is ample evidence that nutrition is a major determinant of drug action. First, abnormal intake of nearly every nutrient modified the activity of the liver microsomal system. Second, modest changes in nutrient intake can produce considerable differences in enzyme activity.

On a chronic basis, it is well established that nutrition can influence the rate of metabolism of foreign chemicals. Furthermore, comparisons of rates of mixed-function oxidation in different metabolic states show that mixed-function oxidation can be regulated acutely by diet. One explanation for this is the influence of diet on various sources of NADPH, because the K_m of cytochrome P-450 reductase for NADPH is of the same order of magnitude as concentrations of free NADPH in the cytosol.[66,77]

i. Pentose Phosphate Pathway. Results of several studies have demonstrated that rates of generation of reducing equivalents via the oxidative enzymes of the pentose phosphate shunt are sufficient to supply the NADPH required for mixed-function oxidation of a variety of substrates in liver.[78,79] With new methods, it has been shown that aminopyrine[80] and organic hydroperoxides[81] elevate the rate of formation of $^{14}CO_2$ from [1-^{14}C]glucose, which demonstrates that substrates for mixed-function oxidation and substances that enhance cytochrome P-450 turnover accelerate flux of sugar phosphates through the pentose phosphate shunt. In one study carried out in isolated hepatocytes, it was demonstrated that rates of pentose phosphate shunt activity provide NADPH at rates in excess of rates of mixed-function oxidation.[78]

It is clear that $NADP^+$ activates and NADPH inhibits activity of the pentose phosphate shunt. Also, the pentose phosphate shunt is stimulated by oxidized glutathione,[82] which is released from perfused liver by aminopyrine.[83] Thus, during high rates of mixed-function oxidation, generation of reducing equivalents via the pentose phosphate shunt in the fed state in which carbohydrate reserves are high would be expected to be accelerated. This possibility is supported by the finding that oxidation of p-nitroanisole in perfused livers from fed animals is accompanied by significant increases in 6-phosphogluconate and ribulose-5-phosphate.[67] It is noteworthy that induction of mixed-function oxidation in rat liver by phenobarbital and 3-methylcholanthrene is accompanied by significant increases in the activity of the oxidative enzymes of the pentose phosphate shunt.[67,84] Phenobarbital treatment also increased the concentration of ribulose-5-phosphate and xylulose-5-phosphate.[67] When these data are considered with a rise in lactate and a decline in fructose 1,6-diphosphate, they support the hypothesis that induction of mixed-function oxidation also increases the activity and carbon flux through the pentose phosphate shunt. This effect of phenobarbital to increase the capacity of the liver to produce reducing equivalents for mixed-function oxidation occurs both by induction of various oxidative enzymes and by alteration of the oxidation–reduction state of NADP.[66] Phenobarbital and 3-methylcholanthrene pretreatment cause the NADP couple to become more oxidized, and this favors increased flux through the pentose phosphate pathway. Such actions may be as significant as the well-known induction of cytochrome P-450 in enhancing rates of mixed-function oxidation in intact cells.

6-Aminonicotinamide, a diabetogen, markedly inhibited metabolism via the oxidative enzymes of the pentose phosphate pathway in the perfused liver from well-fed rats, but did not diminish p-nitroanisole O-demethylation.[66] Under these conditions, 6-phosphogluconate increased over 700-fold in the tissue.[75] Thus, under conditions in which pentose phosphate shunt activity was markedly diminished, mixed-function oxidation was not inhibited. Surprisingly, 6-aminonicotinamide caused a reduction of cytoplasmic $NADP^+$. At present, no explanation exists for this interesting and unexpected observation. One possibility, however, is that 6-aminonicotinamide treatment activates alternative sources of NADPH generation.

   ii. *Role of NADPH of Mitochondrial Origin.* Evidence has been acquired that NADPH formed within mitochondria supports drug metabolism even in the well-fed state. Over two-thirds of the hepatocellular NADPH is located in the mitochondrial space and is actually about -10 mV more reduced than the cytosolic pool.[85] Thus, a flow of reducing equivalents from the mitochondrial to the cytosolic space will occur based simply on thermodynamic considerations. Second, as mentioned above, inhibition of the pentose phosphate shunt in well-fed[66,75] or fasted[74] livers with 6-aminonicotinamide did not diminish rates of *p*-nitrophenol production. Third, rates of mixed-function oxidation in perfused livers[73] or isolated hepatocytes were diminished only slightly by fasting. Fasting depleted glycogen content to less than 2% of control values in 24 hr and markedly diminished activity of the pentose shunt.

   The fasted state is characterized by a lack of substrate for the pentose phosphate shunt.[86] In this condition, mixed-function oxidation, as reflected by oxygen uptake on addition of aminopyrine[72] or hexobarbital,[87] is abolished by inhibitors of mitochondrial oxidations. Thus, mitochondrial oxidations must be major sources of reducing equivalents in the fasted state. Both maximal rates and kinetics of *p*-nitroanisole O-demethylation differed in various metabolic states.[75,88] Maximal rates of drug metabolism were greatest in livers from fasted and refed rats, somewhat lower in livers from fed rats, and slowest in livers from fasted rats. Livers from fasted animals had the ability to sustain elevated rates of mixed-function oxidation for much longer time periods than livers from fed or fasted–refed animals. Further, the rate of decline of *p*-nitroanisole O-demethylation was less in livers from fasted rats than in livers from either of the other two groups.

   Carbohydrate reserves differ in the three metabolic states compared above. Fasted–refed livers contain large stores of glycogen, fed livers contain intermediate stores, and the fasted liver contains only 1–2% of the glycogen present in the fed state.[86] It is unlikely that an intermediate of carbohydrate metabolism such as glucose-6-phosphate has a predominant role in sustaining high rates of mixed-function oxidation, because there was an inverse relationship between the duration of high rates and carbohydrate reserves. Thus, it is difficult to ascribe a major role to the pentose phosphate shunt in providing reducing equivalents for drug oxidations. Further, rates of mixed-function oxidation declined in the presence of high rates of glucose production.[88] The failure of glucose to stimulate *p*-nitroanisole O-demethylation in livers from fed animals, even though ATP levels were sufficient to allow phosphorylation of the sugar,[67] suggests that generation of reducing equivalents from carbohydrate oxidation is not rate-limiting for mixed-function oxidation in the fed state.

It is not altogether clear how reducing equivalents generated in the mitochondrial space move into the extramitochondrial space to support mixed-function oxidation. First, mitochondrial membranes are impermeable to pyridine nucleotides.[89] Also, the citric acid cycle and β-oxidation generate NADH from the oxidation of acetyl-CoA and acyl-CoA, respectively. However, the mixed-function oxidation system functions with highest efficiency when NADPH is the cofactor. Mitochondria can transform NADH into NADPH via an energy-dependent transhydrogenase. Energization of the mitochondria has a profound effect on this reaction and drives it in the direction of NADPH while inhibiting the reverse reaction. Energization drives the apparent equilibrium constant for the transhydrogenase from near unity to about 500 in the direction of NADPH formation.[90] The transhydrogenase is inhibited by acyl-CoA compounds.[91] Further support for the possibility that mitochondria serve as sources of reducing equivalents is the finding that oxidation of aminopyrine by liver slices was stimulated by citric-acid-cycle intermediates.[92,93]

Little information on the role of the transhydrogenase in supplying reducing equivalents for mixed-function oxidation is available. Hoeck and Ernster[90] demonstrated that the energy-linked transhydrogenase was highly sensitive to carbonyl cyanide p-trifluoromethylphenylhydrazone (FCCP), and uncouplers of oxidative phosphorylation (dinitrophenol and FCCP) inhibit mixed-function oxidation of p-nitroanisole in perfused livers from fasted rats while not affecting activity of isolated microsomes.[94]

Another and perhaps more important mechanism for generating cytosolic NADPH from mitochondrial oxidations involves substrate shuttles. The subject of anion transport systems for moving reducing equivalents across the mitochondrial membrane has been reviewed extensively.[95] Two major hydrogen shuttle mechanisms have been proposed to move mitochondrial hydrogen into the cytoplasmic space. One shuttle mechanism involves $NADP^+$-dependent isocitrate dehydrogenases in the mitochondrial and extramitochondrial spaces. $NADP^+$-dependent enzymes are present in both spaces, whereas an NAD^+-dependent enzyme is present only as a component of the citric acid cycle in mitochondria.[96] This latter enzyme is a highly regulated, essentially nonequilibrium system.[97] Thus, mitochondrial NADPH but not NADH may be transported by the isocitrate:2-oxoglutarate shuttle. This location of isocitrate dehydrogenase is predominantly cytosolic,[98] and this activity in liver is higher than other $NADP^+$-dependent dehydrogenases.[67] The participation of the isocitrate:2-oxoglutarate shuttle in providing reducing equivalents for mixed-function oxidation is supported by the finding that when ureagenesis was stimulated in isolated hepatocytes, rates of mixed-function oxidation were diminished slightly.[85] The authors concluded that NADPH of mitochondrial origin was diverted from the isocitrate:2-oxoglutarate shuttle to ureagenesis. There is further support for the involvement of the isocitrate: 2-oxoglutarate shuttle mechanism in mixed-function oxidation. First, ethanol inhibits the citric acid cycle and markedly lowers the intracellular concentrations of 2-oxoglutarate and isocitrate.[99] Ethanol also causes over a 50% inhibition of the O-demethylation of *p*-nitroanisole in the fed and fasted states that can be partially reversed with addition of aspartate or glutamate.[99] Second, in isolated hepatocytes from fed rats, the transaminase inhibitor aminoxyacetate had no effect on $^{14}CO_2$ production from [^{14}C]aminopyrine; however, the production of $^{14}CO_2$ was decreased about 30% in hepatocytes from fasted rats.[100]

Another energy-sensitive shuttle mechanism based on mitochondrial pyruvate carboxylase and malate dehydrogenase and an extramitochondrial malic enzyme has been proposed.[72] This shuttle mechanism differs from the isocitrate:2-oxoglutarate shuttle in that mitochondrial NADH rather than NADPH is the hydrogen donor. Thus, the energy-linked transhydrogenase is not necessary for reducing equivalents to be produced by this mechanism. With this shuttle mechanism, mitochondrial oxaloacetate accepts reducing equivalents from NADH. The malate formed diffuses into the cytosol, where it reacts with malic enzyme to form NADPH and pyruvate. Pyruvate then enters the mitochondria, and an energy-requiring carboxylation regenerates mitochondrial oxoaloacetate to complete the cycle. Substrates for mixed-function oxidation such as aminopyrine may divert malate carbon from the pathway of glucose synthesis in NADPH generation of drug oxidation.[101] As discussed above, aminopyrine was found to suppress maximal rates of glucose synthesis from lactate over 50% in perfused liver from phenobarbital-treated rats; however, submaximal rates of glucose formation with lactate or maximal rates with dihydroxyacetone were only slightly affected. These data suggest that active NADPH-utilizing processes such as the mixed-function oxidation of aminopyrine divert malate away from the pathway of gluconeogenesis for formation of NADPH via malic enzyme, and this leads to a compensatory influx through the pyruvate carboxylase reaction. Thus, gluconeogenesis is suppressed only when pyruvate carboxylation is maximal, indicating that the malic enzyme shuttle is functioning under gluconeogenic conditions in the presence of substrates from mixed-function oxidation.

2.1.2c. Relationship between Energy Metabolism and Mixed-Function Oxidation. There is a small body of information that suggests that an indirect and possibly regulatory role exists between energy metabolism and mixed-function oxidation. For example, a number of drug substrates or products of mixed-function oxidation can act as inhibitors or uncouplers of oxidative phosphorylation in the perfused liver (for a review, see Thurman *et al.*[102]) β-Adrenergic blocking agents (propranolol and alprenolol) have been shown to block mitochondrial respiration at the level of NADH oxidase.[103] Moreover, benzphetamine and its metabolite, norbenzphetamine, are potent uncouplers of oxidative phosphorylation. Conversely, substrates for mixed-function oxidation that decrease the ATP/adenosine diphosphate (ADP) ratio in the cell may actually stimulate their own metabolism.

Hexobarbital[69,104] and aminopyrine[67,100] oxidize cytosolic NADPH when they are metabolized; however, oxidation of NADPH with p-nitroanisole probably does not occur, even though high rates of mixed-function oxidation of this compound were observed in phenobarbital-treated rats. The oxidation of NADPH by aminopyrine could be blocked by addition of an uncoupling agent of oxidative phosphorylation, dinitrophenol.

Both p-nitroanisole alone and aminopyrine plus dinitrophenol uncoupled oxidative phosphorylation as reflected by decreased ATP/ADP ratios.[67] However, neither aminopyrine alone nor hexobarbital alone had any effect. Lowering of the ATP/ADP ratio may be a critical event, because both dehydrogenases of the pentose phosphate pathway[105–108] and isocitrate dehydrogenase and malic enzyme[66] are strongly inhibited by ATP. Inhibitor constants of ATP for the various NADPH-generating enzymes range from 9 μM for malic enzyme to 1.8 mM for glucose-6-phosphate dehydrogenase.[66] Thus, a decrease in the concentration of ATP in the liver by an agent that uncouples oxidative phosphorylation results in the activation of the metabolism of hexose phosphate, malate, and isocitrate, leading to enhanced NADPH generation. During the mixed-function oxidation of a drug such as hexobarbital, the rates of NADPH oxidation probably exceed the capacity of the liver to regenerate NADPH; therefore, the calculated NADP$^+$/NADPH ratio increases. When an uncoupling agent is either present (e.g., dinitrophenol) or generated (e.g., p-nitrophenol), the high capacity of the liver to form NADPH in livers from phenobarbital-treated rats via pentose phosphate, malic enzyme, and isocitrate dehydrogenase is greater, possibly due to a decline of ATP. The rate of NADPH generation may then be equal to or even exceed the rate of NADPH utilization. Thus, mixed-function oxidation of p-nitroanisole to p-nitrophenol leads to reduction of NADP$^+$ rather than to the expected oxidation of NADPH.

There are at least two examples of agents that lower ATP/ADP ratios and stimulate mixed-function oxidation. First, fructose is an active substrate for ketohexokinase and causes a rapid lowering of the ATP/ADP ratio.[66,109,110] The addition of fructose to perfused liver from phenobarbital-treated rats stimulated the O-demethylation of p-nitroanisole, and this was accompanied by a decrease in the NADP$^+$/NADPH ratio.[66] Second, pretreatment with 6-aminonicotinamide elevated p-nitroanisole O-demethylation slightly and lowered the calculated NADP$^+$/NADPH ratio.[75] 6-Aminonicotinamide treatment also caused a decrease in the ATP/ADP ratio.[66] Thus, these examples support the conclusion reached with the *in vitro* systems and suggest that toxic agents that alter the ATP/ADP ratio by inhibiting or uncoupling oxidative phosphorylation stimulate their own metabolism acutely and rapidly by increasing NADPH for the mixed-function oxidation system. Alteration in steady-state concentrations of pyridine and adenine nucleotides occurs rapidly over a period of a few minutes and thus represents a means whereby rates of mixed-function oxidation may be changed long before enzyme components of the system are induced. Zonal differences in regulation of these systems will be considered later in this chapter.

2.1.2d. *Effect of Ethanol.* Ethanol is an agent that has long been known to affect drug metabolism. Most reports indicate that ethanol inhibits drug metabolism. To understand ethanol–drug interactions clearly, it is important to relate ethanol oxidation in the cell to microsomal oxidations. Several papers and reviews have dealt with the controversy surrounding the mechanism of microsomal ethanol oxidation.[111–113] In summary, Orme-Johnson and Ziegler[114] first demonstrated that microsomes incubated with NADPH and oxygen were capable of converting ethanol in acetaldehyde. However, it is not known whether this is due to the direct oxidation of ethanol via cytochrome P-450 or to the action of H_2O_2 with catalase. It has been demonstrated that microsomes can generate H_2O_2.[115] A number of workers have failed to observe ethanol oxidation in purified, reconstituted mixed-function oxidases,[113,116,117] whereas others have observed it.[118,119] In the latter studies, however, the production of acetaldehyde was not accompanied by increases in consumption of either NADPH or oxygen, common requirements for classic mixed-function oxidation reactions.

While the mechanism of microsomal ethanol oxidation remains controversial, the effect of ethanol on mixed-function oxidation *in vitro* is clearer. In a review of this subject, Mezey[120] cited several reports in which it was shown that ethanol inhibited mixed-function oxidation *in vitro*. This action may be dependent on the substrate for mixed-function oxidation, because ethanol has been reported not to affect the metabolism of hexobarbital.[121] In general, very high concentrations of ethanol are required to inhibit drug metabolism *in vitro*. The mechanism for this inhibition is, in all likelihood, direct binding of ethanol to cytochrome P-450 and subsequent displacement of the drug substrate. This mechanism is unlikely to account for inhibition of drug metabolism in whole cells, because the binding constants of ethanol *in vitro* range between 0.5 and 1.3 M for microsomes[122] and the purified cytochrome P-450,[117] respectively. Concentrations of ethanol above 0.1 M are lethal in man. Moreover, *p*-nitroanisole O-demethylation in the perfused liver is half-maximally inhibited by 1–2 mM ethanol.[123] Rubin et al.[121] observed that meprobamate metabolism was inhibited by 10 mM ethanol in liver slices, and Grundin[124] reported that low concentrations of ethanol stimulated alprenolol oxidation in isolated hepatocytes, whereas 10 mM inhibited it. Similar effects of ethanol have been noted with *p*-nitroanisole O-demethylation. Reinke et al.[74,123] observed that low concentrations of ethanol first stimulated and then inhibited *p*-nitroanisole O-demethylation in perfused rat livers. The stimulation was observed only in livers from fasted rats, whereas the inhibition was present in both fed and fasted livers. Stimulation by ethanol corresponded directly to the effect on reduction of NAD^+. Other agents that reduced NAD^+, such as glucose, sorbitol, and xylitol,[125] stimulated *p*-nitroanisole O-demethylation in a manner similar to ethanol. These findings, along with the observation that inhibition of alcohol dehydrogenase by 4-methylpyrazole prevented stimulation by ethanol, suggest that NADH produced from ethanol in all likelihood interacts with NADH-cytochrome b_5 reductase to stimulate mixed-function oxidation in the whole organ in a fashion similar to that described for "NADH-synergism" in isolated microsomes.[126–129] The high amount of NADH formed from glycolysis in the fed state probably explains why infusion of ethanol does not stimulate mixed-function oxidation in this metabolic state. NADH-dependent mixed-function oxidation is probably activated maximally in the fed state.

In another series of experiments, Reinke et al.[74,130] showed that inhibition of mixed-function oxidation of p-nitroanisole by ethanol (K_i = 1–2 mM) was apparently due to acetaldehyde generated from ethanol oxidation. Acetaldehyde apparently enters the mitochondrial space and generates reducing equivalents via aldehyde dehydrogenase, which in turn inhibits the citric acid cycle and depletes key intermediates needed for the movement of reducing equivalents from the mitochondria into the cytosolic space. Evidence for this hypothesis is listed as follows: First, the ethanol inhibition was abolished by 4-methylpyrazole, an inhibitor of alcohol dehydrogenase. This indicates that the ethanol molecule per se is not responsible for the inhibition, but either NADH, acetaldehyde, NADH from acetaldehyde, or acetate is the causative agent. Since sorbitol and xylitol, agents that elevate the cytosolic NADH redox state, do not inhibit mixed-function oxidation, NADH of cytosolic origin can be ruled out as well. Changes in pyridine nucleotide and flavin oxidation–reduction state correlated well with the inhibition of mixed-function oxidation as the concentration of ethanol was increased. Acetaldehyde also inhibited p-nitroanisole O-demethylation at concentrations one to two orders of magnitude lower than those necessary to inhibit microsomal p-nitroanisole O-demethylation in vitro. During ethanol inhibition, levels of α-ketoglutarate and isocitrate declined markedly, possibly below the K_m values for transport of NADPH into the cytosol from the mitochondria via the isocitrate substrate shuttle mechanism, which suggests that ethanol acts to deplete intermediates necessary for this substrate shuttle. This conclusion is supported by the observations that aspartate and glutamate, amino acids that give rise to oxaloacetate and α-ketoglutarate in the cell, both partially reversed the inhibition of p-nitroanisole O-demethylation by ethanol. Taken together, these data strongly support the concept that ethanol interrupts the flow of NADPH of mitochondrial origin into the cytosol. Implicit in this conclusion is that mitochondrial NADPH plays an important role in the normal regulation of mixed-function oxidation in the hepatocyte.

Ethanol can also interact with mixed-function oxidation by inducing components of the drug-metabolizing system. Several groups[131–133] have demonstrated that chronic exposure of animals to ethanol leads to an increase in cytochrome P-450 levels. Often, this is cited as evidence that ethanol is a substrate for the mixed-function oxidase; however, other compounds that bind to cytochrome P-450 (e.g., barbital) but are not metabolized also induce microsomal components.

It has been suggested that the increase in the activity of the microsomal ethanol-oxidizing systems accounts for the well-documented[131] increase in ethanol metabolism after chronic exposure to ethanol in rodents or in man. This argument should be viewed with caution, however, since considerable evidence has accumulated to support the concept that microsomal ethanol oxidation, irrespective of its molecular mechanism, does not operate in whole cells. For example, carbon tetrachloride treatment markedly diminishes microsomal drug and ethanol metabolism, but does not affect the rate of ethanol elimination *in vivo*.[134] Similar conclusions can be drawn from experiments with menadione. Menadione stimulates microsomal H_2O_2 production, but does not alter the rate of ethanol uptake by the perfused rat liver.[116] Finally, Mezey[135] treated rats chronically with ethanol to induce cytochrome P-450 and accelerate the rate of ethanol elimination. However, when the treatment was terminated, ethanol elimination rates returned rapidly to control levels in 48 hr, whereas 2 weeks were required for the decay in elevated cytochrome P-450 levels as well as rates of microsomal ethanol oxidation. Thus, there appears to be no relationship between levels of microsomal mixed-function oxidase components and rates of ethanol elimination in intact cells.

2.2. Intralobular Distributions of Xenobiotic-Metabolizing Enzymes

As indicated above, the findings of numerous investigations conducted during the past several years have demonstrated conclusively that many hepatotoxins undergo metabolic activation before they damage the liver. These findings strongly suggest that metabolism is one of the major factors, if not the primary factor, giving rise to the relatively selective regional injuries that commonly occur within the liver lobule after *in vivo* exposure to a variety of hepatotoxins. The intrahepatic and intralobular distributions of hepatotoxins and differences in the uptake of a given hepatotoxin into cells across the lobule are also unquestionably of great importance in determining the basis for regional selectivity in many chemically induced hepatotoxicities.

The liver differs from most tissues in that it is fairly homogeneous with respect to cell types. However, morphologically similar cells, such as hepatic parenchymal cells (hepatocytes), often exhibit significant and, in some instances, rather marked differences in the contents and activities of certain enzymes. Indeed, results of microchemical and enzyme histochemical analyses have clearly revealed a zonation of metabolic function of parenchymal cells across the liver lobule, especially with respect to carbohydrate homeostasis.[136–144] The intracellular balance between the activation and detoxication of hepatotoxins and other xenobiotics is a critical determinant of the accumulation of metabolites within specific cells. Metabolic zonation or nonuniform distribution of xenobiotic-activating and -detoxicating enzymes across the liver lobule would therefore be expected to contribute very greatly to the relatively selective regional nature of parenchymal cell damage induced by many hepatotoxins. Several different experimental approaches and methodologies have been utilized to describe the distribution of enzymes and xenobiotic biotransformations across the liver lobule. These include: isolated subpopulations of hepatocytes[145–147]; autoradiography to localize covalently bound metabolites of hepatotoxins within the liver lobule[148,149]; *in vivo* exposure to hepatotoxins that produce relatively selective regional toxicities within the liver lobule[150–152]; normal and retrograde perfusions of the liver with substrates for glucuronidation and sulfation[153–157]; enzyme histochemistry[158–162]; microspectrophotometry, i.e., microdensitometry[163–167]; surface microfluorometry[29,31,171]; and immunohistochemistry.[162,169–182] Microspectrophotometric, immunohistochemical, and histochemical findings on the intralobular distributions of several key xenobiotic-metabolizing enzymes are summarized below.

2.2.1. Cytochromes P-450

The endoplasmic reticulum and nuclear envelope of the hepatic parenchymal cell contain a number of isoenzymes of cytochrome P-450 that play pivotal roles in the oxidative metabolism—activation as well as detoxification—of hepatotoxins and other xenobiotics. Primarily because of the prominent roles of these hemeproteins in xenobiotic metabolism, their intralobular distributions have been investigated much more intensively than have those of other xenobiotic-metabolizing enzymes. Insight into the distribution of the cytochromes across the liver lobule has been gained through microspectrophotometric and immunohistochemical technologies.

In 1975, Altman *et al.*[163] described a microspectrophotometric method with which cytochrome P-450 could be detected and quantitated directly within individual cells in unfixed cryostat liver sections. Employing this method, Gooding *et al.*,[164] Chayen *et al.*,[165] and Smith and Wills[166] demonstrated that the concentration of cytochrome P-450 within parenchymal cells varied significantly across the lobule in livers of both control and phenobarbital-treated rats. Cytochrome P-450 concentration was found to decrease in a fairly steady manner from the central vein toward the portal triad. In livers of control rats, centrilobular cells contained approximately 1.6 times as much cytochrome P-450 as did periportal cells. After rats had been treated with phenobarbital, cytochrome P-450 was found to be induced primarily within centrilobular cells, which then contained between 2.8 and 4.0 times as much cytochrome P-450 as did periportal cells. Results of studies conducted with isolated subpopulations of hepatocytes also indicated that phenobarbital induced cytochrome P-450 to significantly greater degrees within centrilobular cells than within periportal cells.[145,147]

While the intralobular distribution of cytochrome P-450 can be investigated quantitatively using the microspectrophotometric technique, this method is not sufficiently sensitive to detect the hemeprotein when it is present at low levels.[164] Since the detection and quantitation of cytochrome P-450 is based solely on the spectral characteristics of the carbon monoxide complex of the reduced hemeprotein, the microspectrophotometric methods cannot discriminate among the various cytochrome P-450 isoenzymes present. All forms of cytochrome P-450 associated with the endoplasmic reticulum, the nucleus, and mitochondria are detected. Although different isoenzymes of hepatic microsomal and nuclear cytochrome P-450 exhibit overlapping substrate specificities, they differ in the efficiency with which they catalyze the monooxygenations of different substrates. Furthermore, different isoenzymes often catalyze the formation of different metabolites from a given substrate molecule. Since one isoenzyme of cytochrome P-450 may catalyze the formation of a highly reactive and cytotoxic electrophile, whereas another isoenzyme may generate nontoxic metabolite(s) from the same parent compound, differences in the intralobular distributions of different cytochrome P-450 isoenzymes may be of critical importance for determining the locations as well as severities of certain chemically induced hepatotoxicities.

As discussed in greater detail in Chapter 4, the application of immunohistochemical and immunocytochemical technologies permits antigens such as enzymes and other proteins to be visualized within tissues and cells. Moreover, these techniques possess exquisite specificity and sensitivity. They can detect not only specific antigens within limited regions of tissues and cells, but also antigens in the overall tissue and cellular levels of which may be too low to be detected using more conventional biochemical and biophysical methodologies. Because of these advantages, immunohistochemical techniques have recently been employed to investigate the intralobular distributions of cytochrome P-450 isoenzymes.[162,169-172,174,175,183-185] To determine whether different cytochrome P-450 isoenzymes are distributed in similar manners across the liver lobule, Baron and his associates.[162,169,170,183-185] initiated qualitative and quantitative immunohistochemical investigations of the intralobular distributions of three isoenzymes, cytochromes P-450 PB-B, MC-B, and PCN-E, in rat liver. These isoenzymes represent the major forms of cytochrome P-450 isolated from hepatic microsomes of rats treated with phenobarbital, 3-methylcholanthrene, and pregnenolone-16α-carbonitrile, respectively.[186-189] Utilizing qualitative immunohistochemical staining techniques, other laboratories have also investigated the intralobular distributions of cytochromes P-450. Koyada[172] and Ohnishi et al.[174] have studied the major phenobarbital-inducible form of cytochrome P-450 in rat liver. A minor form, cytochrome P-450a, has been examined in rat liver. Moody et al.,[175] and Masters et al.,[171] investigated cytochrome P-450 in rat liver using an antibody raised against phenobarbital-induced pig hepatic microsomal cytochrome P-450. Finally, four isoenzymes [forms 2 (P-450$_{LM2}$), 3 (P-450$_{LM3b}$), 4 (P-450$_{LM4}$), and 6] have been studied in rabbit liver by Dees et al.[173]

Two forms of rabbit hepatic microsomal cytochrome P-450, cytochromes P-450$_{LM2}$ and P-450$_{LM3b}$, were found to be distributed quite uniformly across the liver lobule, whereas each of the other cytochromes P-450 studied appeared to be distributed in nonuniform manner across the lobule of livers from control animals. Moreover, centrilobular parenchymal cells appeared to be stained most intensely for each of these hemeproteins, suggesting that centrilobular cells in livers of control animals contain the greatest levels of these cytochromes P-450. Quantitative analyses of immunohistochemical staining intensities revealed, however, that different cytochrome P-450 isoenzymes are distributed in significantly different manners across the lobule in livers of control rats.[162,169,170,184,185] For example, both cytochromes P-450 PB-B and PCN-E decreased steadily from the central vein toward the portal triad. However, although the level of each isoenzyme was determined to be between 1.4 and 1.5 times greater in centrilobular cells than in midzonal cells, the difference in cytochrome P-450 PCN-E levels between centrilobular and periportal cells was significantly more pronounced than that for cytochrome P-450 PB-B; while centrilobular cells contained approximately 2.4 times more cytochrome P-450 PCN-E than did periportal cells, the level of cytochrome P-450 PB-B in centrilobular cells was only about 1.8 times that in cells located near the portal triad.[162,169,170,184] Quantitative immunohistochemical findings on cytochrome P-450 PB-B levels are thus consistent with the difference in total cytochrome P-450 content found between centrilobular and periportal cells in livers of control rats using the microspectrophotometric technique.[164–166] In marked contrast to these observations, midzonal and periportal cells contain similar levels of cytochrome P-450 MC-B, and this was approximately 20% less than that in centrilobular parenchymal cells.[162,169,170,184]

The effects of a number of xenobiotics on cytochromes P-450 within the liver lobule have been investigated utilizing immunohistochemical techniques.[162,170,172–175,185] Although treatment of rabbits with 2,3,7,8-tetrachlorodibenzo-*p*-dioxin did not affect cytochromes P-450 LM2 and LM3b, staining for cytochrome P-450$_{LM4}$ and another isoenzyme (form 6) was found to be enhanced and to become distributed fairly evenly across the liver lobule.[173] Since centrilobular cells were stained most intensely for these two isoenzymes in control rabbit liver, these findings indicate that the hemoproteins were induced to greater extents within midzonal and periportal cells than within centrilobular cells. In contrast to these findings, phenobarbital enhanced staining for the major phenobarbital-inducible cytochrome P-450 isoenzyme to a greater extent around the central vein than around the portal triad in rat liver.[172,174] Staining for cytochrome P-450a in rat liver was also affected more greatly by phenobarbital within centrilobular cells than within periportal cells.[175] Employing a quantitative immunohistochemical method, Baron *et al.*[169,170] investigated the effects of a number of xenobiotics on cytochromes P-450 in rat liver. They found that treatment of rats with phenobarbital enhanced the degree of immunohistochemical staining for cytochrome P-450 PB-B throughout the liver. However, levels of this is-

induction of cytochrome P-450 PB-B were produced within midzonal and periportal cells, while significantly less induction occurred within centrilobular cells.[162] In contrast to the effects of phenobarbital, a gradient in the induction of cytochrome P-450 PB-B was detected across the lobule after rats were treated with *trans*-stilbene oxide. The greatest degree of induction was produced within periportal cells and the least within centrilobular cells.[162] Although cytochrome P-450 PB-B was not affected by β-naphthoflavone, the content of this isoenzyme was decreased significantly, especially within centrilobular cells, after rats had been treated with 3-methylcholanthrene.[162,185] Levels of cytochrome P-450 MC-B were not altered by either phenobarbital or *trans*-stilbene oxide, whereas 3-methylcholanthrene and β-naphthoflavone both induced this isoenzyme within parenchymal cells throughout the lobule.[162,170,185] However, while the two polycyclic aromatic hydrocarbons induced cytochrome P-450 MC-B to similar degrees within midzonal and periportal cells, they produced significantly less induction of this isoenzyme within centrilobular cells.[165,188] Finally, pregnenolone-16α-carbonitrile was found to induce cytochrome P-450 PCN-E to a much greater extent within periportal cells than within either midzonal or centrilobular cells.[162] This observation may provide the explanation for protection against the centrilobular necrosis induced by carbon tetrachloride afforded by pregnenolone-16α-carbonitrile.[189]

2.2.2. NADPH-Cytochrome P-450 Reductase

Koudstaal and Hardonk[159] found that centrilobular parenchymal cells in livers of both control and phenobarbital-treated rats were the most intensely stained for NADPH-tetrazolium reductase activity. Since NADPH-cytochrome P-450 reductase is capable of catalyzing the NADPH-dependent reduction of tetrazolium dyes, this observation suggested that the reductase was localized predominantly within centrilobular cells. However, other enzymes, including certain NADH-linked dehydrogenases supplied with NADH via mitochondrial transhydrogenase activity and the NADPH-dependent flavoprotein dehydrogenase (hepatic ferredoxin reductase) that is associated with mitochondrial cytochrome P-450, could also participate in the histochemical staining reaction for hepatic NADPH-tetrazolium reductase activity. These enzymes, moreover, may not be distributed uniformly across the liver lobule. For this reason, the intralobular distribution of NADPH-cytochrome P-450 reductase has been examined by means of immunohistochemical methodologies.[162,169,170,190–194] Results of these studies demonstrated that the reductase is not distributed uniformly across the lobule in livers of control rats. Amounts of NADPH-cytochrome P-450 reductase within centrilobular and midzonal cells were quite similar, whereas periportal cells contained only about half as much enzyme.[162,169,191,192,194] Smith *et al.*[194] employed scanning and integrating microdensitometry to quantitate the intensities of unlabeled-antibody peroxidase–antiperoxidase staining (see Chapter 4) and were able to determine the distribution of NADPH-cytochrome P-450 reductase across the entire lobule in livers of control rats. Results of these analyses demonstrated that although the content of the reductase was fairly constant within both centrilobular and periportal cells, a considerable degree of variability in this enzyme was found among midzonal cells, especially between those cells adjacent to the centrilobular region and those adjacent to the periportal region (Fig. 2).

The induction of NADPH-cytochrome P-450 reductase across the liver lobule by various xenobiotics has also been investigated.[162,170,192,193] Although 3-methylcholanthrene did not affect the enzyme, both phenobarbital and pregnenolone-16α-carbonitrile induced the reductase within the parenchymal cells throughout the lobule.[162,170,192] However, the two xenobiotics had significantly different effects on NADPH-cytochrome P-450 reductase: Phenobarbital induced the reductase uniformly across the lobule, whereas pregnenolone-16α-carbonitrile affected the enzyme markedly differently within the three regions of the lobule. The greatest induction occurred within periportal cells and the least within midzonal cells.[162,170,192] Thus, not only is NADPH-cytochrome P-450 reductase normally distributed across the liver lobule in a nonuniform pattern (one that differs significantly from those determined for cytochromes P-450 PB-B, MC-B, and PCN-E), but also it is affected in quite different manners within the three regions of the liver lobule by different xenobiotics.

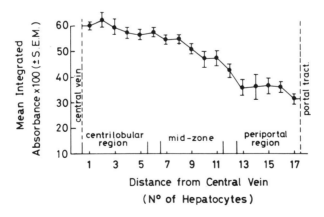

Figure 2.   Intralobular distribution of NADPH-cytochrome P-450 reductase in rat liver as determined by microdensitometry after unlabeled-antibody peroxidase–antiperoxidase staining. The values represent the means ± S.E.M. of at least 16 determinations made using liver sections prepared from 4 rats. Reprinted from Smith *et al.*[194] with permission.

2.2.3. Cytochrome b_5

The distribution of cytochrome b_5 across liver lobules of normal rats has been investigated by means of an immunohistochemical approach.[169,176,177,195] Although Tavassoli et al.[195] reported initially that immunohistochemical staining for cytochrome b_5 was restricted to centrilobular parenchymal cells, subsequent investigations by Franke et al.[177] and Redick et al.[169] demonstrated conclusively that this hemeprotein was present within parenchymal cells throughout the liver lobule. However, quantitative immunohistochemical analyses did reveal that cytochrome b_5 was distributed across the lobule in a nonuniform manner. The level of the hemoprotein decreased from the central vein toward the portal triad. Centrilobular cells contained approximately 12 and 31% more cytochrome b_5 than did midzonal and periportal cells, respectively. Midzonal cells contained approximately 17% more than did periportal cells.[169] Thus, the intralobular distribution of cytochrome b_5 in livers of control rats resembles the distributions determined for cytochromes P-450 PB-B and PCN-E, although the difference in cytochrome b_5 levels between centrilobular and periportal cells was much less pronounced than that determined for either of the two cytochrome P-450 enzymes.

2.2.4. Epoxide Hydrolase

Highly reactive and toxic, electrophilic epoxides are frequently generated during the cytochromes-P-450-catalyzed oxidative metabolism of aromatic and olefinic substances, including a number of hepatotoxins. These reactive metabolites can be inactivated, in part, by conversion to their corresponding trans-dihydrodiols under the influence of the enzyme epoxide hydrolase.[196,197] Although the hydration of epoxides leads to their detoxification, certain isoenzymes of cytochrome P-450, especially those induced by polycyclic aromatic hydrocarbons, e.g., cytochrome P-450 MC-B, may further oxidatively metabolize trans-dihydrodiols to yield highly cytotoxic, mutagenic, and carcinogenic dihydrodiol-epoxides.[198] Thus, the relationship between the epoxide-generating cytochromes-P-450-containing monooxygenase enzyme systems and epoxide hydrolase appears to be a critical factor that regulates intracellular and intratissue levels of potentially cytotoxic epoxide metabolites.

The intralobular distribution of epoxide hydrolase has been investigated immunohistochemically in livers of control as well as xenobiotic-pretreated rats.[162,169,178,179,199–201] Parenchymal cells throughout the lobule in livers of control rats stained for epoxide hydrolase. However, centrilobular parenchymal cells were stained more intensely for the hydrolase than were either midzonal or periportal cells, and results of quantitative immunohistochemical analyses demonstrated that epoxide hydrolase was distributed across the lobule in a manner essentially identical to that determined for cytochrome P-450 MC-B in livers of control rats, i.e., midzonal and periportal cells contained similar amounts of the hydrolase, while between 20 and 30% more enzyme was present within centrilobular cells.[162,169,200,201]

Treatment of rats with 2-acetylaminofluorene, a hepatocarcinogen that initially produces relatively selective injury within periportal cells,[40,41] resulted in an increased intensity of staining for epoxide hydrolase, especially within midzonal and periportal cells.[178,179] This finding suggested that epoxide hydrolase was induced by 2-acetylaminofluorene to the greatest extent within midzonal and periportal cells. Subsequent semiquantitative immunohistochemical analyses demonstrated that epoxide hydrolase was also induced to similar extents within midzonal and periportal cells and to a significantly lesser extent within centrilobular cells after rats had been treated with *trans*-stilbene oxide.[162,200,201] Although 3-methylcholanthrene did not affect epoxide hydrolase significantly, the enzyme was induced by phenobarbital, but the induction occurred nonuniformly across the lobule; the greatest extent of induction was produced within midzonal cells and the least within periportal cells.[186,201] Thus, like various cytochrome P-450 isoenzymes and NADPH-cytochrome P-450 reductase, epoxide hydrolase is distributed nonuniformly across the lobule in livers of control rats. Moreover, levels of epoxide hydrolase can be affected in significantly different manners within the three regions of the liver lobule following the administration of different xenobiotics.

2.3. Sources of Reducing Equivalents in Specific Regions of the Liver Lobule

Reducing equivalents required for mixed-function oxidation are acquired from sources in the cytosol or from mitochondria. Cytosolic reducing equivalents may be generated via the two oxidative enzymes of the pentose phosphate pathway, malic enzyme and isocitrate dehydrogenase.[202] These two enzymes appear to be a major source of reducing equivalents in livers from fed animals.[203] Reducing equivalents generated within the mitochondria must be transferred to the cytosol via specific shuttle transport mechanisms because reduced pyridine nucleotides do not readily cross the inner mitochondrial membrane.[204] There is growing evidence that mechanisms associated with the generation of reducing equivalents are unevenly distributed across the liver lobule. For example, early quantitative histochemical studies indicated that glucose-6-phosphate dehydrogenase[205–207] and isocitrate dehydrogenase[208] are localized in the central portion of the liver lobule. More recent studies by Smith and Wills[166] employing quantitative cytochemical methods confirmed that glucose-6-phosphate dehydrogenase was 2–4 times more active in the centrolobular region of the liver than in the periportal zone. Malic enzyme has also been found to be more heavily concentrated in the pericentral zone of the liver than in the periportal zone.[209,210] Information concerning the intralobular distribution of mitochondria is less definitive than that dealing with the distribution of NADPH-generating enzymes. On the basis of the volume densities of mitochondria per mononuclear hepatocyte, Loud[211] concluded that mitochondria were more densely localized in periportal regions of the liver lobule; however, other investigators using a similar approach[212–214] indicated that there was no zonal gradient of mitochondria across the liver lobule. The staining pattern of succinate dehydrogenase, which is more intense in periportal regions,[215] supports the idea that mitochondria are more concentrated in periportal regions. Possible differences in specific substrate shuttle mechanisms in separate zones of the liver have not been evaluated to date.

Although data on the distribution across the liver lobule indicate that the capacity to generate NADPH via cytosolic enzymes is greater in the pericentral region than in periportal areas of the liver lobule, concentrations of NADPH do not seem to differ across the liver lobule either *in vivo*[215] or in the perfused liver.[216] NADPH represents 80–90% of the NADP content in the liver, and its level is about 1.5 mmoles/kg dry tissue in both zones.[215] The total content of NADP in the isolated perfused liver is essentially the same as in the liver *in situ*[216]; however, it differs from that *in vivo* in that only 30% of the total NADP is in the reduced state in both the periportal and the pericentral zone of the perfused liver. The total content of NADP in the isolated, perfused liver is essentially the same as in the liver *in situ*.[215,216] The distributions of other low-molecular-weight metabolites participating in the generation of NADPH in the two zones of the liver have not been studied extensively. Amounts of glucose-6-phosphate do not appear to differ significantly between cells in the periportal and pericentral regions of the liver lobule.[143]

Steady-state levels of metabolites and NADPH may not differ significantly in the two zones of the liver lobule; however, rates of utilization via mixed-function oxidation vary; thus, the turnover of cofactor must differ. For example, during mixed-function oxidation of 7-ethoxycoumarin, significant oxidation of NADPH occurs in both zones of the liver lobule; however, the oxidation is significantly greater in the periportal than in the pericentral region. Since local rates of drug oxidation of 7-ethoxycoumarin are roughly twice as high in pericentral as in periportal zones of the liver, the generation of NADPH, i.e., turnover, must be greater in pericentral than in periportal regions.[216] The possibility that the generation of NADPH is rate-limiting for high rates of mixed-function oxidation in the two zones of the liver lobule is suggested by the finding that addition of xylitol to the isolated, perfused liver stimulates rates of drug metabolism in both regions of the liver lobule.[216] It is not known whether this limitation by NADPH supply occurs under physiological conditions *in vivo*, in which much lower rates of mixed-function oxidation occur.

2.4. Distribution of Function in Intact Liver Periportal and Pericentral Regions of the Liver

2.4.1. Use of Anterograde and Retrograde Perfusions

In a series of elegant experiments, Ji *et al.*[29,168] showed that micro-light guides could be used to measure mixed-function oxidation noninvasively in periportal and pericentral regions of the liver lobule (see Fig. 3). A new fluorometric method has been developed to measure the relative rates of the 7-ethoxycoumarin O-deethylase activities in periportal and pericentral regions of the liver lobule. The method utilizes a pair of micro-light guides constructed from two strands of 80-μm-diameter glass optical fibers. The micro-light guides

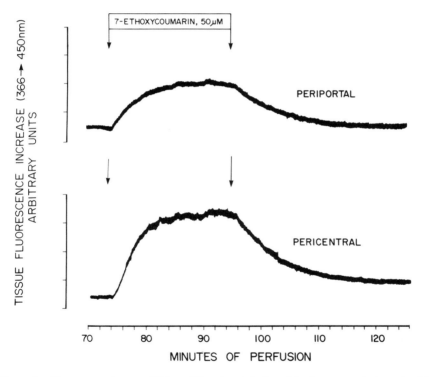

Figure 3. Fluorescence increase (366 → 450 nm) on infusion of 7-ethoxycoumarin in periportal and pericentral regions of the liver lobule in fed, phenobarbital-treated rat. Micro-light guides (tip diameter 170 μm) were placed on two adjacent periportal regions (1–3 mm apart) on the left lateral lobe of the liver. The output voltages (600–650 V) of the photomultipliers were adjusted to give similar anode currents in both channels. Subsequently, one micro-light guide was moved to a pericentral area. (↓) Infusion of 7-ethoxycoumarin.

are placed on periportal and pericentral regions on the surface of the perfused liver. The increase in tissue fluorescence due to 7-hydroxycoumarin formation from 7-ethoxycoumarin is measured in periportal and pericentral regions by illuminating tissue with light at 360 ± 50 nm and measuring fluorescence at 450 ± 50 nm. Since the steady-state tissue fluorescence due to 7-hydroxycoumarin monitored with a large light guide was found to be directly proportional to the steady-state rate of 7-ethoxycoumarin O-deethylation, the sublobular fluorescence of 7-hydroxycoumarin measured by micro-light guides following infusion of 7-ethoxycoumarin allows one to estimate sublobular rates of the mixed-function oxidation of 7-ethoxycoumarin. The results from preliminary studies indicated that the rate of 7-ethoxycoumarin O-deethylation was approximately twice as great in pericentral regions as in periportal areas of the liver.

2.4.2. Studies of Ethoxycoumarin Metabolism with Micro-Light Guides

In a series of experiments, Belinsky et al.[216] studied mixed-function oxidation in periportal and pericentral regions of the liver lobule. In livers from fasted, phenobarbital-treated rats, rates of 7-hydroxycoumarin production were 2.2 and 5.2 μmoles $\times$ g^{-1} $\times$ $^{p-1}$ in periportal and pericentral regions of the liver lobule, respectively. The purpose of the study was to determine whether these differences in rates of mixed-function oxidation could be explained by differences in NADPH supply or in cytochrome P-450 in various zones of the liver lobule.

Although NADPH content was similar in both periportal and pericentral regions, cofactor turnover could differ considerably. If the liver could not regenerate NADPH, rates of 7-hydroxycoumarin formation could be sustained for only 3 min. Thus, the liver must constantly resynthesize NADPH at high rates. If rates of mixed-function oxidation are regulated predominantly by the concentration of cytochrome P-450, which is greater in pericentral hepatocytes, then an increase in NADPH content in the liver should have little effect on local rates of 7-hydroxycoumarin formation. However, addition of xylitol enhanced rates of 7-hydroxycoumarin production from 7-ethoxycoumarin in both periportal and pericentral regions of the liver lobule. This action of xylitol is best explained by an increase in NADPH supply. This conclusion is supported by the observation that sorbitol, which increases NADPH supply, also stimulates mixed-function oxidation, while ethanol, which increases NADH but decreases NADPH, produced inhibition. However, isoenzyme patterns in different regions of the liver lobule could be important as well.

In mammalian liver, xylitol is oxidized predominantly by an NAD$^+$-linked dehydrogenase to form xylulose, which is subsequently phosphorylated and enters intermediary metabolism at the triose phosphate level.[217] In livers from fasted rats, xylitol, which is converted rapidly into glucose,[129,218] which is subsequently phosphorylated to glucose-6-phosphate and generates NADPH for mixed-function oxidation via the pentose phosphate shunt, abolished the stimulation of mixed-function oxidation by sorbitol, a sugar that is metabolized via the same reaction sequence as xylitol.[219] Xylitol caused a significant decrease in the $NADP^+/$ NADPH ratio in both regions of the liver lobule. It also stimulated 7-ethoxy-coumarin metabolism in both periportal and pericentral regions. Thus, it is reasonable to conclude that NADPH supply is a major determinant of rates of mixed-function oxidation in both regions of the liver lobule.

Since NADPH supply is an important rate determinant of mixed-function oxidation, it could account for differences in rates observed in periportal and pericentral regions of the liver lobule. For example, it is possible that NADPH utilization for lipid or cholesterol biosynthesis predominates in periportal cells, allowing less NAPDH to be utilized for mixed-function oxidation. In fact, Smith and Wills[167] observed greater lipid synthesis in periportal than in pericentral hepatocytes. Another possibility is that the supply or turnover of NADPH varies across the liver lobule as a consequence of the heterogeneous distribution of enzymes that generate NADPH.[167] On the basis of the observation by Smith and Wills[167] that glucose-6-phosphate dehydrogenase activity was 4 times greater in pericentral than in periportal hepatocytes of phenobarbital-treated rats, one might argue that enhanced pentose phosphate shunt activity is responsible for higher rates of mixed-function oxidation in pericentral areas of the liver lobule. However, our experiments were performed in livers from fasted rats in which carbon flux over the pentose phosphate pathways is reduced severely[220] due to limiting amounts of the substrate glucose-6-phosphate. Differences in NADPH generation via mitochondrial oxidations could also explain the differences in local rates of mixed-function oxidation observed in this study.

Cytochrome P-450 is distributed unevenly across the liver lobule.[183] The cytochrome P-450 induced by phenobarbital (P-450-PB) is greater in pericentral than in periportal regions, whereas the cytochrome P-450 induced by 3-meth-ylcholanthrene (P-450-MC) is more evenly distributed across the liver lobule.[183] However, even this form is about 30% higher in pericentral than in periportal regions.[182] The highest rate of turnover with 7-ethoxycoumarin as substrate occurs with the P-450-MC isoenzyme[221,222]; however, a substantial amount of this substrate is also metabolized by the isoenzyme induced by phenobarbital. In livers from phenobarbital-treated rats, the concentration of the P-450-PB isoenzyme is 16-fold greater than that of the P-450-MC isoenzyme.[223] Thus, the greater rate of metabolism of 7-ethoxycoumarin in these experiments is likely due to the phenobarbital-inducible form of cytochrome P-450. Differences in the distribution of the cytochrome P-450-PB isoenzyme across the liver lobule could also contribute to the observed differences in rates of 7-hydroxycoumarin formation in pericentral and periportal zones of the liver.

In these studies, evidence has been presented indicating that NADPH supply is a major rate determinant of the mixed-function oxidation of 7-ethoxycoumarin in both periportal and pericentral regions of the liver lobule. However, NADPH supply is not the sole determinant of rates of mixed-function oxidation. Differences in mixed-function oxidation across the liver lobule may also involve the uneven distribution of cytochrome P-450 isoenzymes across the liver lobule.

In another series of experiments, the relative contribution of the pentose cycle and mitochondrial oxidations to NADPH supply for mixed-function oxidation in periportal and pericentral regions of the liver lobule was evaluated in perfused liver.[224] Micro-light guides were placed on periportal and pericentral regions of the liver surface to monitor the conversion of nonfluorescent 7-ethoxycoumarin to fluorescent 7-hydroxycoumarin. Rates of 7-ethoxycoumarin O-deethylation in livers from fed, normal rats were 1.2 μmoles/g per hr in both regions of the liver lobule. In livers from fed, phenobarbital-treated rats, however, rates were 3.6 and 7.0 μmoles/g per hr in periportal and pericentral regions, respectively. Fasting or treatment with 6-aminonicotinamide was employed to inhibit the generation of NADPH by the pentose cycle, and KCN was used to decrease generation of reducing equivalents via mitochondria. Rates of 7-hydroxycoumarin production were approximately 0.9 μmole/g per hr in both periportal and pericentral regions of livers from normal rats following nearly complete inhibition of the pentose cycle with 6-aminonicotinamide treatment. Rates were 2.1 and 3.4 μmoles/g per hr in periportal and pericentral regions, respectively, in livers from phenobarbital-treated rats given 6-aminonicotinamide. Thus, we conclude that the pentose cycle supplies NADPH at rates of 0.3 μmole/g per hr in both regions of the liver lobule in livers from normal rats. In contrast, the pentose cycle supplies 1.5 and 3.6 μmoles NADPH/g per hr in periportal and pericentral regions, respectively, in livers from phenobarbital-treated rats. KCN was a more potent inhibitor of 7-ethoxycoumarin O-deethylation than 6-aminonicotinamide. It decreased rates to approximately 0.6 μmole/g per hr in both regions of the liver lobule in livers from normal rats. After fasting or treatment with 6-aminonicotinamide, rates were around 0.2 μmole/g per hr in the presence of KCN. In livers from fasted, phenobarbital-treated rats, rates of 7-hydroxycoumarin production were 0.3 and 0.7 μmole/g per hr in periportal and pericentral regions, respectively, in the presence of KCN. We conclude that the mitochondria supply 0.7 μmole NADPH/g per hr in both regions in livers from normal rats and 1.3 and 2.7 μmoles NADPH/g per hr in periportal and pericentral regions, respectively, after phenobarbital treatment. Thus, mitochondria supply 50–70% of the reducing equivalents for mixed-function oxidation in both regions of the liver lobule. In general, the sum of KCN- and 6-aminonicotinamide-sensitive rates of 7-ethoxycoumarin metabolism was very close to the actual rate observed in the absence of the inhibitors. Thus, we have determined rates of NADPH generation by the pentose cycle and mitochondria for mixed-function oxidation in periportal and pericentral regions of the liver lobule for the first time.

Treatment of rats with β-naphthoflavone increased rates markedly to around 21 μmoles/g per hr in both regions.[225] Fasting or treatment with 6-aminonicotinamide was employed to inhibit the generation of NADPH by the pentose cycle, while KCN was used to decrease NADPH generation via the mitochondria. Fasting or treatment with 6-aminonicotinamide decreased rates of mixed-function oxidation in both regions of the liver lobule from 1.4 to 0.9 μmole/g per hr in livers from corn oil-treated rats. Rates of 7-hydroxycoumarin production in periportal and pericentral regions were decreased from approximately 21 to 16 μmoles/g per hr following fasting or 6-aminonicotinamide treatment in livers from β-naphthoflavone-treated rats. Thus, pentose cycle activity supplies about 0.5 and 5 μmoles NADPH/g per hr in both regions of the liver lobule for mixed-function oxidation in livers from corn oil- and β-naphthoflavone-treated rats, respectively. KCN decreased rates of 7-ethoxycoumarin O-deethylation to 0.5 μmole/g per hr in both regions of the liver lobule in livers from fed, corn oil-treated rats. In livers from fasted or 6-aminonicotinamide-treated rats, KCN reduced sublobular rates of mixed-function oxidation to 0.2 μmole/g per hr. Infusion of KCN did not alter maximal rates of 7-hydroxycoumarin production significantly in livers from fasted, β-naphthoflavone-treated rats; however, rates declined by 60% to 5 μmoles/g per hr during 30 min of perfusion. With longer perfusions, rates declined to less than 2 μmoles/g per hr. We conclude that in livers from β-naphthoflavone-treated rats, mitochondria supply 15 μmoles NADPH/g per hr in both regions of the liver lobule. Thus, mitochondria play a major role in the supply of reducing equivalents for mixed-function oxidation in both periportal and pericentral regions of the liver lobule after treatment with β-naphthoflavone.

2.4.3. Aryl Hydrocarbon Hydroxylase (Benzo[a]pyrene Hydroxylase) Activity

The first direct proof that xenobiotics are not oxidatively metabolized at uniform rates within parenchymal cells across the liver lobule was provided over 20 years ago by Wattenberg and Leon.[158] Employing a fluorescence histochemical technique, these investigators demonstrated that benzo[a]pyrene and several other polycyclic aromatic hydrocarbons were hydroxylated throughout the lobule in livers of control rats. However, they observed that the oxidative metabolism of these substances occurred most extensively within centrilobular parenchymal cells. Wattenberg and Leong also concluded that 3-methylcholanthrene induced aryl hydrocarbon hydroxylase activity to the greatest degree within centrilobular cells. Although there are numerous problems associated with the fluorescence histochemical assay for aryl hydrocarbon hydroxylase activity, this pioneering study thus demonstrated not only that xenobiotics such as polycyclic aromatic hydrocarbons undergo oxidative metabolism nonuniformly across the lobule, but also that induction of the oxidative metabolism of xenobiotics may not occur uniformly across the liver lobule.

Two major technical problems have severely limited the application of the fluorescence histochemical method that was developed by Wattenberg and Leong. These problems are associated with the diffusion of polar benzo[a]pyrene phenols within the tissue section and the fading of fluorescence due to phenolic metabolites after sections are mounted in an alkaline medium. Recently, Baron *et al.*[162] were able to overcome these difficulties by maintaining tissue sections at 0–4°C after incubation and during microscopy; under these conditions, the intralobular distributions of emitted fluorescence due to both benzo[a]pyrene and its phenolic metabolites (primarily 3-hydroxybenzo[a]pyrene) could be examined quite easily. With this modified fluorescence histochemical technique, benzo[a]pyrene was found to be hydroxylated to the greatest extent within centrilobular cells in livers of control rats (Fig. 4A). Although this finding agreed with the original observation made by Wattenberg and Leong, Baron and co-workers were able to demonstrate further that 3-methylcholanthrene induced aryl hydrocarbon hydroxylase activity to greater extents within periportal and midzonal cells than within centrilobular cells. Moreover, this pattern of intralobular induction caused the cytochrome-P-450-catalyzed monooxygenase activity to become distributed fairly uniformly across the lobule (Fig. 4B). This histochemical observation is thus consistent with the results of immunohistochemical analyses that demonstrated that cytochrome P-450 MC-B was also induced by 3-methylcholanthrene to significantly greater extents within midzonal and periportal cells than within centrilobular cells. Furthermore, cytochrome P-450 MC-B was also found to be distributed quite uniformly across the lobule in livers of rats that had been treated with 3-methylcholanthrene.[162,185] Similar to 3-methylcholanthrene, *trans*-stilbene oxide enhanced aryl hydroxylase activity markedly and caused it to become distributed fairly uniformly across the lobule (Fig. 4C). Thus, it also produced a significantly greater degree of induction of this monooxygenase activity within midzonal and periportal cells than within centrilobular cells. Again, this demonstrated excellent agreement with the results of quantitative immunohistochemical analyses.

Although phenobarbital did not produce a very pronounced increase in aryl hydrocarbon hydroxylase activity, the formation of phenolic metabolites from benzo[a]pyrene was found to be increased throughout the liver, especially within midzonal cells: Comparison of Fig. 4A and D demonstrates that there was a marked difference in the fluorescence emission intensity between centrilobular and periportal regions in sections prepared from the livers of control rats, whereas the fluorescence due to phenolic metabolites in livers of phenobarbital-treated rats extended from the central veins to the edges of the portal triads. Once again, the histochemical observation is consistent with the immunohistochemical finding that phenobarbital induced cytochrome P-450 PB-B to significantly greater degrees within midzonal and periportal cells than within centrilobular cells. Treatment of rats with pregnenolone-16α-carbonitrile was found to result in only a minimal increase in aryl hydrocarbon hydroxylase activity (Fig. 4E). However, the steroid did cause benzo[a]pyrene hydroxylase activity to become distributed quite uniformly across the lobule, indicating that similar to its effects on cyto-

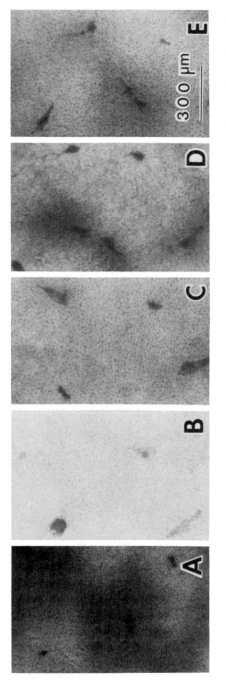

Figure 4. Distribution of benzo[a]pyrene hydroxylase activity within livers of control rats (A) and of rats pretreated with 3-methylcholanthrene (B), *trans*-stilbene oxide (C), phenobarbital (D), and pregnenolone-16α-carbonitrile (E). The photomicrographs show fluorescence due to benzo[a]pyrene phenols emitted from unfixed cryostat sections that had been exposed to 15 ng HPLC-purified benzo[a]pyrene and then incubated at 37°C in potassium phosphate buffer, pH 7.4, containing 1.6 mM glucose-6-phosphate, 0.25 unit glucose-6-phosphate dehydrogenase/ml, 0.58 mM NADPH, and 0.11 mM NADH. After incubation, the sections were rinsed with buffer, mounted in alkaline glycerol, kept at 0–4°C, and examined by incident-light fluorescence microscopy.

chrome P-450 PCN-E, it affected the monooxygenase activity to the greatest extent within periportal cells.

3. CONJUGATION REACTIONS

3.1. General Considerations

The ability of cells to conjugate xenobiotics, products of mixed-function oxidation, and endogenous compounds such as estradiol and bilirubin represents a major mechanism of detoxification.[226] Such reactions have been studied extensively *in vitro*, but only a few studies have been performed *in vivo* or in isolated cells or perfused organs.

Conjugation with glucuronic acid is the major route of removal of products of mixed-function oxidation. Glucuronidation of drug metabolites has been studied primarily in isolated hepatocytes[65] and in the perfused rat liver.[227,228] At least five rate-controlling factors have been identified for glucuronidation in whole cells: substrate supply, uridine diphosphate (UDP) glucuronic acid, $NAD^+/$ NADH redox state, the supply of carbohydrate, and the activity of a group of glucuronyltransferases. In isolated hepatocytes[65,229,230] as well as in the perfused liver,[227] rates of glucuronidation of p-nitrophenol, 4-methylumbelliferone, harmol, phenolphthalein, biphenyl, and β-naphthol were accelerated with increases in drug substrate concentration. Thus, a major factor that regulates glucuronidation is substrate supply. Maximal rates of conjugation of 7-hydroxycoumarin[65] and p-nitrophenol could be enhanced severalfold by pretreatment of the experimental animal with 3-methylcholanthrene or phenobarbital, respectively. In large part, these increases are probably due to enhanced rates of production of hydroxylated products of mixed-function oxidation (i.e., more substrate for conjugation reactions). Alteration of pathways of conjugation with specific inhibitors markedly changes the pathway of benzo[a]pyrene binding in isolated hepatocytes.[229]

Cellular energetics influence glucuronidation via formation of uridine triphosphate (UTP) required to form UDP-glucose. In a recent study, Reinke *et al.*[227] demonstrated that rates of p-nitrophenol glucuronidation varied over 10-fold between livers of fasted and fasted re-fed, phenobarbital-treated rats, but that ATP/ADP ratios were identical. Thus, it appears that cellular energetics do not normally limit glucuronidation. On the other hand, agents that drastically diminish the energy state (e.g., KCN or dinitrophenol) inhibit glucuronidation of p-nitrophenol in the perfused rat liver (L. Reinke and R. G. Thurman, unpublished observations). Moreover, salicylamide (0.5 mM), an agent that interacts with the mitochondrial respiratory chain, markedly inhibits sulfation without diminishing glucuronidation.[65] One possible interpretation of this interesting finding is that sulfation is more dependent on ATP than is glucuronidation. By diminishing the ATP/ADP ratio, carbohydrate supplied for glucuronidation may be enhanced. Data acquired with isolated hepatocytes suggest that conjugation reactions may be more susceptible than hydroxylation to depletion of cellular ATP. Wiebkin et al.[231] examined the effect of menadione, rotenone, and dinitrophenol, inhibitors of mitochondrial function, on the metabolism of biphenyl, 7-ethoxycoumarin, and benzo[a]pyrene in hepatocytes from normal and phenobarbital-treated rats. Although menadione depressed drug hydroxylation to a great extent, possibly via oxidation of NADPH and inhibition of cytochrome P-450 reduction, the other inhibitors of mitochondrial function had little effect on xenobiotic hydroxylation. In contrast, the conjugation of all three xenobiotics was depressed markedly by the inhibitors of mitochondrial function.

UDP-glucose dehydrogenase (E.C.1.1.1.22) is an NAD^+-requiring enzyme; therefore, alteration in the redox state of NAD^+ could influence the rate of glucuronidation by regulating the intracellular concentration of UDP-glucuronic acid. This is exemplified in experiments with ethanol, an agent that markedly increases the intracellular NADH content. Ethanol causes at least 50% inhibition of glucuronidation of morphine[232] and p-nitrophenol (L. Reinke and R. G. Thurman, unpublished observations). However, while redox inhibition of conjugation reactions is easily demonstrated, it does not appear that glucuronidation can be stimulated by increasing the NAD^+ supply with infusion of pyruvate into the perfused liver.

One major regulating factor for glucuronidation appears to be carbohydrate reserves. This is not surprising, since glucuronic acid is derived from glycogen and glucose. In phenobarbital-treated rats, Reinke et al.[227] showed that large differences in rates of conjugation of p-nitrophenol, essentially due to glucuronidation, paralleled carbohydrate reserves and uridine diphosphoglucuronic acid (UDPGA) levels in the livers of animals in different nutritional states. For example, maximal rates of conjugation were observed in livers that had the highest levels of glycogen.[227] Addition of phenobarbital to hepatocytes increased UDPGA levels[233]; however, chronic phenobarbital treatment did not alter UDPGA levels in the perfused rat liver (F. C. Kauffman and R. G. Thurman, unpublished observations).

Glucuronyltransferases are essential, but are probably not rate-controlling factors in intact cells except under extreme conditions. Moreover, these enzymes are often activated during isolation. After nutritional manipulations, maximal rates of glucuronidation in the perfused liver did not correlate with the V_{max} of glucuronyltransferase activities measured in vitro.[227] Thus, it appears that factors that regulate rates of mixed-function oxidation and carbohydrate reserves are primary rate-controlling steps in glucuronidation. Interestingly, rates of mixed-function oxidation are also correlated with carbohydrate reserves, suggesting that mixed-function oxidation and glucuronidation are in some manner coordinately regulated. One mechanism whereby rates of mixed-function oxidation and glucuronidation may be coupled in intact cells involves removal of oxidized products that inhibit the microsomal oxidase system. Fahl et al.[234] observed that addition of UDP-glucuronic acid to isolated microsomes resulted in a marked stimulation of benzo[a]pyrene oxidation. The authors interpreted this as removal of a hydroxylated product that inhibited mixed-function oxidation. A similar stimulation of benzo[a]pyrene oxidation[235] and glucuronyltransferase[236] has been observed with the addition of UDP-N-acetylglucosamine to an isolated microsomal system. Whether such a mechanism operates in intact cells remains to be determined.

Much less is known about factors that regulate sulfation in tissues. Rates of sulfation in the liver exceed those of other tissues such as the gut and the lung.[237] In general, when sulfation is decreased, glucuronidation is increased.[238] Elizabeth and James Miller and their colleagues[239,240] demonstrated that 2-acetylaminofluorine (AAF), a procarcinogen, is hydroxylated via mixed-function oxidation and subsequently sulfated in the liver to a compound that reacts covalently with critical sites in the cell. The formation of the N-sulfate requires the presence of an active sulfotransferase and β-phosphoadenosine-5'-phosphosulfate (PAPS). The sulfate is much more carcinogenic than the parent compound. Thus, sulfation can increase the toxicity of some foreign compounds.

Sulfation in intact cells, in analogy with glucuronidation, could be regulated by the supply of inorganic sulfate, the ATP/ADP ratio, and the activity of a group of sulfotransferases. Sulfation may be much more sensitive to changes in cellular energetics than glucuronidation, because agents that uncouple oxidative phosphorylation inhibit sulfation. Salicylamide,[65] p-chlorophenol, and 2,6-dichlorophenol,[238] all of which decrease sulfation in intact cells, either inhibit or uncouple oxidative phosphorylation.

Because of its well-established role in decreasing acetaminophen toxicity and participating in conjugation of carcinogens, much attention has been given to glutathione conjugation.[241] However, few studies have been designed to identify rate-controlling factors of glutathione conjugation in intact cells. Mercapturic acids have long been recognized in detoxification reactions. For example, naphthalene mercaptide was discovered over 70 years ago. Thirty-five years ago, Boyland[242] argued that polycyclic aromatic hydrocarbon metabolism proceeds via an epoxide intermediate. Recently, in an elegant series of experiments, Mitchell et al.[243,244] have demonstrated that glutathione is involved in protecting the liver against necrosis due to acetaminophen metabolism. Covalent binding of acetaminophen metabolites to tissue occurred only after 60–70% of the intracellular glutathione had been depleted. Metabolites of acetaminophen were conjugated to glutathione and were responsible for this depletion. Subsequently, metabolites of glutathione bound covalently to critical intracellular sites, leading to tissue necrosis.

Agents that increase intracellular glutathione levels, e.g., cysteine and methionine, decrease both covalent binding of acetaminophen metabolites and tissue necrosis.[244,245] Glutathione depletion via conjugation or inhibition of glutathione synthesis has also been implicated in the toxicity of benzene[246] and bromobenzene.[247]

Glutathione conjugates have been described for several oxides of benzo[a]pyrene[248] and styrene oxide.[249] However, little is known about regulation of glutathione conjugation in intact cells. Resolution of the question whether ATP, which is required for glutathione synthesis,[250] substrate supply, or the activity of glutathione-S-transferases are controlling factors in intact cells will also require further work. Moreover, considerable nonenzymatic conjugation could occur with glutathione.

Isolated, perfused organs have been used in a series of studies on conjugation. In perfused livers, [14C]styrene oxide was excreted mainly as the glutathione conjugate.[251] They have studied the oxidation and conjugation of benzo[a]pyrene and the conjugation of styrene oxide. In the isolated, perfused rat liver, the rates of formation of glutathione conjugates and styrene glycol were investigated. At low concentrations of styrene oxide, the glycol conjugate predominated.[252] In the perfused rabbit lung, methylcholanthrene treatment had no effect on aryl hydrocarbon hydroxylase activity or glutathione-S-transferase, but did enhance the activity of epoxide hydrase.[253] Similar results were obtained with benzo[a]pyrene-4,5-oxide in the perfused liver.[254]

3.2. Glucuronidation

The production of glucuronides by the liver is influenced by a variety of factors, including the delivery of drug substrate via the hepatic microcirculation, concentrations of intracellular metabolites such as UDP-glucuronic acid and inhibitors and activators of enzymes involved in the synthesis and degradation of glucuronides, activities of UDP-glucuronosyltransferases and β-glucuronidase, and competing conjugation reactions such as sulfation and mercapturic acid biosynthesis. The current understanding of events that regulate glucuronidation in intact hepatocytes and possible variations in these events across the liver lobule is at a very elementary level. Nevertheless, there is growing evidence that rates of glucuronidation differ in periportal and pericentral regions of the hepatic lobule under physiological conditions. Evidence supporting this possibility has been obtained from pharmokinetic modeling,[156,255,256] studies using hepatotoxins that selectively injure pericentral or periportal hepatocytes,[40,150,257,258] quantitative histochemical determinations of enzymes involved in glucuronidation,[259] and application of noninvasive light guides to quantitate glucuronidation of a fluorescent substrate in periportal and pericentral regions in the liver lobules of intact isolated, perfused livers.[154,260] Information gained using these various approaches is reviewed below.

3.2.1. Zonal Distribution of Conjugating Enzymes

The influence of zonal distribution on sulfation and glucuronidation of acetaminophen[156,255,256] was investigated during retrograde perfusions of isolated rat livers to probe the heterogeneous distribution of drug-conjugating enzymes.

Retrograde perfusions were used to reverse the location of drug-metabolizing enzyme systems with respect to the flow of perfusion fluid. Previous observations indicating that the elimination of [^{14}C]acetaminophen, which was formed from [^{14}C]phenacetin, was slower than that of preformed [^{3}H]acetaminophen in the normal direction of flow but was virtually the same during retrograde perfusion supported the idea of an uneven distribution of enzyme systems associated with oxidation and conjugation of the drug. On the basis of these data, Pang and her colleagues concluded that sulfate conjugation occurred predominantly in periportal hepatocytes, while O-deethylation occurred preferentially in the centrilobular region of the liver.[255] A similar approach applied to investigating the kinetics of harmol conjugation in the perfused liver suggested that the extraction of the drug is greater during retrograde than during anterograde perfusions.[256] Retrograde perfusions also lowered the amount of sulfate conjugate formed relative to the glucuronide, suggesting that the sulfation system is anterior to the glucuronidation system along the normal blood flow path in the liver.

Another indirect approach to studying the uneven distribution of drug-metabolizing systems in the liver is to use hepatotoxins that selectively destroy hepatocytes in specific sublobular zones. Using allyl alcohol and N-hydroxy-2-acetylaminofluorene to destroy periportal hepatocytes, Thorgeirsson et al.[40] concluded that glucuronosyltransferases are localized predominantly in the periportal region. This conclusion was supported by a similar approach in which glucuronidation was preserved after injury of rat liver with carbon tetrachloride, which was presumed to selectively damage pericentral hepatocytes.[258] Use of bromobenzene, an agent assumed to cause midzonal hepatic necrosis, has led to the suggestion that glucuronosyltransferase is located in this zone as well as in pericentral hepatocytes.[258] A major drawback to using hepatotoxins to localize drug-metabolizing enzymes is that conclusions regarding their specificity are based on gross morphological alterations of selected regions of the hepatic lobule. Caution is required in interpreting such studies, because direct measurements of glucuronosyltransferase in microdissected samples and use of micro-light guides to monitor drug conjugation in sublobular zones of the liver indicate that glucuronidation occurs mainly in centrilobular hepatocytes.

Using quantitative histochemical sampling techniques introduced by Lowry and his coworkers,[261,262] we found significantly higher activities of glucuronosyltransferase in pericentral hepatocytes.[259,260] A newly developed ultramicroassay was used to measure UDP-glucuronosyltransferase in microdissected samples of periportal and pericentral regions of livers obtained from normal, phenobarbital-treated, and 3-methylcholanthrene-treated rats. Samples were obtained from 20-μm lyophilized tissue sections and assayed using 7-hydroxycoumarin as substrate. We found the activity of the enzyme to be consistently higher in tissues dissected from pericentral regions than in those obtained from periportal zones. For example, in normal rat liver, glucuronosyltransferase was about 0.7 nmole/mg dry wt. per min in periportal hepatocytes and 1.7 nmoles/mg dry wt. per min in pericentral hepatocytes. Treatment of rats with phenobarbital caused a slight increase (<2-fold) in both zones of the liver; however, 3-methylcholanthrene elevated glucuronosyltransferase 9-fold in periportal regions and about 8-fold in pericentral regions. On the basis of the affinity of the glucuronosyltransferase(s) for UDP-glucuronic acid and the aglycone 7-hydroxycoumarin, the forms of the enzyme appear similar in both zones. The K_m for UDP-glucuronic acid was about 0.2 mM and 55 μM for hydroxycoumarin.[260] 3-Methylcholanthrene appears to induce different forms of the enzyme than are normally present in the two zones, since the K_m's for UDPGA in both zones were elevated significantly after exposure to this carcinogen. Similar findings concerning the sublobular distribution of glucuronosyltransferase in rat liver have been reported by Ullrich et al.[284a]

Rates of glucuronidation in intact hepatocytes as well as in isolated microsomes may reflect the activities of both glucuronosyltransferase(s) and β-glucuronidase, which is also localized in the hepatic endoplasmic reticulum.[263,264] It has been proposed that net glucuronide production by the liver may be determined by a conjugation–deconjugation cycle.[265] In accord with this possibility, we have found that the production of p-nitrophenyl glucuronide by the isolated, perfused liver is inhibited by several agents that elevate cytosolic Ca^{2+} [266] and activate microsomal β-glucuronidase.[267] To date, the possibility that the content of microsomal β-glucuronidase varies across the liver lobule has not been studied. Preliminary studies conducted in our laboratory indicate that the total content of β-glucuronidase does not differ significantly in periportal and pericentral zones of the liver.

3.2.2. Use of Micro-Light Guides to Study Drug Conjugation in Specific Sublobular Zones

Recent development of noninvasive micro-light guides to monitor the fluorescence of drug metabolites now allows direct measurement of rates of conjugation in sublobular zones of the liver. Briefly, this approach involves placing micro-light guides with tip diameters of 150–170 μm on periportal and pericentral regions of hepatic lobules at the liver surface and monitoring the production or disappearance of a fluorescent drug substrate such as 7-hydroxycoumarin. This technique indicated that when small amounts of 7-hydroxycoumarin (<30 μM) were infused into the liver, all the substrate was conjugated in either the pericentral or the periportal region of the liver, depending on the direction of perfusion.[154] Sulfation predominated over glucuronidation when 2–10 μM 7-hydroxycoumarin was infused in the anterograde direction. At concentrations above 20 μM, glucuronidation predominated. When perfusion was in the retrograde direction, glucuronidation and sulfation were about equal with low concentrations of 7-hydroxycoumarin. These findings are in accord with the idea that at low concentrations of substrate, sulfation predominates over glucuronidation in periportal but not in pericentral hepatocytes. With high concentrations of 7-hy-droxycoumarin (>30 μM), the predominant conjugate in both zones of the liver is the glucuronide.

Micro-light guides have also been used to quantitate rates of glucuronidation in sublobular zones of the liver during infusion of high concentrations of substrate (see Fig. 5). This method involves measurement of 7-hydroxycoumarin fluores-cence in livers before and after the induction of complete anoxia in the tissue by perfusion with medium saturated with nitrogen containing 20 mM ethanol.[260] The rationale behind this approach is that induction of anoxia completely inhibits glucuronidation. Thus, the difference in fluorescence from the surface of livers perfused with 7-hydroxycoumarin before and after anoxia is a measure of the fraction of drug conjugated. Perfusions are performed in sulfate-free media to prevent sulfation. Using this method, maximal rates of 7-hydroxycoumarin glu-curonidation were found to be about 10 and 35 μmoles/g per hr in periportal and pericentral regions of livers from phenobarbital-treated rats. This technique also allowed kinetic analysis of drug conjugation in the two zones of intact livers, and it was found that half-maximal rates were obtained with 50 μM 7-hydrox-ycoumarin. This value is remarkably close to the value of 54 μM mentioned above for glucuronosyltransferase in microdissected samples of periportal and pericentral regions of the liver lobule. The maximal activity of the enzyme

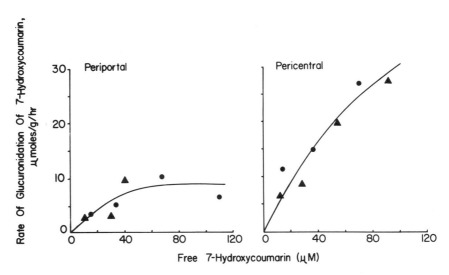

Figure 5. Rates of glucorinidation of 7-hydroxycoumarin in periportal and pericentral regions of perfused rat livers. The concentration of glucuronide conjugates formed in each region during anterograde (●) and retrograde (▲) perfusions was derived from fluorescence measurements of free 7-hydroxycoumarin in the tissue. Rates were calculated using the flow rate and the wet weight of each sublobular region (wet weight/2). Concentrations of substrate are the average of the free 7-hydroxycoumarin entering and leaving each sublobular region.

determined in microdissected samples using 7-hydroxycoumarin as substrate also differed by a factor of 3. Thus, the close correlation between maximal rates of 7-hydroxycoumarin glucuronosyltransferase measured *in vitro* and in the intact liver indicates that activities of this enzyme are important determinants of rates of glucuronidation in the two zones of the liver lobule.

3.2.3. Influence of Carbohydrate and Cofactors on Conjugation Reactions

In addition to enzyme activities, the supply of the cofactor UDPGA, which in turn is regulated by the content of carbohydrate in the liver[153] as well as the oxidation–reduction state of NAD, is an important determinant of rates of glucuronidation. The latter has been shown to influence the rate of UDP-glucose dehydrogenase in intact hepatocytes. The little information available indicates that the oxidation–reduction state of NAD is uniform across the liver lobule.[215] This is based on the measurements of glycerol-3-phosphate/dihydroxyacetone phosphate ratios in the two zones of the liver lobule.[215] No information exists concerning the translobular distribution of UDPGA across the liver lobule; however, studies of rates of 7-hydroxycoumarin conjugation in periportal and pericentral lobules of perfused livers from fasted rats suggest that during high rates of conjugation, UDPGA is rate-limiting.[260]

The content of UDPGA in hepatocytes is influenced by glucose supplied to the liver or derived from glycogenolysis. Thus, variation in glucose transport or glycogenolysis across the liver lobule might indirectly affect intracellular concentrations of UDPGA and conjugation in sublobular zones. Glycogen deposition and degradation appear to differ in periportal and pericentral hepatocytes. At the morphological level, glycogen is deposited as large discrete aggregates in the periportal zones and is dispersed homogeneously within the cytoplasm of pericentral hepatocytes.[211,268] In the presence of carbohydrate supplied in the diet, glycogen is stored initially in the periportal region; however, during glycogenolysis, glycogen disappears from both regions. An early histological study indicated that glycogen use was initially greatest in pericentral regions.[269] This pattern of glycogen synthesis and degradation appears to reflect the zonal distribution of glycogen synthetase and phosphorylase. Glycogen synthetase is concentrated in pericentral hepatocytes.[270] Relating the dynamics of glycogen turnover to drug conjugation in specific sublobular zones warrants further study.

3.3. Sulfation

It is well documented that the enzymes of mixed-function oxidation are unevenly distributed over the liver lobule[29,150,162,169,183]; however, much less information is available on enzyme systems involved in conjugation reactions. One approach has been the selective destruction of periportal or pericentral hepatocytes by site-specific toxins. James *et al.*[150] used allyl alcohol to destroy periportal regions and bromobenzene to damage pericentral areas prior to assaying for microsomal glucuronyltransferase activity. They observed higher specific activity of glucuronyltransferase in microsomes from bromobenzene-treated rats than in those from allyl-alcohol-treated rats, consistent with a predominant periportal localization of glucuronyltransferase activity. However, enzyme distribution in tissue may not determine local rates of glucuronidation *per se,* since the supply of the cofactor UDP-glucuronic acid may be an important determinant of rate.[153,271] With low substrate concentrations under conditions in which sulfation occurs, glucuronidation of 7-hydroxycoumarin in pericentral regions exceeded that in periportal areas. In the absence of sulfate, rates of glucuronidation in the two regions were equivalent. Thus, under these latter conditions, in which 7-hydroxycoumarin is most likely limiting, the lobular distribution of glucuronidation as measured quantitatively in these studies is different from the distribution of glucuronyltransferase activities following treatment with selective hepatotoxins.[150] At higher substrate concentrations (20–30 μM), glucuronidation occurred at about equal rates in both regions of the liver lobule. These studies demonstrate clearly the utillity of the new method described above, since it allows direct determination of rates of conjugation predominantly in pericentral and periportal regions of the liver lobule.

Sulfation has been shown to be a low-capacity, high-affinity system.[153,272] With excess sulfate, the entry of sulfate into the cell is much faster than rates of sulfation.[273] Pang and Terrell[156] utilized the uneven distribution of mixed-function oxidation to study the lobular distribution of sulfation in perfused liver. These studies were based on the reasonable assumption that phenacetin is converted into acetaminophen via mixed-function oxidation to a greater extent in pericentral hepatocytes than in periportal hepatocytes. Under these conditions, more acetaminophen sulfate was detected in the effluent perfusate with retrograde perfusions than with anterograde perfusions,[156] leading the authors to conclude that sulfation occurs to a greater extent in periportal hepatocytes than in pericentral hepatocytes. This conclusion is supported generally by direct measurement of rates of sulfation of 7-hydroxycoumarin in the studies reported here. Rates of sulfation are twice as high in periportal hepatocytes as in pericentral hepatocytes. Thus, these data are consistent with the hypothesis that either sulfotransferases or cofactor supply (e.g., 3′-phosphoadenosine 5′-phosphosulfate or the enzymes needed for its synthesis) predominate in periportal hepatocytes.

3.3.1. Competition between Sulfation and Glucuronidation in Periportal and Pericentral Regions of the Liver.

It is known that sulfation and glucuronidation can compete for substrate.[150] For example, when perfusate was switched from one containing sulfate to one deficient in sulfate, sulfation was rapidly diminished, whereas glucuronidation was enhanced. In these experiments, sulfation markedly exceeded glucuronidation at low concentrations in periportal hepatocytes, but not in pericentral hepatocytes. We therefore asked whether this was due to competition between the two metabolic processes for substrate. Since glucuronidation was significantly greater during perfusion with sulfate-free medium (i.e., in the absence of sulfation), we conclude that the higher rate of sulfation observed in periportal regions is due to competition for substrate. Competition was less dramatic between these two important metabolic systems in pericentral hepatocytes. At present, we cannot explain why the sulfation system is more successful at competing for substrate in periportal regions than in pericentral regions of the liver lobule. However, the sulfation system can compete more successfully for 7-hydroxycoumarin in both regions, since it has a much lower apparent K_m as derived from perfusion experiments (about 8 μM) than does glucuronidation (about 90 μM).

3.3.2. Generation of 7-Hydroxycourmarin via Mixed-Function Oxidation of 7-Ethoxycoumarin

When 7-ethoxycoumarin was added to the liver, about half of it was rapidly converted into 7-hydroxycoumarin conjugates. It is reasonable to assume that the remainder of the 7-ethoxycoumarin infused leaves the liver unmetabolized. Furthermore, perfusion of 7-ethoxycoumarin in the anterograde direction produced 7-hydroxycoumarin fluorescence from periportal regions but not from pericentral regions of the liver lobule. With retrograde perfusion, fluorescence was detected only in pericentral areas. At these low concentrations of 7-hydroxycoumarin formed, we assume that it is conjugated predominantly at the lobular site of generation, since 7-hydroxycoumarin was detected only in the region first exposed to flow. Thus, mixed-function oxidation appears to be rate-limiting for conjugation reactions in both regions when the substrate for conjugation arises via metabolism. It is therefore highly likely that conjugates are formed predominantly in the region of the liver lobule where they are generated. In support of this hypothesis, the patterns of the sulfate/glucuronide ratio were similar in any given lobular region irrespective of whether the substrate was 7-hydroxycoumarin or 7-ethoxycoumarin.

In another series of experiments, Conway et al.[154] studied rates of sulfation and glucuronidation in periportal and pericentral regions of the liver lobule by infusing 7-hydroxycoumarin. During infusion of up to 30 μM 7-hydroxycoumarin, fluorescence of free 7-hydroxycoumarin could be detected only in periportal regions during anterograde perfusion and in pericentral areas during retrograde perfusion. Over 95% of 7-hydroxycoumarin infused was converted into nonfluorescent sulfate and glucuronide conjugates. Thus, under these conditions, rates of sulfation can be studied in the periportal and pericentral regions of the lobule by measuring conjugates of 7-hydroxycoumarin in the effluent perfusate via anterograde or retrograde perfusions. Sulfation predominated over glucuronidation when 2–10 μM 7-hydroxycoumarin was infused in the anterograde direction; however, with 20–30 μM 7-hydroxycoumarin, glucuronidation predominated. In contrast, rates of glucuronidation and sulfation were similar when 2–5 μM 7-hydroxycoumarin was infused in the retrograde direction; however, glucuronidation predominated at higher substrate concentrations. Thus, at low concentrations of 7-hydroxycoumarin, sulfation predominated over glucuronidation in periportal hepatocytes, but not in pericentral hepatocytes. These data indicate that sulfation successfully competes with glucuronidation for 7-hydroxycoumarin at low substrate concentrations. Rates of sulfation were significantly greater (about 3-fold) in periportal regions than in pericentral regions when 7-hydroxycoumarin was infused directly or generated indirectly via mixed-function oxidation.

This method was not appropriate to measure glucuronidation, however, since the K_m of glucuronosyltransferase was an order of magnitude higher than the concentration of 7-hydroxycoumarin infused in the previous study. Therefore, the same authors developed another method to study glucuronidation in periportal and pericentral regions of the liver lobule at relatively high substrate concentrations.

Livers were perfused with sulfate-free buffer under normoxic conditions, and fluorescence of free 7-hydroxycoumarin was monitored in the tissue. The formation of nonfluorescent 7-hydroxycoumarin glucuronide was then inhibited completely by perfusion with N_2-saturated perfusate containing 20 mM ethanol. Under these conditions, fluorescence recorded from the surface of the liver was directly proportional to the concentration of substrate infused. The difference in 7-hydroxycoumarin fluorescence between perfusion with N_2 plus ethanol and normoxic perfusion was due to glucuronidation. Maximal rates of glucuronidation in periportal and pericentral regions of the liver lobule calculated with this new method were 9.6 and 35 μmoles/g per hr, respectively. Glucuronidation was half-maximal with 25–50 μM 7-hydroxycoumarin in both regions. Glucuronosyltransferase activity assayed in microdissected, freeze–dried tissue samples *in vitro* was 3-fold greater in pericentral than in periportal areas. This activity was half-maximal with 0.2 mM UDPGA and 54 μM 7-hydroxycoumarin in both regions of the liver lobule. Thus, the maximal capacity of the glucuronidation system determined *in vitro* is about 3-fold greater in pericentral than in periportal regions of the liver lobule, a difference that correlates well with measured rates of glucuronidation of 7-hydroxycoumarin in the two zones of the lobule in the intact, perfused liver.

3.4. Mercapturic Acid Synthesis

3.4.1. Intralobular Distribution of Glutathione

The tripeptide glutathione (L-γ-glutamyl-L-cysteinyl-glycine) is the most common nonprotein thiol in the liver. In its reduced form, it functions as an intracellular antioxidant, protecting sulfhydryl groups on cellular macromolecules.[274] In addition to this critically important function, reduced glutathione serves a number of important roles in the detoxification of hepatotoxins and other xenobiotics: First, reduced glutathione can inactivate electrophilically reactive metabolites by means of a nonenzymatic interaction with these molecules.[275] Second, it is a cofactor for the glutathione S-transferases, enzymes that inactive electrophiles by catalyzing their conjugation with reduced glutathione.[276] Third, it is also a cofactor for glutathione peroxidase, one of the key enzymes that protect cells from H_2O_2 and organic peroxides, including those produced during lipid peroxidation.[277] Hepatic levels of glutathione can be depleted either by substances, such as diethylmaleate and buthione sulfoximine, that inhibit its synthesis[278,279] or by single or repeated administration of high doses of hepatotoxins and other xenobiotics that require reduced glutathione for their inactivation.[280,281] Depletion of glutathione levels in liver is associated with the increased severities of hepatotoxicities produced by a number of chemicals, including acetaminophen,[280,281] vinyl chloride,[282] and bromobenzene.[283]

Since reduced glutathione is, by itself, so important for the inactivation of electrophilically reactive and toxic metabolites of hepatotoxins, and since the catalytic functions of both glutathione S-transferases and glutathione peroxidase are dependent on this thiol-containing compound, the distribution of reduced glutathione across the liver lobule might be one of the major underlying factors responsible for the relatively selective regional nature of many chemically induced hepatotoxicities. The intralobular distribution of reduced glutathione has been investigated histochemically; however, conflicting results have been reported. Both Asghar *et al.*[284] and Deml and Oesterle[285] observed that histochemical staining for reduced glutathione was dispersed fairly uniformly throughout the lobule in livers of control rats. In contrast to this visual finding, results of quantitative cytochemical analyses conducted by Smith *et al.*[286] revealed that reduced glutathione was distributed nonuniformly across the lobule. Smith and co-workers also demonstrated that centrilobular parenchymal cells contained significantly lower levels of reduced glutathione than did either midzonal or periportal cells. This latter finding may explain, at least in part, why centrilobular cells frequently exhibit a much greater susceptibility to chemically induced toxicities that result from the generation of reactive electrophiles that are inactivated by means of enzymatic and nonenzymatic conjugation with reduced glutathione.

3.4.2. Intralobular Distribution of the Glutathione S- Transferases

The glutathione S-transferases are a family of multifunctional enzymes that play significant roles in the detoxification of both endogenous and exogenous substances.[276,287] Not only are they capable of catalyzing the conjugation of the sulfhydryl group of reduced glutathione with a wide variety of electrophilic substances (this is the first step leading to the formation of water-soluble mercapturic acid derivatives that are readily excreted via the kidney),[276,287] but also they have the capacity to bind a large number of potentially toxic, hydrophobic nonsubstrates such as bilirubin.[53,54,57,276,288] Because of their multiple functions of detoxification, knowledge of how the glutathione S-transferases are distributed across the liver lobule should contribute significantly to an understanding of the basis for the relatively selective regional nature of many chemically induced hepatotoxicities.

The intralobular distributions of the glutathione S-transferases, especially transferase B, which has also been referred to as ligandin and azo-dye-binding protein, have been investigated solely through the application of immunohisto-chemical methodologies.[180–182,287] Conflicting findings have been reported, how-ever, for the distribution of glutathione S-transferase B across the liver lobule. Bannikov et al.[180] initially observed that centrilobular parenchymal cells were stained much more intensely for glutathione S-transferase B than were periportal cells in livers of control rats. Subsequently, Fleischner et al.[181] reported that parenchymal cells throughout the lobule in livers of control rats were stained with essentially equal intensity for this glutathione S-transferase, and Campbell et al.[182] reported similar findings on staining for this enzyme in human liver. More recently, the intralobular distributions of three isoenzymes of glutathione S-transferase, transferases B, C, and E, have been examined employing quali-tative and quantitative immunohistochemical techniques.[162,50] Redick et al.[50] demonstrated that each of these enzymes was present within parenchymal cells throughout the lobule in livers of control rats. In addition, glutathione S-trans-ferases C and E, but not transferase B, were shown to be present within bile-duct epithelial cells. While all parenchymal cells were stained by antibodies raised against the three glutathione S-transferases, staining produced by each antibody was found to be distributed nonuniformly across the lobule: Centrilob-ular cells were stained more intensely by each antibody than were either midzonal or periportal cells. In agreement with this visual observation, the results of quantitative immunohistochemical analyses[162] revealed that the level of each glutathione S-transferase decreased from the central vein toward the portal triad. While these findings have demonstrated that the glutathione S-transferases are not distributed uniformly across the liver lobule and that they are present at higher levels within pericentral parenchymal cells than within periportal cells, it must be appreciated that the catalytic role of these enzymes in the detoxication of chemicals is dependent, in large measure on the content of reduced glutathione within individual hepatic parenchymal cells. As indicated in the previous section, periportal parenchymal cells have been found to contain greater amounts of reduced glutathione than do centrilobular cells.[286] Thus, although reduced glu-tathione and the three glutathione S-transferases each exhibit gradients in their intralobular distributions, their gradients are opposing; that is, levels of the three glutathione S-transferases decrease from the central vein toward the portal triad, whereas reduced glutathione levels decrease from the portal triad toward the central vein. These findings may therefore explain why decreases in the hepatic levels of reduced glutathione lead to an exacerbation of the pericentral necrosis that results from the *in vivo* exposure to high doses of hepatotoxins such as acetaminophen[280,281] and bromobenzene.[282]

3.4.3. Intralobular Distribution of Glutathione Peroxidase

The fact that periportal parenchymal cells contain higher levels of reduced glutathione than do centrilobular cells only partially explains why periportal cells are usually less susceptible that pericentral cells to most chemically induced toxicities. A number of hepatotoxins, e.g., carbon tetrachloride, are considered to exert their deleterious effects on the liver parenchyma primarily, if not solely, by promoting lipid peroxidation.[51] Thus, glutathione peroxidase, the enzyme that catalyzes the breakdown and hence the inactivation of both organic hydroperoxides and H_2O_2,[277] is yet another factor that appears to be of considerable importance in affording protection to cells from chemically induced damage. The distribution of glutathione peroxidase across the liver lobule has recently been investigated. Employing an immunohistochemical approach, Yoshimura *et al.*[52] found that parenchymal cells throughout the lobule in livers of control rats were stained by an antibody raised against glutathione peroxidase. However, these investigators also observed that periportal cells were stained more intensely for this enzyme than were pericentral cells. This finding thus offers still another explanation as to why periportal cells usually exhibit greater resistance to most chemically induced toxicities than do pericentral cells.

4. CONCLUSIONS

Information that is becoming available on isoenzymes from histochemical techniques and on flux rates determined noninvasively with micro-light guides supports the conclusion that few rules about detoxification reactions in different regions of the liver lobule can be written. Rather, because of marked influences of inhibition and induction state on enzyme and cofactor supply, information on specific chemicals should be obtained experimentally.

REFERENCES

1. Zimmerman, H. J., 1978, *Hepatotoxicity,* Appleton-Century-Crofts, New York.
2. Rouiller, C., 1964, Experimental toxic injury of the liver, in: *The Liver,* Vol. II (C. Rouiller, ed.), pp. 335–476. Academic Press, New York.
3. Schoental, R., 1963, Liver disease and natural hepatotoxins, *Bull. W.H.O.* **29**:823–828.
4. Kraybill, H. R., 1974, The toxicology and epidemiology of natural hepatotoxin exposure, *Isr. J. Med. Sci.* **10**:416–430.

5. Klatskin, G., 1975, Toxic and drug-induced hepatitis, in: *Diseases of the Liver* (L. Schiff, ed.), pp. 604–710, J. B. Lippincott, Philadelphia.

6. Schmid, R., 1960, Cutaneous porphyria in Turkey, *N. Engl. J. Med.* **263**:397–400.

7. Von Oettingen, W. F., 1964, *The Halogenated Hydrocarbons of Industrial and Toxicological Importance,* Elsevier, Amsterdam.

8. Sakshqug, J., Sognen, E., Hansen, M. A., and Kippang, N., 1965, Its hepatotoxic effect in sheep and its occurrence in toxic batches of herring meal, *Nature (London)* **206**:1261–1264.

9. Wolff, I. A., and Wasserman, A. E., 1972, Nitrates, nitrites and nitrosamines, *Science* **177**:15–16.

10. Mitchell, J. R., and Jollow, D. J., 1975, Metabolic activation of drugs to toxic substances, *Gastroenterology* **68**:392–402.

11. Recknagel, R. O., and Glinde, E. A., 1973, Carbon tetrachloride hepatoxicity: An example of lethal cleavage, *CRC Crit. Rev. Toxicolol.* **2**:263–300.

12. Mitchell, J. R., Jollow, D. J., Gillette, J. R., and Brodie, B. B., 1973, Drug metabolism as a cause of drug toxicity, in *Drug Metab. Dispos.* **1**:418–438.

13. Miller, J. A., 1970, Carcinogenesis by chemicals, *Cancer Res.* **30**:559–570.

14. Magee, P. N., 1966, Toxic liver necrosis, *Lab Invest.* **15**:111–120.

15. Rees, K. R., and Tarlow, M. J., 1967, The hepatotoxic action of allyl formate, *Biochem. J.* **104**:757–762.

16. Mitchell, J. R., Thorgeirrson, U. P., and Black, M., 1975, Increased incidence of isoniazid hepatitis in rapid acetylators: Possible relation to hydrazine metabolites, *Clin. Pharmacol. Ther.* **18**:70–75.

17. Edmonson, H. A., and Schiff, L., 1975, Needle biopsy of the liver, in: *Diseases of the Liver* (L. Schiff, ed.), pp. 247–271, J. B. Lippincott, Philadelphia.

18. Farber, E., 1975, Some fundamental aspects of liver injury, in: *Alcohol Liver Pathology* (J. M. Khanna, Y. Israel, and H. Kalant, eds.), pp. 289–303, Addiction Research Foundation of Ontario, Toronto.

19. Judah, J. D., McLean, A. E. M., and McLean, E. K., 1970, Biochemical mechanisms of drug injury, *Am. J. Med.* **49**:609–614.

20. Glyn, L. E., and Himsworth, H. P., 1948, Intralobular circulation in acute liver injury by carbon tetrachloride, *Clin. Sci.* **19**:63–67.

21. Seneviratne, R. D., 1949, Physiological and pathological responses in blood vessels of the liver, *Q. J. Exp. Physiol.* **35**:77–82.

22. Christe, G. S., and Judah, J. D., 1954, Mechanisms of action of carbon tetrachloride, *Proc. R. Soc. London* **142**:241–249.

23. Kerr, J. F. R., 1973, Some lysosome functions in liver cells reacting to sublethal injury, in: *Lysosomes in Biology and Pathology* (J. Dingle, ed.), pp. 365–394, American Elsevier, New York.

24. Kamath, J. A., and Rubin, E., 1974, Effect of carbon tetrachloride and phenobarbital on plasma membranes: Enzymes and phospholipid transfer, *Lab. Invest.* **30**:494–499.

25. Govindan, V. M., Faulstich, H., Wieland, T., Agostini, B., and Hasselbach, W., 1972, *In vitro* effect of phalloidin on a plasma membrane preparation from rat liver, *Naturwissenschaften* **59**:521–528.

26. Farber, J. L., and El-Mofty, S. K., 1975, The biochemical pathology of liver cell necrosis, *Am. J. Pathol.* **81**:237–250.

27. Smith, M., Thor, T., and Orrenius, S., 1981, Toxic injury to isolated hepatocytes is not dependent on extracellular calcium, *Science* **213**:1257–1259.

28. Mitchell, J. R., Potter, W. Z., and Hinson, J. A., 1975, Toxic drug reactions, in: *Concepts in Biochemical Pharmacology* (J. R. Gillette ed.), pp. 383–419, Springer-Verlag, Berlin.

29. Ji, S., Lemasters, J. J., and Thurman, R. G., 1981, A fluorometric method to measure sublobular rates of mixed-function oxidation in the hemoglobin-free perfused rat liver, *Mol. Pharmacol.* **19**:513–516.

30. Matsumura, T., and Thurman, R. G., 1983, Measuring rates of O_2 uptake in periportal and pericentral regions of liver lobule: Stop-flow experiments with perfused liver, *Am. J. Physol.* **244**:G656–G659.

31. Ji, S., Lemasters, J. J., Christenson, V., and Thurman, R. G., 1982, Periportal and pericentral pyridine nucleotide fluorescence from the surface of the perfused liver: Evaluation of the hypothesis that chronic treatment with ethanol produces pericentral hypoxia, *Proc. Natl. Acad. Sci. U.S.A.* **79**:5415–5419.

32. Rees, K. R., and Tarlow, M. J., 1967, The hepatoxic action of allyl formate, in *Biochem. J.* **104**:757–761.

33. Serafini-Cessi, F., 1972, Conversion of allyl alcohol into acrolein by rat liver, *Biochem. J.* **128**:1103–1107.

34. Patel, J. M., Wood, J. C., and Leibman, K. C., 1980, The biotransformation of allyl alcohol and acrolein in rat liver and lung preparations, *Drug Metab. Dispos.* **8**:305–308.

35. Reid, W. D., 1972, Mechanism of allyl alcohol-induced hepatic necrosis, *Experientia* **28**:1058–1061.

36. Piazza, J. G., 1915, Toxicity of allyl formate, *Z. Exp. Pathol. Ther.* **17**:318–325.

37. Greenberger, N. J., Cohen, R. B., and Isselbacher, K. J., 1965, The effect of chronic ethanol administration on liver alcohol dehydrogenase activity in the rat, *Lab. Invest.* **14**:264–271.

38. Belinsky, S. A., Matsumura, T., Kauffman, F. C., and Thurman, R. G., 1984, Rates of allyl alcohol metabolism in periportal and pericentral regions of the liver lobule, *Mol. Pharmacol.* **25**:158–164.

39. Matsumura, T., and Thurman, R. G., 1983, A new method to measure rates of oxygen uptake in periportal and pericentral regions of the liver lobule, *Am. J. Physiol.* **6**:656–659.

40. Thorgeirsson, S. S., Mitchell, J. R., Sasame, H. A., and Potter, W. Z., 1976, Biochemical changes after hepatic injury by allyl alcohol and *N*-hydroxy-2-acetylaminofluorene, *Chem.-Biol. Interact.* **15**:139–147.

41. Meerman, J. H. N., and Mulder, G. J., 1981, Prevention of the hepatotoxic action of *N*-hydroxy-2-acetylaminofluorene in the rat by inhibition of N,O-sulfation by pentachlorophenol, *Life Sci.* **28**:2361–2365.

42. Miller, E. C., 1978, Some current perspectives on chemical carcinogenesis in humans and experimental animals, *Cancer Res.* **38**:1469–1496.

43. Zimmerman, H. J., 1968, The spectrum of hepatotoxicity, *Perspect. Biol. Med.* **12**:135.

44. Recknagel, R. O., and Glende, E. A., Jr., 1973, Carbon tetrachloride hepatotoxicity: An example of lethal cleavage, *CRC Crit. Rev. Toxicol.* **2**:263.

45. Slater, T. F., 1972, *Free Radical Mechanisms in Tissue Injury,* pp. 118–163, Arrowsmith, Bristol.

46. Reynolds, E. S., 1972, Comparison of early injury to liver endoplasmic reticulum by halo-methanes, hexachloroethane, benezene, toluene, bromobenzene, ethionine, thioacetamide and dimethylnitrosamine, *Biochem. Pharmacol.* **21**:2555.

47. Brauer, R. W., Leong, G. F., and Holloway, R. J., 1961, Liver injury in isolated perfused rat liver preparation exposed to chloroform, *Am. J. Physiol.* **200**:548.

48. Butler, T. C., 1961, Reduction of carbon tetrachloride *in vivo* and reduction of carbon tetrachloride and chloroform *in vitro* by tissue homogenates, *J. Pharmacol. Exp. Ther.* **134**:311.

49. Calligaro, A., and Vannini, V., 1975, Electron spin resonance study of homolytic cleavage of carbon tetrachloride in rat liver: Trichloromethyl free radicals, *Pharmacol. Res. Commun.* **7**:323.

50. Redick, J. A., Jakoby, W. B., and Baron, J., 1983, Immunohistochemical localization of glutathione S-transferases in livers of untreated rats, *J. Biol. Chem.* **257**:15,200–15,203.

51. Recknagel, R. O., Glende, E. A., Waller, R. L., and Lowrey, K., 1982, Lipid peroxidation: Biochemistry, measurements, and significance in liver cell injury, in: *Toxicology of the Liver* (G. Plaa and W. R. Hewitt, eds.), pp. 213–241, Raven Press, New York.

52. Yoshimura, S., Komatsu, N., and Watanabe, K., 1980, Purification and immunohistochemical localization of rat liver glutathione peroxidase, *Biochim. Biophys. Acta* **621:**130–137.
53. Wolkoff, A. W., Weisiger, R. A., and Jakoby, W. B., 1979, The multiple roles of the glutathione transferases (ligandins), in: *Progress in Liver Diseases,* Vol. 6 (H. Popper and F. Schaffner, eds.), pp. 213–224, Grune and Stratton, New York.
54. Vander Jagt, D. L., Wilson, S. P., Dean, V. L., and Simons, P. C., 1982, Bilirubin binding to rat liver ligandins (glutathione S-transferases A and B), *J. Biol. Chem.* **257:**1997–2001.
55. Drill, V. A., 1952, Hepatotoxic agents: Mechanism of action and dietary relationship, *Pharmacol. Rev.* **4:**1.
56. Mitchell, J. R., Thorgeirsson, S. S., Potter, W. Z., Jollow, D. J., and Keiser, H., 1974, Acetaminophen-induced hepatic injury: Protective role of glutathione in man and rationale for therapy, *Clin. Pharmacol. Ther.* **16:**676.
57. Smith, G. J., Ohl, V. S., and Litwack, G., 1977, Ligandin, the glutathione S-transferases, and chemically-induced hepatocarcinogenesis: A review, *Cancer Res.* **37:**8–14.
58. Björkhem, I., 1977, Rate-limiting step in microsomal cytochrome P-450 catalyzed hydroxylations, *Pharmacol. Ther.* **1:**327–348.
59. Cooper, D. Y., Levin, S., Narasimihulu, S., Rosenthal, O., and Estabrook, R. W., 1965, Photochemical action spectrum of the terminal oxidase of mixed-function oxidase systems, *Science* **147:**400–402.
60. Estabrook, R. W., and Werringloer, J., 1977, Cytochrome P-450—its role in oxygen activation for drug metabolism, in: *Drug Metabolism Concepts* (D. M. Jerina, ed.), pp. 16–26, American Chemical Society, Washington, D.C.
61. Lu, A. Y. H., and Levin, W., 1974, The resolution and reconstitution of the liver microsomal hydroxylation system, *Biochim. Biophys. Acta* **344:**205–240.
62. Omura, T., and Sato, R., 1964, The carbon monoxide-binding pigment of liver microsomes. I. Evidence for its hemoprotein nature, *J. Biol. Chem.* **239:**2370–2378.
63. Omura, T., and Sato, R., 1964, The carbon monoxide-binding pigment of liver microsomes. II. Solubilization, purification and properties, *J. Biol. Chem.* **239:**2379–2385.
64. Coon, M. J., Ballou, D. P., Haugen, D. A., Kzezoski, S. O., Nordblom, G. D., and White, R. E., 1977, Purification of membrane-bound oxygenases: Isolation of two electrophoretically homogenous forms of liver microsomal cytochrome P-450, in: *Microsomes and Drug Oxidations* (V. Ullrich, A. Hildebrandt, I. Roots, R. W. Estabrook, and A. H. Conney, eds.), pp. 82–84, Pergamon Press, New York.
65. Orrenius, S., Andersson, B., Jernström, B., and Moldeus, P., 1978, Isolated hepatocytes as an experimental tool in the study of drug conjugation reactions, in: *Conjugation Reactions in Drug Biotransformation* (A. Aitio, ed.), pp. 273–282, Elsevier/North-Holland, Amsterdam.
66. Kauffman, F. C., Evans, R. K., Reinke, L. A., and Thurman, R. G., 1979, Regulation of *p*-nitroanisole O-demethylation in perfused rat liver: Adenine nucleotide inhibition of NADP$^+$-dependent dehydrogenases and NADPH-cytochrome *c* reductase, *Biochem. J.* **184:**675–681.
67. Kauffman, F. C., Evans, R. K., and Thurman, R. G., 1977, Alterations in nicotinamide and adenine nucleotide systems during mixed-function oxidation of *p*-nitroanisole in perfused liver from normal and phenobarbital-treated rats, *Biochem. J.* **167:**583–592.
68. Campbell, T. C., and Hayes, J. R., 1976, The effect of quantity and quality of dietary protein on drug metabolism, *Fed. Proc. Fed. Am. Soc. Exp. Biol.* **35:**2470–2474.
69. Imai, Y., Sato, R., and Iyanagi, T., 1977, Rate-limiting step in the reconstituted microsomal drug hydroxylase system in *J. Biochem. (Tokyo)* **82:**1237–1246.
70. Guengerich, F. P., Ballou, D. P., and Coon, M. J., 1975, Purified liver microsomal cytochrome P-450: Electron-accepting properties and oxidation–reduction potential, *J. Biol. Chem.* **250:**7405–7414.
71. Matsubara, T., Baron, J., Peterson, L. L., and Peterson, J. A., 1976, NADPH-cytochrome P-450 reductase, *Arch. Biochem. Biophys.* **172:**463–469.

72. Thurman, R. G., and Scholz, R., 1969, Mixed-function oxidation in perfused rat liver: The effect of aminopyrine on oxygen uptake, *Eur. J. Biochem.* **10:**459–467.

73. Thurman, R. G., Marazzo, D. P., and Scholz, R., 1975, Mixed-function oxidation and intermediary metabolism: Metabolic interdependences in the liver, in *Cytochrome P-450 and b_5* (D. Y. Cooper, O. Rosenthal, R. Snyder, and C. Witmer, eds), pp. 355–370, Plenum Press, New York.

74. Reinke, L. A., Danis, M., Belinsky, S. A., Thurman, R. G., and Kauffman, F. C., 1980, Interactions between energy metabolism and mixed-function oxidation in perfused rat liver, in: *Microsomes, Drug Oxidations and Chemical Carcinogenesis,* Vol. II (M. J. Coon, A. H. Conney, R. W. Estabrook, U. V. Gelboin, J. R. Gillette, and P. J. O'Brien, eds.), pp. 953–957, Academic Press, New York.

75. Thurman, R. G., Lunguin, M., Evans, R., and Kauffman, F. C., 1977, The role of reducing equivalents generated in mitochondria in hepatic mixed-function oxidation, in *Microsomes and Drug Oxidation* (V. Ullrich, ed.), pp. 315–322, Pergamon Press, New York.

76. Campbell, T. C., and Hayes, J. R., 1974, Role of nutrition in the drug metabolizing enzyme system, *Pharmacol. Rev.* **26:**171–197.

77. Vermillion, J. L., and Coon, M. J., 1978, Purified liver microsomal NADPH-cytochrome P-450 reductase: Spectral characterization of oxidation–reduction states, *J. Biol. Chem.* **253:**2694–2704.

78. Junge, O., and Brand, K., 1975, Mixed-function oxidation of hexobarbital and generation of NADPH by the hexose monophosphate shunt in isolated rat liver cells, *Arch. Biochem. Biophys.* **171:**398–406.

79. Sies, H., Weigl, K., and Waydhaus, C., 1979, Metabolic consequences of drug oxidations in perfused liver and in isolated hepatocytes from phenobarbital-pretreated rats, in: *The Induction of Drug Metabolism* (R. W. Estabrook and E. L. Lindenlaub, eds.), pp. 381–400, F. K. Shattsuer Verlag, Stuttgart and New York.

80. Busch, U., 1975, Untersuchungen zur Regulation der Fettsäuresynthese in der perfundierten Rattenleber, Thesis, Medical Faculty of the University of Munich.

81. Sies, H., and Summer, K.-H., 1975, Hydroperoxide-metabolizing systems in rat liver, *Eur. J. Biochem,* **57:**503–512.

82. Eggleston, L. V., and Krebs, H. A., 1974, Regulation of the pentose phosphate cycle, *Biochem. J.* **138:**425–435.

83. Oshino, N., and Chance, B., 1977, Properties of glutathione release observed during reduction of organic hydroperoxides, demethylation of aminopyrine and oxidation of some substances in perfused rat liver, *Biochem. J.* **162:**509–525.

84. Kauffman, F. C., Evans, R. K., Reinke, L. A., Belinsky, S. A., Ballow, C., and Thurman, R. G., 1980, Effects of 3-methylcholanthrene on oxidized NADP-dependent dehydrogenases and selected metabolites in perfused rat liver, *Biochem. Pharmacol.* **29:**697–700.

85. Sies, H., Akerboom, T. P. M., and Tager, J. M., 1977, Mitochondrial and cytosolic NADPH systems and isocitrate dehydrogenase indicator metabolites during ureogenesis from ammonia in isolated rat hepatocytes, *Eur. J. Biochem.* **72:**301–307.

86. Tepperman, H. M., and Tepperman, J., 1964, Patterns of dietary and hormonal induction of certain NADP-linked liver enzymes, *Am. J. Physiol.* **206:**357–361.

87. Sies, H., and Brauser, B., 1970, Interaction of mixed-function oxidase with its substrates and associated redox transitions of cytochrome P-450 and pyridine nucleotides in perfused rat liver, *Eur. J. Biochem.* **15:**531–540.

88. Thurman, R. G., Marazzo, D. R., Jones, L. S., and Kauffman, F. C., 1977, The continuous kinetic determination of *p*-nitroanisole O-demethylation in hemoglobin-free perfused rat liver, *J. Pharmacol. Exp. Ther.* **201:**498–506.

89. Lehninger, A. L., 1951, Phosphorylation coupled to oxidation of dihydrodiphosphopyridine nucleotide, *J. Biol. Chem.* **190:**345–359.

90. Hoek, J. B., and Ernster, L., 1974, Mitochondrial transhydrogenase and the regulation of cytosolic reducing power, in: *Alcohol and Aldehyde Metabolizing Systems* (R. G. Thurman, T. Yonetani, J. R. Williamson, and R. Chance, eds.), pp. 351–364, Academic Press, New York.

91. Rydstrom, J., 1972, Site-specific inhibitors of mitochondrial nicotinamide-nucleotide transhydrogenase, *Eur. J. Biochem.* **31:**496–504.

92. Cinti, D. L., Ritchie, A., and Schenkman, J. B., 1972, Hepatic organelle interaction. II. Effect of tricarboxylic acid cycle intermediates on N-demethylation and hydroxylation reactions in rat liver, *Mol. Pharmacol.* **8:**338–344.

93. Cinti, D. L., and Schenkman, J. B., 1972, Hepatic organelle interaction. I. Spectral investigation during drug biotransformation, *Mol. Pharmacol.* **8:**338–344.

94. Belinsky, S. A., Reinke, L. A., Kauffman, F. C., and Thurman, R. G., 1980, Inhibition of mixed-function oxidation of p-nitroanisole and conjugation of p-nitrophenol in perfused rat liver by 2,4-dinitrophenol, *Arch. Biochem. Biophys.* **204:**207–213.

95. Williamson, D. H., Ellington, E. V., Illic, V., and Saal, J., 1973, Hepatic effects of saturated and unsaturated short-chain fatty acids and the control of ketogenesis *in vivo,* in: *Regulation of Hepatic Metabolism* (F. Lundquist and N. Tygstrup, eds.), pp. 191–206, Academic Press, New York.

96. Plaut, G. W. E., 1970, DPN-linked isocitrate dehydrogenase of animal tissue, *Curr. Top. Cell. Regul.* **2:**1–27.

97. Goebell, H., and Klingenberg, M., 1964, DPN-spezifische Isocitrat-dehydrogenase der Mitochondrien, *Biochem Z.* **340:**441–464.

98. Pette, D., 1965, Mitochondrial enzyme activities in regulation of metabolic processes in mitochondria, in: *Regulation of Metabolic Processes in Mitochondria,* Vol. VII (J. M. Tager, S. Papa, E. Quagliariello, and E. C. Slater, eds.), pp. 28–50, Elsevier, New York.

99. Reinke, L., Belinsky, S. A., Thurman, R. G., and Kauffman, F. C., 1980, A mechanism of inhibition of mixed-function oxidation by ethanol, in: *Alcohol and Aldehyde Metabolizing Systems,* Vol. IV (R. G. Thurman, ed.), pp. 151–162, Plenum Press, New York.

100. Weigl, K., and Sies, H., 1977, Drug oxidations dependent on cytochrome P-450 in isolated hepatocytes, *Eur. J. Biochem.* **77:**401–408.

101. Thurman, R. G., and Scholz, R., 1973, Interaction of mixed-function oxidation with biosynthetic processes. 2. Inhibition of lipogenesis by aminopyrine in perfused rat liver, *Eur. J. Biochem.* **38:**73–78.

102. Thurman, R. G., Reinke, L. A., and Kauffman, F. C., 1979, The isolated perfused liver: A model to define biochemical mechanisms of chemical toxicity, *Biochem. Toxicol.* **1:**249–285.

103. Grundin, R., Moldéus, P., Vadi, H., Orrenius, S., Von Bahr, C., Bäckström, D., and Ehrenberg, A., 1975, Drug metabolism in isolated rat liver cells, *Adv. Exp. Med. Biol.* **58:** 251–269.

104. Sies, H., and Kandel, M., 1970, Positive increase of redox potential of the extramitochondrial NADP(H) system by mixed-function oxidations in hemoglobin-free perfused rat liver, *FEBS Lett.* **9:**205–208.

105. Afolayan, A., 1972, Regulation and kinetics of glucose-6-phosphate dehydrogenase from *Candida utilis, Biochemistry* **11:**4172–4178.

106. Avigad, G., 1966, Inhibition of glucose-6-phosphate dehydrogenase by adenosine 5′-triphosphate, *Proc. Nat. Acad. Sci. U.S.A.* **56:**1543–1547.

107. Kauffman, F. C., and Johnson, E. C., 1970, Regulatory properties of 6-P-gluconate dehydrogenase from mammalian brain, *Fed Proc.* **29:**892.

108. Passonneau, J. V., Schultz, D., and Lowry, O. H., 1966, The kinetics of glucose-6-P-dehydrogenase, *Fed Proc.* **25:**219 (Abstract 167).

109. Maenpaa, P. H., Raivio, K. O., and Kekomaki, M. P., 1968, Liver adenine nucleotides: Fructose-induced depletion and its effect on protein synthesis, *Science* **161:**1253–1254.

110. Woods, H. F., Eggleston, L. V., and Krebs, H. A., 1970, The cause of hepatic accumulation of fructose 1-phosphate on fructose loading, *Biochem. J.* **119**:501–510.
111. Roach, M. K., 1975, Microsomal ethanol oxidation: Activity *in vitro* and *in vivo*, in: *Biochemical Pharmacology of Ethanol* (E. Majchrowicz, ed.), pp. 33–56, Plenum Press, New York.
112. Thurman, R. G., 1977, Hepatic alcohol oxidation and its metabolic liability, *Fed. Proc.* **36**:1640–1646.
113. Thurman, R. G., Reinke, L. A., Belinsky, S. A., and Kauffman, F. C., 1980, The influence of the nutritional state in rates of *p*-nitroanisole O-demethylation and *p*-nitrophenol conjugation in perfused rat liver, in: *Microsomes, Drug Oxidations and Chemical Carcinogenesis*, Vol. II (M. J. Coon, A. H. Conney, R. W. Estabrook, H. V. Gelboin, J. R. Gillette, and P. J. O'Brien, eds.), pp. 913–916, Academic Press, New York.
114. Orme-Johnson, W. H., and Ziegler, D. M., 1965, Alcohol mixed-function oxidation activity of mammalian liver microsomes, *Biochem. Biophys. Res. Commun.* **21**:78–82.
115. Thurman, R. G., Ley, H. G., and Scholz, R., 1972, Hepatic microsomal ethanol oxidation, *Eur. J. Biochem.* **25**:420–43.
116. Thurman, R. G., and Scholz, R., 1973, The role of hydrogen peroxide and catalase in hepatic microsomal ethanol oxidation, *Drug Metab. Dispos.* **1**:441–448.
117. Vatsis, K. P., and Coon, M. J., 1977, On the question of whether cytochrome P-450 catalyzes ethanol oxidation: Studies with purfied forms of the cytochrome from rabbit liver microsomes, in: *Alcohol and Aldehyde Metabolizing Systems*, Vol. II (R. G. Thurman, J. R. Williamson, H. Drott, and B. Chance, eds.), pp. 307–322, Academic Press, New York.
118. Miwa, G. T., Levin, W., Thomas, P. F., and Lu, A. Y. H., 1977, Evidence for the direct involvement of hepatic cytochrome P-450 in ethanol metabolism, in: *Alcohol and Aldehyde Metabolizing Systems*, Vol. II (R. G. Thurman, J. R. Williamson, H. Drott, and B. Chance, eds.), pp. 323–340, Academic Press, New York.
119. Ohnishi, K., and Lieber, C. A., 1977, Reconstitution of the hepatic microsomal ethanol oxidizing system (MEOS) in control rats after ethanol feeding, in: *Alcohol and Aldehyde Metabolizing Systems*, Vol. II (R. G. Thurman, J. R. Williamson, H. Drott, and B. Chance, eds.), pp. 341–350, Academic Press, New York.
120. Mezey, E., 1976, Ethanol metabolism and ethanol–drug interactions, *Biochem. Pharmacol.* **25**:869–875.
121. Rubin, E., Gang, A., Misra, P. S., and Lieber, C. S., 1970, Inhibition of drug metabolism by acute ethanol intoxication, *Am. J. Med.* **49**:801–806.
122. Imai, Y., and Sato, R., 1967, Studies on the substrate interactions with P-450 in drug hydroxylation by liver microsomes, *J. Biochem. (Tokyo)* **82**:1237–1246.
123. Reinke, L. A., Kauffman, F. C., and Thurman, R. G., 1979, Stimulation of *p*-nitroanisole O-demethylation in perfused livers from fasted rats, *J. Pharmacol. Exp. Ther.* **211**:133–139.
124. Grundin, R., 1975, Metabolic interaction of ethanol and alprenolol in isolated liver cells, *Acta Pharmacol. Toxicol.* **37**:185–200.
125. Reinke, L. A., Kauffman, F. C., and Thurman, R. G., 1980, Stimulation of *p*-nitroanisole O-demethylation in perfused rat livers by xylitol and sorbitol, *Biochem. Pharmacol.* **28**:813–819.
126. Correia, M. A., and Mannering, G. J., 1973, Reduced diphosphopyridine nucleotide synergism of the reduced triphosphopyridine nucleotide-dependent mixed-function oxidase system of hepatic microsomes. I. Effects of activation and inhibition of the fatty acyl coenzyme A desaturation system, *Mol. Pharmacol.* **9**:455–469.
127. Mannering, G. J., 1973, Microsomal enzyme systems which catalyze drug metabolism, in: *Fundamentals of Drug Metabolism and Drug Disposition* (B. N. La Du, H. G. Mandel, and E. C. Way, eds.), pp. 206–214, Williams & Wilkins, Baltimore.
128. Raj, H. G., and Venkitasubramanian, T. A., 1974, Carbohydrate metabolism in aflatoxin B_1 toxicity, *Environ. Physiol. Biochem.* **4**:181–187.

129. Hildebrandt, A., and Estabrook, R. W., 1971, Evidence for the participation of cytochrome b_5 in hepatic microsomal mixed-function oxidation reactions, *Arch. Biochem. Biophys.* **143:**66–79.

130. Reinke, L. A., Kauffman, F. C., Belinsky, S. A., and Thurman, R. G., 1980, Interactions between ethanol metabolism and mixed-function oxidation in perfused rat liver: Inhibition of p-nitroanisole O-demethylation, *J. Pharmacol Exp. Ther.* **213:**70–78.

131. Lieber, C. A., and Decarli, L. M., 1970, Reduced nicotinamide-adenine dinucleotide phosphate oxidase: Activity enhanced by ethanol consumption, *Science* **170:**78–79.

132. Thurman, R. G., 1973, Induction of hepatic microsomal reduced nicotinamide adenine dinucleotide phosphate-dependent production of hydrogen peroxide by chronic prior treatment with ethanol, *Mol. Pharmacol.* **9:**670–675.

133. Tobon, F., and Mezey, E., 1971, Effect of ethanol administration on hepatic ethanol and drug-metabolizing enzymes on rates of ethanol degradation, *J. Lab. Clin. Med.* **77:**110–121.

134. Khanna, J. M., Kalant, H., Lin, G., and Bustos, G. O., 1971, Effect of carbon tetrachloride treatment on ethanol metabolism, *Biochem. Pharmacol.* **20:**3269–3279.

135. Mezey, E., 1972, Duration of the enhanced activity of the microsomal ethanol-oxidizing enzyme system and rate of ethanol degradation in ethanol-fed rats after withdrawal, *Biochem. Pharmacol.* **21:**137–142.

136. Novikoff, A. B., 1959, Cell heterogeneity within the hepatic lobule of the rat (staining reactions), *J. Histochem. Cytochem.* **7:**240–244.

137. Novikoff, A. B., and Essner, E., 1960, The liver cell: Some new approaches to its study, *Am. J. Med.* **29:**102–131.

138. Katz, N., and Jungermann, K., 1976, Autoregulatory shift from fructolysis to lactate gluconeogenesis in rat hepatocyte suspensions: The problem of metabolic zonation of liver parenchyma, *Hoppe-Seyler's Z. Physiol. Chem.* **357:**359–375.

139. Jungermann, K., and Sasse, D., 1978, Heterogeneity of liver parenchymal cells, *Trends Biochem. Sci.* **3:**198–202.

140. Rappaport, A. M., 1979, Physioanatomical basis of toxic liver injury, in: *Toxic Injury of the Liver,* Part A (E. Farber and M. M. Fisher, eds.), pp. 1–57, Marcel Dekker, New York.

141. Jungermann, K., Heilbronn, R., Katz, N., and Sasse, D., 1982, The glucose–glucose-6-phosphate cycle in the periportal and perivenous zones of rat liver, *Eur. J. Biochem.* **123:**429–436.

142. Andersen, B., Nath, A., and Jungermann, K., 1982, Heterogeneous distribution of phosphoenolpyruvate carboxykinase in rat liver parenchyma, isolated, and cultured hepatocytes, *Eur. J. Cell Biol.* **28:**47–53.

143. Jungermann, K., and Katz, N., 1982, Functional hepatocellular heterogeneity, *Hepatology* **2:**385–395.

144. Katz, N. R., Fischer, W., and Ick, M., 1983, Heterogeneous distribution of ATP citrate lyase in rat-liver parenchyma: Microradiochemical determination in microdissected periportal and perivenous liver tissue, *Eur. J. Biochem.* **130:**297–301.

145. Gumucio, J. J., DeMason, L. J., Miller, D. L., Krezoski, S. O., and Keener, M., 1978, Induction of cytochrome P-450 in a selective subpopulation of hepatocytes, *Am. J. Physiol.* **234:**C102–C109.

146. Sweeney, G. D., Garfield, R. E., Jones, K. G., and Latham, A. N., 1978, Studies using sedimentation velocity on heterogeneity of size and function of hepatocytes from mature male rats, *J. Lab. Clin. Med.* **91:**432–443.

147. Tonda, K., Hasegawa, T., and Hirata, M., 1983, Effects of phenobarbital and 3-methylcholanthrene pretreatments on monooxygenase activities and proportions of isolated rat hepatocyte populations, *Mol. Pharmacol.* **23:**235–343.

148. Brodie, B. B., Reid, W. D., Cho, A. K., Sipes, G., Krishna, G., and Gillette, J. R., 1971, Possible mechanism of liver necrosis caused by aromatic organic compounds, *Proc. Natl. Acad. Sci. U.S.A.* **68:**160–164.

149. Jollow, D. J., Mitchell, J. R., Potter, W. Z., Davis, D. C., Gillette, J. R., and Brodie, B.

B., 1973, Acetaminophen-induced hepatic necrosis. II. Role of covalent binding *in vivo, J. Pharmacol. Exp. Ther.* **187**:185–202.

150. James, R., Desmond, P., Kupfer, A., Schenker, S., and Branch, R. A., 1981, The differential localization of various drug metabolizing systems within the rat liver lobule as determined by the hepatotoxins allyl alcohol, carbon tetrachloride and bromobenzene, *J. Pharmacol. Exp. Ther.* **217**:127–132.

151. Willson, R. A., and Hart, J. R., 1981, *In vivo* drug metabolism and liver lobule heterogeneity in the rat, *Gastroenterology* **81**:563–569.

152. Gumbrecht, J. R., and Franklin, M. R., 1983, The alteration of hepatic cytochrome P-450 subpopulations of phenobarbital-induced and uninduced rat by regioselective hepatotoxins, *Drug Metab. Dispos.* **11**:312–318.

153. Reinke, L. A., Belinsky, S. A., Evans, R. K., Kauffman, F. C., and Thurman, R. G., 1981, Conjugation of *p*-nitrophenol in the perfused rat liver: The effect of substrate concentration and carbohydrate reserves, *J. Pharmacol. Exp. Ther.* **217**:863–870.

154. Conway, J. G., Kauffman, F. C., Ji, S., and Thurman, R. G., 1982, Rates of sulfation and glucuronidation of 7-hydroxycoumarin in periportal and pericentral regions of the liver lobule, *Mol. Pharmacol.* **22**:509–516.

155. Pang, K. S., Koster, H., Halsema, I. C. M., Scholtens, E., and Mulder, G. J., 1981, Aberrant pharmocokinetics of harmol in the perfused rat liver preparation: Sulfate and glucuronide conjugations, *J. Pharmacol. Exp. Ther.* **219**:134–140.

156. Pang, K. S., and Terrell, J. A., 1981, Retrograde perfusion to probe the heterogeneous distribution of hepatic drug metabolizing enzymes in rats, *J. Pharmacol. Exp. Ther.* **216**:339–346.

157. Pang, K. S., Koster, H., Halsema, I. C. M., Scholtens, E., Mulder, G. J., and Stillwell, R. N., 1983, Normal and retrograde perfusion to probe the zonal distribution of sulfation and glucuronidation activities of harmol in the perfused rat liver preparation, *J. Pharmacol Exp. Ther.* **224**:647–653.

158. Wattenberg, L. W., and Leong, J. L., 1962, Histochemical demonstration of reduced pyridine nucleotide dependent polycyclic hydrocarbon metabolizing systems, *J. Histochem. Cytochem.* **10**:412–420.

159. Koudstaal, J., and Hardonk, M. J., 1969, Histochemical demonstration of enzymes related to NADPH-dependent hydroxylating systems in rat liver after phenobarbital treatment, *Histochemie* **20**:68–77.

160. Gangolli, S., and Wright, M., 1971, The histochemical demonstration of aniline hydroxylase activity in rat liver, *Histochem. J.* **3**:107–116.

161. Grasso, P., Williams, M., Hodgson, R., Wright, M. G., and Gangolli, S. D., 1971, The histochemical distribution of aniline hydroxylase in rat tissues, *Histochem. J.* **3**:117–126.

162. Baron, J., Kawabata, T. T., Knapp, S. A., Voigt, J. M., Redick, J. A., Jakoby, W. B., and Guengerich, F. P., 1984, Intrahepatic distribution of xenobiotic-metabolizing enzymes, in: *Foreign Compound Metabolism* (J. Caldwell and G. D. Paulson, eds.), pp. 17–36, Taylor & Francis, London.

163. Altman, F. P., Moore, D. S., and Chayen, J., 1975, The direct measurement of cytochrome P-450 in unfixed tissue sections, *Histochemistry* **41**:227–232.

164. Gooding, P. E., Chayen, J., Sawyer, B., and Slater, T. F., 1978, Cytochrome P-450 distribution in rat liver and the effect of sodium phenobarbitone administration, *Chem.-Biol. Interact.* **20**:299–310.

165. Chayen, J., Bitensky, L., Johnstone, J. J., Gooding, P. E., and Slater, T. F., 1979, The application of microspectrophotometry to the measurement of cytochrome P-450, in: *Quantitative Cytochemistry and Its Applications* (J. R. Pattison, L. Bitensky, and J. Chayen, eds.), pp. 129–137, Academic Press, New York.

166. Smith, M. T., and Wills, E. D., 1981, Effects of dietary lipid and phenobarbitone on the

distribution and concentration of cytochrome P-450 in the liver studied by quantitative cytochemistry, *FEBS Lett.* **127**:33–36.

167. Smith, M. T., and Wills, E. D., 1981, The effects of dietary lipid and phenobarbitone on the production and utilization of NADPH in the liver: A combined biochemical and quantitative cytochemical study, *Biochem. J.* **200**:691–699.

168. Ji, S., Lemasters, J. J., and Thurman, R. G., 1980, A non-invasive method to study metabolic events within sublobular regions of hemoglobin-free perfused liver, *FEBS Lett.* **113**:37–41.

169. Redick, J. A., Kawabata, T. T., Guengerich, F. P., Krieter, P. A., Shires, T. K., and Baron, J., 1980, Distributions of monooxygenase components and epoxide hydratase within the livers of untreated male rats, *Life Sci.* **27**:2465–2470.

170. Baron, J., Taira, Y., Redick, J. A., Greenspan, P., Kapke, G. F., and Guengerich, F. P., 1980, Effects of xenobiotics on the distributions of monooxygenase components in liver, in: *Microsomes, Drug Oxidations and Chemical Carcinogenesis*, Vol. II (M. J. Coon, A. H. Conney, R. W. Estabrook, H. V. Gelboin, J. R. Gillette, and P. J. O'Brien, eds.), pp. 501–504, Academic Press, New York.

171. Masters, B. S. S., Yasukochi, Y., Okita, R. T., Parkhill, L. K., Taniguchi, H., and Dees, J. H., 1980, Laurate hydroxylation and drug metabolism in pig liver and kidney, in *Microsomes, Drug Oxidations and Chemical Carcinogenesis*, Vol. II (M. J. Coon, A. H. Conney, R. W. Estabrook, H. V. Gelboin, J. R. Gillette, and P. J. O'Brien, eds.), pp. 709–719, Academic Press, New York.

172. Koyada, A. Yu., 1981, Immunohistochemical localization of cytochrome P-450 in rat liver during phenobarbital induction, *Bull. Exp. Biol. Med.* **92**:994–996.

173. Dees, J. H., Masters, B. S. S., Muller-Eberhard, U., and Johnson, E. F., 1982, Effect of 2,3,7,8-tetrachlorodibenzo-*p*-dioxin and phenobarbital on the occurrence and distribution of four cytochrome P-450 isozymes in rabbit kidney, lung, and liver, in *Cancer Res.* **42**:4123–4132.

174. Ohnishi, K., Mishima, A., and Okuda, K., 1982, Immunofluorescence of phenobarbital inducible cytochrome P-450 in the hepatic lobule of normal and phenobarbital inducible cytochrome P-450 in the hepatic lobule of normal and phenobarbital-treated rats, *Hepatology* **2**:849–855.

175. Moody, D. E., Taylor, L. A., Smuckler, E. A., Levin, W., and Thomas, P. E., 1983, Immunohistochemical localization of cytochrome P-450a in liver sections from untreated rats and rats treated with phenobarbital or 3-methylcholanthrene, *Drug Metab. Dispos.* **11**:339–343.

176. Muller-Eberhard, U., Yam, L., Tavassoli, M., Cox, K., and Ozols, J., 1974, Immunohistochemical demonstration of cytochrome b_5 and hemopexin in rat liver parenchymal cells using horseradish peroxidase, *Biochem. Biophys. Res. Commun.* **61**:983–988.

177. Franke, W. W., Fink, A., and Schmid, E., 1978, Demonstration of the display of components of the endoplasmic reticulum by indirect fluorescence microscopy using antibodies against cytochrome b_5 from rat liver microsomes, *Cell Biol. Int. Rep.* **2**:465–474.

178. Bentley, P., Waechter, F., Oesch, F., and Staubli, W., 1979, Immunochemical localization of epoxide hydratase in rat liver: Effects of 2 acetylaminofluorene, *Biochem. Biophys. Res. Commun.* **91**:1101–1108.

179. Enomoto, K., Ying, T. S., Griffin, M. J., and Farber, E., 1981, Immunohistochemical study of epoxide hydrolase during experimental liver carcinogenesis, *Cancer Res.* **41**:3281–3287.

180. Bannikov, G. A., Guelstein, V. I., and Tchipsheva, T. A., 1973, Distribution of basic azo dye binding protein in normal rat tissues and carcinogen-induced liver tumors, *Int. J. Cancer* **11**:398–411.

181. Fleischner, G. M., Robbins, J. B., and Arias, I. M., 1977, Cellular localization of ligandin in rat, hamster, and man, *Biochem. Biophys. Res. Commun.* **74**:992–1000.

182. Campbell, J. A. H., Bass, N. M., and Kirsch, R. E., 1980, Immunohistological localization of ligandin in human tissues, *Cancer* **45**:503–510.

183. Baron, J., Redick, J. A., and Guengerich, F. P., 1978, Immunohistochemical localizations of cytochromes P-450 in rat liver, *Life Sci.* **23**:2627–2632.

184. Baron, J., Redick, J. A., and Guengerich, F. P., 1981, An immunohistochemical study on the localizations and distributions of phenobarbital and 3-methylcholanthrene-inducible cytochromes P-450 within the livers of untreated rats, *J. Biol. Chem.* **256:**5931–5937.

185. Baron, J., Redick, J. A., and Guengerich, F. P., 1982, Effects of 3-methylcholanthrene, β-naphthoflavone, and phenobarbital on the 3-methylcholanthrene-inducible isozymes of cytochrome P-450 within centrilobular, midzonal, and periportal hepatocytes, *J. Biol. Chem.* **257:**953–957.

186. Guengerich, F. P., 1977, Separation and purification of multiple forms of microsomal cytochrome P-450: Activities of different forms of cytochrome P-450 towards several compounds of environmental interest, *J. Biol. Chem.* **252:**3970–3979.

187. Guengerich, F. P., 1978, Separation and purification of multiple forms of microsomal cytochrome P-450: Partial characterization of three apparently homogeneous cytochromes P-450 prepared from livers of phenobarbital and 3-methylcholanthrene-treated rats, *J. Biol. Chem.* **253:**7931–7979.

188. Guengerich, F. P., Danna, G. A., Wright, S. T., Martin, M. V., and Kaminsky, L. S., 1982, Purification and characterization of liver microsomal cytochromes P-450: Electrophoretic, spectral, catalytic, and immunochemical properties and inducibility of eight isozymes isolated from rats treated with phenobarbital and β-naphthoflavone, *Biochemistry* **21:** 6019–6030.

189. Tuchweber, G., Werringloer, J., and Kourounakis, P., 1974, Effect of phenobarbital or pregnenolone-16-α-carbonitrile (PCN) pretreatment on acute carbon tetrachloride hepatotoxicity in rats, *Biochem. Pharmacol.* **23:**513–518.

190. Baron, J., Redick, J. A., Greenspan, P., and Taira, Y., 1978, Immunohistochemical localization of NADPH-cytochrome *c* reductase in rat liver, *Life Sci.* **22:**1097–1102.

191. Taira, Y., Redick, J. A., and Baron, J., 1980, An immunohistochemical study on the localization and distribution of NADPH-cytochrome *c* (P-450) reductase in rat liver, *Mol. Pharmacol.* **17:**374–381.

192. Taira, Y., Greenspan, P., Kapke, G. F., Redick, J. A., and Baron, J., 1980, Effects of phenobarbital, pregnenolone-16-α-carbonitrile and 3-methylcholanthrene pretreatments on the distributions of NADPH-cytochrome *c* (P-450) reductase within the liver lobule, *Mol. Pharmacol.* **18:**304–312.

193. Dees, J. H., Coe, L. D., Yasukochi, Y., and Masters, B. S. S., 1980, Immunofluorescence of NADPH-cytochrome *c* (P-450) reductase in rat and guinea pig tissues injected with phenobarbital, *Science* **208:**1473–1475.

194. Smith, M. T., Redick, J. A., and Baron, J., 1983, Quantitative immunohistochemistry: A comparison of microdensitometric analysis of unlabeled antibody staining and of microfluorometric analysis of indirect fluorescent antibody staining for nicotinamide adenosine dinucleotide phosphate (NADPH)-cytochrome *c* (P-450) reductase in rat liver, *J. Histochem. Cytochem.* **31:**1183–1189.

195. Tavassoli, M., Ozols, J. Sugimoto, G., Cox, K. H., and Muller-Eberhard, U., 1976, Localization of cytochrome b_5 in rat organs and tissues by immunohistochemistry, *Biochem. Biophys. Res. Commun.* **72:**281–287.

196. Jerina, D. M., and Daly, J. W., 1974, Arene oxides: A new aspect of drug metabolism, *Science* **185:**573–582.

197. Oesch, F., 1973, Mammalian epoxide hydratases: Inducible enzymes catalyzing the inactivation of carcinogenic and cytotoxic metabolites derived from aromatic and olefinic compounds, *Xenobiotica* **3:**305–340.

198. Huberman, E., Sachs, L., Yang, S. K., and Gelboin, H. V., 1976, Identification of mutagenic metabolites of benzo[a]pyrene in mammalian cells, *Proc. Natl. Acad. Sci. U.S.A.* **73:** 607–611.

199. Baron, J., Redick, J. A., and Guengerich, F. P., 1980, Immunohistochemical localization of epoxide hydratase in rat liver, *Life Sci.* **26:**489–493.

200. Kawabata, T. T., Guengerich, F. P., and Baron, J., 1981, An immunohistochemical study on the localization and distribution of epoxide hydrolase within livers of untreated rats, *Mol. Pharmacol.* **20**:709–714.

201. Kawabata, T. T., Guengerich, F. P., and Baron, J., 1983, Effects of phenobarbital, trans-stilbene oxide, and 3-methycholanthrene on epoxide hydrolase within centrilobular, midzonal, and periportal regions of rat liver, *J. Biol. Chem.* **258**:7767–7773.

202. Thurman, R. G., and Kauffman, F. C., 1980, Factors regulating drug metabolism in intact hepatocytes, *Pharmacol. Rev.* **31**:229–251.

203. Junge, O., and Brand, K., 1975, Mixed-function oxidation of hexobarbital and generation of NADPH by the hexose monophosphate shunt in isolated rat liver cells, *Arch. Biochem. Biophys.* **171**:398–406.

204. Purvis, J. L., and Lowenstein, J. M., 1961, The relation between intra- and extramitochondrial pyridine nucleotides, *J. Biol. Chem.* **236**:2794–2803.

205. Shank, R. E., Morrison, G., Cheng, C. H., Karl, J., and Schwartz, R., 1959, Cell heterogeneity within the hepatic lobule (quantitative histochemistry), *J. Histochem. Cytochem.* **7**:237–239.

206. Welsh, F. A., 1972, Changes in distribution of enzymes within the liver lobule during adaptive increases, *J. Histochem. Cytochem.* **20**:107–111.

207. Wimmer, M., and Pette, D., 1979, Microphotometric studies on intraacinar enzyme distribution in a rat liver, *Histochemistry* **64**:23–33.

208. Morrison, G. R., Brock, F. E., and Karl, J. E., 1965, Quantitative analysis of regenerating and degenerating areas in the liver lobule of the carbon tetrachloride, *Arch. Biochem. Biophys.* **111**:448–460.

209. Rieder, H., 1981, NADP-dependent dehydrogenases in rat liver parenchyma. III. The description of a liponeogenic area on the basis of histochemically demonstrated enzyme activities and the neutral fat content during fasting and refeeding, *Histochemistry* **72**:579–615.

210. Schwarz, G., 1978, Quantitative investigations of the zonal distribution of SDH, G6Pase and malic enzyme activity in liver parenchyma, *Acta Histochem.* **62**:133–141.

211. Loud, A. V., 1968, A quantitative stereological description of the ultrastructure of normal rat liver parenchyma cells, *J. Cell Biol.* **37**:27–46.

212. Jones, A. L., Schmucker, D. L., Mooney, J. S., Adler, R. D., and Ockner, R. K., 1976, Morphometric analysis of rat hepatocytes after total biliary obstruction, *Gastroenterology* **71**:1050–1060.

213. Jones, A. L., Schmucker, D. L., Mooney, J. S., Adler, R. D., and Ockner, R. K., 1978, The quantitative analysis of hepatic ultrastructure in rats during enhanced bile secretion, *Anat. Rec.* **192**:1277–288.

214. Schmucker, D. L., Mooney, J. S., and Jones, A. L., 1978, Stereological analysis of hepatic fine structure in the Fisher 344 rat: Influence of sublobular location and animal age, *J. Cell Biol.* **78**:319–337.

215. Ghosh, A. K., Finegold, D., White, W., Zawalich, K., and Matscinsky, F. M., 1982, Quantitative histochemical resolution of oxidation–reduction and phosphate potentials within the simple hepatic acinus, *J. Biol. Chem.* **257**:5476–5481.

216. Belinsky, S. A., Kauffman, F. C., Ji, S., Lemasters, J. J., and Thurman, R. G., 1983, Stimulation of mixed-function oxidation of 7-ethoxycoumarin in periportal and pericentral regions of the perfused rat liver by xylitol, *Eur. J. Biochem.* **137**:1–6.

217. Jakob, A., Williamson, J. R., and Asakura, T., 1971, Xylitol metabolism in perfused liver: Interactions with gluconeogenesis and ketogenesis, *J. Biol. Chem.* **246**:7623–7631.

218. Correia, M. A., and Mannering, G. J., 1973, DPNA synergism of TPNH-dependent mixed-function oxidase reactions, *Drug Metab. Dispos.* **1**:139–146.

219. Reinke, L. A., Belinsky, S. A., Kauffman, F. C., Evans, R. K., and Thurman, R. G., 1982, Regulation of NADPH-dependent mixed-function oxidation in perfused livers: Comparative studies with sorbitol and ethanol, *Biochem. Pharmacol.* **31**:1621–1624.

220. Belinsky, S. A., Reinke, L. A., Kauffman, F. C., Scholz, R., and Thurman, R. G., 1981, Metabolism of *p*-nitroanisole in perfused rat liver in absence of NADPH generation from the pentose phosphate shunt, *Fed. Proc. Fed. Am. Soc. Exp. Biol.* **40:**2874.

221. Thomas, P. E., Reik, L. M., Ryan, D. E., and Levin, W., 1981, Regulation of three forms of cytochrome P-450 and epoxide hydrolise in rat liver microsomes, *J. Biol. Chem.* **256:**1044–1052.

222. Ryan, D. E., Thomas, D. E., Korzeniowski, D., and Levin, W., 1979, Separation and characterization of highly perfused forms of microsomal cytochrome P-450 from rats treated with polychlorinated biphenyls, phenoborbital, and 3-methylcholanthrene, *J. Biol. Chem.* **254:**1365–1374.

223. Dannan, G. A., Guengerich, F. P., Kaminsky, O. S., and Aust, S. O., 1983, Regulation of cytochrome P-450, *J. Biol. Chem.* **258:**1282–1288.

224. Belinsky, S. A., Kauffman, F. C., and Thurman, R. G., 1984, Reducing equivalents for mixed-function oxidation in periportal and pericentral regions of the liver lobule in perfused livers from normal and phenobarbital-treated rats, *Mol. Pharmacol.* **26:**574–581.

225. Belinsky, S. A., Kauffman, F. C., and Thurman, R. G., 1983, Mixed-function oxidation of 7-ethoxycoumarin in β-naphthoflavone-treated rats: Sources of reducing equivalents in periportal and pericentral regions of the liver lobule, *Fed. Proc. Fed. Am. Soc. Exp. Biol.* **42:**1141.

226. Aitio, A., 1978, *Conjugation Reactions in Drug Biotransformations*, Elsevier/North Holland, Amsterdam.

227. Reinke, L. A., Kauffman, F. C., Evans, R. K., Belinsky, S. A., and Thurman, R. G., 1979, *p*-Nitrophenol conjugation in perfused livers from normal and phenobarbital-treated rats: Influence of nutritional state, *Res. Commun. Chem. Pathol. Pharmacol.* **23:**813–819.

228. Thurman, R. G., Reinke, L. A., Belinsky, S. A., and Kauffman, F. C., 1980, The influence of the nutritional state on rates of *p*-nitroanisole O-demethylation and *p*-nitrophenol conjugation in perfused rat livers, in: *Microsomes, Drug Oxidations and Chemical Carcinogenesis*, Vol. II (M. J. Coon, A. H. Conney, R. W. Estabrook, H. V. Gelboin, J. R. Gillette, and P. J. O'Brien, eds.), pp. 913–916, Academic Press, New York.

229. Burke, M. D., Vadi, H., Jernström, B., and Orrenius, S., 1977, Metabolism of benzo[a]pyrene with isolated hepatocytes and the formation and degradation of DNA-binding derivatives, *J. Biol. Chem.* **252:**6421–6431.

230. Wiebkin, P., Fry, J. R., Jones, C. A., Lowing, R. K., and Bridges, J. W., 1978, Biphenyl metabolism in isolated rat hepatocytes: Effect of induction and nature of the conjugates, *Biochem. Pharmacol.* **27:**1899–1907.

231. Wiebkin, P., Parker, G. L., Fry, J. R., and Bridges, J. W., 1979, Effect of various metabolic inhibitors on biphenyl metabolism in isolated rat hepatocytes, *Biochem. Pharmacol.* **28:**3315–3321.

232. Del Villar, E., Sanchez, E., and Tephley, T. R., 1977, Morphine metabolism. V. Isolation of separation glucuronyltransferase activities for morphine and *p*-nitrophenol from rabbit liver microsomes, *Drug Metab. Dispos.* **5:**273–278.

233. Notten, W. R. F., Henderson, P. T., and Kuyper, C. M. A., 1975, Stimulation of the glucuronic acid pathway in isolated rat liver cells by phenobarbital, *Int. J. Biochem.* **6:**713–718.

234. Fahl, W. E., Shen, A. L., and Jefcoate, C. R., 1978, UDP-glucuronyl transferase and the conjugation and benzo[a]pyrene metabolites to DNA, *Biochem. Biophys. Res. Commun.* **85:**891–899.

235. Bock, K. W., 1978, Increase of liver microsomal benzo[a]pyrene monooxygenase activity by subsequent glucuronidation, *Naunyn-Schmiedeberg's Arch. Pharmacol.* **304:**77–79.

236. Berry, C. S., 1979, Critical evaluation of UDP-*N*-acetyl-glucosamine and product glucuronides as allosteric effectors of UDP-glucuronyl transferase, in: *Conjugation Reactions in Drug Biotransformation* (A. Aitio, ed.), pp. 233–246, Elsevier/North-Holland, Amsterdam.

237. Powell, G. M., and Curtis, C. C., 1978, Sites of sulfation and the fates of sulfate esters, in: *Conjugation Reactions in Drug Biotransformation* (A. Aitio, ed.), pp. 409–416, Elsevier/North-Holland, Amsterdam.

238. Mulder, G. J., and Meerman, J. H. N., 1978, Glucuronidation and sulfation *in vivo* and *in vitro:* Selective inhibition of sulfation by drugs and deficiency of inorganic sulfate, in: *Conjugation Reactions in Drug Biotransformation* (A. Aitio, ed.), pp. 389–397, Elsevier/North-Holland, Amsterdam.

239. Maher, V. M., Miller, E. C., Miller, J. A., and Szybalski, W., 1968, Mutations and decreases in density of transforming DNA produced by derivatives of the carcinogens 2-acetylaminofluorene and *N*-methyl-4 aminoazobenzene, *Mol. Pharmacol.* **4:**411–426.

240. Miller, J. A., 1970, Carcinogens by chemicals: An overview, *Cancer Res.* **30:**559–576.

241. Arias, I. M., and Jakoby, W. B., (eds.), 1976, *Glutathione: Metabolism and Function,* Raven Press, New York.

242. Boyland, E., 1950, The biological significance of metabolism of polycyclic compounds, *Biochem. Soc. Symp.* **5:**40–54.

243. Mitchell, J. R., Hinson, J. A., and Nelson, S. D., Glutathione and drug-induced tissue lesions, in: *Glutathione: Metabolism and Function* (I. M. Arias and W. B. Jakoby, eds.), pp. 357–365, Raven Press, New York.

244. Mithell, J. R., Thorgeirsson, S. S., Potter, W. Z., Jahow, D. J., and Keiser, H., 1974, Acetaminophen-induced hepatic injury: Protective role of glutathione in man and rationale for therapy, *Clin. Pharmacol. Ther.* **16:**676–687.

245. Boyland, E., and Chasseaud, L. F., 1967, Enzyme-catalysed conjugations of glutathione with unsaturated compounds, *Biochem. J.* **104:**95–102.

246. Longacre, S. L., Kocsis, J. J., and Snyder, S., 1980, Benzene metabolism and toxicity in CD-1, C57/B6 and DBA/2N mice, in: *Microsomes, Drug Oxidations and Chemical Carcinogenesis,* Vol. II (M. J. Coon, A. H. Conney, R. W. Estabrook, H. V. Gelboin, J. R. Gillette, and P. J. O'Brien, eds.), pp. 897–902, Academic Press, New York.

247. Thor, H. P., Thorold, S., and Orrenius, S., 1980, Mechanisms of cytochrome P-450-mediated cytotoxicity studied in isolated hepatocytes, in: *Microsomes and Drug Oxidations* (M. J. Coon, ed.), pp. 907–911, Academic Press, New York.

248. Gelboin, H. V., Selkirk, J. K., Yang, S. K., Wiehel, F. J., and Nemoto, N., 1976, Benzo[a]pyrene metabolism by mixed-function oxygenase, hydratases, and glutathione S-transferses: Analysis by high pressure liquid chromatography, in: *Glutathione: Metabolism and Function* (I. M. Arias and W. B. Jakoby, eds.), pp. 339–356, Raven Press, New York.

249. Van Anda, J., Bend, J. R., and Fouts, J. R., 1978, Effect of diethyl maleate pretreatment on metabolism and toxicity of ^{14}C-styrene oxide in the isolated perfused rat liver, *Pharmacologist* **20:**200.

250. Meister, A., 1977, Glutathione and the γ-glutamyl cycle, in: *Glutathione: Metabolism and Function* (I. M., Arias and W. Jakoby, eds.), pp. 35–43, Raven Press, New York.

251. Ryan, A. J., and Bend, J. R., 1977, The metabolism of styrene oxide in the isolated perfused liver, *Drug. Metab. Dispos.* **5:**363–367.

252. Van Anda, J., Smith, B. R., and Bend, J. R., 1979, Concentration-dependent metabolism and toxicity of [^{14}C]styrene oxide in the isolated perfused rat liver, *J. Pharmacol. Exp. Ther.* **211:**207–212.

253. Smith, B. R., Philpot, R. M., and Bend, J. R., 1978, Metabolism of benzo[a]pyrene by the isolated perfused rabbit lung, *Drug Metab. Dispos.* **6:**425–431.

254. Smith, B. R., and Bend, J. R., 1979, Metabolism and excretion of benzo[a]pyrene 4,5-oxide by the isolated perfused rat liver, *Cancer Res.* **39:**2051–2056.

255. Pang, K. S., and Terrell, J. A., 1981, Conjugation kinetics of acetaminophen by the perfused rat liver preparation, *Biochem. Pharmacol.* **30:**1959–1965.

256. Pang, K. S., Koster, H., Halsema, I. C. M., Scholtens, E., Mulder, G. J., and Stillwell, R. N., 1983, Normal and retrograde perfusion to probe the zonal distribution of sulfation and glucuronidation activities of harmol in the perfused rat liver preparation, *J. Pharmacol. Exp. Ther.* **224:**647–653.

257. De Baun, J. R., Smith, J. Y., Miller, E. C., and Miller, J. A., 1970, Reactivity *in vivo* of the carcinogen *N*-hydroxy-2-acetylaminofluorene: Increases by sulfate ion, in *Science* **167**:184–186.

258. Desmond, P. V., James, R., Schenker, S., Gerkens, J. F., and Branch, R. A., 1981, Preservation of glucuronidation in carbon tetrachloride-induced acute liver injury in the rat, *Biochem. Pharmacol.* **30**:993–999.

259. Tsukuda, T., Thurman, R. G., and Kauffman, F. C., 1983, Effect of reducing agents on distribution and kinetic properties of UDP-glucuronyl transferase in periportal and pericentral zones of rat liver, *Fed. Proc.* **49**:912.

260. Conway, J. G., Kauffman, F. C., Tsukuda, T., and Thurman, R. G., 1984, Glucuronidation of 7-hydroxycoumarin in periportal and pericentral regions of the liver lobule, *Mol. Pharmacol.* **25**:158–164.

261. Lowry, O. H., 1953, The quantitative histochemistry of the brain: Histological sampling, *J. Histochem. Cytochem.* **1**:420–428.

262. Lowry, O. H., and Passonneau, J. V., 1972, *A Flexible System of Enzymatic Analysis,* Academic Press, New York.

263. Owens, J. W., and Stahl, P., 1976, Purification and characterization of rat liver microsomal β-glucuronidase, *Biochim. Biophys. Act.* **438**:474–476.

264. Paigen, K., 1979, Acid Hydrolyses as models of genetic control, *Annu. Rev. Genetics* **13**:417–466.

265. Schöllhammer, I., Poll, D. S., and Bischell, M. H., 1975, Liver microsomal β-glucuronidase and UDP-glucuronyltransferase, *Enzyme* **20**:269–275.

266. Belinsky, S. A., Kauffman, F. C., Sokolove, P. M., Tsukuda, T., and Thurman, R. G., 1984, Calcium-mediated inhibition of glucuronidation by epinephrine in the perfused rat liver, *J. Biol. Chem.* **259**:7705–7711.

267. Sokolove, P. M., Wilcox, M. A., Thurman, R. G., and Kauffman, F. C., 1984, Stimulation of hepatic microsomal β-glucuronidase by calcium, *Biochem. Biophys. Res. Comm* **121**:897–993.

268. Miller, D. L., Harasin, J. M., and Gumucio, J. J., 1978, Bromobenzene-induced zonal necrosis in hepatic acinus, *Exp. Mol. Pathol.* **29**:358–370.

269. Deane, H. W., 1944, A cytological study of the diurnal cycle of the liver of the mouse in relation to storage and secretion, *Anat. Rec.* **88**:39–65.

270. Sasse, D., 1975, Dynamics of liver glycogen, *Histochemistry* **45**:237–254.

271. Thurman, R. G., Reinke, L. A., Belinsky, S. A., Evans, R. K., and Kauffman, F. C., 1981, Co-regulation of mixed-function oxidation and glucuronidation of *p*-nitrophenol in the perfused rat liver by carbohydrate reserves, *Arch. Biochem. Biophys.* **209**:137–142.

272. Moldeus, P., Anderson, B., and Gergely, V., 1979, Regulation of glucuronidation and sulfate conjugation in isolated hepatocytes, *Drug Metab. Dispos.* **7**:416–417.

273. Mulder, G. J., and Scholtens, E., 1978, The availability of inorganic sulphate in blood for sulphate conjugation of drugs in rat liver *in vivo:* (S^{35})Sulphate incorporation into harmol sulphate, *Biochem. J.* **172**:247–251.

274. Kosower, E. M., 1976, Chemical properties of glutathione, in: *Glutathione: Metabolism and Function* (I. M. Arias and W. B. Jakoby, eds.), pp. 1–16, Raven Press, New York.

275. Ketterer, B., 1982, The role of nonenzymatic reactions of glutathione in xenobiotic metabolism, *Drug Metab. Rev.* **13**:161–187.

276. Jakoby, W. B., 1978, The glutathione S-transferases: A group of multifunctional detoxification proteins, *Adv. Enzymol.* **46**:383–414.

277. Lawrence, R. A., and Burk, R. F., 1976, Glutathione peroxidase activity in selenium-deficient rat liver, *Biochem. Biophys. Res. Commun.* **71**:952–958.

278. Boyland, E., and Chasseaud, L. F., 1970, The effect of some carbonyl compounds on rat liver glutathione levels, *Biochem. Pharmacol.* **19**:1526–1528.

279. Williamson, J. M., Boettcher, B., and Meister, A., 1982, Intracellular cysteine delivery system that protects against toxicity by promoting glutathione synthesis, *Proc. Natl. Acad. Sci. U.S.A.* **79**:6246–6249.

280. Davis, D. C., Potter, W. Z., Jollow, D. J., and Mitchell, J. R., 1974, Species differences in hepatic glutathione depletion, covalent binding and hepatic necrosis after acetaminophen, *Life Sci.* **14:**2099–2109.

281. Potter, W. Z., Thorgeirsson, S. S., Jollow, D. J., and Mitchell, J. R., 1974, Acetaminophen-induced hepatic necrosis. V. Correlation in hepatic necrosis, covalent binding and glutathione depletion in hamsters, *Pharmacology* **12:**129–143.

282. Connolly, R. B., and Jaeger, R. J., 1979, Acute hepatotoxicity of vinyl chloride and ethylene: Modification by trichloropropene oxide, diethylmaleate, and cysteine, *Toxicol. Appl. Pharmacol.* **50:**523–531.

283. Reid, W. D., Christie, B., Krishna, G., Mitchell, J. R., Moskowitz, J., and Brodie, B. B., 1971, Bromobenzene metabolism and hepatic necrosis, *Pharmacology* **6:**41–55.

284. Asghar, K., Reddy, B. G., and Krishna, G., 1975, Histochemical localization of glutathione in tissues, *J. Histochem. Cytochem.* **23:**774–779.

284a. Ullrich, D., Fischer, G., Katz, N., and Bock, K. W., 1984, Intralobular distribution of UDP-glucuronosyltransferase in liver from untreated, 3-methylcholanthrene- and phenobarbital-treated rats. *Chem.-Biochem. Interact.* **48:**181–190.

285. Deml, E., and Oesterle, D., 1980, Histochemical demonstration of enhanced glutathione content in enzyme altered islands induced by carcinogens in rat liver, *Cancer Res.* **40:**490–491.

286. Smith, M. T., Loveridge, N. Wills, E. D., and Chayen, J., 1979, The distribution of glutathione in the rat liver lobule, *Biochem. J.* **182:**1103–108.

287. Boyland, E., and Chasseaud, L. F., 1969, The role of glutathione and glutathione S-transferases in mercapturic acid biosynthesis, *Adv. Enzymol.* **32:**173–219.

288. Ketley, J. N., Habig, W. H., and Jakoby, W. B., 1975, Binding of nonsubstrate ligands to the glutathione S-transferases, *J. Biol. Chem.* **250:**8670–8673.

Chapter 14

Protein Synthesis and Secretion

A. V. LeBouton

1. INTRODUCTION

From a biochemical viewpoint, protein synthesis has probably been investigated more intensively in the liver than in any other organ. Unfortunately, the same cannot be said for studies at the tissue level within the simple liver acinus (see Chapter 1 for anatomical considerations).

The purpose of this chapter is to review the role of the liver in overall body protein metabolism, the regulation of hepatic protein synthesis and secretion, and its location within the simple liver acinus. At times, discussion and subsequent interpretation of results will be deliberately speculative in order to stimulate further research in this area.

2. INTERORGAN RELATIONSHIPS

In the human, the liver makes plasma proteins at the rate of about 100 g/day,[1] which is almost one third of total hepatic protein synthesis.[2] Most interactions that the liver has with other organs are mediated by plasma proteins.

A. V. LeBouton • Department of Anatomy, College of Medicine, University of Arizona, Tucson, Arizona 85724.

Some of these relationships include bulk pinocytosis of plasma as a nonspecific source of amino acids, transport of specific ligands for receptor-mediated endocytosis, inactivation of proteolytic extracellular enzymes, and catalysis of clot formation. Some of these proteins and their functions are listed in Table I.

Ligands for albumin are not listed in Table I because they are too numerous, ranging from inorganic ions, various metabolites, enzymes, bile intermediates,[3] and drugs to hormones.[4] Albumin is the most concentrated protein in plasma (60% of all protein), requiring nearly 15% of total hepatic protein synthesis.[5] Ceruloplasmin transports copper, which is used in cells as a prosthetic group in cytochrome oxidase. The haptoglobin–hemoglobin complex that is degraded by macrophages is the initial step in reutilization of iron for hemoglobin synthesis in developing erythrocytes. Hemopexin, when complexed with porphyrin heme, undergoes endocytosis in hepatocytes, where the heme is further metabolized to bilirubin and its iron either complexed with an apoprotein and stored as ferritin or transported to the bone marrow by transferrin.

In bone marrow, developing erythroblasts do not degrade transferrin taken up via endocytosis. Instead, they remove its two iron atoms and release it by exocytosis, which allows it to recirculate to the liver for more iron. Although all cells possess the genes for establishing cholesterol synthesis, few do so.

Table I. Characteristics of Some Liver-Derived Plasma Proteins

Protein	Ligand	Function	Half-life Human	Half-life Rat
Albumin	Numerous	Transport, osmotic pressure	19.0 days	2.5 days
Ceruloplasmin	Copper	Transport to body cells	6.0 days	13.0 hr
Haptoglobin	Hemoglobin	Transport to macrophages	3.8 days	—
Hemopexin	Heme	Transport to liver	7.0 days	—
Transferrin	Iron	Transport to bone marrow	8.5 days	4.0 days
Thyroxine-binding globulin	Thyroxine	Transport to body cells	—	—
Transcobalamin	Vitamin B_{12}	Transport to body cells	—	—
Low-density lipoprotein	Cholesterol	Transport to body cells	3.2 days	—
Transcortin	Cortisol	Transport to body cells	—	—
Retinol-binding protein	Vitamin A	Transport to retina	—	—
High-density lipoprotein	Lipids	Transport to body cells	4.5 days	—
α_1-Antitrypsin	None	Inhibits proteases	5.5 days	5.5 days
α_2-Macroglobulin	None	Inhibits proteases	—	—
Prothrombin	None	Proenzyme of thrombin	—	—
Fibrinogen	None	Substrate of thrombin	5.8 days	1.3 days
Antithrombin	None	Inhibits thrombin	2.8 days	—
α_1-Acid glycoprotein	None	Increased in inflammation	5.2 days	29.0 hr
α-Fetoprotein	None	Unknown	—	—

Instead, the cholesterol they need for membranes is transported to them as a complex with low-density lipoproteins derived from the liver.[3]

Under certain conditions, proteolytic enzymes such as trypsin, elastase, and collagenase can reach the extracellular compartment, where their effects would be disastrous if it were not for the presence of α_1-antitrypsin from the liver, which inactivates them. The final two steps in the cascade of reactions leading to blood-clot formation include two proteins formed by the liver: the conversion of prothrombin to thrombin and the thrombin-dependent conversion of fibrinogen to fibrin. Finally, during inflammation, fever, or trauma, the liver produces copious amounts of C-reactive protein and α_1-acid glycoprotein, the functions of which are unknown.

Thus, hegemony over practically every cell in the body is achieved by the liver through its plasma proteins. Many factors and conditions impinge on the liver to regulate the synthesis and secretion of these plasma proteins.

3. REGULATION OF HEPATIC PROTEIN SYNTHESIS BY EXTRAHEPATIC AND HEPATIC FACTORS

3.1. Photoperiod

Periods of activity of both humans and other animals are synchronized with times of illumination and darkness. Such activity patterns profoundly affect hepatic protein synthesis.[6] In rats, which are nocturnal, overall hepatic protein synthesis is cyclic and peaks during the dark period.[7,8] Consistent with this is the observation that there is a daily rhythm in the concentration of circulating rat plasma proteins of nearly 17%, with a high point near the end of the dark phase and a low point toward the end of the light phase.[9]

3.2. Nutrition

Normally, food intake and the photoperiod are linked; humans eat most of their food during daylight, whereas rats ingest most of their food in the first half of darkness.[10] Hepatic protein synthesis in rats and dogs is most rapid shortly after a meal[8,11] and, among other factors, is regulated directly by changes in amount and kind of amino acids that enter the liver through the portal vein.[12,13] It has been observed, however, that increased rates of protein synthesis still occur in the dark phase even if food is removed at its beginning.[14]

Not surprisingly, deprivation of food adversely affects hepatic protein synthesis. Fasting rats for 2 days decreases total protein content by nearly 20%.[15] Even the standard overnight fast, which is done to remove particulate glycogen from microsomal fractions, is deleterious to hepatic protein synthesis. Thus, total protein synthesis in livers of overnight-starved rats is decreased by 33%.[16] The effects of a brief overnight fast are also detrimental to the synthesis of specific plasma proteins such as albumin (60% decrease)[17] and transferrin (27% decrease).[18]

3.3. Osmotic Pressure

Plasma oncotic pressure is also a factor in the regulation of hepatic protein synthesis. When isolated rat livers were perfused with erythrocytes suspended in saline only, the incorporation of [^{14}C]leucine into total protein was nearly double the value from control livers perfused with whole blood.[19] This finding is reflected by individual proteins such as albumin, the synthetic rate of which is nearly doubled during perfusion conditions of lowered osmotic pressure and, conversely, exhibits a 47% decrease in synthetic rate when the osmotic pressure of the perfusion medium is elevated above normal.[20] Related to this phenomenon is the finding that when plasma proteins, mainly albumin, are lost from the kidney due to nephrosis, the synthetic rates of total hepatic protein and albumin are elevated.[16] Currently, it is thought that plasma protein synthesis is regulated more by total plasma oncotic pressure than by the plasma concentration of any particular protein.

3.4. Hormones

In general, the regulatory effect of most hormones on hepatic protein synthesis is positive. If a hormone is absent due to prior hypophysectomy, thyroidectomy, or diabetes mellitus, protein synthesis is decreased and can be restored by injection of the missing hormone. Thus, hypophysectomy decreases albumin synthesis by 50%,[21] and diabetic rats have low rates of albumin synthesis.[22] Both are returned to normal values by injection of the appropriate hormone. Insulin stimulates lipoprotein secretion as well.[23]

After injection into normal animals, thyroxine increases the incorporation of [^{14}C]leucine into albumin by 252% and into transferrin by 166%.[18] Both cortisol and growth hormone stimulate fibrinogen synthesis in rat hepatocytes.[24,25] Finally, estradiol has been shown to elevate the serum content of antithrombin by 20%, presumably as a result of increased synthesis.[26] Hormonal regulation is accomplished by: increased messenger RNA (mRNA) transcription,[27] increased survival of mRNA,[28] or decreased synthesis time at the ribosome.[29]

3.5. Age

With increasing age, protein synthesis in the liver declines by 40–70%.[30–33] The age-related decrease is thought to be regulated at the rough endoplasmic reticulum (RER), since addition of cytosol from young rats to microsomes from old rats does not increase the microsomal synthetic rate.[34]

The aging phenomenon is not confined solely to later postnatal life. All organisms begin to age from the moment of their inception. In this regard, regulation of fetal and early postnatal protein synthesis is important, especially with respect to α-fetoprotein, which is formed during fetal life and early postnatal life, and by hepatomas at any age.[35] Studies with hybridization kinetics of mRNA for α-fetoprotein indicate regulation at transcription,[36] whereas others have found evidence of hormonal regulation at translation.[37]

3.6. Polyploidy

An age-associated phenomenon that results in increased hepatic protein synthesis is ploidy formation (see Chapter 1), the production of multiple copies of the entire genome from diploid through tetraploid and octaploid cells.[38] Rat liver cells produce albumin at a rate that is directly correlated with their degree of ploidy.[39] The majority of ploidy formation is completed in the liver by young adulthood, however.[40,41] Thus, ploidy would not be expected to ameliorate the deleterious effects of aging on protein synthesis. In this regard, it has been found that transcription levels increase in octaploid cells by a factor only 1.1 times that of tetraploid cells, and the rate of RNA synthesis declines in all ploidy classes with age.[42]

3.7. Stress

The liver responds to various forms of stress by regulating production of certain plasma proteins. During inflammation, α_1-antitrypsin, ceruloplasmin, haptoglobin, and fibrinogen are increased in amount, as are proteins with normally low plasma levels, such as C-reactive protein and α_1-acid glycoprotein.[43–45] The synthesis of fibrinogen is also increased after partial hepatectomy.[46] In addition, the secretion time (i.e., the interval from injection of a radioisotope-labeled protein precursor to first appearance of labeled protein outside the cell) of albumin drops from 15 to 10 min in rats 48 hr after partial hepatectomy.[47]

Hemorrhage has been shown to cause a 263% increase in the incorporation of [^{14}C]leucine into transferrin.[18] In this case, it is difficult to separate the regulatory effects of plasma oncotic pressure from other forms of stimulation provided by the need for more erythrocytes. When rabbits are subjected to an increased ambient temperature, their rate of albumin synthesis drops by 62%, whereas cold has no effect.[48] The drop in synthesis is considered to be due partly to a lowered nitrogen intake (nutrition) and to decreased thyroid activity (hormones).

3.8. Genetic Diseases

Analbuminemia in the rat is due to a regulatory defect in processing of heterogenous nuclear RNA. With complementary DNA (cDNA) to albumin mRNA as a probe, it was found that primary transcripts of albumin mRNA are processed incompletely and therefore never leave the nucleus.[49]

In α_1-antitrypsin deficiency, the defect is somewhere between the RER and the Golgi complex because no nascent antitrypsin enters transition vesicles. Consequently, the cisternae of the RER become engorged with the protein.[50]

3.9. Blood Flow

Blood reaches the liver by two routes: the hepatic artery and the portal vein (see Chapters 1 and 2). Almost 80% of total hepatic blood flow is carried by the portal vein, which drains the intestines, pancreas, and spleen. Under certain conditions, blood from one organ does not mix with blood from another organ by turbulence; instead, it remains as a longitudinal stream from the organ all the way to the liver. There is evidence for this phenomenon in prone, anesthetized rats. In this case, the majority of [^{3}H]leucine injected directly into the spleen was found in protein in the right liver lobes, whereas radioactivity injected into the jejunum entered primarily the left hepatic lobes.[51] This is a case of laminar flow that crosses over. Also, the distribution of copper within the liver has been found to be nonrandom, with more found in the right lobes.[52] Thus, due to the possibility of laminar blood flow in the portal vein, protein synthesis within various portions of the liver could be regulated differently. In active rats, however, when adequate mixing occurs by injection of [^{3}H]leucine into a peripheral vein, there is nearly identical protein metabolism among the various liver lobes.[51]

3.10. Turnover

The concept of turnover is that proteins have a finite life-span; they are continuously lost by degradation and replaced by newer molecules. Turnover is a steady state or balance between loss and replacement.[53] It is also expressed as half-life—the time required for a radioactively labeled protein to decrease to half its initial highest value. Inherent in this concept is loss of labeled molecules by degradation and dilution of remaining labeled molecules by newly made unlabeled ones.

Turnover of total hepatic proteins in the rat requires nearly 18 hr.[16] Of 17 hepatocellular soluble protein fractions separated by electrophoresis, 13 had half-lives greater than 12 hr and 4 turned over in less than 1 hr.[54] The half-life of hepatic mitochondria has been estimated at 10 days.[55] Various mitochondrial components have different turnovers: outer membrane, 7.0 days; inner membrane, 8.4 days; soluble matrix, 6.78 days.[56] The half-lives of ribosomal RNA and protein are identical at 4–5 days, suggesting that rat liver ribosomes turn over as intact units.[57]

In the plasma, fates and half-lives of liver-derived proteins are variable (Table I). An important concept displayed by the data in Table I is that with the exception of α_1-antitrypsin, plasma proteins turn over faster in rats than their counterparts do in humans. This is mostly due to the larger surface-to-volume ratio of rats, which allows more energy to be lost as radiant heat and hence requires a faster metabolic rate.[58]

4. REGULATION OF HEPATIC PROTEIN SYNTHESIS AT THE SUBCELLULAR LEVEL

The intracellular route that is known to be taken by all proteins listed in Table I is: RER, smooth ER (SER) (primarily transition vesicles), Golgi complex, and export from the cell into the blood.[59] Regulation can occur at many locations along this sequence.

4.1. Transcription

In rat liver responding to inflammation, mRNA for fibrinogen increases 7-fold, while albumin mRNA decreases by one half.[60] This agrees with the finding that the secretion time of α_1-acid glycoprotein remains unchanged at 15 min even though synthesis of the protein increases greatly during inflammation.[61] Evidently, more mRNA coding for α_1-acid glycoprotein becomes available.

4.2. Competition for Ribosomes

Plasma proteins are synthesized on membrane-bound polysomes, whereas nonsecreted proteins are formed on free polysomes.[62] Since all polysomes are considered to be derived from a common pool of monosomes, it is possible that competition between various species of mRNA could be a regulatory event.[63]

4.3. Translation

The time required from addition of a radioactively labeled amino acid to the first appearance of labeled protein within the RER is the translation time. Normally, *in vivo*, amino acids are added to growing polypeptides at the rate of six to seven per second. The reason for observed differences between the translation time of albumin (1.5 min)[64] and that of apolipoprotein B (10 min)[65] is apparently a function of molecular size: Larger proteins contain more amino acids and therefore take longer to polymerize. Specific regulation at translation has been proposed, however. When the N-terminal hexapeptide of proalbumin is added to isolated hepatocytes, albumin synthesis decreases.[66] This is thought to be the result of local negative feedback by the N-terminal hexapeptide at the ribosome.

4.4. Transport

Recent evidence shows that there may be regulation at the transport step from RER to the Golgi complex. The half-times of transport of proteins between these two organelles are: albumin, 14 min; transferrin, 73 min; retinol-binding protein, 137 min. This implies that transfer of proteins by transition vesicles may not be due to bulk-phase movement, but instead could be the result of a specific receptor-mediated process.[67]

4.5. Secretion

Secretion times for proteins are variable: albumin, 15 min[68]; transferrin, 21 min[68]; α_1-acid glycoprotein, 15 min[61]; α_1-antitrypsin, 30 min[69]; apolipoprotein B, 30 min.[65] Since secretion time includes transit time, these differences are also due to polypeptide length as well as degree of glycosylation. The extent of coupling between synthesis and secretion must also be a regulatory factor, since there is no appreciable storage of fibrinogen (tightly coupled synthesis and secretion), whereas only 20–40% of secreted albumin is freshly synthesized (loose coupling).[70]

5. INTRAACINAR LOCALIZATION

Any attempt to study the synthesis and distribution of proteins in the liver acinus requires, at some point, the production of histological sections (see Chapter 3). Primarily, two techniques have been applied to liver sections: radioautography and immunohistology (Chapter 4).[71]

Radioautography gives information about *all* nascent hepatic proteins—enzymatic, structural, and secretory. In combination with the parameter of time, radioautography can yield kinetic information.

Immunohistology, on the other hand, can provide knowledge about the synthesis and distribution of a specific protein. When immunohistology is coupled with pharmacological or physiological manipulations, more dynamic results can be obtained from what is basically a qualitative technique.

5.1. Radioautography

5.1.1. Kinetics

To date, only one detailed radioautographic study of general protein synthesis in the simple liver acinus has been performed.[72] In this work, fed young adult male rats were given an intravenous injection of [³H]leucine and killed at various times thereafter. Radioautograms from the livers of these rats were analyzed for each time by scoring the number of silver grains over hepatocytes in the straightest plate of cells traversing the three acinar zones (Fig. 1).

Results of the grain counts showed that radioactivity in zone I peaked at nearly 60 grains/cell by 15 min (Fig. 2). This was about 40% higher than that in cells of zones II and III. On the other hand, radioactivity in zones II and III was not highest until 45 min to 1 hr, when it reached only 46 grains/cell. At 1 hr, zone III hepatocytes were about 18% more radioactive than those of zone I (Fig. 2), and they remained more radioactive even until 12 hr, when they were found to be nearly 43% higher.[73] The rise and fall of radioactivity in zone I cells is discernible even without laborious grain counts (Fig. 3).

These data are interpreted to mean that a decreasing gradient of general protein metabolism exists across the acinus, with cells of zone I having the fastest rate. If all liver cells metabolized proteins at identical rates, then the higher radioactivity of zone I cells was simply because they received more [³H]leucine. If this is true, then peak radioactivity should have occurred simultaneously in all three zones, and at that time, zone I should have had the most, zone III the least, and zone II an intermediate value. Also, this relationship should have remained during the entire experiment.

Zone I is where hepatic arterial and portal venous blood mix before they begin to flow into the other acinar zones.[74] It is also where the plates of hepatocytes are thicker and more irregular, as though to act as baffles against the incoming blood.[75] The microenvironment in zone I is known to be higher in oxygen and nutrients.[76,77] and these cells consistently display greater activity of many oxidative enzymes (see Chapters 9 and 16). It is therefore not unexpected that general protein metabolism of zone I cells might operate at a higher level. Schreiber et al.[78] were able to accentuate the higher protein metabolism of acinar zone I cells by intraportal injections of [³H]leucine.

5.1.2. Distribution

In the radioautographic study just described, acinar zonal radioactivity was obtained by scoring silver grains over each hepatocyte in a pass across the width of the simple acinus. Although this approach yielded data about the faster kinetics of protein metabolism in hepatocytes of zone I, it gave no indication of the size

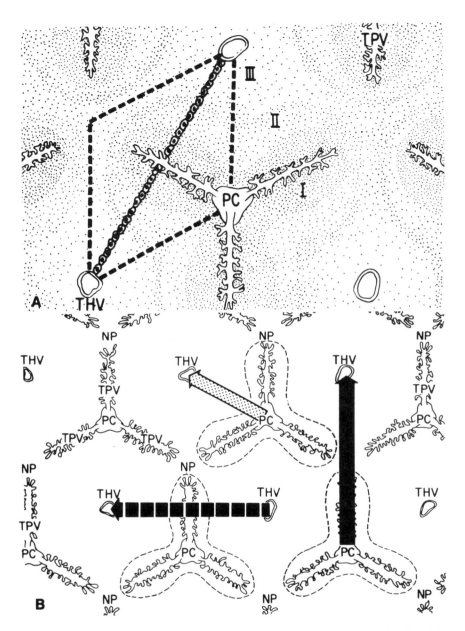

Figure 1. Diagrams of areas of rat liver used for radioautographic analysis of zonal radioactivity (A) and zonal size (B). Landmarks are the portal canal (PC), terminal portal venule (TPV), terminal hepatic venule (THV), and nodal point (NP), where TPVs meet in anastomosis. (A) A simple liver acinus outlined by the dashed line contains the arbitrary metabolic zones, I, II, and III. Scoring of grains per cell was done on the straightest plate of cells across the width of the acinus. (B) The areas of higher protein metabolism are outlined by dashed lines. Pathways followed to obtain the data in Fig. 4 are: dashed arrow, THV to THV analysis; stippled arrow, PC to THV analysis; solid arros, PC through NP to THV analysis. Reproduced from LeBouton[72.79] with permission of Elsevier Biomedical Press.

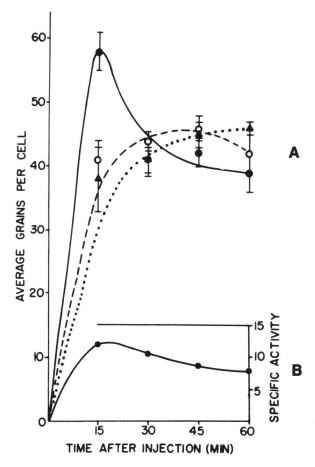

Figure 2. (A) Cellular radioactivity in zones of the rat liver acinus at various times after injection of [³H]leucine. (●----●) Zone I. (O----O) zone II; (▲....▲) zone III. The vertical brackets at the data points denote S.E.M. (B) Specific activity (cpm/μg protein) of soluble intracellular proteins at times after injection of [³H]leucine. Reproduced from LeBouton[72] with permission of Elsevier Biomedical Press.

of this area. This type of data was obtained by using a variety of microscopic scoring passes (as in Fig. 1) designed to reveal the two-dimensional extent of the area of higher protein metabolism.[79] In other words, was this area smaller than, larger than, or equal to the size of acinar zone I, which is arbitrarily one third of the acinus? The data were plotted as overlapping triplet values to minimize individual cellular variation (Fig. 4).

The zone of increased protein metabolism was found to be nearly eight cells wide and ten cells long and to extend out from portal canals about four to five

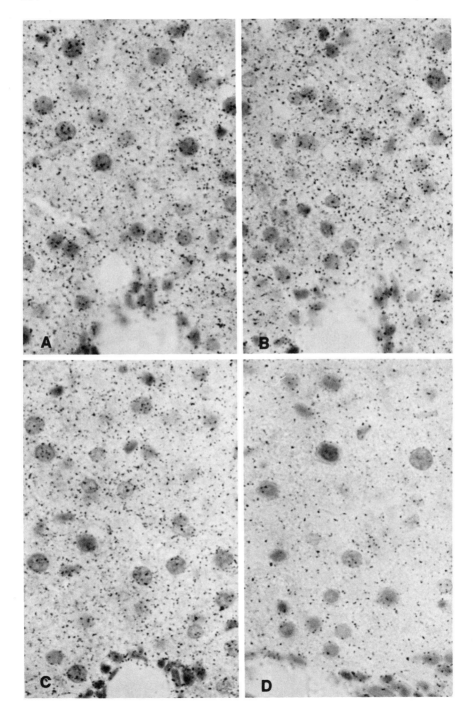

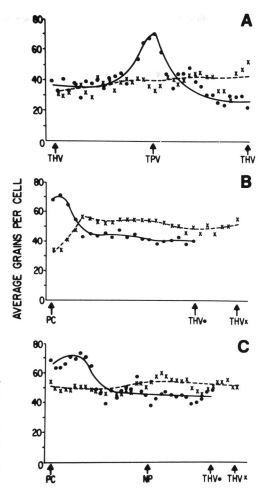

Figure 4. Plots of the distribution of average grains/cell from the pathways in Fig. 1. Time after [³H]leucine injection: (●----●) 15 min; (×----×) 30 min. Abbreviations as in Fig. 1. (A) THV to THV analysis; (B) PC to THV analysis; (C) PC through NP to THV analysis. Reproduced from LeBouton[79] with permission of Elsevier Biomedical Press.

cells. These dimensions are nearly identical to the two-dimensional extent of the arbitrary acinar zone 1 described by Rappaport.[80]

5.2. Immunohistology

In the past, it was erroneously thought either that hepatocytes go through asynchronous stages of synthesis, storage, and release of plasma proteins[81] or

Figure 3. Radioautograms of rat hepatocytes in acinar zone I at various times after injection of [³H]leucine (15 μCi/g): (A) 10 min; (B) 20 min; (C) 1 hr; (D) 4 hr. A portal venule is at the bottom of each photograph.

that there are fixed populations that synthesize only one plasma protein.[82] This misconception arose from numerous reports of immunofluorescence or immunoperoxidase preparations that showed cells positive for a given plasma protein scattered randomly throughout the acinus (Fig. 5). Preparations such as these have been shown to be artifactual and are therefore not valid.[83–88]

The problem arises from the unique situation of the hepatocyte: Much of its surface is in contact with a moderately concentrated colloidal suspension (plasma) of the same proteins that it synthesizes and secretes. Thus, any conditions that allow plasma to pass through the hepatocyte plasma membrane and enter the cytosol will result in cells that are artifactually immunopositive for *any* plasma proteins, including gamma globulins, that are not synthesized by liver cells.[82,89,90]

Such conditions occur when liver samples or biopsies are fixed via immersion while their sinusoids are still filled with whole blood. This means that the space of Disse contains plasma that can, under appropriate conditions, leak back into adjacent hepatocytes.

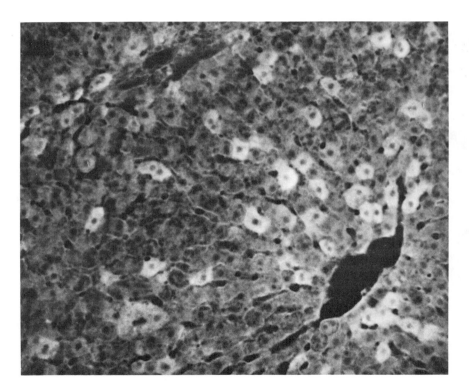

Figure 5. Immunofluorescence staining for albumin in rat hepatocytes from a liver that was immersion-fixed while filled with blood. The intense artifactually positive cells are scattered randomly within the acinus. The space of Disse is seen to contain the source of the artifactual albumin as a thin white line adjacent to many cells. It is especially evident at center left.

Liver cells that artifactually take in plasma proteins are apparently those that have a relatively high glycogen content.[89-91] Presumably, in the time between cessation of blood flow and termination of metabolism by fixation, hepatocytes that are high in glycogen catabolize it anaerobically into organic acids. The presence of these excess acids lowers intracellular pH to the point where the integrity of the plasma membrane is compromised. Nearby plasma proteins then diffuse through the plasma membrane driven only by a simple concentration gradient. Yet the physical chemistry of the situation appears to modulate this artifactual movement of proteins through the plasma membrane in that smaller (low-molecular-weight), more negatively charged (low-isoelectric-point) molecules apparently enter liver cells more easily.[90]

Conditions that produce the artifact can be avoided if plasma is flushed rapidly from the space of Disse with saline introduced through the portal vein before immersion-fixation or if perfusion–fixation immediately follows the flush.[71,89,90,92] Using this simple precaution, LeBouton and Masse[89,90] have shown that *all* hepatocytes in the liver acinus of fed adult male rats simultaneously produce all liver-based plasma proteins, such as fibrinogen (Fig. 6) and albumin (Fig. 7). This observation has subsequently been confirmed with preflushed livers

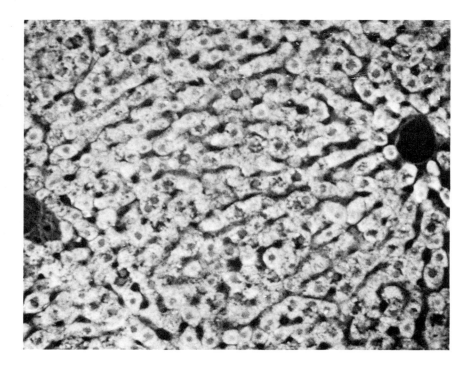

Figure 6. Immunofluorescence staining for fibrinogen in cells of a rat liver acinus after flushing of blood followed by immersion-fixation. All hepatocytes fluoresce with nearly identical intensity.

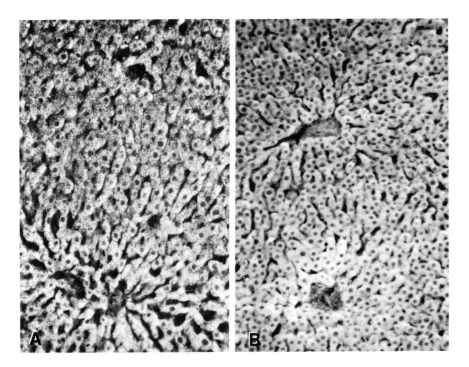

Figure 7. Immunofluorescence staining of albumin in cells of the rat liver acinus after flushing out blood prior to fixation. (A) Immersion-fixation, fed rat. All hepatocytes contain albumin, and those in zone I (bottom) contain more. (B) Perfusion fixation, 5 days' starvation. All hepatocytes contain albumin, and those in zone I contain more.

by Yokata and Fahimi,[93] Geuze *et al.*,[94] and Guillouzo *et al.*[95] All the preceding studies were antedated by that of Schreiber *et al.*,[78] who demonstrated, with a radioautographic approach, that all hepatocytes synthesize albumin. Unfortunately, their experimental design is difficult to understand, and as a result the work has not been cited adequately.

5.2.1. Age

When the albumin content of hepatocytes is observed in 6-week-old pubescent rats (Fig. 8A)[96] and in 11-week-old adult rats (Fig. 8B),[97] all cells in the acinus contain albumin. If, however, the relative amount of specific reaction product in the cells is compared *between* the age groups, hepatocytes in the older rats contain more albumin. This difference could be due to slower movement of nascent albumin through older liver cells. This implies that in older rats, hepatocytes should contain more protein and the rate of entry of albumin into their plasma should also be slower. Accordingly, after an injection of [^{3}H]leucine,

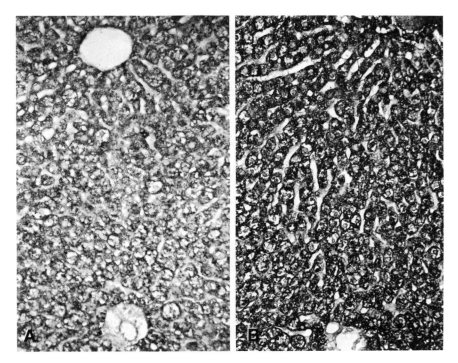

Figure 8. Immunoperoxidase staining for albumin in liver cells of rats at different ages. Fed male rats were killed at 9:30 A.M., and livers were flushed free of blood before immersion-fixation. (A) 6-Week-old rat. All hepatocytes contain a moderate amount of reaction product for albumin. (B) 11-Week-old rat. All hepatocytes contain an abundant amount of reaction product for albumin. (A) Reproduced from LeBouton[97] with permission of Alan R. Liss, Inc. (B) Reproduced from LeBouton[96] with permission of Springer-Verlag.

the rate of appearance of labeled albumin of old rats in plasma is slower, and the amount of protein per gram of liver is 21% higher.[98]

5.2.2. Nutrition

It has been shown by immunocytochemistry that overnight fasting depletes hepatocytes of albumin in a nonuniform way that is age-dependent.[96,97] Overnight starvation (16 hr) of 11-week-old rats results in a profound cellular depletion of albumin in areas roughly equal to acinar zones I and II (Fig. 9A).[96] When the duration of the fast is increased to 48 hr, the depletion of hepatocellular albumin extends to include cells of zone III (Fig. 9B). Thus, it appears that during an overnight fast of older rats, the vector for the decrease in hepatocyte albumin content is directed from zone I toward zone III.

If younger rats ($5\frac{1}{2}$ weeks old) are starved overnight, cells in all acinar zones

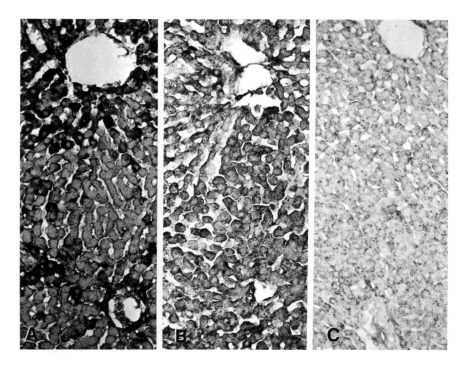

Figure 9. Immunoperoxidase staining for albumin in liver cells of male rats of different ages that were fed or starved overnight. All rats were killed at 9:30 A.M., and livers were flushed free of blood before immersion-fixation. (A) 11-Week-old rat that was starved overnight (16 hr). Most hepatocytes in acinar zones I and II are negative for reaction product for albumin. (B) 11-Week-old rat that was starved for 48 hr. All hepatocytes contain a minimal amount of albumin. (C) 6-Week-old rat that was starved overnight (16) hr. All hepatocytes contain only a small amount fo reaction product for albumin. (A, B) Reproduced from LeBouton[96] with permission of Springer-Verlag. (C) Reproduced from LeBouton[97] with permission of Alan R. Liss.

become depleted of albumin (Fig. 9C).[97] From these findings, it can be concluded that since young rats have a higher basal metabolic rate,[99] their response to the same length of fast is more rapid than that of older rats.

Apparently, the decreased amount of amino acids in the blood during a fast somehow down-regulates protein synthesis in cells of zone I first. With increasing duration of the fast, the decrease in protein synthesis appears to recruit more hepatocytes in the direction of zone III. It would be interesting to know if, at first, this was only modulation of protein synthesis at the translational level, which would mean that a full complement of mRNA species would still be present, or whether there was an actual loss of mRNA. *In situ* hybridization with a labeled cDNA probe might give the answer.

Extensive starvation (5 days) accentuates the normally slightly higher level of protein synthesis in zone I cells, since they come to contain more albumin (see Fig. 7).

5.2.3. Photoperiod

Most biochemical studies indicate that plasma proteins, such as albumin, are probably synthesized and secreted at a faster rate during the night, which means that hepatic albumin content should be low in the daytime and high at night. Yet when the immunohistochemical distribution of albumin within the liver acinus is studied over a 24-hr period, the results appear to be in conflict with biochemical and physiological predictions.[97] Hepatocellular albumin content is highest during the first half of the light period, from 6 A.M. (Fig. 10A) to noon (Fig. 10B). In the first half of the dark phase, from 9 P.M. (Fig. 10C) to midnight (Fig. 10D), hepatocytes generally contain a lower amount of albumin, with certain cells exhibiting a pronounced depletion similar to those seen after a 16-hr fast (see Fig. 9). Specifically, the small population of cells that appear nearly depleted of albumin first appear at 6 P.M. in zone I (Fig. 10C). These hepatocytes usually contain a few discrete albumin-positive granules that have been shown to be in the Golgi apparatus, since it is the only organelle in which albumin is concentrated.[59,93,94] The majority of cells still have a uniform distribution of albumin, but it is the least intense of all times studied. The appearance of albumin-depleted cells at 6 P.M. also coincides with the low points of plasma albumin content in circulating blood and total hepatic protein synthesis.[8]

By midnight, the subpopulation of hepatocytes that are depleted of albumin increases to include cells in zone II (Fig. 10D). Also, the pancytoplasmic albumin in the majority of hepatocytes at midnight is more concentrated than at 6 P.M.

The direction of the appearance of the hepatocytes that become depleted of albumin during the dark phase thus appears to be from zone I toward zone III, the same direction that hepatocellular albumin depletion takes during an overnight fast. In other words, the gross depletion of albumin in zones I and II as the result of an overnight fast could be the exaggeration of a more subtle response on the part of fewer cells to the self-imposed fast that occurs normally during the light phase.

Apparently, the inertia of this subtle wave of lowered albumin content of certain hepatocytes lasts at least up to midnight in the dark phase. But due to the increase of incoming amino acids that stimulates synthesis, by 6 A.M. all hepatocytes again contain moderate to heavy amounts of pancytoplasmic albumin. Thus, the appearance of cells depleted of albumin is not in direct coincidence with the times of light and dark, but instead is shifted somewhat, beginning before the end of the light phase and ending before the end of the dark phase.

This proposed wave of synthesis followed by one of depletion may also explain why hepatocytes are immunohistochemically high in albumin during the

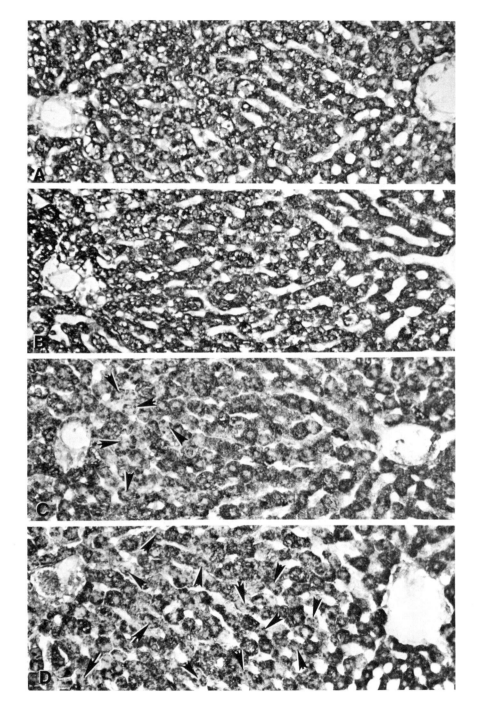

day, the time at which biochemical findings indicate that synthesis is slowest.[16] It is possible that the albumin that is synthesized and collected in secretion vesicles during increased synthesis in the preceding dark phase is of such magnitude that it carries over into the light phase. In other words, coupling of synthesis and secretion could be regulated, and the equivalent of a storage phase would occur in hepatocytes during the dark phase when the cytoplasm becomes filled with secretion vesicles. These vesicles would then be released slowly during the daylight, first by certain cells in zone I, followed by others in zone II.

It is not known why only particular hepatocytes become depleted of albumin in a normal diurnal cycle, but it is probably due to variations in their own rates of metabolism. In this regard, it is interesting to discuss the polyploidy-related findings of LeRumeur *et al.*,[39] who found that diploid hepatocytes synthesize and secrete albumin at roughly half the rate of tetrapoid cells. Thus, it is also possible that the cells that initially become depleted of albumin are diploid.

5.2.4. Stress

Inflammation produced by subcutaneous injection of turpentine recruits all hepatocytes into synthesis of α_1-acid glycoprotein, haptoglobin, α_2-macroglobulin, and fibrinogen.[100] With time after turpentine, recruitment begins in zone I (10 hr), then progresses to zone II (16 hr), and finally all hepatocytes are involved when zone III cells begin synthesis (24 hr). The level of regulation that is most likely involved here is transcription.

6. INTRACELLULAR LOCALIZATION

Most immuno-electron-microscopic studies of nascent plasma proteins demonstrate that they are associated with organelles known to be responsible for their synthesis and secretion: RER, SER, Golgi complex, and secretion vesicles. This is not unexpected. With respect to the RER, however, what *is* unexpected is the finding that bound ribosomes are positive. This means that antigenic determinants (epitopes) of nascent plasma proteins are located on the surface of

---

Figure 10. Immunoperoxidase staining for albumin in liver cells of 6-week-old fed male rats over a 24-hr diurnal cycle. The photoperiod was a 12 hr–12 hr light–dark cycle with lights on at 6 A.M. and off at 6 P.M. Livers were flushed free of blood before immersion-fixation. Vacuoles represent loss of glycogen and lipid during processing. Terminal portal venules are on the left. (A) 6 A.M. All hepatocytes contain a moderate to abundant amount of reaction product for albumin. (B) Noon. All hepatocytes contain an abundant amount of reaction product for albumin. (C) 6 P.M. A few cells in zone I contain only a few discrete granules of reaction product for albumin ($\rightarrow$). (D) Midnight. Hepatocytes with only a few granules of reaction product for albumin have increased in number by extending into zone II ($\rightarrow$). Reproduced from LeBouton[97] with permission of Alan R. Liss, Inc.

bound ribosomes. This has been shown for albumin,[82,89,101] fibrinogen,[100,102,103] transferrin,[104] hemopexin,[104] haptoglobin,[100] α_1-acid glycoprotein,[100] and α_2-macroglobulin.[100]

That the surface of bound ribosomes is where nascent plasma proteins could expose their epitopes to the cytosol does not agree with the signal hypothesis, which states that growing polypeptides are kept sequestered within a deep groove or tunnel in the large ribosomal subunit until they attain the lumen of the RER, where they can fold and acquire antigenicity.[105] To explain this discrepancy, a model has been proposed in which polypeptide folding occurs on the surface of, and is even assisted by, bound ribosomes. Then, favored by entropy changes in a situation in which nonequilibrium thermodynamics prevail, the folded polypeptide loses most of its cage of bound water as it partitions through the membrane of the ER.[106]

7. SUMMARY

Almost one third of all proteins synthesized by the liver are plasma proteins. This large amount of protein is needed by the liver to mediate its extensive interactions with nearly all body cells. These relationships include transport of trace metals and various metabolites, inactivation of proteolytic enzymes, clot formation, and participation in the response to inflammation.

Protein synthesis and secretion are regulated by many factors outside and inside the liver. The photoperiod primarily dictates when food will be eaten, which directly stimulates protein synthesis. Most hormones increase hepatic protein synthesis, as does a decrease in the oncotic pressure of blood plasma. There is a generalized decline of plasma protein synthesis with age. The liver usually responds to many forms of stress by an increase in protein synthesis. Genetic diseases that exhibit total absence of particular proteins in plasma are due to either inadequate processing of mRNA transcripts in the nucleus or an inability to transfer protein from the RER to the Golgi complex. Finally, the lifetime of each plasma protein is different, ranging from hours to days.

Hepatic protein synthesis is regulated mainly at transcription and at the transition from the RER to the Golgi complex. Protein translation times vary, but this is due primarily to molecular size.

General protein metabolism within cells of the simple liver acinus exists as a gradient of decreasing activity, with cells in acinar zone I operating at a moderately higher rate. The two-dimensional extent of this area of higher protein metabolism coincides almost exactly with acinar zone I.

The synthesis and secretion of liver-derived plasma proteins occur simultaneously within all hepatocytes at any given time. In the case of plasma proteins, the gradient of general protein metabolism becomes evident under certain conditions, such as 5 days of starvation, when hepatocytes in zone I contain slightly more albumin.

Primarily as a result of generally overall slower metabolism, all hepatocytes in acini of older rats contain more plasma proteins. This is probably due to slower movement of nascent proteins through the cells.

An overnight fast lowers hepatocyte albumin content drastically. Due to their slower metabolism, older rats lose albumin only from acinar zones I and II, whereas all three acinar zones become depleted in young rats.

Finally, there is a circadian rhythm of immunocytochemically detectable albumin in the liver acinus. All hepatocytes contain a large amount of albumin during the first half of the light period. Some time toward the end of the light period, and carrying over into the latter half of the dark phase, some hepatocytes become depleted of albumin. These cells first appear in zone I and, with time, begin to appear in zone II. The loss of albumin from all cells in zones I and II after an overnight fast of older rats is considered to be an exaggeration of this more subtle diurnal rhythm.

REFERENCES

1. Guyton, A. C., 1971, *Textbook of Medical Physiology,* p. 816, W. B. Saunders, Philadelphia.
2. Scornik, O. A., and Botbol, V., 1976, Role of changes in protein degradation in the growth of regenerating livers, *J. Biol. Chem.* **251:**2891–2897.
3. Brown, M. S., Anderson, R. G. W., Basu, S. K., and Goldstein, J. L., 1981, Recycling of cell-surface receptors: Observations from the LDL receptor system, *Cold Spring Harbor Symp. Quant. Biol.* **46:**713–721.
4. Benhold, H., 1966, Transport function of the serum proteins, in: *Transport Function of Plasma Proteins* (P. Desgrez and P. M. DeTraverse, eds.), pp. 1–12, Elsevier, Amsterdam.
5. Zakim, D., and Boyer, T. D., 1982, *Hepatology: A Textbook of Liver Disease,* W. B. Saunders, Philadelphia.
6. Wurtman, R. J., 1970, Diurnal rhythms in mammalian protein metabolism, in: *Mammalian Protein Metabolism,* V. IV (H. N. Munro, ed.), pp. 445–479, Academic Press, New York.
7. Hardeland, R., Hohmann, D., and Rensing, L., 1973, The rhythmic organization of rat liver, *J. Interdiscip. Cyclic Res.* **4:**89–118.
8. LeBouton, A. V., and Handler, S. D., 1970, Diurnal incorporation of ^{3}H-leucine into liver protein, *FEBS Lett.* **10:**78–80.
9. Scheving, L. E., Pauly, J. E., and Tsai, T. H., 1968, Circadian fluctuations in plasma proteins of the rat, *Am. J. Physiol.* **215:**1096–1101.
10. Zucker, I., 1971, Light–dark rhythms in rat eating and drinking behavior, *Physiol. Behav.* **6:**115–126.
11. Elwyn, D. H., Parikh, H. C., and Shoemaker, W. C., 1968, Amino acid movements between gut, liver, and periphery in unanesthetized dogs, *Am. J. Physiol.* **215:**1260–1275.
12. Ehrhardt, V., and Rensing, L., 1974, Circadian rhythmic changes of amino acid concentrations in rat liver, *Int. J. Chronobiol.* **2:**367–371.
13. Lardeux, B., Bourdel, G., and Girard-Globa, A., 1978, Regulation of hepatic synthesis of proteins by the chronology of protein ingestion, *Biochim. Biophys. Acta.* **518:**113–124.

14. LeBouton, A. V., and Handler, S. D., 1971, Persistent circadian rhythmicity of protein synthesis in the liver of starved rats, *Experientia* **27:**1031–1032.
15. Addis, T., Poo, L. J., and Lew, W., 1936, The quantities of protein lost by the various organs and tissues of the body during a fast, *J. Biol. Chem.* **115:**111–116.
16. Peters, T., Jr., and Peters, J. C., 1972, The biosynthesis of rat serum albumin. VI. Intracellular transport of albumin and rates of albumin and liver protein synthesis *in vivo* under various physiological conditions, *J. Biol. Chem.* **247:**3858–3863.
17. Peters, T., Jr., 1973, The biosynthesis of rat serum albumin. VII. Effects observed in liver slices, *J. Biol. Chem.* **224:**1363–1368.
18. Morgan, E. H., 1969, Factors affecting the synthesis of transferrin by rat tissue slices, *J. Biol. Chem.* **244:**4193–4199.
19. Tracht, M. E., Tallal, L., and Tracht, D. G., 1967, Intrinsic hepatic control of plasma albumin concentration, *Life Sci.* **6:**2621–2628.
20. Rothschild, M. A., Oratz, M., Mongelli, J., and Schreiber, S. S., 1969, Effect of albumin concentration on albumin synthesis in the perfused liver, *Am. J. Physiol.* **216:**1127–1130.
21. Keller, G. H., and Taylor, J. M., 1976, Effect of hypophysectomy on the synthesis of rat liver albumin, *J. Biol. Chem.* **251:** 3768–3773.
22. Peavy, D. E., Taylor, J. M., and Jefferson, L. S., 1978, Correlation of albumin production rates and albumin mRNA levels in livers of normal, diabetic and insulin-treated rats, *Proc. Natl. Acad. Sci. U.S.A.* **75:**5879–5883.
23. Olefsky, J. M., Farquar, J. W., and Reaven, G. M., 1974, Reappraisal of the role of insulin in hypertriglyceridemia, *Am. J. Med.* **57:**551–560.
24. Crane, L. J., and Miller, D. L., 1977, Plasma protein synthesis by isolated rat hepatocytes, *J. Biol. Chem.* **72:**11–25.
25. Jeejeebhoy, K. N., Bruce-Robertson, A., Sodke, U., and Foley, M., 1970, The effect of growth hormone on fibrinogen synthesis, *Biochem. J.* **119:**243–249.
26. Kobayashi, N., and Takeda, Y., 1977, Studies of the effects of estradiol, progesterone, cortisol, thrombophlebitis, and typhoid vaccine on synthesis and catabolism of antithrombin III in the dog, *Thromb. Ademost.* **37:**111–122.
27. Tata, J. R., and Williams, A., 1967, Effects of growth hormone and tri-iodothyronine on amino acid incorporation by microsomal subfractions from rat liver, *Eur. J. Biochem.* **2:**366–374.
28. Roy, A. K., Chatterjee, B., Demyan, W. F., Nath, T. S., and Motwani, N. M., 1982, Pretranslation regulation of alpha-2μ-globulin in rat liver by growth hormone, *J. Biol. Chem.* **257:**7834–7838.
29. Gehrke, L., Bast, R. E., and Ilan, J., 1981, An analysis of rates of polypeptide chain elongation in avian liver explants following *in vivo* estrogen treatment, *J. Biol. Chem.* **256:**2522–2530.
30. Buetow, D. E., and Gandhi, P. S., 1973, Decreased protein synthesis by microsomes isolated from senescent rat liver, *Exp. Gerontol.* **8:**243–249.
31. Buetow, D. E., Moudgil, P. G., Eicholz, R. L., and Cook, J. R., 1977, Protein synthesis in senescent liver, in: *Liver and Aging* (D. Platt, ed.), pp. 211–224, F. K. Schattauer Verlag, Stuttgart.
32. Makrides, S. C., 1983, Protein synthesis and degradation during aging and senescence, *Biol. Rev.* **58:**343–422.
33. Viskup, R. W., Baker, M., Holbrook, J. P., and Penniall, R., 1979, Age-associated changes in activities of rat hepatocytes. I. Protein synthesis, *Exp. Aging Res.* **5:**487–496.
34. Mainwaring, W. I. P., 1969, The effect of age on protein synthesis in mouse liver, *Biochemistry* **113:**869–878.
35. Sell, S., and Becker, F. F., 1978, Alpha-fetoprotein, *J. Natl. Cancer Inst.* **60:**9–26.
36. Sala-Trepat, J. M., Dever, J., Sargent, T. D., Thomas, K., Sell, S., and Bonner, J., 1979, Changes in expression of albumin and alpha-fetoprotein genes during rat liver development and neoplasia, *Biochemistry* **18:**2167–2178.

37. Belanger, L., Hamel, D., Lachance, L., Dufour, D., Tremblay, M., and Gagnon, P. M., 1975, Hormonal regulation of alpha-fetoprotein, *Nature (London)* **256:**657–659.

38. Ordahl, C. P., 1977, Reassociation kinetics of polyploid hepatocyte DNA, *Biochim. Biophys. Acta* **474:**17–29.

39. LeRemeur, E., Beaumont, C., Guillouzo, C., Rissel, M., and Guillouzo, A., 1981, All normal hepatocytes produce albumin at a rate related to their degree of ploidy, *Biochem. Biophys. Res. Commun.* **101:**1038–1046.

40. Carriere, R., 1969, The growth of liver parenchymal nuclei and its endocrine regulation, *Int. Rev. Cytol.* **25:**201–277.

41. Doljanski, F., 1960, The growth of the liver with special reference to mammals, *Int. Rev. Cytol.* **10:**217–241.

42. Collins, J. M., 1978, RNA synthesis in rat liver cells with different DNA contents, *J. Biol. Chem.* **253:**5769–5773.

43. Jamieson, J. C., Morrison, K. E., Molasky, D., and Turchen, B., 1975, Studies on acute phase proteins of rat serum. V. Effect of induced inflammation on the synthesis of albumin and alpha-1-acid glycoprotein by liver slices, *Can. J. Biochem.* **53:**401–414.

44. Schumer, W., Molnar, J., Dowling, J., and Winzler, R. J., 1967, Biosynthesis of glycoproteins: Effect of injury on seromucoid fraction of rat plasma, *Am. J. Physiol.* **212:**186–190.

45. Werner, M., 1969, Serum protein changes during the acute phase reaction, *Clin. Chim. Acta* **25:**299–305.

46. Majumdar, C., Tsukada, K., and Lieberman, I., 1967, Liver protein synthesis after partial hepatectomy and acute stress, *J. Biol. Chem.* **242:**700–704.

47. Schreiber, G., Urban, J., Zähringer, J., Reutter, W., and Frosch, U., 1971, The secretion of serum protein and the synthesis of albumin and total protein in regenerating rat liver, *J. Biol. Chem.* **246:**4531–4538.

48. Oratz, M., Walker, C., Schreiber, S. S., Gros, S., and Rothschild, M. A., 1967, Albumin and fibrinogen metabolism in heat- and cold-stressed rabbits, *Am. J. Physiol.* **213:**1341–1349.

49. Esumi, H., Takahashi, Y., Sekiya, T., Sato, S., Nagase, S., and Sugimura, T., 1982, Presence of albumin mRNA precursors in nuclei of analbuminemic rat liver lacking cytoplasmic albumin mRNA, *Proc. Natl. Acad. Sci. U.S.A.* **79:**734–738.

50. Bahn, A. T., Grand, R. J., Colten, H. R., and Alper, C. A., 1976, Liver in alpha$_1$-antitrypsin deficiency: Morphologic observations and *in vitro* synthesis of alpha$_1$-antitrypsin, *Pediatr. Res.* **10:**35–40.

51. LeBouton, A. V., and Hoffman, T. E., 1969, Protein metabolism among lobes of the rat liver in relation to site of radioisotope injection, *Proc. Soc. Exp. Biol. Med.* **132:**15–19.

52. Haywood, S., 1981, The non-random distribution of copper within the liver of rats, *Br. J. Nutr.* **45:**295–300.

53. Schultze, H. E., and Heremans, J. F., 1966, *Molecular Biology of Human Proteins,* Vol. 1, *Nature and Metabolism of Extracellular Proteins,* Elsevier, Amsterdam.

54. LeBouton, A. V., 1969, A study of soluble intracellular proteins, *Cytologia* **32:**345–350.

55. Fletcher, M. J., and Sanadi, D. R., 1961, Turnover of rat liver mitochondria, *Biochim. Biophys. Acta* **51:**356–360.

56. Beattie, D. S., 1969, The turnover of the protein components of the inner and outer membrane fractions of rat liver mitochondria, *Biochem. Biophys. Res. Commun.* **35:**721–727.

57. Retz, K. C., and Steele, W. J., 1980, Ribosome turnover in rat brain and liver, *Life Sci.* **27:**2601–2604.

58. Munro, H. N., and Downie, E. D., 1964, Relationship of liver composition to intensity of protein metabolism in different mammals, *Nature (London)* **203:**603–604.

59. Peters, T., Jr., Fleischer, B., and Fleischer, S., 1971, The biosynthesis of rat serum albumin. IV. Apparent passage of albumin through the Golgi apparatus during secretion, *J. Biol. Chem.* **244:**4308–4315.

60. Princen, J. M. G., Nieuwenhuizen, W., Mol-Backx, G. P. B. M., and Yap, S. H., 1981, Direct evidence of transcriptional control of fibrinogen and albumin synthesis in rat liver during the acute phase response, *Biochem. Biophys. Res. Commun.* **102:**717–723.

61. Jamieson, J. C., and Ashton, F. E., Studies on acute phase proteins of rat serum. IV. Pathway of secretion of albumin and alpha$_1$-acid glycoprotein from liver, *Can. J. Biochem.* **51:**1281–1291.

62. Redman, C., 1969, Biosynthesis of serum proteins and ferritin by free and attached ribosomes of rat liver, *J. Biol. Chem.* **244:**4308–4315.

63. Drysdale, J. W., Olafdottir, E., and Munro, H. N., 1968, Effect of ribonucleic acid depletion on ferritin induction in rat liver, *J. Biol. Chem.* **243:**552–555.

64. Peters, T., Jr., and Davidson, L. K., 1982, The biosynthesis of rat serum albumin: *In vivo* studies on the formation of the disulfide bonds, *J. Biol. Chem.* **257:**8847–8853.

65. Siuta-Mangano, P., Howard, S. C., Lennarz, W. J., and Lane, M. D., 1982, Synthesis, processing, and secretion of apolipoprotein B by the chick liver cell, *J. Biol. Chem.* **257:**4292–4300.

66. Weigand, K., Schmid, M., Villringer, A., Birr, C., and Heinrich, P. C., 1982, Hexa- and pentapeptide extension of proalbumin: Feedback inhibition of albumin synthesis by its pro-peptide in isolated hepatocytes and in the cell-free system, *Biochemistry* **24:**6053–6059.

67. Fries, E., Gustafsson, L., and Peterson, P. A., 1984, Four secretory proteins synthesized by hepatocytes are transported from endoplasmic reticulum to Golgi complex at different rates, *EMBO J.* **3:**147–152.

68. Schreiber, G., Drybirgh, H., Millership, A., Matsuda, Y., Inglis, A., Phillips, J., Edwards, K., and Maggs, J., 1979, The synthesis and secretion of rat transferrin, *J. Biol. Chem.* **254:**12,013–12,019.

69. Carlson, J., and Stenflo, J., 1982, The biosynthesis of rat alpha$_1$-antitrypsin, *J. Biol. Chem.* **257:**12,987–12,994.

70. Crane, L. J., and Miller, D. L., 1974, Synthesis and secretion of fibrinogen and albumin by isolated rat hepatocytes, *Biochem. Biophys. Res. Commun.* **60:**1269–1277.

71. LeBouton, A. V., 1983, Immunohistochemistry and radioautography of hepatic secretory proteins, in: *Plasma Protein Secretion by the Liver* (H. Glaumann, T. Peters, Jr., and C. Redman, eds.), pp. 195–234, Academic Press, London.

72. LeBouton, A. V., 1968, Heterogeneity of protein metabolism between liver cells as studied by radioautography, *Curr. Mod. Biol.* **2:**111–114.

73. LeBouton, A. V., 1966, Autoradiography and radiobiochemistry of protein synthesis in the rat liver, Doctoral dissertation, University of California, Los Angeles.

74. Rappaport, A. M., 1976, The microcirculatory acinar concept of normal and pathological hepatic structure, *Beitr. Pathol.* **157:**215–243.

75. LeBouton, A. V., 1974, Growth, mitosis, and morphogenesis of the simple liver acinus in neonatal rats, *Dev. Biol.* **41:**22–30.

76. Ji, S., LeMasters, J. J., Christenson, V., and Thurman, R. G., 1982, Periportal and pericentral pyridine nucleotide fluorescence from the surface of the perfused liver: Evaluation of the hypothesis that chronic treatment with ethanol produces pericentral hypoxia, *Proc. Natl. Acad. Sci. U.S.A.* **79:**5415–5419.

77. Wimmer, M., and Pette, D., 1979, Microphotometric studies on intraacinar enzyme distribution in rat liver, *Histochemistry* **64:**23–33.

78. Schreiber, G., Lesch, R., Weinssen, U., and Zähringer, J., 1970, The distribution of albumin synthesis throughout the liver lobule, *J. Cell. Biol.* **47:**285–289.

79. LeBouton, A. V., 1969, Relations and extent of the zone of intensified protein metabolism in the liver acinus, *Curr. Mod. Biol.* **3:**4–8.

80. Rappaport, A. M., 1963, Acinar units and the pathophysiology of the liver, in: *The Liver*, Vol. I (C. Rouiller, ed.), pp. 266–328, Academic Press, New York.

81. Barnhart, M. 1., 1960, Cellular site for prothrombin synthesis, *Am. J. Physiol.* **199:**360–366.

82. Feldmann, G., Penaud-Laurencin, J., Crassous, J., and Benhamou, J. P., 1972, Albumin synthesis by human liver cells: Its morphological demonstration, *Gastroenterology* **63**:1036–1048.
83. Barnhart, M. I., 1965, Prothrombin synthesis: An example of hepatic function, *J. Histochem. Cytochem.* **13**:740–751.
84. Guillouzo, A., Belanger, L., Beaumont, C., Valet, J. P., Briggs, R., and Chiu, J. F., 1978, Cellular and subcellular immunolocalization of alpha fetoprotein and albumin in rat liver: Reevaluation of various experimental conditions, *J. Histochem. Cytochem.* **26**:948–959.
85. Hamashima, Y., Harter, J. G., and Coons, A. H., 1964, The localization of albumin and fibrinogen in human liver cells, *J. Cell Biol.* **20**:271–279.
86. Lane, R. S., 1968, Transferrin synthesis in the rat: A study using the fluorescent antibody, *Br. J. Haematol.* **15**:355–364.
87. Lin, C. T., and Chang, J. P., 1975, Electron microscopy of albumin synthesis, *Science* **190**:465–467.
88. Roy, A. K., and Raben, D. L., 1972, Immunofluorescent localization of alpha-2μ-globulin in the hepatic and renal tissues of rat, *J. Histochem. Cytochem.* **20**:89–96.
89. LeBouton, A. V., and Masse, J. P., 1980, A random arrangement of albumin-containing hepatocytes seen with histo-immunologic methods. I. Verification of the artifact, *Anat. Rec.* **197**:183–194.
90. LeBouton, A. V., and Masse, J. P., 1980, A random arrangement of albumin-containing hepatocytes seen with histo-immunologic methods. II. Conditions that produce the artifact, *Anat. Rec.* **197**:195–203.
91. Brozman, M., 1971, The localization of serum albumin in human liver cells, *Acta Histochem.* **39**:89–100.
92. LeBouton, A. V., 1983, Immuno-identification of plasma proteins in hepatocytes, *J. Histochem. Cytochem.* **31**:847.
93. Yokata, S., and Fahimi, H. D., 1981, Immunocytochemical localization of albumin in the secretory apparatus of rat liver parenchymal cells, *Proc. Natl. Acad. Sci. U.S.A.* **78**:4970–4974.
94. Geuze, J. J., Slot, J. W., and Brands, R., 1981, The occurrence of albumin in the rat liver: A light and electron microscope immunocytochemical study, *Cell Biol. Int. Rep.* **5**:463.
95. Guillouzo, A., Beaumont, C., LeRumeur, E., Rissel, M., Latinier, M. F., Gugen-Guillouzo, C., and Bourel, M., 1982, New findings of immunolocalization of albumin in rat hepatocytes, *Biol. Cell* **43**:163–172.
96. LeBouton, A. V., 1982, Routine overnight starvation and immunocytochemistry of hepatocyte albumin content, *Cell Tissue Res.* **227**:423–427.
97. LeBouton, A. V., 1984, Immunocytochemistry of albumin in hepatocytes after overnight starvation and during a diurnal cycle in young rats, *Anat. Rec.* **209**:67–75.
98. Ove, R., Obenrader, M., and Lansing, A., 1972, Synthesis and degradation of liver proteins in young and old rats, *Biochem. Biophys. Acta.* **277**:211–221.
99. Spector, W. S., 1956, *Handbook of Biological Data*, p. 258, W. B. Saunders, Philadelphia.
100. Courtoy, P. J., Lombart, C., Feldmann, G., Monguilevsky, N., and Rogier, M. S., 1981, Synchronous increase of four acute phase proteins synthesized by the same hepatocytes during the inflammatory reaction, *Lab. Invest.* **44**:105–115.
101. Kraemer, M., Vassy, J., Foucrier, J., Rigaut, J. P., and Chalumeau, M. T., 1981, Subcellular localization of transferrin and albumin synthesis in the same rat hepatocyte by immunoenzymatic, immunoferritin and image analysis methods, *Biol. Cell* **40**:103–108.
102. Antakly, T. W., Tanaka, S., Ohkawa, K., and Bernhard, W., 1979, Cytochemical localization of peroxidase and peroxidase-labelled antibodies in ultrathin frozen sections, *Cell. Mol. Biol.* **24**:205–212.
103. Feldmann, G., Maurice, M., Sapin, C., and Benhamou, J. P., 1975, Inhibition by colchicine of fibrinogen translocation in hepatocytes, *J. Cell Biol.* **67**:237–243.

104. Foucrier, J., Kraemer, M., Vassy, J., and Chalumeau, M. T., 1979, Demonstration of the simultaneous presence of transferrin, hemopexin, and albumin in the same adult rat hepatocyte, *Cell Differ.* **8:**39–48.
105. Blobel, G., 1977, Synthesis and segregation of secretory proteins: The signal hypothesis, in: *International Cell Biology* (B. R. Brinkley and K. R. Porter, eds.), pp. 318–325, The Rockefeller University Press, New York.
106. LeBouton, A. V., and Masse, J. P., 1981, Ultrastructural immunocytochemistry of nascent albumin topology: Proposed cytosolic folding and membrane transit of the protein, *Anat. Rec.* **201:**203–223.

Chapter 15

Bile Acid Metabolism

Jorge J. Gumucio, William F. Balistreri, and Fred J. Suchy

1. INTRODUCTION

Transport and metabolism of bile acids by the liver have been the subject of several recent reviews.[1-3] In this chapter, however, the problem is analyzed in a different context. An attempt is made to integrate the development of these functions in the fetal and newborn liver with the transport and metabolic regulation of bile acids observed in the adult liver. Moreover, these processes are analyzed in the context of the functional heterogeneity of the hepatic parenchyma observed in both the fetal and the adult liver. While significant progress has been made recently in this area, the available data are still scarce. Many more questions can be raised than answers given in dealing with the transport and metabolism of bile acids by the functional units of the fetal liver or by the zones of the adult hepatic acinus. We hope this review will stimulate research in these areas.

JORGE J. GUMUCIO • Veterans Administration Hospital, University of Michigan, Ann Arbor, Michigan 48103.   WILLIAM F. BALISTRERI and FRED J. SUCHY • Children's Hospital, University of Cincinnati, Cincinnati, Ohio 45229.

2. FUNCTIONAL UNITS

2.1. Mature Liver

All hepatocytes comprising the hepatic acinus receive blood from a common source, the terminal portal venule and hepatic arteriole. The hepatic acinus, therefore, and not the hepatic lobule, represents the structural and functional unit of hepatic parenchyma.[4] This microcirculatory unit, the acinus, is described in detail in Chapter 1.

2.2. Developing Liver

The liver develops within the vitelline sinusoids surrounding the gut. Initially, in humans, blood coming from the placenta distributes into the right and left umbilical veins. Later, the right umbilical vein involutes, while the left umbilical vein continues to perfuse the vitelline plexus of the left liver. The relatively poorly oxygenated fetal blood returns to the placenta via the umbilical arteries. In the placenta, blood is reoxygenated and returns to the liver via the umbilical vein(s). This vein perfuses mainly the left lobe of the fetal liver. The right lobe is perfused almost entirely by the fetal portal vein. In addition, the ductus venosus connecting the umbilical vein with the inferior vena cava regulates the flow of oxygenated blood directly into the heart, thus bypassing the liver sinusoids.[6–8]

The fetal liver is therefore formed by two distinct units, the right and left liver lobes, each of which receives blood containing different concentrations of oxygen, and possibly different concentrations of hormones and other substrates. Consequently, hepatocytes of the right and left fetal liver lobes are exposed to different microenvironments, a circumstance that may result, as in the adult liver, in morphological and functional heterogeneity of the hepatic parenchyma. In fact, Emery[8,9] found that the left fetal lobe was larger than the right. The right/left lobe size ratio was about 0.89. Moreover, he showed that a greater number of hematopoeitic foci existed in the right lobe and proposed that a functional asymmetry exists in both the fetal and the newborn liver. In addition to the studies in humans,[8,9] experiments performed in nonhuman primates,[5] lambs,[6,7] and guinea pigs[10] have also shown differences in blood supply to the right and left liver lobes.

Edelstone *et al.*[6] showed that in fetal lambs *in utero* the pO_2 of the umbilical vein was about 33 torr, while the pO_2 in the portal vein was about 18 torr. Similarly, the pCO_2 was 37 and 45 torr in the umbilical and portal veins, respectively. These authors also showed that the blood flow supplied by the portal vein to the right fetal lobe was about 43 ml/min and that to the left lobe 1 ml/min. In contrast, blood flow supplied by the umbilical vein was about 116 ml/min to the left lobe and about 100 ml/min to the right lobe. The hepatic artery contributed less than 10% of the total blood flow to each lobe.[11] In experiments performed by Gumucio et al.[10] in pregnant guinea pigs, the pO_2 in umbilical vein blood was about 42 torr, while that of the portal vein blood was about 21 torr. In these studies, ^{51}Cr-radioactive microspheres were injected into either the umbilical or the portal vein of fetal guinea pigs near term. About 72% of the radioactivity was distributed in the left lobe after umbilical vein injection, and a similar percentage was found in the right lobe following injection via the portal vein.

Additional support for the proposal that the fetal liver is indeed formed by two distinct functional units has been provided by Mihaly et al.,[12] who measured propranolol disposition in pregnant sheep. In these studies, the hepatic extraction of propranolol from fetal portal blood was almost zero. In contrast, it was estimated that the extraction ratio of propranolol by the left fetal lobe was about 0.35 at all dosages studied, suggesting that the fetal liver does not act as a homogeneous organ with respect to the biotransformation of drugs.

As discussed below, most of our knowledge of the maturation of bile acid metabolism has been gained through use of the entire fetal liver as though it were a homogeneous organ. Studies on the metabolism of bile acids, taking into consideration that the right and left fetal liver lobes represent two distinct functional units, may provide important information on the role of the microenvironment in the maturation of processes involved in bile acid transport and metabolism. At the time of birth, new and sudden changes occur in the hepatic circulation. Blood flow through the umbilical vein is interrupted, and all lobes are then perfused via the portal vein and the hepatic artery. Moreover, the rate of perfusion through the portal vein and particularly via the hepatic artery increases substantially above the rates observed during fetal life.[11] Concomitantly, the left lobe undergoes partial involution.[8,9] Therefore, rapid adjustments occur in the hepatic parenchyma of the newborn in response to this new microenvironment. Later, the lobar heterogeneity of the fetal liver seems to cease, and the heterogeneity of the adult hepatic parenchyma is expressed best at the level of the hepatic acinus.[13–15]

3. BILE ACID TRANSPORT

3.1. Enterohepatic Circulation

An efficient mechanism for bile acid conservation is made possible by the restriction of bile acids to the enterohepatic circulation. The anatomical localization of bile acid molecules in the hepatocyte, biliary tract, intestinal tract, and portal venous system allows continuous recycling of these physiologically important compounds. Specific transport and metabolic processing of bile acids within the various locations of the enterohepatic circulation serve as efficient regulatory mechanisms to ensure homeostasis. A recent excellent review[16] has analyzed the enterohepatic circulation of bile acids in detail.

3.2. Unidirectional Perfusion of Bile Acids

Following intestinal reabsorption, bile acids return to the liver via the portal vein. In man, the concentration of bile acids in portal vein blood varies between 8 μM during fasting and about 32 μM 30–45 min after a meal.[1] These bile acids come into contact with the hepatic parenchyma at the level of the liver acinus.[17]

The hepatic acinus, the microcirculatory unit of liver parenchyma,[4] is a three-dimensional mass of tissue perfused from an axial core formed by the terminal portal venule and the hepatic arteriole. From this core, portal blood flows into the hepatic sinusoids, establishing contact with the hepatic parenchyma. Blood then perfuses the liver unidirectionally from this axial core toward the periphery of this three-dimensional structure. Having perfused the acinus, blood is drained into the systemic circulation by two or more hepatic venules. While there is considerable turbulence in hepatic sinusoids created by the intermittent opening of the arterial vessels as well as a merry-go-round perfusion of some hepatocytes,[4] there is no evidence for significant retrograde flow from the periphery to the central core of the acinus. Therefore, bile acids reaching the acinus will be in contact first with hepatocytes in zone 1, located around terminal portal venules, and subsequently with hepatocytes of zones 2 and 3. The transport of bile acids by hepatocytes of each of these zones during this unidirectional perfusion will depend not only on the direction of perfusion, but also on the distribution and kinetic characteristics of the bile acid transport system in each zone, as well as on the binding of bile acids to serum proteins.[17]

3.3. Mechanisms of Bile Acid Uptake

Data generated by studies using intact animals,[18,19] perfused livers,[20] isolated hepatocytes,[21] hepatocytes in culture,[22] liver cell plasma membranes,[23] and plasma membrane vesicles[24] have provided evidence that bile acids such as taurocholate, glycocholate, cholate, and glycochenodeoxycholate are taken up by hepatocytes in a process characterized as secondary active transport.[22,25] This involves a carrier-mediated, sodium-coupled process that derives its energy from the hydrolysis of ATP by an Na^+, K^+-ATPase located in the basolateral segments of the liver cell plasma membrane.[26,27] The characteristics and regulation of this transport system have been reviewed recently.[28]

3.4. Zonal Uptake of Bile Acids

3.4.1. Acinar Distribution

How are bile acids, which return to the liver via the portal vein, distributed within hepatocytes of the acinus? Two recent studies have used autoradiography to provide a direct visual demonstration of the uptake of bile acids by hepatocytes in each acinar zone. Jones et al.[30] determined by quantitative autoradiography that the transport of a bile acid analogue, [3H]cholylglycylhistamine, was carried out predominantly by hepatocytes of zones 1 and 2 when injected into the portal vein of rats. Recently, Groothuis et al.[31] successfully overcame the technical difficulties imposed by autoradiography of water-soluble compounds and showed that a tracer dose (7 nmoles) of [3H]taurocholate was transported predominantly by hepatocytes of zones 1. As shown in Fig. 1, a profile of decreasing concen-

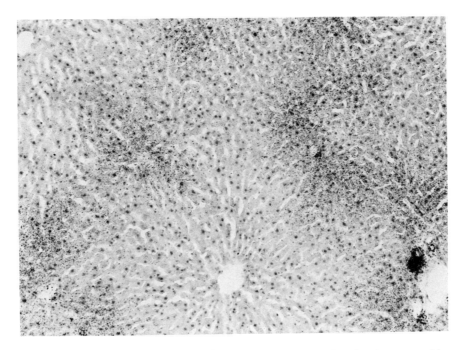

Figure 1.   Distribution of a low dose of [3H]taurocholate within the hepatic acinus assessed by autoradiography. After the administration of 7 nmoles [3H]taurocholate via the portal vein, grains were distributed mainly around hepatocytes surrounding terminal portal venules in acinar zone 1. As can be seen at the center of the micrograph, hepatocytes surrounding terminal hepatic venules (zone 3) weredevoid of grains. Reproduced from Groothuis et al.[31] by permission of the author and of the American Physiological Society.

tration of grains, from zone 1 to zone 3, was observed. In contrast, the injection of a high dose of [³H]taurocholate into the portal vein (8 μmoles in 0.5 ml 0.9% NaCl) resulted in homogeneous distribution of the label throughout hepatocytes of all zones (Fig. 2). Therefore, the contribution of hepatocytes of zones 1, 2, and 3 to taurocholate transport depends on the concentration of the incoming load of bile acids.[32,33] At high loads, there is a sequential recruitment of hepatocytes in zone 2 and later in zone 3 for transport, suggesting that the capacity to transport bile acids is distributed throughout the acinus. Earlier studies[32,33] attempted to approach this problem of bile acid receptor distribution within the acinus either by producing zonal toxic damage or by measuring the changes in the cross-diameter of the bile canaliculus in response to bile acid infusions. Both studies proposed that the capacity for bile acid transport was indeed distributed in all acinar hepatocytes and that the predominant contribution of zone 1 was due mainly to the fact that these hepatocytes are the first perfused. A more direct demonstration that hepatocytes of zone 3 can transport bile acids was provided by Groothuis *et al.*[31] As shown in Fig. 3, the injection of a tracer dose of

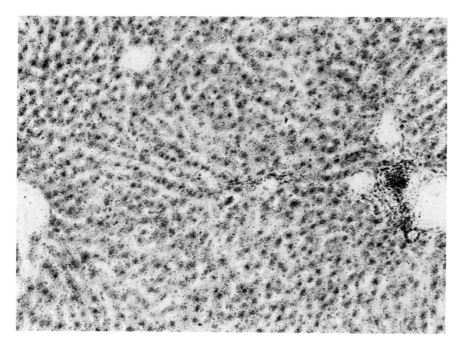

Figure 2. Distribution of a large dose of [³H]taurocholate within the hepatic acinus. Following administration of 8 μmoles [³H]taurocholate via the portal vein, grains were distributed in all acinar zones. Reproduced from Groothuis *et al.*[31] by permission of the author and of the American Physiological Society.

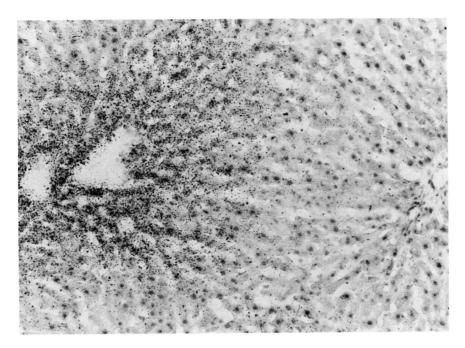

Figure 3. Retrograde injection of [³H]taurocholate via the inferior vena cava. After the injection of a low dose of [³H]taurocholate via the inferior vena cava, grains were distributed mainly in hepatocytes surrounding a terminal hepatic venule (zone 3). At the right of the micrograph, a small portal space can be seen. Hepatocytes surrounding this portal space (zone 1) are devoid of grains. Reproduced from Groothuis *et al.*[31] by permission of the author and of the American Physiological Society.

[³H]taurocholate via the inferior vena cava cannula during retrograde perfusion of the liver (i.e., from hepatic vein to portal vein) resulted in the predominant distribution of grains in hepatocytes of zone 3. These data demonstrate that the direction of perfusion, rather than receptor distribution, plays a major role in the contribution of specific hepatocytes to taurocholate transport. However, the role that possible differences in the kinetics of bile acid receptors play in these results cannot be assessed by these experiments. Moreover, similar studies have not been performed either in humans or in animals with a gallbladder. While it seems plausible that hepatocytes of zone 1 will transport most of the load of taurocholate during fasting, the zonal distribution of bile acids after a meal remains to be established.

The data analyzed above dealt with two bile acids, sodium taurocholate, a water-soluble compound, and cholylglycylhistamine, a poorly soluble bile acid analogue. In both cases, the fraction of these compounds extracted by the hepatocytes first exposed to them was high; therefore, a decreasing concentration gradient develops within the acinus. Can we predict the zonal distribution of other bile acids on the basis of these results?

In general terms, the development of concentration gradients for any solute will depend on the fraction extracted in a single pass by hepatocytes of zone 1. If the fraction of a solute extracted by these hepatocytes is high, a pattern of decreasing concentration of the solute in zones 2 and 3 will occur. In the experiments of Groothuis et al.,[31] the fraction of taurocholate extracted when the bile acid was injected in trace amounts was 96%, and gradients were detected. In contrast, following the administration of taurocholate in high doses (8 μmoles), the fraction extracted was about 45%, and the distribution of the label throughout the acinus was homogeneous.

3.4.2. Role of Conjugation and the Number of Hydroxyl Groups

Smallwood et al.,[34] in experiments using rats with a bile fistula, found that the hepatic extraction fraction was highest for taurocholate, followed in decreasing order by glycocholate, cholate, deoxycholate, and chenodeoxycholate. Aldini et al.[35] raised the question whether these differences in hepatic extraction of bile acids were due to differences in the binding affinity of each bile acid either for the postulated plasma membrane receptor or for serum albumin. Using the isolated rat liver perfusion system, they showed that the hepatic extraction of taurocholate was about 74% compared to 63% for glycocholate and about 53% for cholate. The hepatic extraction of cholate, however, was higher than that of 7-ketolithocholate, ursodeoxycholate, and chenodeoxycholate. These authors[35] also observed that conjugation with either taurine or glycine increased the hepatic extraction over that of the unconjugated forms without a measurable change in the percentage of bile acids bound to albumin. These results suggested, in agreement with other proposals,[34,36,37] that conjugation, the number of hydroxyl groups in the molecule, and the binding affinities of each bile acid for albumin play a role in determining the hepatic extraction of bile acids. These data, however, must now be interpreted in the light of more recent evidence provided by experiments with cultured hepatocytes. Van Dyke et al.[22] showed that while the uptake of taurocholate, glycocholate, cholate, and glycochenodeoxycholate occurred via a saturable, sodium-coupled mechanism, the uptake of other bile acids (chenodeoxycholate, deoxycholate, lithocholate, cholylglycylhistamine) occurred via a nonsaturable sodium-independent mechanism. Moreover, the sodium-coupled transport system exhibited substrate specificity. Thus, the removal of either of the hydroxyl groups in the ring or of the conjugating amino acid reduced transport via this sodium-coupled system. Therefore, the interpretation of results measuring hepatic extraction must now take into account that bile acids, depending on molecular characteristics, are taken up by two distinct mechanisms: a secondary active transport system and, most likely, by simple diffusion.[22]

3.4.3. Role of Albumin

Bile acid binding to serum albumin seems to modify bile acid uptake by at least two mechanisms. First, it decreases the extraction fraction of bile acids in a single pass. As a consequence, it influences the concentration of bile acids in each acinar zone. Second, the concentration of the bile acid–albumin complex in the space of Disse seems to regulate the rate of bile acid uptake. Unfortunately, studies of the effect of albumin binding on the zonal distribution of bile acids have not been performed. However, data are available for other organic anions. In experiments performed using the *in situ* perfused rat liver,[38] in the absence of albumin in the perfusate, the hepatic extraction fraction of a 1×10^{-5} M sulfobromophthalein (BSP) solution in a single pass was about 0.99. Under these conditions, gradients of decreasing concentration of BSP between hepatocytes of zones 1 and 3 were demonstrated visually. The addition of either 1 or 4.5% albumin to the perfusate resulted in a decrease of the hepatic extraction fraction of BSP to about 0.20. Concomitantly, BSP was distributed homogeneously throughout all acinar hepatocytes.[38] Thus, binding to albumin seems to offset the effects of the unidirectional perfusion of the acinus by distributing bound solutes in a more homogeneous manner. If these observations can be extrapolated to bile acids, it is likely that the higher the affinity of a bile acid for albumin, the lower will be the extraction fraction in a single pass and the more homogeneous will be its distribution throughout the acinus. In contrast, bile acids with a lower affinity for albumin and a high affinity for the plasma membrane receptor will have a high extraction fraction in a single pass if carrier-mediated transport is operative. Under these conditions, a clear-cut gradient of decreasing bile acid concentration should be observed between zones 1 and 3 of the acinus. For bile acids taken up by simple diffusion (see above), the unidirectional perfusion of the acinus will tend to deliver these molecules mainly into the hepatocytes of zone 1; however, the actual zonal distribution will also depend on the affinity of the bile acid molecule for albumin.

The second effect of bile acid binding to albumin is on the rate of bile acid uptake. The traditional view has been that the rate of uptake of bile acids, as well as that of other organic anions, is determined exclusively by the concentration of the free or unbound fraction of the anion in sinusoidal blood. Recent studies, indicate, however, that the rate of bile acid uptake is regulated by the concentration of the bile acid–albumin complex in the space of Disse. In 1966, Baker and Bradley[39] noted that the free fraction of BSP was so small under clinical conditions that the "hepatic extraction of BSP may entail a substantial uptake directly from plasma albumin." Forker and Luxon[40,41] observed that the rate of bile acid uptake in the perfused liver was faster than the rate of uptake that can be calculated from the concentration of the free bile acid fraction measured *in vitro* by equilibrium dialysis. Similar findings[42–44] have been observed for the uptake of fatty acids, bilirubin, and BSP. It should be noted, however, that direct measurement of the rate of dissociation of the bile acid–albumin complex in the space of Disse has not been achieved. In summary, these studies indicate that binding of bile acids to albumin results in decreased extraction, the magnitude of which depends on the binding affinity of the individual bile acid for albumin. In addition, the rate of bile acid uptake is faster than the rate calculated from the concentration of the free bile acid fraction, suggesting that the concentration of the bile acid–albumin complex determines the rate of bile acid uptake. These observations by no means deny that under experimental conditions, organic anions can be taken up by the liver very efficiently in the absence of albumin. As mentioned, bile acids and BSP are extracted more efficiently from the medium in the absence than in the presence of albumin. Actually, the efficient extraction of compounds such as bile acids and BSP by hepatocytes in zone 1 in the absence of albumin may result in toxic damage.[32,38] Binding to albumin by decreasing the fraction extracted by hepatocytes in zone 1 distributes the incoming load of bile acids or BSP in a more equilibrated manner, thus diminishing the concentration of potentially toxic anions delivered to a few hepatocytes.[38]

In the discussion presented above as well as in most experimental designs, it has been assumed that bile acids are physiologically bound to serum albumin. In the last few years, however, it has been shown that bile acids in blood are bound to albumin as well as to high-density lipoproteins (HDL).[45] Indeed, the relative distribution of bile acids between albumin and HDL was dependent on the molecular structure of each bile acid. Moreover, it has been observed that 64% of *N*-cholylglycine appears after electrophoresis in the α-$_2$-globulin fraction.[37,46] The β-lipoprotein fraction contained significant amounts of conjugated bile acids, which are increased in hyperlipidemic individuals.[46] What, then, is the relative distribution of bile acids among serum proteins in portal vein blood under physiological conditions? These data have yet to be obtained.

4. INTRACELLULAR METABOLISM OF BILE ACIDS IN THE MATURE LIVER

4.1. Bile Acid Synthesis

4.1.1. Mechanisms

The sequence of events by which the primary bile acids, cholic and chenodeoxycholic acid, are formed in the liver from obligatory precursor, unesterified cholesterol, remains somewhat conjectural.[47–50] There are data, however, that suggest that compartmentalization of cholesterol into "functional pools" occurs. Endogenous and exogenous precursor cholesterol undergo different modes of incorporation into bile acids.[51,52] In addition, cholesterol bound to HDL seemingly undergoes greater side-chain oxidation than does low-density-lipoprotein–cholesterol in the intact rat.[53] The transformation to bile acids involves a sequence of reactions (Fig. 4) including: (1) epimerization of the 3β-OH group, (2) reduction of the Δ5 double bond, (3) introduction of α-OH groups at C-3, C-7, or C-12, and (4) oxidative degradation (loss of 3 carbons) of the side chain. The traditional concepts held that the initial modification of the cholesterol

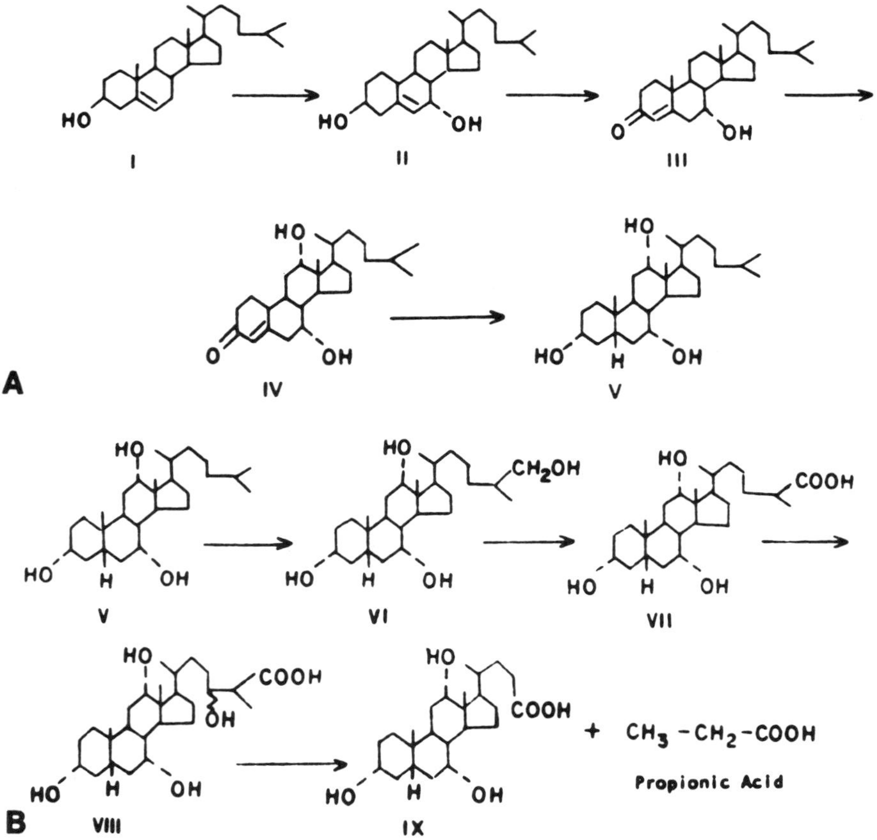

Figure 4. Key reactions evaluated in the transformation of the cyclopentanophenathrene nucleus (A) and in side-chain oxidation (B).[142] (I) Cholesterol; (II) 7α-hydroxycholesterol; (III) 7α-hydroxy-4-cholesten-3-one; (IV) 7α,12α-dihydroxy-4-cholesten-3-one; (V) 5β-cholestane-3α,7α,12α-triol; (VI) 5β-cholestane-3α,7α,12α,26-tetrol; (VII) 3α,7α,12α-trihydroxy-5β-cholestanoic acid; (VIII) varanic acid; (IX) cholic acid.

molecule involves hydroxylation at the C-7 position of the steroid skeleton (Fig. 4), a reaction catalyzed by mixed-function oxidase in the smooth endoplasmic reticulum under the activity of 7α-hydroxylase. This reaction, which forms 7α-hydroxy cholesterol, is seemingly rate-limiting in overall bile acid synthesis.[54–56] This step and the subsequent fate of the next intermediate compound, 7α-hydroxy-cholest-4-ene-3-one, are the subject of some controversy. This compound may serve as a common denominator and provide a branch point leading to synthesis of either cholic or chenodeoxycholic acid. Cholic acid synthesis requires 12α-hydroxylation, followed by reduction of the C-3 ketone and the double bond to form 5β-cholestane-3α,7α,12α-triol. Chenodeoxycholate synthesis follows reduction of 7α-OH-cholest-4-ene-3-one at C-4,5 and C-3 to form 5β-cholestane-3α,7α-diol. It is unclear whether the 12α-hydroxylase plays a significant role in the regulation of the ratio between the primary bile acids in human bile.[57] In the most frequently studied model, the rat, it appears that mitochondrial or microsomal enzymes modify the hydrocarbon side chain (26-hydroxylation) of the cholestane nucleus to form C-24 steroids. There are several alternate hypotheses. Shefer and colleagues suggest that oxidation of the side chain of 5β-cholestane-3α,7α,12α-triol does not involve intermediates hydroxylated at C-26. The proposed 25-hydroxylation pathway has been demonstrated in both rat and human liver.[58–60]

An alternative concept suggests that a quantitatively important pathway to chenodeoxycholate synthesis involves initial side-chain oxidation before nuclear biotransformation occurs.[49] This alternative concept has received further impetus from studies that suggest that in the human liver, there is an absence of microsomal enzyme activity directed toward the oxidation of the cholesterol side chain. This observation suggests that mitochondrial C-27 sterol 26-hydroxylase is an important rate-limiting step in humans.[58,59] Recent work by Bostrom and Wikvall[61] has isolated subfractions from cytochrome P-450$_{LM4}$ with different amino acid compositions and with different specificities toward substrates in bile acid biosynthesis. A question for future study is to define the physiological importance of the apparent peroxisomal formation of cholic acid.[62,63]

4.1.2. Regulation and Modulation

Modulation of bile acid pool size and synthetic rate appears to occur, at least partially, via feedback control of 7α-hydroxylase activity by bile acids returning to the liver. Hydroxymethylglutaryl (HMG)-CoA reductase, and possibly 7α-hydroxylase, may exist in an inactive and an active form, depending on the state of phosphorylation.[64] Therefore, short-term modulation of enzyme activity may occur via this activation–inactivation mechanism. There are different sensitivities of the feedback inhibition mechanism for individual bile acids; e.g., in the rat, taurocholate is a more effective inhibitor than cholate.[65] Several studies have documented an inverse correlation between the recycling frequency of the pool and the magnitude of bile acid pool size.[66–68] These studies suggest that the smaller the bile acid pool size, the more rapid the recycling frequency, and vice versa. It has further been suggested that an increase in intestinal motility accelerates the delivery of bile acids to the ileum for absorption.[66] This results in a decreased synthesis rate and a diminution of the bile acid pool size. Prolongation of intestinal transit time will similarly increase bile acid pool size in the face of a decreased fractional turnover rate and an increased rate of synthesis. However, fasting is associated with a decrease in the rate of synthesis of bile acids and decreased 7α-hydroxylase activity. Since there is a decrease flux of bile acids through the liver, it is postulated that additional regulatory mechanisms exist.[69–71]

Synthesis of bile acids in the rat has been shown to fluctuate in a diurnal pattern, with peak rates occurring during the dark or feeding phase.[71] Further elucidation of the role of these physiological factors in the subcellular regulation of 7α-hydroxylase is needed. The rhythmic, diurnal variation in bile acid pool size and bile acid secretion rate may be related to the migrating myoelectric complex or "interdigestive housekeeper," which serves to deliver bile acids to the ileum even in the fasting state.[72]

4.1.3. Metabolic Compartmentation

The subcellular distribution of bile acids *in vivo* may not only relate to the modulation of various metabolic processes, but also govern transhepatic transport. The physical, chemical, and physiological events in the intrahepatic transport of bile acids are poorly understood. It has been suggested that the intrahepatic concentration of total bile acids such as cholate and chenodeoxycholate in the rat liver is approximately 0.2 mM.[73,74] In the study of Okishio and Nair,[73] approximately 70% of the bile acids were found in the cystosol, with the nuclear, microsomal, and mitochondrial fractions each containing 10%. These data may be reasonable estimates; however, they provide no knowledge regarding the percentage of bile acid present in free solution. Further, this study seemingly did not take into account redistribution of bile acids during homogenization, extraction, and dilution.

Strange and colleagues have sought specific bile acid binding proteins in liver cytosol following subcellular fractionation.[74–79] They have suggested the existence of wide variability in the relative affinity and number of binding sites in each of the subcellular organelles. Using lithocholate binding as a marker, they isolated two binding proteins from cytosol, one of which was subsequently identified as ligandin.[74,75,77,79] The authors concluded that bile acid binding may therefore play a role in transport, may govern metabolism, and may possibly exert a protective effect. However, the true physiological significance of bile acid binding by ligandin or other cytosolic proteins, such as glutathione-*S*-transferase, remains to be determined.

Partitioning of bile acid into subcellular organelles may also account for the observed association with subcellular fractions. In the studies of Strange *et al.*[76,78] substantial amounts of cholate, chenodeoxycholate, and lithocholate were found in the nuclei as well as in other subcellular fractions examined (Table I).

4.2. Bile Acid Conjugation

Cholic and chenodeoxycholic acids are conjugated, as *N*-acyl conjugates, in a peptide linkage with either glycine or taurine by enzymes localized predominantly in the endoplasmic reticulum prior to secretion. The interaction is initiated by the microsomal enzyme cholyl-CoA ligase, forming a bile acid–Co A thioester.[25,80,81] This intermediate combines with taurine or glycine in a reaction catalyzed in the cytosol by bile acid-CoA: amino acid *N*-acyltransferase to produce the conjugated product.[80,81] It is possible that conjugation itself may be a rate-limiting step in bile secretion.[25,82]

4.3. Intracellular Transport

The role of intracellular organelles in hepatobiliary transport remains uncertain. Tracer studies indicate that the smooth endoplasmic reticulum (SER) is involved in the production of phospholipids that are destined for biliary excretion.[83] The volume density of both the SER and the Golgi aparatus of rat liver increases during taurocholate-induced choleresis.[84] Recent autoradiographic studies using bile acid analogues showed prominent labeling of the SER and the Golgi apparatus during transcellular transport.[85,86] The SER may be also facilitate transport of compounds such as bile acids by conjugation.

Table I. Distribution of Cholate Conjugates, Chenodeoxycholate Conjugates, and Lithocholate in Rat Liver

Location	Cholate conjugates (%)	Chenodeoxycholate conjugates (%)	Lithocholate (%)
Nuclei	41.2	28.6	17.2
Microsomes	16.8	19.5	11.1
Mitochondria	9.5	14.6	2.9
Protein-bound in cytosol	21.6	33.2	68.0
Free solution in cytosol	10.8	4.1	0.8

4.4. Biliary Secretion

4.4.1. General Process

The rate at which various bile acids are excreted into bile by the rat liver is quite variable. For example, taurocholate is excreted much more rapidly than cholate.[34] Glycocholate is excreted into rat bile more rapidly than lithocholate.[78] These differences may be due partially to the intrahepatic fate of the bile acids and are presumably compatible with the hypothesis that bile acids cross the liver in free solution; therefore, the rate of passage depends on the relative proportions present in free solution.

It remains to be determined how bile acids traverse the canaliculus. These studies are limited, however, since canalicular bile is not readily available for direct sampling. However, several lines of evidence suggest that this process may be carrier-mediated.[25] Saturability may be present; a T_m exists, and there is a nonlinear relationship between the intracellular concentration and the excretion rate. It is unclear whether the process is energy-dependent or whether the driving force is a chemical and electrical gradient into the canaliculus. The seemingly large bile acid concentration gradient between liver cells (0.1–0.3 mM) and bile (up to 100 mM) may be accounted for by either an active transport system or passive facilitated diffusion followed by incorporation into micelles. The presence of vesicles in the pericanalicular cytoplasm following taurocholate-induced choleresis raises the question of the overall importance of Golgi-derived vesicles in bile secretion.

The end result, however, is that once bile acid reaches the canaliculus, osmotic and electrical gradients favor movement of Na^+ and obligated water from the intercellular space across the junctional complex into the lumen, thereby providing a motive force for bile formation.

4.4.2. Zonal Contribution to the Biliary Secretion of Bile Acids

Since available data indicate that hepatocytes in zones 1 and 2 take up most of the incoming load of bile acids, these acinar zones should also contribute predominantly to the biliary secretion of bile acids.[30–33] However, between the zonal binding of bile acids to sinusoidal plasma membranes and canalicular secretion of bile acids, there is a series of steps regarding which there are insufficient data to date. For instance, little is known about either the characteristics of the bile acid receptor in sinusoidal membranes[23] or the process of bile acid translocation. Moreover, there are no data on the zonal contribution to bile acid conjugation. Indeed, very few studies have dealt with the zonal capabilities to conjugate solutes. To date, only the zonal conjugation of BSP with glutathione[87] and the O-diethylation and sulfation of acetaminophen[88,89] have been directly probed.

Regarding the zonal contribution to bile acid secretion, Groothuis et al.,[31] showed that there are differences in the kinetics of secretion of taurocholate into bile by hepatocytes in zones 1 and 3. The rate of biliary secretion of taurocholate by hepatocytes in zone 3 was slower than the rate of secretion by those in zone 1. A similar observation has been made during perfusions of BSP–glutathione.[87] These findings raise the possibility that the number of receptor sites in the canalicular membrane in each zone may be different. If this is correct, study of the zonal differences may provide an interesting model to define the factors that regulate the number of receptor sites in each zone.

5. HEPATOCELLULAR METABOLISM AND TRANSPORT OF BILE ACIDS DURING LIVER DEVELOPMENT

5.1. Concept of "Physiological Cholestasis" in Infancy

Efficient uptake by the hepatocyte of a variety of compounds from portal blood, their transcellular movement, and their excretion across the canalicular membrane into bile are essential for postnatal adaptation to the extrauterine environment. In newborns and infants of most mammalian species, the efficiency of hepatic transport of bile acids, other organic anions, organic cations, and neutral compounds is often decreased in comparison with that of the adult.[90,91] Immaturity of hepatic transport functions may lead to dangerous accumulation of some drugs in plama, retention of endogenous toxins such as bilirubin, and increased susceptibility to cholestatic liver disease.[92] Numerous studies support the hypothesis that the human infant and suckling rat undergo a period of "physiological cholestasis" due to decreased hepatic transport of bile acids.[93] Recent advances in our understanding of liver physiology and application of newer techniques in hepatocyte and membrane isolation have allowed some insight to be gained into the cellular determinants of hepatic transport during development.

5.1.1. Evidence for Impaired Bile Acid Transport during Early Life

Of the potential ratelimiting steps in overall hepatic transport during development, the uptake process has been examined most thoroughly. Specific clearance studies have provided much information regarding hepatic uptake capacity. Hepatic uptakes of labeled digoxin, digitoxin, eosin, ouabain, indocyanine green (ICG), BSP, and bile acids are all decreased in several fetal and suckling mammals in comparison with the adult.[90] Klassen[94] observed that the plasma disappearance and biliary excretion of taurocholate occurred at a much slower rate in suckling 7-day-old rats than in adults. He also noted complete inability of the neonatal rat liver to concentrate ouabain; the liver of the adult was able to concentrate this compound about 30-fold over the level in plasma.[95] In the newborn rhesus monkey, hepatic clearance of bilirubin was decreased during the first few days of life.[96] Recent studies have also shown that serum cholic acid conjugates are markedly elevated in the serum of suckling rats, indirectly suggesting impaired clearance.[97] The high levels of bile acids in serum are all the more striking in light of the fact that the circulating pool of bile acids is low and active ileal reabsorption of bile acids is absent during the suckling period.[98,99] The concept of decreased hepatic uptake of a relatively smaller bile acid "load" is further supported by comparison of bile acid levels in portal and peripheral blood.[100] Although the portal vein concentration of cholic acid conjugates in the 14-day-old rat pup was significantly lower than concentrations found in the adult rat, levels in peripheral serum of pups were 2-fold higher than in the adult. The peripheral/portal vein serum ratio of cholic acid conjugates was higher in pups than in adult rats. Immaturity of hepatic bile acid clearance is most dramatically demonstrated at weaning, when serum bile acid concentrations reach their peak (Fig. 5); this peak probably occurs as a result of an expansion of the pool size and the appearance of active ileal transport of bile acids.[97–99]

There have understandably been few direct studies of hepatic clearance in human infants. The observation of high serum concentrations of drugs and en-

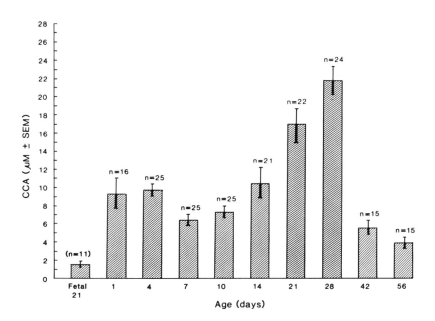

Figure 5. Serum concentration of conjugates of cholate (CCA) in developing rats (n = number of animals.)[7]

dogenous compounds, such as bilirubin, has indicated that hepatic metabolism and transport of many substrates may be immature at birth.[100] Alterations in the rate of disposition of digitalis, propanolol, and bilirubin in various animal models suggest that impaired hepatic uptake may contribute to the abnormal accumulation of these compounds in serum in the human neonate.[91,101,102]

BSP has been used over the last 40 years by several investigators to evaluate liver function in the neonate.[103–105] When tested at birth, normal full-term and premature infants have delayed clearance of BSP in comparison with adults when given a 5 mg/kg dose of BSP intravenously. Decreased uptake has been mentioned as only one of several factors in addition to conjugation and secretion that lead to altered disposition of BSP during the perinatal period. Progressive improvement in the ability of infants to remove BSP from the circulation takes place during the first 3–4 weeks of life.[103,106] Similarly, the clearance of ICG was decreased markedly in a group of normal newborns.[107] The authors noted that the low rate of elimination of ICG and the low affinity constant in comparison with older infants could be related to altered hepatic blood flow or the intrinsic clearance capacity of the liver or both. These kinetic parameters were further reduced in a group of infants with nonhemolytic hyperbilirubinemia.[108] This observation adds additional evidence to the concept that ICG and bilirbuin may utilize the same carrier for uptake into the hepatocyte.

Recent studies have indicated that hepatic transport of bile acids is also decreased in infants during the first year of life. Cord-blood concentrations of the conjugates of cholic acid and chenodeoxycholic acid are not different from levels in maternal blood.[93,109] Itoh et al.,[110] in fact, noted a lower mean concentration in umbilical blood than in maternal blood. The levels of the bile acid conjugates in serum from the umbilical artery were found to be significantly higher than in umbilical venous blood, suggesting that fetal serum bile acid concentrations were maintained at low levels by net placental transfer to the mother. Suchy et al.[93] showed that after birth, conjugates of both cholate and chenodeoxycholate increased progressively in serum during the first week of life. Unlike the transient physiological hyperbilirubinemia of the newborn, serum bile acid levels remained elevated to a similar degree in infants 6–8 weeks old; there was a gradual decline to adult levels after the first 4–6 months of life. An additional 12 infants (mean age 22 weeks) were studied while fasting and at 30-min intervals for 3 hr after a standard liquid feeding; both the baseline and the maximum postprandial concentration of cholic acid conjugates were significantly higher than in older children. This exaggerated postprandial response and the significantly greater integrated area under the meal-response curve suggested defective clearance of bile acids by the liver.

5.1.2. Implications: Susceptibility to Pathological Cholestasis

These findings suggest, on balance, that the infantile liver has a tendency toward cholestasis and that any additional insult could lead to a marked decrease in bile flow. The clinical correlate of this physiological propensity is illustrated most dramatically in infants who manifest conjugated hyperbilirubinemia during an episode of sepsis, during infusion of nutrient amino acid solutions, and during other insults (e.g., hypoxia, hypoperfusion) that commonly occur in early life in infants with low birth weight.[98]

5.2. Bile Acid Metabolism

5.2.1. Control of Bile Acid Synthesis

In view of the prime importance of bile acid synthesis, not only as a "choleretic force" but also as a major pathway for cholesterol degradation and elimination, attention has been devoted to the development of cholesterol metabolic and bile acid synthetic pathways in early life. Early studies sought to determine the development of the bile acid pool in various animal models. For example, Lambiotte et al.[111] described an increase of greater than 20-fold in the amount of cholic acid found in rat fetuses on the 22nd day, from less than 10 μg prior to 21 days of age. This group further noted marked increases in bile acid pool size following the termination of gestation. Similar data have been obtained in other species. Little et al.[112] described qualitative and quantitative changes in the bile acid pool size of the rat fetus; in addition, they noted a shift of the pool size from an intrahepatic localization in the fetus. Cholic acid was detected in rat fetuses on the 15th day of gestation. There were also significant amounts of chenodeoxycholate, deoxycholate, and β-muricholate in the rat fetus; following birth, however, cholic acid predominated. More than 80% of the taurocholate pool was then found in the intestine. In other species, such as the rabbit, deoxycholate was found in the fetus, suggesting transfer of this bile acid from the mother.[113]

Coincident with the marked postnatal increase in bile acid pool size, there is a concomitant decrease in cholesterol levels, which may be markedly elevated in early life, as in the neonatal guinea pig.[114] Li et al.[119] have shown that the activity of the presumed rate-controlling enzyme, cholesterol 7α-hydroxylase, is less in neonatal liver than in the adult. Comparable activity of hepatic HMG-CoA reductase is present. Perinatal modulation has been suggested by Naseem et al.[116] since hepatic cholesterol 7α-hydroxylase was higher in pups of mothers who had received cholesterol during their pregnancy. These data suggest that an increased fetal cholesterol pool might stimulate pathways of bile acid biogenesis.

5.2.2. Intracellular Metabolism

There are large interspecies differences in the major conjugate formed in early life. In the neonatal rat, human, and rabbit, taurine conjugates predominate.[117] In humans, glycine conjugation becomes the predominant pathway later in life as a reflection of the alterations of dietary intake.

As discussed previously, the exact events involved in intracellular metabolism of bile acids are unknown; however, it is possible that binding to cytosolic proteins, e.g., the glutathione-S-transferase class, is an important process.[118] This step may modulate transport and metabolism through the hepatocyte. There are no data on age-related changes in these proteins, however. Conjugation may also serve as a rate-limiting step, and various studies have suggested that the overall conjugation capacity is limited in early life.[83,98,99] Specific activities of the individual enzymes involved in bile acid conjugation, namely, cholyl-CoA ligase and N-acetyltransferase, are lower in early life than in mature species. In addition, activity of bile acid sulfotransferase is reduced in rat pups in comparison to adult rats.[119] Whether these apparently inefficient biotransformation pathways play a role in bile acid transport remains to be determined.

5.3. Bile Acid Transport

5.3.1. Structural Features of the Developing Liver That Could Influence Uptake

Many changes occur in the hepatocyte during the final days of gestation to prepare the liver for the enhanced synthetic rate and transport function required after birth. Neonatal rat hepatocytes are smaller, with a surface area of 0.476 ± 0.018 cm^2/cm^3 vs. 0.825 ± 0.020 cm^2/cm^3 in the adult rat; at both ages, however, hepatocytes approach 80% of adult parenchymal volume.[120–122] Although the surface area of the sinusoidal space is also smaller in the neonate, it comprises a percentage ($\approx 10\%$) of liver volume similar to that in the adult rat.[123] It is not known whether the surface area of the sinusoidal membranes is increased in zone 1 as compared to zone 3 of neonatal liver. This structured feature has been described in adult rat liver and may contribute to the more avid uptake in zone 1 of certain compounds such as bile acids.[124,125] Liver cell plates are often several hepatocytes thick in livers of human infants, which might result in less of the hepatocyte surface being exposed to portal blood. The dynamics of the perinatal portal circulation have recently been the subject of excellent reviews.[6,7] Current evidence supports the notion that the ductus venosus closes shortly after birth in most mammals, including man. There is no evidence that significant shunting of blood occurs after functional closure of this structure. However, a recent study utilizing an isolated, perfused suckling rat liver model suggests that an increased volume of distribution may contribute to low rates of bile acid uptake observed prior to weaning.[126]

The acinar heterogeneity of many metabolic and transport systems has been well recognized in the liver.[13–15,125,127] For example, several groups have utilized radioautographic techniques to demonstrate that there is a distinct zone-1-to-zone-3 gradient for bile acid uptake in the adult rat liver.[30,31] An acinar distribution for uptake is possible only with compounds that are very efficiently extracted from portal blood.[17,38] Groothuis et al.[128] were unable to demonstrate an acinar gradient for the uptake of dibromosulfophthalein, which has an extraction efficiency of about 40%. Likewise, Suchy et al.[86,100] proposed that the decreased clearance of bile acids by the developing liver might result in an acinar distribution for bile acid uptake that differed from that of the adult. On light-microscopic radioautography, there was a distinct zone-1-to-zone-3 gradient for the uptake of the bile acid analogue [^{125}I]cholylglycyltyrosine (CGT) in the adult rat liver. Silver grains were localized primarily in zone 1 hepatocytes. In contrast, there was no acinar gradient for CGT uptake visible in the 14-day-old suckling rat. The pattern was quite similar to that observed in adult rat liver during bile acid infusion, which causes progressive recruitment of hepatocytes within the liver acinus. We concluded that the entire hepatic acinus, including the normal "reserve" function of the zone 3 hepatocytes, participates in the transport of bile acids during development even under basal conditions. However, despite recruitment, overall clearance is not sufficient to compensate for decreased uptake in the 14-day-old rat, and bile acids spill over from the portal into the systemic circulation.

5.3.2. Uptake of Bile Acids during Development

Suchy and Balistreri[90] have recently studied the development of the bile acid transport system using isolated hepatocytes. Uptake of taurocholate was decreased markedly in hepatocytes isolated from suckling rats. There was a progressive increase in taurocholate uptake between 7 and 56 days of age. The uptake process exhibited saturable kinetics in every age group (Fig. 6). At 7

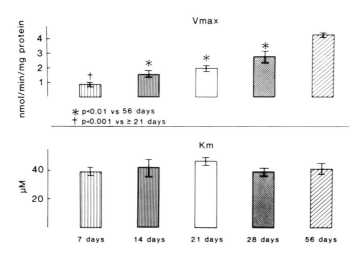

Figure 6. Rate constant for uptake of taurocholate by hepatocytes isolated from developing rats.[86] Each bar represents the mean ± S.E. of data obtained from animals.

days of age, the V_{max} was only 23% of that attained in the adult rat; a 2-fold increment in V_{max} occurred between weaning (21 days) and 56 days. In contrast, there were no significant differences in K_m values for taurocholate uptake between any of the age groups studied. These data suggest that the affinity of the liver cell plasma membrane for taurocholate remains constant during this period of development. However, the 4-fold increase in V_{max} may reflect an increase in the number of functional bile acid carriers. Qualitatively similar developmental changes in taurocholate uptake were described recently in the isolated, perfused suckling rat liver.[126]

In more intact systems such as isolated hepatocytes and the perfused rat liver, the actual forces that drive bile acid uptake may potentially be obscured by age-related changes in variables such as cellular metabolism, sodium-pump activity, and intracellular compartmentation. For this reason, Suchy *et al.*[129] also studied taurocholate uptake utilizing basolateral liver plasma membrane vesicles isolated from 14-day-old rats. These membranes were 28- to 30-fold enriched in the basolateral membrane marker Na^+, K^+-ATPase activity; interestingly, there was no difference in the activity of Na^+,K^+-ATPase between suckling and adult rat membranes. In this system, however, energy for the sodium pump is not provided and bile acid transport is driven by an artifical sodium gradient. Although actual Na^+ pumping activity remains to be examined *in vivo*, these data suggest that developmental differences in bile acid uptake cannot be explained on the basis of differences in Na^+,K^+-ATPase activity. The presence of a well-developed sodium pump in suckling rat liver is not surprising in light of its essential role in the maintenance of cell homeostasis. Data obtained from uptake studies using membrane vesicles isolated from 14-day-old rats were quite similar to data derived from isolated hepatocytes. The V_{max} for taurocholate uptake in the suckling rat was only 30% of that found in the adult. There were no difference in the K_m for taurocholate uptake. Preliminary experiments using basolateral liver membrane vesicles isolated from neonatal rats indicate that saturable, sodium-dependent uptake of taurocholate is present at birth.

Several additional factors that could also influence bile acid uptake should be mentioned briefly. Several studies have indicated that albumin binding of certain ligands is an important determinant of the rate of solute uptake.[41–44] Bile acid uptake by adult liver plasma membrane vesicles is actually accelerated in the presence of low concentrations of albumin.[130] The mechanism of this albumin effect is not known, but may involve binding of an albumin–ligand complex to the plasma membrane, allowing more efficient presentation of the ligand to its carrier. Determination of the possible developmental significance of this effect awaits further studies of the ontogeny of albumin binding of ligands such as bile acids.

Bile acid uptake could also be retarded by the uptake of substrates such as amino acids, that utilize sodium symport systems.[131] Decreased uptake would then occur because of dissipation of the transmembrane sodium gradient, rather than by competition for the same carrier. This inhibition may assume particular significance in the fetal and suckling rat, in which higher circulating levels of amino acids are found.

5.3.3. Transcellular Transport: Structural Features of the Developing Liver That Could Influence Transcellular and Canalicular Transport

Morphometric studies have demonstrated that major changes occur during development in the volume density of organelles tha may comprise the bile secretory apparatus. The Golgi apparatus appears to be well developed at birth, but volume density per milliliter of tissue and SER volume per hepatocyte are markedly less in the neonatal compared with the adult rat liver.[122] A rapid proliferation of SER leads to values in excess of those in the adult by the 8th postnatal day.[121-123]

The bile canaliculi of neonatal rat liver comprise 1.4% of liver volume compared to 0.43% of adult liver.[123] However, the canalicular morphology and histochemical profile suggest an immaturity of secretory function in the perinatal rat. DeWolf-Peeters et al.[132,133] noted that at birth, bile canaliculi were large and irregular in form and showed several plump, short side branches and very large saccular dilatations at the points of mutual junction. These structural features were associated with a very intense canalicular staining reaction for alkaline phosphatase over the entire acinus. By 10 days of age, canaliculi had become thinner and more regular in form, and the alkaline phosphatase reaction was weakly positive only in zone 1 hepatocytes. The authors noted that similar changes can be found in the adult rat liver during experimental cholestasis.[132,133]

An undefined factor in overall hepatic excretory function may be the contribution of the cytoskeletal elements. Actin microfilaments may effect secretion and serve an additional site at which developmental immaturity may be manifest. Preliminary studies by Miyairi and Phillips[134] utilizing cultured fetal rat hepatocytes, have shown a decreased frequency and force of bile canalicular contraction compared to adult cells. Qualitative and quantitative differences in microfilament structure and function in early life needs to be defined.

5.3.4. Canalicular Transport during Development

Little is known about the transcellular movement of most organic ions and their subsequent transport across the bile canalicular membrane in either mature or immature animals. Further studies are necessary, focusing on the role of intracellular binding proteins, such as compounds of the gluthathione-S-transferase class, in the transport of organic anions. Specific carriers for active transport may exist in the canalicular membrane.[23,135] Although decreased hepatic uptake during development has been well documented for multiple substrates, biliary excretion is thought to be the rate-limiting step in hepatocellular transport.[25,136] The maximal hepatic transport capacity (T_m) for organic anions such as bilirubin, eosin, BSP, and ICG reflects this final stage in transport; this capacity is, in fact, lower in newborn animals than in adults.[90,136–140] Vest[104] observed that it was predominantly the second half of the plasma BSP disappearance curve that was prolonged in the human neonate and suggested further that this part of the curve reflects the rate at which the dye passes from the liver into bile. Decreased storage capacity for BSP and ICG in developing animals can also be inferred from plasma clearance studies, but liver storage capacity is always higher than excretory capacity in the mature and immature liver.[91,94] Insight into mechanisms of canalicular transport may come from use of isolated bile canalicular membrane vesicles.[24,135,141]

6. SUMMARY

Hepatocellular heterogeneity is present in both the mature and the developing liver. While the heterogeneity of the adult liver is expressed best at the level of the hepatic acinus, that of the developing liver is manifested between the right and left liver lobes. Alterations in bile acid uptake and elevated serum levels of bile acids have been demonstrated in the newborn liver, suggesting that a step of physiological cholestasis occurs during liver maturation. Due to the decreased fraction of bile acids extracted by the newborn liver, bile acids tend to distribute more homoegeneously through the hepatocytes of the acinus than in the mature liver. In contrast, hepatocytes in zones 1 and 2 of the liver acinus take up most of the incoming load of bile acids in the adult liver and thus contribute predominantly to the biliary secretion of these compounds. While the mechanisms of hepatic uptake of bile acids comprise a secondary active transport system for certain bile acids and apparently simple diffusion for others, the processes of translocation, intracellular transport, and canalicular secretion are still poorly understood. Similarly, the zonation of bile acid synthesis has not been defined. We propose that transport and metabolic regulation of bile acid synthesis be studied at the level of the functional units of the fetal liver (right and left liver lobes) and at the level of the hepatic acinus in the adult liver.

REFERENCES

1. Palmer, R. H., 1982, Bile salts and the liver, in: *Progress in Liver Diseases*, Vol. VII (H. Popper and F. Schaffner, eds.), pp. 221–242, Grune and Stratton, New York.
2. Nair, P., and Kritchevsky, D., eds., 1971, *The Bile Acids*, Plenum Press, New York.
3. Bjorkheim, I., and Danielson, H., 1976, Biosynthesis and metabolism of bile acids in man, in: *Progress in Liver Diseases*, Vol. V (H. Popper and F. Schaffner, eds.), pp. 215–231, Grune and Stratton, New York.
4. Rappaport, A. M., Borowy, Z. J., Lougheed, W. M., and Lotto, W. N., 1954, Subdivision of hexagonal liver lobules into a structural and functional unit, *Anat. Rec.* **1119**:11–27.

5. Dvorchick, B. H., Stenger, V. G., and Onattropain, S. L., 1974, Fetal hepatic drug metabolism in the nonhuman primate, *Macaca arctoides, Drug Metab. Dispos.* **2:**539–546.

6. Edelstone, D., Rudolph, A., and Heyman, M., 1978, Liver and ductus venous blood flows in fetal lambs *in utero, Circ. Dis.* **42:**426–432.

7. Rudolph, A. M., 1983, Hepatic and ductus venous blood flow in fetal liver, *Hepatology* **3:**254–258.

8. Emery, J. L., 1955, Asymmetrical liver disease in infancy, *J. Pathol. Bacteriol.* **69:**219–224.

9. Emery, J. L., 1963, Functional asymmetry of the liver, *Ann. N. Y. Acad. Sci.* **111:**37–44.

10. Gumucio, J. J., Functional units of the developing guinea pig liver (in prep.).

11. Zink, J., 1981, The fetal and neonatal hepatic circulation, in: *Hepatic Circulation in Health and Disease* (W. W. Lautt, ed.), pp. 227–248, Raven Press, New York.

12. Mihaly, G. W., Morgan, D. J., Smallwood, R., and Haroy, K. J., 1982, The developing liver: The steady-state disposition of propranolol in pregnant sheep, *Hepatology* **2:**344–349.

13. Gumucio, J. J., and Miller, D. L., 1981, Functional implications of liver cell heterogeneity, *Gastroenterology* **80:**393–403.

14. Jungermann, K., and Katz, N., 1982, Functional hepatocellular heterogeneity, *Hepatology* **2:**385–395.

15. Gumucio, J. J., and Miller, D. L., 1982, Liver cell heterogeneity, in: *The Liver: Biology and Pathobiology* (I. Arias, H. Popper, D. Schachter, and D. A. Shafritz, eds.), pp. 647–673, Raven Press, New York.

16. Carey, M. C., 1982, The enterohepatic circulation, in: *The Liver: Biology and Pathobiology* (I. Arias, H. Popper, D. Schachter, and D. A. Shafritz, eds.), pp. 429–465, Raven Press, New York.

17. Gumucio, J. J., and Miller, D. L., 1982, Zonal hepatic function: Solute–hepatocyte interactions within the liver acinus, in: *Progress in Liver Diseases,* Vol. VII (H. Popper and F. Schaffner, eds.), pp. 17–30, Grune and Stratton, New York.

18. Glasinovic, J. C., Dumont, M., Duval, M., and Erlinger, S., 1975, Hepatocellular uptake of taurocholate in the dog, *J. Clin. Invest.* **55:**419–426.

19. Scharschmidt, B. F., Waggoner, J. G., and Berk, P. D., 1976, Hepatic organic anion uptake in the rat, *J. Clin. Invest.* **56:**1280–1292.

20. Reicher, J., and Paumgartner, G., 1975, Kinetics of taurocholate uptake by the perfused rat liver, *Gastroenterology* **68:**132–136.

21. Schwarz, L. R., Burr, R., Schwenk, M., Pfaff, E., and Greim, H., 1975, Uptake of taurocholic acid into isolated rat liver cells, *Eur. J. Biochem.* **55:**617–623.

22. Van Dyke, R. W., Stephens, J. E., and Scharschmidt, B. F., 1982, Bile acid transport in cultured rat hepatocytes, *Am. J. Physiol.* **243:**G484–G492.

23. Accatino, L., and Simon, F. R., 1976, Identification and characterization of a bile acid receptor in isolated liver surface membranes, *J. Clin. Invest.* **57:**496–508.

24. Inoue, M., Kinne, R., Tran, T., Biempica, L., and Arias, I. M., 1983, Rat liver canalicular membrane vesicles: Isolation and topological characterization, *J. Biol. Chem.* **258:**5183–5188.

25. Erlinger, S., 1981, Hepatocyte bile secretion: Current views and controversies, *Hepatology* **1:**352–359.

26. Blitzer, B. L., and Boyer, J. L., 1978, Cytochemical localization of Na^+, K^+-ATPase in the rat hepatocyte, *J. Clin Invest.* **62:**1104–1108.

27. Latham, P. S., and Kashgariam, M., 1979, The ultrastructural localization of transport ATPase in rat liver at nonbile canalicular plasma membranes, *Gastroenterology* **76:**988–996.

28. Scharschmidt, B. F., and Van Dyke, R. W., 1983, Mechanisms of hepatic electrolyte transport, *Gastroenterology* **85:**1199–1216.

29. Reicher, J., Preisig, R., and Paumgartner, G., 1977, Influence of chemical structure on hepatocellular uptake of bile acids, in: *Bile and Metabolism in Health and Disease* (G. Paumgartner and A. Stiehl, eds.), pp. 113–123, MTP Press, Lancaster.

30. Jones, A. L., Hrodek, G. T., Renston, R. H., Wong, K. Y., Karlagaris, G., and Paumgartner, G., 1980, Autoradiographic evidence for hepatic lobular concentration gradient of bile acid derivative, *Am. J. Physiol.* **238:**G233–G237.

31. Groothuis, G. M. M., Hardonk, M. J., Karleman, K. P. T., Miervenhuis, P., and Meijer, D. K. F., 1981, Autoradiographic and kinetic demonstration of acinar heterogeneity of taurocholate transport, *Am. J. Physiol.* **243:**G455–G462.

32. Gumucio, J. J., and Katz, M. E., 1978, The acinar organization for bile salt transport, in: *The Liver: Quantitative Aspects of Structure and Function* (R. Preisig and J. Bircher, eds.), pp. 179–184, Editio Cantor Aulendorf, Berne.

33. Layden, T. J., and Boyer, J. L., 1978, Influence of bile acids on bile canalicular membrane morphology and the lobular gradient in canalicular size, *Lab. Invest.* **39:**110–119.

34. Smallwood, R. A., Iser, J. H., and Hofmann, N. E., 1974, in: *Advances in Bile Acid Research* (S. Matern, J. Hackenschmidt, P. Back, and W. Gerok, eds.), pp. 229–232, Schattauer-Verlag GmbH, Stuttgart.

35. Aldini, R., Roda, A., Labati, A. M. M., Cappelleri, G., Roda, E., and Barbara, L., 1982, Hepatic bile acid uptake: Effect of conjugation, hydroxyl and keto groups, and albumin binding, *J. Lipid Res.* **23:**1167–1173.

36. Rudman, D., and Kendall, F. E., 1957, Bile acid content of human serum. II. The binding of cholanic acids by human plasma protein, *J. Clin. Invest.* **36:**538–542.

37. Kramer, W., Buscher, H. P., Gerok, W., and Kurz, G., 1979, Bile salt binding to serum components: Taurocholate incorporation into high-density lipoproteins revealed by photoaffinity labelling, *Eur. J. Biochem.* **102:**1–9.

38. Gumucio, D. L., Gumucio, J. J., Wilson, J. A. P., Cutter, C., Krauss, M., Caldwell, R., and Chen, E., Albumin influences sulfobromophthalein transport by hepatocytes of each acinar zone, *Am. J. Physiol.* **246:**G86–G95.

39. Baker, K., and Bradley, S. E., 1966, Binding of sulfobromophthalein (BSP) sodium by plasma albumin: Its role in hepatic BSP extraction, *J. Clin. Invest.* **45:**281–287.

40. Forker, E. L., and Luxon, B. A., 1981, Albumin helps mediate removal of taurocholate by rat liver, *J. Clin. Invest.* **67:**1517–1522.

41. Forker, E. L., and Luxon, B. A., 1978, Hepatic transport kinetics and plasma disappearance curves: Distributed modeling versus conventional approach, *Am. J. Physiol.* **235:**648–660.

42. Weisinger, R. A., Gollan, J., and Ockner, R., 1981, Receptor for albumin in the liver cell surface may mediate uptake of fatty acids and other albumin-bound substances, *Science* **211:**1048–1050.

43. Weisinger, R. A., Gollan, J., and Ockner, R., 1982, The role of albumin in hepatic uptake processes, in: *Progress in Liver Diseases,* Vol. VII (H. Popper and F. Schaffner, eds.), pp. 71–85, Grune and Stratton, New York.

44. Ockner, R., Weisinger, R. A., and Gollan, J. L., 1983, Hepatic uptake of albumin-bound substances: Albumin receptor concept, *Am. J. Physiol.* **245:**G13–G18.

45. Middlehoff, G., Mordasini, R., Shiehl, A., and Greten, H., 1979, A bile-rich high density lipoprotein (HDL) in acute hepatitis, *Scand. J. Gastroenterol.* **14:**267–272.

46. Delahunty, T., and Feldkamp, C., 1980, Studies of endogenous *N*-cholylglycine distribution among serum proteins using radioimmunoassay, *Steroids* **36:**439–449.

47. Danielsson, H., 1973, Mechanism of bile acid synthesis, in: *The Bile Acids,* Vol. 3 (P. P. Nair and D. Kritchevsky, eds.), pp. 1–32, Plenum Press, New York.

48. Danielsson, H., and Sjovall, J., 1975, Bile acid metabolism, *Annu. Rev. Biochem.* **44:**233–253.

49. Swell, L., Gustaffson, J., Schwartz, C. C., Halloran, L. G., Danielsson, H., and Vlahcevic, Z. R., 1980, An *in vivo* evaluation of the quantitative significance of several potential pathways to cholic and chenodeoxycholic acids from cholesterol in man, *J. Lipid Res.* **21:**455–466.

50. Vlahcevic, Z. R., Schwartz, C. C., Gustaffson, J., Halloran, L. G., Danielsson, H., and Swell, L., 1980, Biosynthesis of bile acids in man: Multiple pathways to cholic and chenodeoxycholic acid, *J. Biol. Chem.* **255:**2925–2933.
51. Ayaki, Y., Tsuma-Date, T., Endo, S., and Ogura, M., 1981, Role of endogenous and exogenous cholesterol in liver as the precursor for bile acids in rats, *Steroids* **38:**495–509.
52. Kempen, H. J., Vos-van Holstein, M., and de Lange, J., 1983, Bile acids and lipids in isolated rat hepatocytes. II. Source of cholesterol used for bile acid formation, estimated by incorporation of tritium from tritiated water, and by the effect of ML-236 B, *J. Lipid Res.* **24:**316–323.
53. Miller, L. K., Tiell, L., Paul, I., Spaet, T. H., and Rosenfeld, R. S., 1982, Side-chain oxidation of lipoprotin-bound 24,25-^{3}H cholesterol in the rat: Comparison of HDL and LDL and implications for bile acid synthesis, *J. Lipid Res.* **23:**335–344.
54. Dowling, R. H., Mack, E., Small, D. M., and Picott, J., 1970, Effects of controlled interruption of the enterohepatic circulation of bile salts by biliary diversion and by ileal resection on bile salt secretion, synthesis and pool size in the rhesus monkey, *J. Clin. Invest.* **49:**232–242.
55. Shefer, S., Hauser, S., Berkersky, I., and Mosbach, E. H., 1969, Feedback regulation of bile acid biosynthesis in the rat, *J. Lipid Res.* **10:**646–655.
56. Shefer, S., Hauser, S., Berkersky, I., and Mosbach, E. H., 1970, Biochemical site of regulation of bile acid biosynthesis in the rat, *J. Lipid Res.* **11:**404–411.
57. Bjorkhem, I., Eriksson, M., and Eniarsson, K., 1983, Evidence for a lack of regulatory importance of the 12α-hydroxylase in formation of bile acids in man: An *in vivo* study, *J. Lipid Res.* **24:**1451–1456.
58. Bjorkhem, I., Gustafsson, J., Johansson, G., and Persson, B., 1975, Biosynthesis of bile acids in man, *J. Clin. Invest.* **55:**478.
59. Cronholm, T., and Johansson, G., 1970, Oxidation of 5β-cholestane-3α,7α,12α-triol by rat liver microsomes, *Eur. J. Biochem.* **16:**373.
60. Shefer, S., Chen, F. W., Dayal, B., Hauser, S., Tint, G. S., Salen, G., and Mosbach, E. H., 1975, A 25-hydroxylation pathway of cholic acid biosynthesis in man and rat, *J. Clin. Invest.* **57:**897–903.
61. Bostrom, H., and Wikvall, K., 1982, Hydroylations in biosynthesis of bile acids: Isolation of subfractions with different substrate specificity from cytochrome P-450$_{LM4}$, *J. Biol. Chem.* **257:**11,755–11,759.
62. Kase, F., Bjorkhem, I., and Pedersen, J. I., 1983, Formation of cholic acid from 3α,7α,12α-trihydroxy-5β-cholestanoic acid by rat liver peroxisomes, *J. Lipid Res.* **24:**1560–1567.
63. Pederson, J. I., and Gustafsson, J., 1980, Conversion of 3α,7α,12α-trihydroxy-5β-cholestanoic acid into cholic acid by rat liver peroxisomes, *FEBS Lett.* **121:**345–348.
64. Sanghvi, A., Grassi, E., Warty, V., Diven, W., Wight, C., and Lester, R., 1981, Reversible activation–inactivation of cholesterol 7α-hydroxylase possibly due to phosphorylation–dephosphorylation, *Biochem. Biophys. Res. Commun.* **103:**886–892.
65. Pries, J. M., Gustafson, A., Wiegand, D., and Duane, W. C., 1983, Taurocholate is more potent than cholate in suppression of bile salt synthesis in the rat, *J. Lipid Res.* **24:**141–146.
66. Duane, W. C., 1978, Simulation of the defect of bile acid metabolism associated with cholesterol cholelithiasis by sorbitol ingestion in man, *J. Lab. Clin. Med.* **91:**969–978.
67. Mok, H. Y. I., von Bergmann, K., and Grundy, S. M., 1977, Regulation of pool size of bile acids in man, *Gastroenterology* **73:**684–690.
68. Mok, H. Y. I., von Bergman, L., and Grundy, S. M., 1980, Kinetics of the enterohepatic circulation during fasting: Biliary lipid secretion and gall bladder storage, *Gastroenterology* **78:**1023–1033.
69. Duane, W. C., Gilberstadt, M. L., and Wiegand, D. M., 1979, Diurnal rhythms of bile acid production in the rat, *Am. J. Physiol.* **237:**R175–R179.
70. Duane, W. C., Ginsberg, R. L., and Bennion, L. J., 1976, Effects of fasting on bile acid metabolism and biliary lipid composition in man, *J. Lipid Res.* **17:**211–219.

71. Duane, W. C., Levitt, D. G., Mueller, S. M., and Behrens, J. C., 1983, Regulation of bile acid synthesis in man: Presence of a diurnal rhythm, *J. Clin. Invest.* **72:**1930–1936.

72. Scott, R. B., Strasberg, S. M., El-Sharkawy, T. Y., and Diamant, N. E., 1983, Regulation of the fasting enterohepatic circulation of bile acids by the migrating myoelectric complex in dogs, *J. Clin. Invest.* **71:**644–654.

73. Okishio, T., and Nair, P. P., 1966, Studies on bile acids: Some observations on the intracellular localization of major bile acids in rat liver, *Biochemistry* **5:**3662–3668.

74. Strange, R. C., Beckett, G. J., and Percy-Robb, I. W., 1979, Nuclear and cytosolic distribution of conjugated cholic acid and radiolabelled glycocholic acid in rat liver, *Biochem. J.* **178:**71–78.

75. Hayes, J. D., Strange, R. C., and Percy-Robb, I. W., 1979, Identification of two lithocholic acid-binding proteins: Separation of ligandin from glutathione-S-transferase B, *Biochem J.* **181:**699–708.

76. Strange, R. C., Chapman, B. J., Johnston, J. D., Nimmo, I. A., and Percy-Robb, I. W., 1979, Partitioning of bile acids into subcellular organelles and the *in vivo* distribution of bile acids in rat liver, *Biochim. Biophys. Acta* **573:**535–545.

77. Strange, R. C., Cramb, R., Hayes, J. D., and Percy-Robb, I. W., 1977, Partial purification of two lithocholic acid-binding proteins from rat liver 100,000 *g* supernatants, *Biochem. J.* **165:**425–429.

78. Strange, R. C., Nimmo, I. A., and Percy-Robb, I. W., 1979, Studies in the rat on the hepatic subcellular distribution and biliary excretion of lithocholic acid, *Biochim. Biophys. Acta* **588:**70–80.

79. Strange, R. C., Nimmo, I. A., and Percy-Robb, I. W., 1977, Binding of bile acids by 100,000 *g* supernatants from rat liver, *Biochem. J.* **162:**659–664.

80. Simion, F. A., Fleischer, B., and Fleischer, S., 1983, Subcellular distribution of cholic acids: Coenzyme A ligase and deoxycholic acid activities in rat liver, *Biochemistry* **22:**5029–5034.

81. Vessey, D. A., Whitney, J., and Gollan, J. L., 1983, The role of conjugation reactions in enhancing biliary secretion of bile acids, *Biochem. J.* **214:**923–927.

82. Zouboulis-Vafiadis, I., Dumont, M., and Erlinger, S., 1983, Conjugation is rate limiting in hepatic transport of ursodeoxycholate in the rat, *Am. J. Physiol.* **243:**G208–G213.

83. Gregory, D. H., Vlahcevic, Z. R., Schatzki, P., and Swell, L., 1975, Mechanism of secretion of biliary lipids. I. Role of bile canalicular and microsomal membranes in the synthesis and transport of biliary lecithin and cholesterol, *J. Clin. Invest.* **55:**105–114.

84. Jones, A. L., Schmucker, D. L., Mooney, J. S., Ockner, R. K., and Adler, R. D., 1979, Alterations in hepatic pericanalicular cytoplasm during enhanced bile secretory activity, *Lab. Invest.* **40:**512–517.

85. Goldsmith, M. A., and Huling, S., 1982, Effect of estradiol on hepatocyte handling of horseradish peroxidase and bile salts, *Gastroenterology* **82:**1255A.

86. Suchy, F. J., Balistreri, W. F., Hung, J., Miller, P., and Garfield, S. A., 1983, Intracellular bile acid transport in rat liver as visualized by electron microscope autoradiography using a bile acid analogue, *Am. J. Physiol.* **245:**G681–G689.

87. Chen, E., Gumucio, J. J., and Ho, H., 1984, Hepatocytes of zones 1 and 3 of the liver acinus conjugate BSP with glutathione, *Hepatology* **4:**467–476.

88. Pang, K. S., and Gillette, J. R., 1980, Kinetics of metabolite formation and elimination in the perfused rat liver preparation: Differences between the elimination of preformed acetaminophen and acetaminophen formed from phenacetin, *J. Pharmacol. Exp. Ther.* **207:**178–194.

89. Pang, L. S., and Terrell, J. A., 1981, Retrograde perfusion to probe the heterogeneous distribution of hepatic drug metabolizing enzymes in rats, *J. Pharmacol. Exp. Ther.* **216:**339–346.

90. Suchy, F. J., and Balistreri, W. F., 1982, Uptake of taurocholate in hepatocytes isolated from developing rats, *Pediatr. Res.* **16:**282–285.

91. Klinger, W., 1982, Biotransformation of drugs and other xenobiotics during postnatal development, *Pharmacol. Ther.* **16:**377–429.

92. Lester, R., 1980, Physiologic cholestasis, *Gastroenterology* **78:**864–870.

93. Suchy, F. J., Balistreri, W. F., Heubi, J. E., Searchy, J. E., and Levin, R. S., 1981, Physiologic cholestasis: Elevation of the primary serum bile acid concentrations in normal infants, *Gastroenterology* **80**:1037–1041.

94. Klaassen, C. D., 1978, Independence of bile acid ouabain hepatic uptake: Studies in the new born rat, *Proc. Soc. Exp. Biol. Med.* **157**:66–69.

95. Klaassen, C. D., 1975, Hepatic uptake of cardiac glycosides in new born rats, rabbits and dogs, *Biochem. Pharmacol.* **24**:923–925.

96. Gartner, L. M., Lee, K. S., Vaismans, L., Lane, D., and Zarafu, I., 1977, Development of bilirubin transport and metabolism in the newborn rhesus monkey, *J. Pediatr.* **90**:513–531.

97. Belknap, W. M., Balistreri, W. F., Suchy, F. J., and Miller, P., 1981, Physiologic cholestasis. II. Serum bile acids reflect the development of the enterohepatic circulation in rats, *Hepatology* **1**:613–616.

98. Balistreri, W. F., Heubi, J. E., and Suchy, F. J., 1983, Immaturity of the enterohepatic circulation in early life: Factors predisposing to "physiologic" maldigestion and cholestasis, *J. Pediatr. Gastroenterol. Nutr.* **2**:346–354.

99. Suchy, F. J., Heubi, J. E., Balistreri, W. F., and Belknap, W. M., 1981, The enterohepatic circulation of bile acids in suckling and weaning rats, *Gastroenterology* **80**:1351A.

100. Suchy, F. J., Balistreri, W. F., Shockey, J. R., and Garfield, S. A., 1983, Absence of a hepatic lobular gradient on bile acid uptake in the suckling rat, *Hepatology* **3**:847A.

101. Marshall, A. W., Milhaly, G. W., Smallwood, R. A., Morgan, D. J., and Hardy, K. J., 1981, Fetal hepatic function: The disposition of propranolol in the pregnant sheep, *Res. Commun. Chem. Pathol. Pharmacol.* **32**:3–25.

102. Tatsuji, G. A., and Klaassen, C. D., 1982, Age-related pharmacokinetics of ouabain in rats, *Proc. Soc. Exp. Biol. Med.* **170**:59–62.

103. Sussman, S., Carbone, J. V., Grodsky, G., Hjelte, V., and Miller, P., 1962, Sulfobromophthalein sodium metabolism in newborn infants, *Pediatrics* **29**:899–906.

104. Vest, M. F., 1962, Conjugation of sulfobromophthalein in newborn infants and children, *J. Clin. Invest.* **41**:1013–1020.

105. Yudkin, S., and Bells, S. S., 1949, Liver function in newborn infants with special reference to excretion of bromsulfophthalein, *Arch. Dis. Child.* **24**:12–14.

106. Oppe, T. E., and Gibbs, I. E., 1959, Sulfobromophthalein excretion in premature infants, *Arch. Dis. Child.* **34**:125–130.

107. Heimann, G., Roth, B., and Gladtke, E., 1977, Indocyanin-Grün-Kinetik beim Neugeborenen mit transitorischen Hyperbilirubinämie, *Klin. Wochenschr.* **55**:451–456.

108. Roth, B., Statz, A., Heinisch, H. M., and Gladtke, E., 1981, Elimination of indocyanine green by the liver of infants with hypertrophic pyloric stenosis and the icteropyloric syndrome, *J. Pediatr.* **99**:240–243.

109. Barbara, L., Lazzavi, R., Roda, A., Adlini, R., Festi, D., Sama, C., Morselli, A. M., Collina, A., Bazzoli, F., Mazzella, G., and Roda, E., 1980, Serum bile acids in newborns and children, *Pediatr. Res.* **14**:1222–1225.

110. Itoh, S., Onishi, S., Isobe, K., Manabe, M., and Inukai, K., 1982, Foetal maternal relationships of bile acid pattern estimated by high-pressure liquid chromatography, *Biochem. J.* **204**:1411–1415.

111. Lambiotte, M., Vorbrodt, A., and Benedetti, E. L., 1973, Expression of differentiation of rat foetal hepatocytes in cellular culture under the action of glucocorticoids: Appearance of bile canaliculi, *Cell. Differ.* **2**:43–53.

112. Little, J. M., Richey, J. E., Van Thiel, D. H., and Lester, R., 1979, Taurocholate pool size and distribution in the fetal rat, *J. Clin. Invest.* **63**:1042–1049.

113. Subbiah, M. T. R., Marai, L., Dinh, D. M., and Penner, J. W., 1977, Sterol and bile acid metabolism during development. 1. Studies on the gallbladder and intestinal bile acids of newborn and fetal rabbit, *Steroids* **29**:83–92.

114. Li, J. R., Dinh, D. M., Ellefsson, R. D., and Subbiah, M. T. R., 1979, Sterol and bile acid metabolism during development. 3. Occurrence of neonatal hypercholesterolemia in guinea pig and its possible relation to bile acid pool, *Metabolism* **28**:151–156.
115. Li, J. R., Subbiah, M. T. R., and Kottke, B. A., 1979, Hepatic 3-hydroxyl-3-methylglutaryl coenzyme A reductase activity and cholesterol 7α-hydroxylase activity in neonatal guinea pig, *Steroids* **34**:47–55.
116. Naseem, S. M., Kahn, M. A., Heald, F. P., and Nair, P. P., 1980, The influence of cholesterol and fat in maternal diet of rats on the development of hepatic cholesterol metabolism in the offspring, *Atherosclerosis* **36**:1–8.
117. Subbiah, M. T. R., and Hassan, A. S., 1982, Development of bile acid biogenesis and its significance in cholesterol homeostasis, *Adv. Lipid Res.* **19**:137–161.
118. Sugiyama, Y., Yamada, T., and Kaplowitz, N., 1982, Newly identified organic anion-binding proteins in rat liver cytosol, *Biochim. Biophys. Acta* **709**:342–352.
119. Balistreri, W. F., Zimmer, L., Suchy, F. J., and Bove, K. E., Bile salt sulfotransferase: Alterations during maturation and non-inducibility during substrate ingestion, *J. Lipid Res.* **25**:228–235.
120. Blovin, A., Bolender, R. P., and Weibel, E. R., Distribution of organelles and membranes between hepatocytes and nonhepatocytes in the rat liver parenchyma, *J. Cell Biol.* **72**:441–455.
121. Greengard, O., Federman, M., and Knox, W. E., 1972, Cytomorphometry of developing rat liver and its application to enzyme differentiation, *J. Cell Biol.* **52**:261–272.
122. Rohr, H. P., Wirz, A., Henning, L. C., Riede, U. N., and Biandi, L., 1971, Morphometric analysis of the rat liver cell in the perinatal period, *Lab. Invest.* **24**:128–139.
123. Daimon, T., David, H., Zglinicki, T. V., and Marx, E., 1982, Correlated ultrastructural and morphometric studies on the liver during perinatal development of rats, *Exp. Pathol.* **21**:237–250.
124. Miller, D. L., Zanolli, C. S., and Gumucio, J. J., 1979, Quantitative morphology of the sinusoids of the hepatic acinus, *Gastroenterology* **76**:965–969.
125. Gumucio, J. J., 1983, Functional and anatomical heterogeneity in the liver acinus: Impact on transport, *Am. J. Physiol.* **244**:G578–G582.
126. Sunaryo, F. P., Watkins, J. B., and Ling, S., 1982, Neonatal hepatic function: Changes in vascular volume of distribution influence bile acid uptake, *Gastroenterology* **82**:1247A.
127. Gumucio, J. J., Balabaud, C., Miller, D. L., Demason, L. J., Appleman, H. D., Stoecker, T. J., and Franzblau, D. R., 1978, Bile secretion and liver cell heterogeneity in the rat, *J. Lab. Clin. Med.* **91**:350–362.
128. Groothuis, G. M. M., Keulemans, K. P. T., Hardonk, M. J., and Meijer, D. K. F., 1983, Acinar heterogeneity in hepatic transport of dibromosulfophthalein and ouabain studied by autoradiography, normal and retrograde perfusions and computer simulation, *Biochem. Pharmacol.* **32**:3069–3078.
129. Suchy, F. J., Bueler, R. L., and Blitzer, B. L., 1983, Impaired taurocholate uptake by liver plasma membrane vesicles isolated from suckling rats, *Gastroenterology* **84**:1399A.
130. Blitzer, B. L., and Lyons, L., 1983, Direct demonstration of enhancement of taurocholate uptake by albumin in basolateral liver plasma membrane vesicles, *Hepatology* **3**:850A.
131. Blitzer, B. L., Ratoosh, S. L., and Donovan, C. B., 1983, Amino acid inhibition of bile acid uptake by isolated rat hepatocytes: Relationship to dissipation of the transmembrane Na^+ gradient, *Am. J. Physiol.* **245**:G399–G403.
132. DeWolf-Peeters, C., DeVos, R., and Desmet, V., 1971, Histochemical evidence of a cholestatic period in neonatal rats, *Pediatr. Res.* **5**:704–709.
133. DeWolf-Peeters, C., DeVos, R., and Desmet, V., 1977, Electron microscopy and histochemistry of canalicular differentiation in fetal and neonatal rat liver, *Tissue Cell* **4**:379–388.
134. Miyairi, M., and Phillips, M. J., 1982, Motility behavior of isolated fetal rat hepatocytes in culture, *Hepatology* **2**:706A.

135. Blitzer, B. L., and Boyer, J. L., 1982, Cellular mechanisms of bile formation, *Gastroenterology* **82:**346–357.

136. Hardison, W. G. M., Hatoff, D. E., Miyai, K., and Weiner, R. G., 1981, Nature of bile acid maximum secretory rate in the rat, *Am. J. Physiol.* **241:**G337–G343.

137. Hwang, S. W., and Dixon, R. L., 1973, Perinatal development of indocyanine green biliary excretion in guinea pigs, *Am. J. Physiol.* **225:**1454–1459.

138. Klaassen, C. D., 1975, Hepatic excretory function in the neborn rat, *J. Pharmacol. Exp. Ther.* **184:**721–728.

139. Varga, F., and Fischer, E., Age dependent changes in blood supply of the liver and in the biliary excretion of eosine in rats, in: *Liver and Aging* (K. Kitami, ed.), pp. 327–340, Elsevier, Amsterdam.

140. Fischer, E., Barth, A., Varga, F., and Klinger, W., 1979, Age-dependence of transport in control and phenobarbital pretreated rats, *Life Sci.* **24:**557–562.

141. Meijer, P. J., and Boyer, J. L., 1983, The electrical membrane potential in a driving force for taurocholate (TC) excretion into bile canaliculi, *Hepatology* **3:**860(A-250).

142. Salen, G., and Shefer, S., 1983, Bile acid synthesis, *Annu. Rev. Physiol.* **45:**679–685.

IV

Induction of Liver Cell Heterogeneity

Chapter 16

Zonal Signal Heterogeneity and Induction of Hepatocyte Heterogeneity

Kurt Jungermann

1. INTRODUCTION

Hepatocytes in the periportal (afferent) and perivenous (efferent) zones of the liver parenchyma differ in their enzyme activities and subcellular structures. This heterogeneity has been known for many years, first on a descriptive[1,2], and then increasingly on a functional level.[3–5]. On the assumption that the distribution of a key enzyme indicates the predominant localization of the corresponding metabolic function, the model of "metabolic zonation" was proposed[6] and developed (Table I). The available evidence indicates that the different metabolic *capacities* of the two zones are indeed reflected as different metabolic rates or *activities* (see Chapters 9–15).

All hepatocytes have, of course, the same genome. Its heterogeneous expression is most likely due to zonal differences in (1) the signals that control cellular functions such as oxygen, substrate, and hormone concentrations and cellular innervation and (2) the signal transmission via ecto- or intracellular receptors. This chapter first summarizes the present knowledge of the zonal heterogeneity of signals and signal transmission and then reviews how zonal changes of major signals influence the induction of key enzymes.

KURT JUNGERMANN • Institut für Biochemie, Universität Göttingen, D-3400 Göttingen, Federal Republic of Germany.

Table I. Model of Metabolic Zonation of Liver Parenchyma[a]

Periportal zone	Perivenous zone
Glucose release	Glucose uptake
Glyconeogenesis	Glycolysis
Glycogen synthesis	Glycogen synthesis
from lactate	from glucose
Glycogen degradation	Glycogen
from glucose	degradation
	to lactate
Oxidative energy metabolism	Liponeogenesis
Fatty acid oxidation	
Citrate cycle	
Respiratory chain	
Amino acid utilization	
Amino acid conversion to glucose	
Amino acid degradation	
Ureagenesis from amino acid nitrogen	

NH₃ detoxification

Urea formation	Glutamine formation
Oxidation protection	Biotransformation
Cholic acid excretion	
Bilirubin excretion	

[a] The table indicates predominant localization of major functions as indicated by the zonal distribution of key enzymes.[3-5]

2. ZONAL HETEROGENEITY OF SIGNALS AND SIGNAL TRANSMISSION

During the passage of blood through the liver acinus, concentration gradients of substrates and hormones are established. The autonomic innervation and the hormone receptors of the periportal and perivenous zone may be different.

2.1. Oxygen

The liver is supplied by a varying mixture of arterial and portovenous blood, normally 25% : 75%[7] (See Chapter 2). The oxygen tension corresponding to the free oxygen concentration is 95 mm Hg = 135 μmoles/liter in arteries, 40 mm Hg = 57 μmoles/liter in large veins, 45–55 mm Hg = 65–78 μmoles/liter in the portal vein, and 30–35 mm Hg = 43–50 μmoles/liter in the hepatic vein.[7,8]. Thus, the O_2 tension falls from about 65 mm Hg in *periportal* areas, which is mixed arterial and portal blood, to about 35 mm Hg in *perivenous*, i.e., hepatovenous blood. The oxygen gradient, then, is about 2-fold across the liver lobule.

2.2. Carbon Substrates

2.2.1. Glucose and Lactate

Depending on the metabolic situation, glucose and lactate are taken up or released by the liver. Thus, decreasing or increasing periportal-to-perivenous concentration gradients are established[9–13]; during a normal feeding cycle, they will hardly exceed 25% (Table II). Although glucose can induce enzymes in the absence of hormones (e.g., insulin), such as the "perivenous" ATP-dependent citrate lyase[14] and acetyl-CoA carboxylase,[15] the importance of the small glucose gradients for the heterogeneous induction of enzymes in the liver parenchyma is probably small.

2.2.2. Amino Acids and Ammonia

The liver is the main organ of amino acid metabolism. During a normal feeding cycle with the usual carbohydrate-rich food, it extracts amino acids from the portal blood, creating a decreasing periportal-to-perivenous gradient between 20 and 60%[12,13,16,17] (Table II). Depending on the situation (see Chapter 11), the organ takes up or releases glutamine so that positive or negative gradients do not normally exceed 30% (Table II). It is not known whether these gradients are involved in heterogeneous acinar gene expression; however, the possibility seems unlikely in view of the fact that amino acids are taken up by hepatocytes via active transport processes so that the intracellular concentrations will not necessarily reflect the extracellular levels. The liver detoxifies portal NH_3 coming from the intestine by synthesizing urea; a steep, almost 10-fold periportal-to-perivenous gradient exists for NH_3, but the regulatory importance of this gradient for gene expression has not been assessed[16] (Table II).

2.2.3. Fatty Acids, Glycerol, and Ketone Bodies

The liver takes up fatty acids for energy and ketone body production and glycerol for reesterification and gluconeogenesis. During normal feeding, periportal-to-perivenous gradients of 50–100% for glycerol, of 50% for free fatty acids, and of 50% for acetate are established. The gradient for propionate or butyrate is more than 10-fold[13] (Table II). Since the liver synthesizes ketone bodies, conversely, perivenous-to-periportal gradients on the order of 55–130% are established[13] (Table II). It is not known, however, whether these gradients are of regulatory significance for the control of gene expression.

2.2.4. Miscellaneous Substrates

Of the large number of substrates exchanged by the liver, the bile acids and their conjugates should be given special attention because they are extracted

Table II. Substrate Concentrations in Portal and Hepatovenous Blood of Rats in Different Metabolic States

Substrate	Metabolic state[a]	Blood concentration (mmoles/liter)		Portal/hepatovenous ratio[b]	Ref. Nos.
		Portal	Hepatovenous		
Glucose	Eating	9.5 (10.2)[g]	7.2 (8.9)	1.32 (1.15)	9 (12)
	Fed	5.9 (6.2)	6.0 (6.3)	0.98 (0.98)	11 (13)
	Fasted	5.0 (4.5, 4.6)	5.5 (5.3, 5.5)	0.91 (0.85, 0.84)	
Lactate	Eating	1.8 —	2.1 —	0.86 —	[c]
	Fed	2.1 (1.7)	1.8 (1.4)	1.17 (1.21)	[c](13)
	Fasted	1.3 (1.2)	0.8 (0.5)	1.63 (2.40)	[c](13)
Amino acids					
Alanine	Eating	0.59 (1.14, 1.29)	0.35 (0.87, 0.85)	1.69 (1.31, 1.52)	[c](12, 16)
	Eating PR	1.34 (2.09)	0.79 (0.87)	1.69 (2.40)	17 (16)
	Fed	0.44 (0.78)	0.35 (0.45)	1.25 (1.73)	[c](13)
	Fasted	0.29 (0.38, 0.48)	0.13 (0.23, 0.19)	2.23 (1.65, 2.52)	[c](12, 13)
Serine	Eating	0.21 (0.41, 0.47)	0.15 (0.36, 0.38)	1.40 (1.14, 1.24)	[c](12, 16)
	Eating PR	0.47 (0.90)	0.25 (0.37)	1.88 (2.43)	[c]17 (16)
	Fed	0.14 —	0.12 —	1.17 —	[c]
	Fasted	0.19 (0.29)	0.12 (0.22)	1.58 (1.32)	[c](12)
Threonine	Eating	0.18 (0.50, 0.57)	0.14 (0.47, 0.51)	1.29 (1.06, 1.12)	[c](12, 16)
	Eating PR	0.52 (0.94)	0.38 (0.51)	1.37 (1.84)	[c]17 (16)
	Fed	0.23 —	0.14 —	1.64 —	[c]
	Fasted	0.16 (0.31)	0.14 (0.29)	1.14 (1.07)	[c](12)
Glycine	Eating	0.39 (0.26, 0.29)	0.24 (0.20, 0.20)	1.63 (1.30, 1.45)	[c](12, 16)
	Eating PR	0.29 (0.48)	0.12 (0.18)	2.42 (2.67)	[c]17 (16)
	Fed	0.41 —	0.25 —	1.64 —	[c]
	Fasted	0.40 (0.30)	0.39 (0.25)	1.02 (1.20)	[c](12)
Lysine	Eating	0.24 (0.85)	0.19 (0.75)	1.26 (1.17)	[c](16)
	Eating PR	0.75 (1.58)	0.50 (1.04)	1.50 (1.51)	17 (16)
	Fed	0.20 —	0.21 —	0.95 —	[c]
	Fasted	0.29 —	0.27 —	1.07 —	[c]
Glutamine	Eating	0.46 (0.60)	0.57 (0.70)	0.80 (0.86)	[c] (16)
	Eating PR	0.67 (1.11)	0.48 (0.67)	1.39 (1.66)	17 (16)
	Fed	0.50 (0.55)	0.39 (0.56)	1.28 (0.98)	[c](13)
	Fasted	0.51 (0.51)	0.83 (0.65)	0.61 (0.78)	[c](13)
Ammonia	Eating	0.12 —	0.02 —	6 —	16
	Eating PR	0.22 —	0.02 —	11 —	16
Glycerol	Eating	0.35 —	0.16 —	2.19 —	[c]
	Fed	0.29 —	0.19 —	1.52 —	[c]
	Fasted	0.28 —	0.10 —	2.80 —	[c]
Free fatty acids	Fed	0.38 —	0.25 —	1.52 —	13
	Fasted	0.92 —	0.45 —	2.04 —	13
Acetate	Fed	0.74 —	0.40 —	1.85 —	13
	Fasted	0.30 —	0.24 —	1.25 —	13
Propionate	Fed	0.24 —	0.01 —	24 —	13
	Fasted	0.09 —	0.01 —	9 —	13

(Continued)

Table II. (*Continued*)

Substrate	Metabolic state[a]	Blood concentration (mmoles/liter)		Portal/hepatovenous ratio[b]	Ref. Nos.
		Portal	Hepatovenous		
Butyrate	Fed	0.15 —	0.01 —	15 —	13
	Fasted	0.04 —	0.01 —	4 —	13
Acetoacetate	Fed	0.05 —	0.09 —	0.56 —	13
	Fasted	0.42 —	0.99 —	0.42 —	13
β-Hydrozybutyrate	Fed	0.10 —	0.16 —	0.63 —	13
	Fasted	0.62 —	1.05 —	0.59 —	13
		(μmoles/liter)			
Cholate[d]	Fed	48 —	— —	— —	19
	Fasted	150[e] —	2[f] —	— —	20
Chenodeoxycholate[d]	Fed	4 —	— —	— —	19
	Fasted	1[e] —	0.02[f] —	— —	20
Deoxycholate[d]	Fed	4 —	— —	— —	19
	Fasted	30[e] —	0.5[f] —	— —	20

[a] Eating: 5–8 hr after a normal carbohydrate-rich but protein-containing (15%) meal; Eating PR: 2–4 hr after a protein-rich (30–50%) meal; Fed: 1–3 hr after withdrawal of food; Fasted: 24 or 48 hr after withdrawal of food.
[b] Values >1 = uptake, <1 = release.
[c] Balks and Jungermann (unpublished).
[d] Total equals conjugated and unconjugated, on average 85 and 15%, respectively.
[e] Values may be too high due to sampling technique (see Chronholm and Nair[19]).
[f] Peripheral, not hepatovenous.
[g] Values in parentheses are those published in references in parentheses.

almost completely during one pass through the liver,[18–20] so that steep concentration gradients are created (Table II).

2.3. Hormones

Hormones such as insulin, glucagon, catecholamines, and corticosteroids are degraded during passage through the liver, so that hormone concentration gradients decreasing from the periportal to the perivenous area are formed. Conversely, the liver might release regulatory molecules or mediators such as adenosine so that concentration gradients increasing from the periportal to the perivenous zone are established. If the rate of degradation or release is different for the single hormones or mediators, the hormone/mediator ratio changes from the afferent to the efferent area. Thus, it is clear that depending on the metabolic situation, the combination of signals in the periportal zone might be quite different from that in the perivenous zone.

2.3.1. Insulin and Glucagon

The degradation of insulin and glucagon by the liver was studied in the rat during a normal 24-hr feeding cycle (Fig. 1). The hormone concentrations were measured in portal and hepatovenous blood.[9] The removal of insulin and glucagon by the liver was not constant, but was regulated independently. At the end of the daily fasting period, 52% of portal insulin was removed during a single pass, while only 19% was extracted in the middle of the eating phase at night. The variation in the hepatic removal of glucagon was much smaller than, and not in phase with, that of insulin. Thus, during meals, the perivenous zone, compared to the periportal zone, received a higher insulin/glucagon signal favoring glucose utilization via both short- and long-term regulation. During fasting a lower insulin/glucagon signal exists, leading to sparing of glucose (Fig. 1).

The results cited above are in agreement with the finding that in a perfused pancreas–liver preparation of the rat, the degradation of endogenous insulin was almost zero in the fed and 45% in the fasted state.[21] Also, the hepatic extraction of insulin in dog and man appears to be diminished after the ingestion of food (references in Balks and Jungermann[9]).

2.3.2. Adrenaline and Noradrenaline

The hepatic removal of noradrenaline was studied in fasted dogs[22]; 85% of the portal concentration was removed during a single pass. Catecholamine degradation was also investigated in the perfused rat liver (Beckh, Balks, and Jungermann, unpublished) (Fig. 2). Livers of fed animals removed 80% of adrenaline and 50% of noradrenaline, while livers of fasted animals removed 50% of each catecholamine. Again, the perivenous zone receives quite a different concentration of catecholamines than the periportal zone. Since insulin, on one hand, and

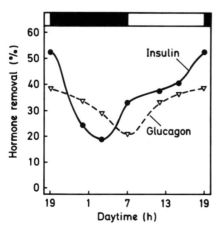

Figure 1. Dynamics of the extraction of insulin and glucagon by rat livers in a single pass *in vivo*. The hormone concentration was measured with standard radioimmunoassays in portal and hepatovenous blood taken from pentobarbital-anesthetized rats during a normal feeding rhythm. The dark period (access to food) is indicated by the black bar. The percentage "portal" extraction, as given by (portal − hepatovenous concentration) × 100/(portal concentration), is shown. These values should be regarded as a first approximation of the "overall" extraction, which occurs from a mixture, in general 3 : 1, of portal and arterial blood. For all pancreatic hormones, the percentage "overall" extraction is therefore smaller than the "portal" extraction shown. Data are from Balks and Jungermann.[9]

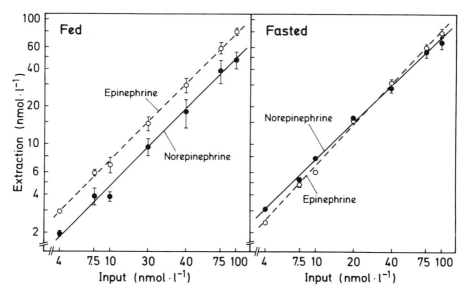

Figure 2. Extraction of adrenaline and noradrenaline by the perfused livers of fed and fasted rats in a single passage. Livers were perfused with Krebs–Henseleit–bicarbonate buffer containing erythrocytes (hematocrit 25%), 5 mM glucose, and 2 mM lactate equilibrated with 13% (vol./vol.) oxygen without recirculation. Catecholamine concentrations were quantitated radiochemically[23] after enzymatic methylation with S-[^{3}H]adenosylmethionine, conversion to [^{3}H]metanephrine, and separation by thin-layer chromatography. Extraction is the difference between the influent and effluent concentrations. Data are from Beckh, Balks, and Jungermann (unpublished results).

glucagon plus catecholamines, on the other, are in general antagonists, the perivenous zone is under control of a much higher insulin/(glucagon + adrenaline + noradrenaline) ratio than the periportal zone. This should favor glucose utilization in the perivenous area in accord with the model of metabolic zonation with regard not only to short-term but also to long-term effects.

2.3.3. Miscellaneous Hormones and Mediators

Hormones other than insulin, glucagon, and catecholamines are also removed during a single pass through the liver. Hepatic extraction of glucocorticoids is about 40–50% in dog and sheep,[24,25] yet only about 10% in guinea pig and man[26,27]; cortisone extraction appears to be higher than 90%. The percentage removal of corticosterone, which is the glucocorticoid of rats, is not known. In man, removal of the mineralocorticoid aldosterone exceeds 90%.[27,28] In addition, with testosterone, estradiol, thyroxine, or gastrointestinal factors, the perivenous zone receives a "lower" signal than the periportal zone. Yet the perivenous zone receives a "higher" signal from adenosine. The adenosine concentration in the hepatic vein was found to be 10-fold higher than levels in the portal vein.[29] Adenosine can function as an inhibitor of adenylate cyclase, as an antagonist of sympathetic nerve action, and as a synergist of insulin effects.[30–32] Thus, adenosine release by the liver can be expected to further increase the prevalence of insulin over its antagonists glucagon and catecholamines in the perivenous zone. The normalized (insulin + adenosine)/(glucagon + adrenaline + noradrenaline) ratio is increased in the fed state from 0.37 in the periportal to 1.15 in the perivenous zone (Fig. 3).

    In conclusion, there can be no doubt that periportal hepatocytes in general receive quite different hormonal signals than those in the perivenous zone (Fig. 3). This signal heterogeneity could provide the basis via long-term induction effects for the zonal heterogeneity of enzymes and subcellular structures, i.e., of the metabolic capacities, and via short-term effects for independent modulation of the different zonal capacities.

2.4. Nerves

    The autonomic innervation of the periportal and perivenous zones may be different and thus contribute via trophic effects to the induction of metabolic zonation. In rat and mouse, sympathetic nerves appear to reach only the outer periportal cells, from which a signal might be propagated through gap junctions via electronic coupling; in guinea pig, rabbit, cat, dog, and man, almost all hepatocytes exhibit nerve contacts.[33–36]

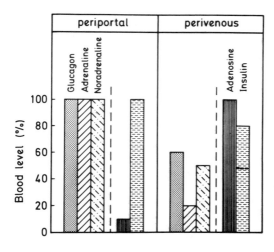

Figure 3. Zonal signal heterogeneity. The higher hormone concentration, in either the portal or the hepatic vein, was set equal to 100%. Data are from fed animals, except that for insulin, which is from eating animals; the value for fed animals is indicated additionally by the dashed line within the bar. Since glucagon and the catecholamines are antagonists of insulin and adenosine, a normalized ratio was calculated using the percentage levels in the two zones: (insulin + adenosine)/(glucagon + adrenaline + noradrenaline). This ratio in the fed state amounts to (100 + 10)/(100 + 100 + 100) = 0.37 in the periportal zone and to (50 + 100)/(60 + 20 + 50) = 1.15 in the perivenous zone. References are given in the text.

2.5. Hormone Receptors

The zonal distribution of the ectocellular receptors for insulin, glucagon, and catecholamines or of the intracellular receptors for glucocorticoids is not known. It is feasible that periportal cells have a lower and perivenous cells a higher density of, for example, insulin receptors due to down-regulation. The distribution of the adenylate cyclase system has recently been studied[37]; it was found that in the fed state, the basal and glucagon-, NaF-, and forskolin-stimulated activities were equally distributed in the two zones, while in the fasted state, the glucagon-stimulated activities showed a gradient with higher levels in the perivenous zone (Fig. 4). Due to the lack of sufficient data, the possible role of heterogeneous distribution of hormone receptors in zonal hepatocyte heterogeneity cannot be assessed at present.

3. INDUCTION OF HEPATOCELLULAR HETEROGENEITY

The effects of oxygen and hormone gradients on enzyme induction have been studied directly in hepatocyte culture, and the actions of the nervous system indirectly *in vivo*. Indirect information is also available from the dynamic nature

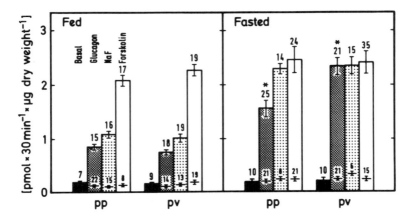

Figure 4.   Distribution of adenylate cyclase activity in periportal and perivenous liver tissue of fed and fasted rats. The activity was measured in microdissected periportal (pp) and perivenous (pv) areas. Only about 60% of the tissue samples could be stimulated by the effectors indicated; the remaining 40% did not respond. The difference between responsive and nonresponsive samples is probably not due to an artifact. Columns represent means ± S.E.M. of basal and glucagon-, NaF-, and forskolin-stimulated activities in responsive samples. Bars within the columns give means ± S.E.M. of samples nonresponsive toward the stimulating agent. The number of determinations is given at the tops of the columns. The periportal and perivenous values were compared by Student's *t* test; $p < 0.01$ for the glucagon-stimulated activities in fasted rats. Data are from Zierz and Jungermann.[37]

of zonal enzyme heterogeneity; the zonation changes on longer-lasting alterations of the metabolic situation which are accompanied by changes in the hormonal or nervous system.

3.1. Modulation of Enzyme Induction by Oxygen

The influence of oxygen on the induction of enzymes was studied using primary cultures of rat hepatocytes. The hepatic oxygen supply via the hepatic artery and the portal vein was mimicked using experimental gas atmospheres with up to 20% (vol./vol.) oxygen, 13% (vol/vol) first approximation to arterial and 6% (vol/vol) to venous concentrations.

3.1.1. Glucagon-Dependent Induction of Phosphoenolpyruvate Carboxykinase and Tyrosine Aminotransferase

In hepatocyte cultures, the activities of the "periportal" enzymes phosphoenolpyruvate carboxykinase (PEPCK) and tyrosine aminotransferase (TAT) were increased by glucagon within 4 hr to higher levels under 13% O_2 than under 6% O_2[38] (Fig.5). Enzyme induction showed a sigmoidal rather than a linear dependence on oxygen. The range of highest sensitivity was between 8 and 11% O_2. Half-maximal induction was obtained with less than 10% O_2 in the gas phase, which corresponds to about 70 mm Hg at the medium surface and, due to the concentration gradient required for diffusion from the medium surface to the cell, to about 50 mm Hg at the cell surface. This concentration lies in the middle of the physiological range of blood levels during passage through the liver. Oxygen ranges from 65 mm Hg in the periportal zone to 35 mm Hg in the perivenous zone. It is very probable that the oxygen dependence of PEPCK and TAT induction is specific and does not reflect a general impairment of energy metabolism, since adenine nucleotides, energy charge, oxygen consumption, and leucine incorporation into cellular protein were not significantly different in hepatocytes cultured under either 6 or 13% O_2.[38]

3.1.2. Insulin-Dependent Induction of Glucokinase and Pyruvate Kinase

Culturing hepatocytes for 48 hr under different physiological oxygen concentrations resulted in different levels of key glycolytic enzymes.[63] Cells cultured under hepatovenous O_2 tensions with insulin as the major hormone displayed 35% higher activities of glucokinase and pyruvate kinase than cells maintained under arterial tensions. The differences in enzyme levels led to differences in metabolic rates. Glycolysis was almost 3-fold higher in cells cultured under hepatovenous O_2 tensions, while gluconeogenesis was increased by about 1.4-fold in cells maintained under arterial O_2 concentrations.

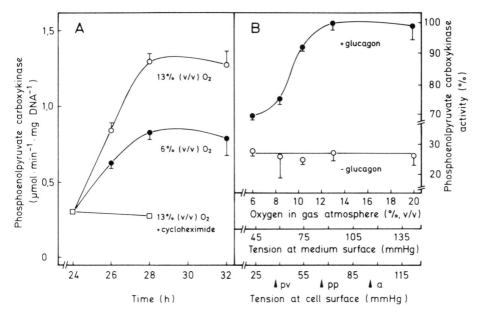

Figure 5. Induction of phosphoenolpyruvate carboxykinase in primary cultures of rat hepatocytes by glucagon under a gas atmosphere with different oxygen tensions.[38] Liver parenchymal cells were cultured under standard conditions in the presence of insulin (1 nM) and dexamethasone (10 nM) under 13% (vol./vol.) O_2. At 4 and 24 hr after plating, the medium was changed. At 24 hr, glucagon (100 nM) and, where indicated, cycloheximide (10 µg/ml) were added, and the culture was continued under different oxygen tensions. Enzyme activity was measured at the time points indicated (A) or at 28 hr (B). The oxygen concentration difference between medium surface and cell surface is required for the diffusion of the gas. The perivenous (pv) situation is mimicked approximately by 8% (vol./vol.) $O_2 \approx 35$ mm Hg ≈ 50 µmoles/liter at the cell surface; the periportal (pp) situation, by 12% (vol./vol.) $O_2 \approx 65$ mm Hg ≈ 90 µmoles/liter at the cell surface; the arterial (a) situation, by 16% (vol./vol.) $O_2 \approx 95$ mm Hg ≈ 130 µmoles/liter at the cell surface.[38] Values are means ± S.E.M. of 6 cultures from two representative experiments.

Thus, the opposite long-term effects of oxygen on the levels of gluconeo-genic and glycolytic enzymes and metabolic rates are consistent with the hypothesis that oxygen is involved in the regulation of gene expression and thus in the induction of parenchymal zonation.

3.2. Insulin–Glucagon Antagonism in Enzyme Induction

Hormones such as insulin, glucagon, catecholamines, and corticosteroids are degraded during passage through the liver (cf. Section 2.3), so that a concentration gradient decreasing from a periportal to the perivenous areas is formed for each hormone. This gradient would offer a ready explanation for the preferential induction of enzymes in the periportal but not in the perivenous zone. Predominant induction in the perivenous zone can be explained only if the antagonism between two hormones or signals rather than one hormone or signal governs gene expression and if the ratio of these two antagonistic signals changes such that the agonist for the "perivenous" enzyme is increased during liver passage relative to the antagonist. Insulin and glucagon are such antagonists in the induction of "perivenous" glucokinase by insulin and of "periportal" PEPCK by glucagon.

3.2.1. Insulin-Dependent Induction of Glucokinase

In hepatocyte cultures, glucokinase is induced by insulin under the permissive action of glucocorticoids, which is inhibited strongly by glucagon[39] (Fig. 6). The higher level of the enzyme in the perivenous area could be effected by an increase of the insulin/glucagon ratio during passage of blood through the liver. This has indeed been observed in the rat under certain conditions (cf. Section 2.3 and Fig. 3). However, the antagonism between the two hormones has been observed with unphysiological concentrations; the question whether it is also effective *in vivo* must therefore remain open.

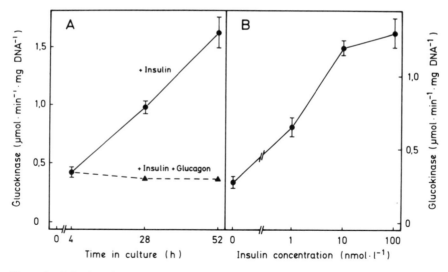

Figure 6. Induction of glucokinase in primary cultures of rat hepatocytes by insulin in the presence of dexamethasone.[39] Liver parenchymal cells were cultured under standard conditions as described in the caption Fig. 5 caption. At 4 and 28 hr after plating, the medium was changed. Insulin (100 nM) with or without glucagon (200 nM) (A) or insulin at the concentrations indicated (B) was added with each medium change. Enzyme activity was measured at the time points indicated (A) or at 52 hr (B). Values are means ± S.E.M. of 6 cultures from two representative experiments.

3.2.2. Glucagon-Dependent Induction of Phosphoenolpyruvate Carboxykinase

The glucagon–insulin antagonism was studied in more detail with the induction of PEPCK and its modulation by glucocorticoids in hepatocyte cultures.[40] In cells cultured with dexamethasone, the antagonism between the hormones was pronounced at physiological hormone concentrations (Fig. 7A). When both hormones were present in equimolar concentrations, they became equally powerful antagonists in the low physiological concentration range between 0.01 and 0.1 nM (Fig. 7C). At high equimolar doses, glucagon became the dominant hormone. The glucagon–insulin antagonism was modulated by glucocorticoids (Fig. 7B). Omission of dexamethasone from the culture shifted the effective insulin and glucagon doses into a high, unphysiological concentration range. Dexamethasone therefore acted to sensitize the cell to low levels of glucagon and insulin.

These results indicate that the glucagon–insulin antagonism should also be operative *in vivo* and that besides other factors, a change in the insulin/glucagon gradient during liver passage (cf. Section 2.3 and Fig. 3) should be involved in differential acinar gene expression. This conclusion is corroborated by the findings that after 48 hr in culture with glucagon as the major hormone, hepatocytes possessed gluconeogenic and glycolytic enzyme activities that to a first approximation were similar to those of periportal cells *in vivo,* and, conversely, that

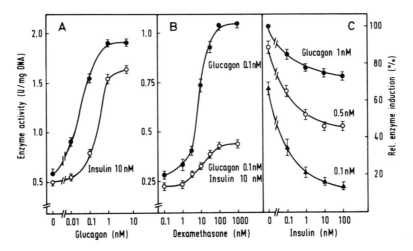

Figure 7.   Induction of phosphoenolypyruvate carboxykinase by glucagon. The graphs indicate the antagonistic action of insulin and the permissive effect of dexamethasone. Cells were cultured for 24 hr with 0.5 nM insulin and with either 0.1 μM dexamethasone (A, C) or different dexamethasone concentrations as shown (B). Glucagon ± insulin was added at 24 hr, and enzyme activity was measured at 28 hr. Relative enzyme induction (C) from 0 to 100% corresponds to uninduced and fully induced enzyme activity (0.6–1.9 U/mg DNA). Values are means ± S.E.M. of 9 dishes from three different cell preparations for each panel. For details, see Probst and Jungermann.[40]

with insulin as the major hormone, the cells had an enzyme content resembling that of perivenous cells.[41] Hepatocytes cultured for 48 hr appeared to be homogeneous in their enzyme content in contrast to cells cultured for 1 hr,[42] which were heterogeneous and thus mirrored the heterogeneity *in vivo* directly (Fig. 8).

3.3. Role of the Hepatic Nerves in Enzyme Induction

The nervous system in general has been shown to exert trophic effects.[43] It is therefore feasible that the hepatic nerves (cf. Section 2.4) are involved in enzyme induction and that a possible heterogeneous innervation of the parenchymal zones contributes to zonal hepatocyte heterogeneity. Electrical stimulation of the ventromedial hypothalamus and thus of the sympathetic system led after 4 hr to an increase of PEPCK and to a decrease of pyruvate kinase (PK) activity, while stimulation of the lateral hypothalamus and the parasympathetic system resulted in a decrease of PEPCK without a change of PK activity.[44] These studies, however, do not allow one to distinguish whether the nervous system acted directly or indirectly, e.g., via the release of glucagon from the pancreas or of epinephrine/norepinephrine from the adrenals.

The induction of PEPCK by sympathetic agents was studied in cell culture.[45] It was found that epinephrine and norepinephrine induced the enzyme via β-receptors. Induction by catecholamines was different in its concentration dependence. With epinephrine, induction was possible with concentrations that just reached the physiological range of blood levels[46]; with norepinephrine, induction could be effected only by concentrations that were far outside that range. These findings may indicate that epinephrine could act as a circulating hormone, while norepinephrine may operate as a neurotransmitter, since in a synapse, neurotransmitter concentrations in the range of $0.1-1$ mM seem to be necessary.[47] Although the findings on enzyme induction after hypothalamic stimulation and in cell culture are suggestive, convincing evidence for a long-term direct neural control of gene expression in liver is still lacking.

3.4. Dynamics of Zonal Hepatocyte Heterogeneity

Zonal heterogeneity is dynamic or functional, rather than static or structural. Zonation may change on longer-lasting changes of the metabolic situation or on pathological alterations of the liver. This dynamic behavior is the strongest *in vivo* evidence for a functional significance of zonal cell heterogeneity. It must be caused by changes in the hormonal or nervous system accompanying the metabolic alterations and should therefore be a valuable indirect indicator of the role of both systems in the induction of heterogeneity.

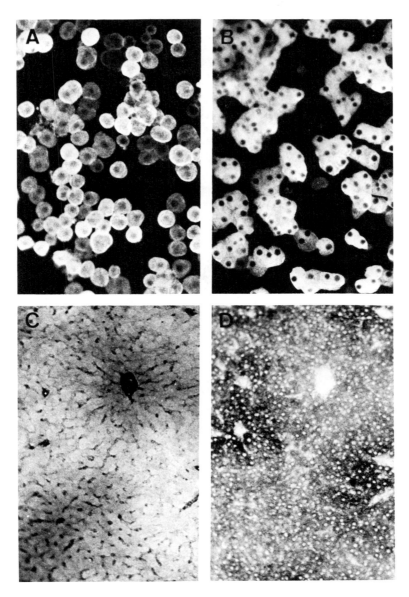

Figure 8. Distribution of phosphoenolypyruvate carboxykinase in hepatocytes cultured for 1 hr under basic conditions (A) and for 48 hr under inducing conditions (10 nM glucagon from 24 to 48 hr) (B), as well as in liver parenchyma of fed rats (C). The parenchymal distribution of succinate dehydrogenase is shown in a parallel section (D). The culture, immunofluorescence, and histochemical techniques were described previously.[41,42] After 1 hr of culture, the hepatocytes still possessed different amounts of enzyme. After 48 hr under inducing conditions, all cells contained essentially the same levels of enzyme; slight differences in fluorescence intensity are due to the varying depth of the cultured cells.

3.4.1. Perinatal Development

Hepatocyte heterogeneity is not an inherent property of liver parenchyma *per se;* in the rat, it develops only gradually during the 2nd week of life before the intake of carbohydrate-rich food. In the fetal phase, the energy supply is maintained by maternal glucose; prenatal liver is not involved in the glucose supply of other organs.[48–50] Therefore, gluconeogenic enzymes are absent; the liver catalyzes glycolysis only. In the suckling phase, the constant glucose-rich nutrition via the maternal blood is replaced by fat- and protein-rich but carbohydrate-poor nutrition via the maternal milk. The neonatal liver then has the function of maintaining the glucose supply to other organs. Gluconeogenesis becomes an increasingly important source of glucose; the key gluconeogenic enzymes are induced at birth. The liver catalyzes predominantly, if not exclusively, gluconeogenesis. In the weaning phase, nutrition again becomes carbohydrate-rich; the liver acquires the function of a glucostat. The diurnal rhythm of glycogen synthesis, glycolysis, and liponeogenesis during the absorptive phase and glycogen degradation and gluconeogenesis during the postabsorptive phase develops. The "nonregulatory" glycolytic isoenzymes hexokinase and PK type M are replaced by the "regulatory" isoenzymes glucokinase and PK type L.

The parenchymal distribution of microsomal glucose-6-phosphatase (G6Pase), cytosolic PEPCK, and mitochondrial succinate dehydrogenase (SDH) was studied with histochemical and immunohistochemical techniques during the perinatal period.[50,51] G6Pase and PEPCK were not detectable before birth; G6Pase showed the first signs of zonal heterogeneity at around 5 and PEPCK at day 1. Zonal heterogeneity of G6Pase and PEPCK became developed fully during the 2nd week. SDH was disseminated heterogeneously before and after birth; zonal heterogeneity also developed during the 2nd week of life.

Thus, zonation of PEPCK, G6Pase, and SDH became fully expressed before the weaning period, i.e., before it would be functionally required according to the model of metabolic zonation, which links zonation with the glucostat function. Therefore, zonal heterogeneity cannot be induced by the nutritional change itself; rather, it must be brought about by a "program" anticipating the nutritional change to come. It is not known how this "program" is linked to changes in the hormonal and nervous system. An important part of the "program" may be that the fetal circulation via the umbilical vessels is changed abruptly in the newborn to a circulation via the hepatic artery and portal vein and that this change allows the differentiation of functional periportal and perivenous areas.

3.4.2. Starvation

After 24 hr of starvation, the key gluconeogenic enzymes PEPCK[52] and G6Pase[53] were increased in rat liver to over 200% in the periportal zone and to 365 and 270%, respectively, in the perivenous zone. Conversely, pyruvate kinase type L $(PK_L)^{54}$ was decreased to 75% in the periportal areas and to 60% in the perivenous area. Glucokinase $(GK)^{55,56}$ did not show any major change, nor did the citrate cycle enzyme SDH. Thus, both with the glucose/glucose-6-phosphate cycle and with the phosphoenolpyruvate/pyruvate cycle, starvation increases the predominance of gluconeogenic over glycolytic enzymes in the periportal zone, while in the perivenous zone, it changes the normal pattern of glycolytic over gluconeogenic enzymes to a prevalance of gluconeogenic over glycolytic enzymes (Fig. 9). Apparently, the major function of the perivenous zone is changed during starvation from glucose uptake to glucose release, which is in accord

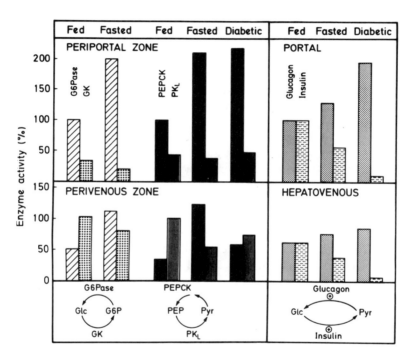

Figure 9. Dynamics of zonal enzyme heterogeneity. Distributions of key enzymes of gluconeogenesis and glycolysis over the liver parenchyma as well as portal and hepatovenous levels of glucoregulatory hormones in fed, fasted, and alloxan-diabetic rats. Enzyme activities were determined in microdissected liver tissue with microbiochemical techniques. Hormone levels were determined with standard radioimmunoassays.[9] To facilitate comparison, the originally measured enzyme activities were all extrapolated to 37°C assuming a doubling of activity per 10°C temperature increase and converted from dry to wet weight using a factor of 0.3; the following values (μmoles $\times$ min^{-1} $\times$ g^{-1}, 37°C) were set equal to 100%: glucokinase (GK), 3.0[56]; glucose-6-phosphatase (G6Pase), 10.7[53]; pyruvate kinase L (PK$_L$), 52[54]; phosphoenolypyruvate carboxykinase (PEPCK), 7.7.[52] The following hormone values (nM) were set equal to 100%: insulin, 1.6; glucagon, 0.07.[9] Enzyme levels of fed and fasted animals are from Guder and Schmidt,[52] Katz et al.,[53] Zierz et al.,[54] and Fischer et al.[56]; the hormone levels are from Balks and Jungermann[9] and Balks and Jungermann (unpublished findings). Enzyme and hormone levels of diabetic rats are from Miethke et al.[64]

with the increased glucose requirement of the organism and with the missing need to "buffer" excess nutritional glucose.

The changes of the zonal levels of the key enzymes in the fasting state are in line with the observed increase of the portal glucagon/insulin ratio (Balks and Jungermann, unpublished) (Fig. 9). These findings corroborate the thesis that the insulin–glucagon antagonism must be important for the induction of liver cell heterogeneity, at least with respect to carbohydrate metabolism.

3.4.3. Diabetes

Severe diabetes was induced in the rat after 48 hr of alloxan treatment, with blood glucose and ketone bodies elevated by more than 5-fold and with portal insulin reduced to below 10% and glucagon increased to almost 200%.[64] PEPCK was increased to 220% in the periportal area and to 180% in the perivenous zone; conversely, PK_L remained unchanged in the periportal zone, but was reduced to 75% in the perivenous area. The zonal distribution of SDH remained unchanged. Thus, diabetes similar to starvation increased the predominance of gluconeogenic over glycolytic key enzymes in the periportal zone, while in the perivenous zone, in contrast to starvation, it diminished rather than reversed the prevalence of the glycolytic over the gluconeogenic enzymes (Fig. 9). Thus, the major function of the perivenous zone, glucose uptake, is not changed entirely to glucose release during starvation, which would be in line with the requirement persisting in diabetes to "buffer" excess nutritional glucose at least in part.

The changes of the zonal levels of the key enzymes in the diabetic state may be at variance with the 20-fold increase of the portal glucagon/insulin ratio observed (Fig. 9). Because of the drastic decrease in the insulin level, a much more pronounced increase of PEPCK and decrease of PK_L in the perivenous zone would have been expected. Since this was not the case, other factors besides the insulin–glucagon antagonism must be involved in the heterogeneous induction of the key enzymes of carbohydrate metabolism. One important factor could be the oxygen gradient, which, of course, is not changed in the diabetic state.

3.4.4. Regeneration after Partial Hepatectomy

After two-third partial hepatectomy in the rat, the specific activity of PEPCK was elevated to about 200%[57,58], that of PK_L, the glucoregulatory isoenzyme of adult parenchymal cells[65] was lowered to about 65% and that of GK to below 30%.[59] Thus, total liver PEPCK activity was restored much faster and total PK_L as well as GK were restored much slower to their preoperational levels than was liver weight. The gluconeogenic capacity was clearly increased and the glycolytic capacity decreased because the liver remnant should also secure the glucose supply of the brain and the erythrocytes. Apparently, the increase of the gluconeogenic capacity of the liver was not sufficient, since the glucose-forming capacity of the kidney was also elevated after partial hepatectomy.[59]

After partial hepatectomy, PEPCK lost its periportal-to-perivenous gradient, as shown by immunohistochemical techniques[58]; the activity was increased in the periportal and even more so in the perivenous zone. Conversely, PK_L also lost its perivenous-to-periportal gradient, as measured in microdissected tissue samples; the activity was reduced only in the perivenous zone.[65] Thus, partial hepatectomy increased the prevalence of the gluconeogenic over the glycolytic enzymes in the periportal zone similar to starvation, while it reversed the prevalence of glycolytic over gluconeogenic enzymes to a predominance of gluconeogenic over glycolytic enzymes in the perivenous zone. In conclusion, the decrease of GK and PK_L and the reciprocal increase of PEPCK after partial hepatectomy and the loss of the normal zonation of PEPCK and PK_L support the notion that the liver was converted from a "bifunctional" gluconeogenic–glycolytic to a "unifunctional" gluconeogenic organ by partial hepatectomy.

The alteration of the zonal contents of the key enzymes after partial hepatectomy would be in accord with a decrease of portal insulin and an increase of portal glucagon levels.[60,61] The findings therefore indicate that after partial hepatectomy, the insulin–glucagon antagonism should be operative in the alteration of zonal enzyme heterogeneity.

3.4.5. Cirrhosis

Cirrhosis was induced experimentally in the rat with thioacetamide.[62] As studied with histochemical techniques, nearly all cirrhotic nodules possessed in their centers a high content of glycogen and high activities of glycogen phosphorylase, G6Pase, and SDH, while in their marginal parts, they had a low content of glycogen and low activities of phosphorylase and G6Pase, but high levels of SDH and glucose-6-phosphate dehydrogenase. Thus, the normal heterogeneity of carbohydrate metabolism was preserved in nearly all cirrhotic nodules, in which the centers correspond to the periportal zone. It was concluded that the heterogeneity is required for the regulatory "altruistic" functions of the organ as a "metabolitostat." In some nodules, the heterogeneity was lost. This was interpreted as the first step in the direction of malignancy, i.e., "autistic" functions.[62]

It is not clear at present how the maintenance of the normal heterogeneity in the vast majority of nodules and the loss of heterogeneity in some nodules are regulated by hormones or other signals.

3.4.6. Portocaval Anastomosis

After end-to-side portocaval anastomosis in the rat, the specific activity of PEPCK remained the same after a transient 2-fold increase during the first few days following surgery, while the activity of PK_L was lowered to about 70%. The periportal-to-perivenous gradient of PEPCK measured after microdissection was essentially preserved, although at different activity levels, during all periods after portocaval anastomosis; the perivenous-to-periportal gradient of PK_L was diminished slightly.[66] Thus, the liver remained the same "bifunctional" gluconeogenic–glycolytic organ as before portocaval anastomosis. Only during the transient postoperative period, during which the animals consumed less than 30% of the normal amounts of food and which is therefore similar to starvation did the liver become predominantly gluconeogenic. Although the "portal" hormones insulin and glucagon cannot reach the liver directly after portocaval anastomosis, the usual zonation of key enzymes of carbohydrate metabolism appears to be maintained. This might indicate that the insulin–glucagon gradients built up by the liver starting from the arterial input only must be similar to those built up starting from the joint portal and arterial input. The finding might also indicate that the insulin–glucagon antagonism may be less important for heterogeneous acinar gene expression than the oxygen gradient, which in animals with portocaval anastomosis can be expected to be steeper than in unoperated controls.

3.5. Conclusion

Direct studies on enzyme induction in hepatocyte culture and indirect investigations on enzyme levels investigating the dynamics of the zonal differences have shown that the oxygen gradient and the insulin–glucagon gradient are important for the establishment of zonal heterogeneity, at least with respect to carbohydrate metabolism. These studies have also revealed that there must be other factors involved. The matter is apparently very complex and is far from being understood.

4. SUMMARY

Periportal and perivenous hepatocytes differ in their enzyme activities and subcellular structures. However, all hepatocytes have, of course, the same genome. The heterogeneous expression of this genome is primarily due to the zonal heterogeneity of signals and signal transmission.

Periportal and perivenous hepatocytes receive different signals in the form of different substrate and hormone concentrations and possibly different autonomic innervation. Due to the metabolism by the liver, the concentration of oxygen is higher in periportal than in perivenous blood by 2-fold; that of most carbon substrates such as glucose, lactate, amino acids, and free fatty acids is normally higher (or lower), however, only by 1.1- to 1.5-fold, while that of some substrates, e.g., propionate, butyrate, ammonia, and cholic acids, is higher by more than 6-fold. The levels of most hormones in the periportal zone exceed those in the perivenous zone; e.g., levels of insulin are only 1.15-fold higher during a meal, but are 2-fold higher during a fast. Glucagon (1.4-fold), adrenaline (5- to 6-fold), and noradrenaline (2-fold) are all higher in periportal zones. Conversely, the concentration of some mediators is clearly higher in the perivenous than in the periportal area (e.g., adenosine is 10-fold higher in perivenous zones).

Signal transmission, i.e., the hormone receptors and receptor-linked enzyme systems of the cells, may also be different. The zonal distribution of the ectocellular receptors for insulin, glucagon, and catecholamines or of the intracellular receptors for glucocorticoids is not known. The glucagon-stimulated adenylate cyclase appears to be evenly distributed in the fed state and located predominantly in the perivenous zone in the fasted state.

As shown in studies of enzyme induction in hepatocyte cultures, the oxygen gradient and the insulin–glucagon gradient are important for the establishment of zonal hepatocyte heterogeneity, at least with respect to carbohydrate metabolism; the role of substrate gradients other than oxygen is at present unknown. Phosphoenolpyruvate carboxykinase, a "periportal" enzyme, is induced by glucagon to higher levels under periportal than under perivenous oxygen tensions. Conversely, glucokinase, a "perivenous" enzyme, is increased by insulin to higher values under perivenous than under periportal oxygen concentrations. The induction of phosphoenolpyruvate carboxykinase by glucagon is anatagonized effectively by insulin and modulated by glucocorticoids in a way consistent with the predominant periportal localization of the enzyme. Some evidence points to a direct role of the hepatic nerves in the induction of zonal differences; however, convincing data are still lacking.

The zonal heterogeneity is dynamic. It changes on longer-lasting alterations of the metabolic situation in health and disease such as starvation, diabetes, regeneration after partial hepatectomy, portocaval anastomosis, or cirrhosis. Studies of the dynamics of zonation have revealed that many factors besides the oxygen and insulin–glucagon gradients must be involved in the establishment of zonal heterogeneity. The matter is apparently very complex and is far from being understood.

ACKNOWLEDGMENTS. This work was supported by grants from the Deutsche Forschungsgemeinschaft, Bonn. Thanks are due to Drs. Balks, Chatzipanagiotou, Katz, Miethke, Probst, Wittig, Wölfle, and Zierz for their cooperation during various stages of the investigations.

REFERENCES

1. Novikoff, A. B., 1959, Cell heterogeneity within the hepatic lobule of the rat (staining reactions), *J. Histochem. Cytochem.* **7**:240–244.
2. Rappaport, A. M., 1960, Betrachtungen zur Pathophysiologie der Leberstruktur, *Klin. Wochenschr.* **38**:561–577.
3. Jungermann, K., and Sasse, D., 1978, Heterogeneity of liver parenchymal cells, *Trends Biochem. Sci.* **3**:198–202.
4. Gumucio, J. J., and Miller, D. L., 1981, Functional implications of liver cell heterogeneity, *Gastroenterology* **80**:393–403.
5. Jungermann, K., and Katz, N., 1982, Functional hepatocellular heterogeneity, *Hepatology* **2**:385–395.
6. Katz, N., and Jungermann, K., 1976, Autoregulatory shift from fructolysis to lactate gluconeogenesis in rat hepatocyte suspensions: The problem of metabolic zonation of liver parenchyma, *Hoppe-Seyler's Z. Physiol. Chem.* **357**:359–375.
7. Grote, J., 1980, Gewebsatmung, in: *Physiologie des Menschen,* 20th ed. (R. F. Schmidt and G. Thews, eds.), p. 560, Springer-Verlag, Berlin, Heidelberg, and New York.
8. Thews, O. G., 1980, Atemgastransport und Säure-Basen-Status des Blutes, in: *Physiologie des Menschen,* 20th ed. (R. F. Schmidt and G. Thews, eds.), p. 543, Springer-Verlag, Berlin, Heidelberg, and New York.
9. Balks, H. J., and Jungermann, K., 1984, Regulation of the peripheral insulin/glucagon ratio by the liver, *Eur. J. Biochem.* **141**:645- 650.
10. Strubbe, J. H., and Steffens, A. B., 1977, Blood glucose levels in portal and peripheral circulation and their relation to food intake in the rat, *Physiol. Behav.* **19**:303–307.
11. Jungermann, K., Heilbronn, R., Katz, N., and Sasse, D., 1982, The glucose/glucose-6-phosphate cycle in the periportal and perivenous zone of rat liver, *Eur. J. Biochem.* **123**:429–436.
12. Remesy, C., Fafournoux, P., and Demigne, C., 1983, Control of hepatic utilization of serine, glycine and threonine in fed and starved rats, *J. Nutr.* **113**:28–39.
13. Remesy, C., and Demigne C., 1983, Changes in availability of glucogenic and ketogenic substrates and liver metabolism in fed or starved rats, *Ann. Nutr. Metab.* **27**:57–70.
14. Katz, N., and Giffhorn, S., 1983, Glucose- and insulin-dependent induction of ATP citrate lyase in primary cultures of rat hepatocytes, *Biochem. J.* **212**:65–71.
15. Katz, N., and Ick, M., 1981, Induction of acetyl-CoA carboxylase in primary rat hepatocyte cultures by glucose and insulin, *Biochem. Biophys. Res. Commun.* **100**:703–709.
16. Remesy, C., and Demigne C., and Aufrere, J., 1978, Interorgan relationships between glucose, lactate and amino acids in rats fed on high carbohydrate or high protein diets, *Biochem. J.* **170**:321–329.
17. Yamamoto, H., Aikawa, T., Matsutaka, H., Okuda, T., and Ishikawa, E., 1974, Interorganal relationships of amino acid metabolism in fed rats, *Am. J. Physiol.* **226**:1428–1433.
18. Hofmann, A. F., Molino, G., Milanese, M., and Belforte, G., 1983, Description and simulation of a physiological pharmacokinetic model for the metabolism and enterohepatic circulation of bile acids in man, *J. Clin. Invest.* **71**:1003–1022.
19. Cronholm, T., and Sjövall, J., 1967, Bile acids in portal blood of rats fed different diets and cholestyramine, *Eur. J. Biochem.* **2**:375–383.
20. Okishio, T., and Nair, P. P., 1966, Studies on bile acids: Some observations on the intracellular localization of major bile acids in rat liver, *Biochemistry* **5**:3662–3668.
21. Striffler, J. S., and Curry, D. L., 1979, Effect of fasting on insulin removal by liver of perfused liver–pancreas, *Am. J. Physiol.* **237**:E349–E355.
22. Yamaguchi, N., and Garceau, D., 1980, Correlations between hemodynamic parameters of the liver and norepinephrine release upon hepatic nerve stimulation in the dog, *Can. J. Physiol. Pharmacol.* **58**:1347–1355.

23. Thiede, H. M., and Kehr, W., 1981, Conjoint radioenzymatic measurements of catecholamines, their catechol metabolites and DOPA in biological samples, *Naunyn-Schmiedeberg's Arch. Pharmacol.* **318:**19–28.

24. McCormick, J. R., Herman, A. M., Lien, W. M., and Egdahl, R. H., 1974, Hydrocortisone metabolism in the adrenalectomized dog: The quantitative significance of each organ system in the total metabolic clearance of hydrocortisone, *Endocrinology* **94:**17–26.

25. Paterson, N., and Harrison, M., 1972, The splanchnic and hepatic uptake of cortisol in conscious and anaesthetized sheep, *J. Endocrinol.* **55:**335–350.

26. Manin, M., Tournaire, C., and Delost, P., 1983, The splanchnic removal of cortisol from plasma of anaesthetized guinea pigs, *J. Endocrinol.* **96:**273–280.

27. Zipser, R.D., Speckart, P.F., Zia, P.K., Edmiston, W.A., Lau, F.Y., and Horton, R., 1976, The effect of ACTH and cortisol on aldosterone and cortisol clearance and distribution in plasma and whole blood, *J. Clin. Endocrinol. Metab.* **43:**1101–1109.

28. Chavarri, M., Lütscher, J. A., Dowdy, A. J., and Ganguly, A., 1977, The effects of temperature and plasma cortisol on distribution of aldosterone between plasma and red blood cells: Influence on metabolic clearance rate and on hepatic and renal extraction of aldosterone, *J. Clin. Endocrinol. Metab.* **44:**752–759.

29. Pritchard, J. B., O'Connor, N., Oliver, J. M., and Berlin, R. D., 1975, Uptake and supply of purine compounds by the liver, *Am. J. Physiol.* **229:**967–972.

30. Newby, A. C., 1984, Adenosine and the concept of "retaliatory metabolites," *Trends Biochem. Sci.* **9:**42–44.

31. Westfall, T. C., 1977, Local regulation of adrenergic neurotransmission, *Physiol. Rev.* **57:**659–728.

32. Joost, H. G., and Steinfelder, H. J., 1983, Modulation of insulin sensitivity by adenosine: Effects on glucose transport, lipid synthesis, and insulin receptors of the adipocyte, *Mol. Pharmacol.* **22:**614–618.

33. Lautt, W. W., 1980, Hepatic nerves, *Can. J. Physiol. Pharmacol.* **58:**105–123.

34. Forssmann, W. G., 1980, Introduction and historical remarks on the innervation of the liver, in: *Communication of Liver Cells* (H. Popper, L. Bianchi, F. Gudat, and W. Reutter, eds), pp. 109–114, MTP Press, Lancaster.

35. McCuskey, R. S., 1980, Intrahepatic distribution of nerves: A review, in: *Coummunication of Liver Cells* (H. Popper, L. Bianchi, F. Gudat, and W. Reutter, eds), pp. 115–120, MTP Press, Lancaster.

36. Shimazu, T., 1981, Central nervous system regulation of liver and adipose tissue metabolism, *Diabetologia* **20:**343–356.

37. Zierz, S., and Jungermann, K., 1984, Alteration with the dietary state of the activity and zonal distribution of the glucagon-, fluoride- and forskolin-stimulated adenylate cyclase in micro-dissected rat liver tissue, *Eur. J. Biochem.* **145:**499–504.

38. Nauck, M., Wölfle, D., Katz, N., and Jungermann, K., 1981, Modulation of the glucagon-dependent induction of phosphoenolpyruvate carboxykinase and tyrosine aminotransferase by arterial and venous oxygen concentrations in hepatocyte cultures, *Eur. J. Biochem.* **119:**657–661.

39. Katz, N., Nauck, M., and Wilson, P., 1979, Induction of glucokinase by insulin under the permissive action of dexamethasone in primary rat hepatocyte cultures, *Biochem. Biophys. Res. Commun.* **88:**23–29.

40. Probst, I., and Jungermann, K., 1983, The glucagon–insulin antagonism and gluca-gon–dexamethasone synergism in the induction of phospho*enol*pyruvate carboxykinase in cultured rat hepatocytes, *Hoppe-Seyler's Z. Physiol. Chem.* **364:**1739–1746.

41. Probst, I., Schwartz, P., and Jungermann, K., 1982, Induction in primary culture of "gluconeogenic" and "glycolytic" hepatocytes resembling periportal and perivenous cells, *Eur. J. Biochem.* **126:**271–278.

42. Andersen, B., Nath, A., and Jungermann, K., 1982, Heterogeneous distribution of phosphoen-*ol*pyruvate carboxykinase in rat liver parenchyma, isolated and cultured hepatocytes, *Eur. J. Cell Biol.* **28:**47–53.

43. Harris, A. J., 1974, Inductive functions of the nervous system, *Annu. Rev. Physiol.* **36**:251–305.
44. Shimazu, T., and Ogasawara, S., 1975, Effects of hypothalamic stimulation on gluconeogenesis and glycolysis in rat liver, *Am. J. Physiol.* **228**:1787–1793.
45. Wölfle, D., Hartmann, H., and Jungermann, K., 1981, Induction of phospho*enol*pyruvate carboxykinase by sympathetic agents in primary cultures of adult rat hepatocytes, *Biochem. Biophys. Res. Commun.* **98**:1084–1090.
46. Bühler, H. V., Da Prada, M., Haefely, W., and Picotty, G. B., 1978, Plasma adrenaline, noradrenaline and dopamine in man and different animal species, *J. Physiol.* **276**:311–320.
47. Wathey, J. C., Nass, M. M., and Lester, H. A., 1979, Numerical reconstruction of the quantal event at nicotinic synapses, *Biophys. J.* **27**:145–164.
48. Bittner, R., Böhme, H. J., Didt, L., Goltzsch, W., Hofmann, E., Levin, M. J., and Sparmann, G., 1979, Developmental changes in the levels of hepatic enzymes and their relation to metabolic functions, *Adv. Enzyme Reg.* **17**:37–57.
49. Walker, P. R., Bonney, R. J., and Potter, V. R., 1974, Diurnal rhythm of hepatic carbohydrate metabolism during development in the rat, *Biochem. J.* **140**:523–529.
50. Katz, N., Teutsch, H. F., Jungermann, K., and Sasse, D., 1976, Perinatal development of the metabolic zonation of hamster liver parenchyma, *FEBS Lett.* **69**:23–28.
51. Andersen, B., Zierz, S., and Jungermann, K., 1983, Perinatal development of the distributions of phospho*enol*pyruvate carboxykinase and succinate dehydrogenase in rat liver parenchyma, *Eur. J. Cell Biol.* **30**:126–131.
52. Guder, W., and Schmidt, U., 1976, Liver cell heterogeneity: The distribution of pyruvate kinase and phospho*enol*pyruvate carboxykinase in the liver lobule of fed and starved rats, *Hoppe-Seyler's Z. Physiol. Chem.* **357**:1793–1800.
53. Katz, N., Teutsch, H., Sasse, D., and Jungermann, K., 1977, Heterogeneous distribution of glucose-6-phosphatase in microdissected periportal and perivenous rat liver tissue, *FEBS Lett.* **76**:226–230.
54. Zierz, S., Katz, N., and Jungermann, K., 1983, Distribution of pyruvate kinase type L and M2 in microdissected periportal and perivenous rat liver tissue with different dietary states, *Hoppe-Seyler's Z. Physiol. Chem.* **364**:1447–1453.
55. Katz, N., Teutsch, H., Jungermann, K., and Sasse, D., 1977, Heterogenous reciprocal localization of fructose-1,6-bisphosphatase and of glucokinase in microdissected periportal and perivenous rat liver tissue, *FEBS Lett.* **83**:272–276.
56. Fischer, W., Ick, M., and Katz, N., 1982, Reciprocal distribution of hexokinase and glucokinase in the periportal and perivenous zone of the rat liver acinus, *Hoppe-Seyler's Z. Physiol. Chem.* **363**:375–380.
57. Brinkmann, A., Katz, N., Sasse, D., and Jungermann, K., 1978, Increase of the gluconeogenic and decrease of the glycolytic capacity of rat liver with a change of the metabolic zonation after partial hepatectomy, *Hoppe-Seyler's Z. Physiol. Chem.* **359**:1561–1571.
58. Andersen, B., Zierz, S., and Jungermann, K., 1984, Alteration in zonation of succinate dehydrogenase, phospho*enol*pyruvate carboxykinase and glucose-6-phosphatase in regenerating rat liver, *Histochemistry* **80**:97–101.
59. Katz, N., Brinkmann, A, and Jungermann, K., 1979, Compensatory increase of the gluconeogenic capacity of rat kidney after partial hepatectomy, *Hoppe-Seyler's Z. Physiol. Chem.* **360**:51–57.
60. Bakewicz, D., and Piro, M., 1981, Changing hormonal levels during the process of rat liver regeneration, *J. Cell Biol.* **91**:9a.
61. Leffert, H. L., Koch, K. S., Moran, T., and Rubalcava, B., 1979, Hormonal control of rat liver regeneration, *Gastroenterology* **76**:1470–1482.
62. Nuber, R., Teutsch, H. F., and Sasse, D., 1980, Metabolic zonation in thioacetamide-induced liver cirrhosis, *Histochemistry* **69**:277–288.
63. Wölfle, D., and Jungermann, K., 1985, Long-term effects of physiological oxygen concentrations on glycolysis and gluconeogenesis in hepatocyte cultures, *Eur. J. Biochem.* **151**:299–303.

64. Miethke, H., Wittig, B., Nath, A., Zierz, S., and Jungermann, K., 1985, Metabolic zonation in liver of diabetic rats. *Biol. Chem. Hoppe-Seyler,* **366:**493–501.
65. Chatzipanagiotou, S., Nath, A., Vogt, B. and Jungermann, K., 1985, Alteration in the capacities as well as in the zonal and cellular distribution of pyruvate kinase L_1 and M_2 in regenerating rat liver, *Biol. Chem. Hoppe-Seyler* **366:**271–280.
66. Wittig, B., Zierz, S., Gubernatis, G., Nath, A., and Jungermann, K., 1985, Glucostat capacity and metabolic zonation in rat liver after portocaval anastomosis, *Biol. Chem. Hoppe-Seyler* **366:**713–722.

V

Speculation and Directions for the Future

Challenges for the Future

Recent work reported in this volume supports the concept that many physiological and metabolic events are compartmented in different regions of the liver lobule. New insights into the structure and regulation of metabolism in the liver are presented. Chapters in this volume have illustrated state of the art methodology being employed to describe the nature of the biochemical microheterogeneity of the liver lobule. Mechanisms underlying the development of this microheterogeneity and its physiological significance are beginning to be studied with methods presented above. Challenges for the future involve refinement of these methodologies to gather more descriptive information as well as the design of meaningful experiments to better understand the role of microheterogeneity in normal hepatic function as well as derangements which occur with pathological states.

Challenges for the immediate future involve the application of anatomical techniques to describe the *innervation* of the liver and to gather further information on the targets for the innervation. Great strides have been made in applying immunocytochemical techniques in neurobiology that have not yet been applied with such sophistication to studies in the liver. Methods have been introduced recently that can be applied to localizing specific types of neurotransmitters in very discrete histological zones. Application of such methods will shed new insights into the distribution of autonomic innervation in the liver as well as evaluate the possible participation of other forms of innervation, *e.g.*, peptidergic and purinergic. Another immediate goal in refinement of methodology involves further development of *methods to separate viable specific cell types* in bulk. Although progress has been made in these areas, there is a great need to improve the purity of isolated cells as well as maintain them in a state suitable for meaningful experiments under nearly physiological conditions. Until further progress is made in cell separation techniques, experiments to probe the physiological significance of microheterogeneity will require the use of noninvasive techniques such as microlight guides and miniature oxygen electrodes described above. There is a need to correlate data obtained with these noninvasive techniques with information gathered from microchemical and immunohistochemical analyses. A final area that requires attention is the critical *evaluation of primary cell cultures* being employed to study the behavior of specific cell types under well-defined conditions *in vitro*. There is an urgent need to describe the similarities and differences of various cell types that are currently being maintained *in vitro* to their counterparts in the intact organ. The likelihood that substantial progress will be made in refining techniques to describe and understand the microheterogeneity of the liver is very high based on the exciting progress that has been made in modern biomedical research.

Further work involving measurement of flux rates of metabolic processes in periportal and pericentral regions of the liver lobule using *noninvasive techniques* is needed. Metabolism in many pathways in different regions of the liver lobule is under short-term dynamic control. New methods described in this volume allow this dynamic regulation to be studied under nearly physiological conditions. Insight into the regulation of metabolic processes in various regions in the liver lobule comes from comparison of the predominance of a given pathway in a particular zone when perfusion is in the retrograde and anterograde directions. Metabolic flux in the various pathways is far below maximal capacity and is regulated by a gradient of nutrients and oxygen across the liver lobule by mechanisms that require elucidation. Other processes such as glucuronidation and monooxygenation in livers of phenobarbital-treated rats do not appear to be under the control of gradients established by the direction of flow across the liver lobule. Both glucuronidation and monooxygenation are localized predominantly in pericentral areas of the liver lobule irrespective of the direction of flow. In some cases such as oxygen uptake, gluconeogenesis and glycolysis, predictions regarding zonation based on enzyme distribution fit data from measured flux rates. Since several hepatic metabolic systems may be switched to the opposite direction rapidly by perfusion in the retrograde direction, it is unlikely that the distribution of enzyme activities is the only determinant in the short-term regulation of hepatic oxygen, carbohydrate and nitrogen metabolism. Further work on the mechanism for the change in these rates from one zone to another when the direction of liver perfusion is altered should be one of the immediate goals of research in the future.

Future problems that will require greater commitment over the long term involve such things as understanding the nature of biochemical *signal hetero-*

geneity across the liver lobule. Recent evidence indicates that receptor distribution for a small number of neurotransmitters (*e.g.*, catecholamines) may differ in different regions of the liver lobule. The possible heterogeneous distribution of various receptors for other neurohumoral agents needs to be evaluated. This work will require refinement of techniques to map receptor densities in different regions of the liver lobule. Understanding biochemical signalling heterogeneity in the liver lobule may provide an understanding of the phenotypic expression of specific enzymes in different regions of the liver lobule. The relationship of the direction of flow through the liver lobule of nutrients and hormones to the expression of enzyme activities as well as acute changes in the regulation of specific metabolic pathways requires additional attention.

Alterations in the physiological state of the liver by various hormones or pharmacological agents needs to be reevaluated in terms of the effects of these agents on specific domains of the hepatic lobule. The role of microheterogeneity in certain pathological states such as centrilobular necrosis in chronic alcoholics, alterations in the processing of specific substrates and hormones in diabetics, and the mechanisms of cirrhosis, may all be better understood as progress is made in the areas identified above.

Considerable progress has been made in biomedical engineering and has led to the development of *non-invasive imaging techniques* employing NMR, ESR, and CAT scanning. Although the resolution of these methods is not great enough to study the heterogeneity of the liver lobule, the potential for applying imaging techniques in the future to study heterogeneity in the intact functioning organ *in vivo* is an exciting prospect.

A major problem facing investigators in this field over the next decade will be to explain how different enzymes exist in periportal and pericentral regions of the liver lobule. While the oxygen gradient and hormone gradient could be important determinants in enzyme distribution, evidence supporting this comes only from cultured cells grown in the presence of various hormones. One approach which has been applied successfully is the surgical implantation of the liver on a long-term basis in the retrograde direction in the neck of an experimental animal. The possibilities for interaction between surgeons and basic scientists interested in long-term regulation of metabolic events in different regions of the liver lobule in the future would be most exciting. In view of progress described in this volume, continued studies of the biochemical microheterogeneity of the liver lobule and its role in health and disease should prove to be a very rewarding enterprise for biomedical scientists in a variety of disciplines.

Index